# The Kidney

To
B. E. Miles, P. J. Little, E. M. Clarkson,
R. W. Schrier, J. B. Eastwood,
G. A. MacGregor and Clarisse Neiman

# The Kidney

## AN OUTLINE OF NORMAL AND ABNORMAL FUNCTION

## H. E. de Wardener

CBE, MBE (Mly), MD(Lond), MD(Hon) Pierre et
Marie Curie, Paris, FRCP
Emeritus Professor of Medicine in the University of
London (Charing Cross Hospital Medical School);
Membre de l'Académie Nationale de Medécine

FIFTH EDITION

CHURCHILL LIVINGSTONE

EDINBURGH LONDON MELBOURNE AND NEW YORK 1985

CHURCHILL LIVINGSTONE
Medical Division of Longman Group Limited

Distributed in the United States of America by
Churchill Livingstone Inc., 1560 Broadway, New York,
N.Y. 10036, and by associated companies, branches
and representatives throughout the world.

First edition 1958
Second edition 1961
Third edition 1967
Fourth edition 1973
Fifth edition 1985

ISBN 0 443 02841 9

British Library Cataloguing in Publication Data
Wardener, H. E. de
    The Kidney. — 5th ed.
    1. Kidneys — Diseases
    I. Title
    616.6'1      RC902

Library of Congress Cataloging in Publication Data
De Wardener, H. E. (Hugh Edward)
    The kidney: an outline of normal and abnormal function.
    Includes bibliographical references and index.
    1. Kidneys — Diseases.   I. Title.   [DNLM: 1. Kidney.
2. Kidney Diseases.   WJ 300 D515k]
RC902.D4   1984        616.6'1        84-7729

Printed in Singapore by
Champion Office Supplies Pte Ltd

# Preface to the fifth edition

It is ten years since the fourth edition. This edition, therefore, has needed more revision than is usual. I have added two new chapters (15, 18) and extensively rewritten many others so that about two thirds of the script is new, as are about half the figures. As many people, including those in the United States, use traditional units of measurements, I have given most of the measurements in both S.I. units and traditional units. When the book first appeared in 1958, it was the first on clinical nephrology. It was difficult then, and it is no easier now, to decide what and how much to include. I thought it was important to have large sections on normal physiology and pathophysiological syndromes. It was noticeable, however, that the reviews from physiologists tended to praise the clinical parts of the book but to deplore the perfunctory approach to physiology; whereas reviews from clinicians, while praising the physiology, thought that more could have been included on certain aspects of renal disease. One could either conclude that the book had achieved the right balance or that one should not attempt to write a small book on the kidney.

When writing the first edition, much of my information, particularly on the clinical aspect of nephrology, came from my own very limited experience and from original papers. Now there are numerous books on the kidney. Some are encyclopaedic, multi-author volumes, e.g. Brenner & Rector's *The Kidney*, which weighs 3.5 kg, while others are so concise that they can be carried in the pocket, like Gower's *Nephrology* which weighs only 200 g. My task in writing this edition, therefore, has been much easier than when writing the first. Though I still prefer original papers, these excellent compendiums of information written by one's friends have been an immense help, and because of them I need no longer worry about those aspects of nephrology which I have not included here.

This book lies between the two extremes mentioned above. It is certainly not encyclopaedic and it is too big to carry in the pocket. It is still aimed at 'those who are interested in the subject', particularly those who are trying to explore its fascination for the first time. A single author book is one man's view of a subject. Therefore, its content reflects how he sees things. I am particularly interested in mechanisms and in those aspects of nephrology in which I have done some research. Certain aspects of the book, therefore, such as urinary infection, the control of sodium excretion and blood pressure, urinary concentrating mechanisms, calcium metabolism and maintenance haemodialysis are written with more intimate knowledge than some others. It is inevitable that the book must be biased. I can only hope that this does not obtrude, and that where it is noticeable, the obtrusion will not be too antigenic.

I am very grateful to Dr Malcolm Phillips for reading large sections of the manuscript and proofs and particularly for his synoptic view of tubular disorders which greatly eased the burden of writing that particular chapter. I am also obliged to Drs J. Curtis, J. B. Eastwood, E. Brown, G. MacGregor, R. Jewkes and J. L. H. Laity for their help in writing or reviewing the rest of the manuscript. I am also indebted to Mr G. Carter and Mrs P. Howard for their contribution to Appendix 2 and 3; Mrs A. Besterman for once again drawing many of the diagrams; Miss Marion Hudson and her colleagues in the Department of Medical Illustrations for their well-tried patience and willing cooperation; and Mrs E. Bylenksa for her meticulous attention to the references. I cannot thank Mrs Joy Lyall adequately for her relentless and cheerful assistance with the manuscript.

1985                                                          H. E. de W.

# Preface to the first edition

The purpose of this book is to present an outline of renal structure and function; and the methods used to obtain information about each are discussed. There then follows a description of the four main syndromes about the subject.

At the beginning there is a short description of normal structure and function; and the methods used to obtain information about each are discussed. There then follows a description of the four main syndromes which occur in renal disease, i.e. the nephrotic syndrome, acute renal failure, chronic renal failure, and the acute nephritic syndrome; there is also a section on the relationship between disturbances of renal function and electrolyte disorders. The second half of the book consists principally of an account of renal diseases, including the renal manifestations of some generalised diseases. These are discussed in terms of the patterns of functional disturbance which have been described in the previous sections. Unless, therefore, the reader is already familiar with the subject it is best that he should start at the beginning or at least read the sections on the four syndromes and electrolyte disturbances before those on specific renal disorders.

For the sake of clarity, I have to confess that I have over-simplified many controversial subjects and in some instances given only one explanation where several exist. I have not attempted a comprehensive classification of renal disease, for in the present state of knowledge I doubt whether it is possible to arrive at a classification whose subdivisions are at the same time mutually exclusive and collectively exhaustive. Renal tuberculosis, hydronephrosis, calculi, renal tumours and certain other predominantly surgical conditions have been excluded.

I am indebted to the many workers and writers who have preceded me and I should like particularly to mention the following sources of information: Homer Smith's textbooks of renal physiology; A. C. Allen's histological textbook, *The Kidney*; A. M. Fishberg's *Hypertension and Nephritis*; T. Addis' *Glomerular Nephritis*; R. W. Lippman's *Urine and the Urinary Sediment*; G. W. Pickering's *High Blood Pressure*; as a guide to more detailed reading there is a list of references at the end of each section.

I am grateful to Drs B. E. Miles, R. R. McSwiney, D. M. Nutbourne, F. del Greco, R. D. Grainger, A. Herxheimer, Mr K. E. D. Shuttleworth, Mr R. D. de Vere, and Miss I. Maureen Young for their generous help with the manuscript and for giving me the benefit of their advice. I am also indebted to Drs A. C. Dornhorst and M. S. R. Hutt, and Mr M. Williams for their most helpful comments and for scrutinising the proofs. I wish to thank Miss J. Dewe and Miss P. Leicester for the patience and care with which they drew Figs 1, 2, 4, 5, 6, 71 to 74, and Figs 51, 53 to 60, and 68, respectively; and Mr A. L. Wooding and Mr B. Kentish for the photographs of the figures. I am also glad to acknowledge the help of Mr F. A. Tubbs, Miss M. E. Warner, Miss M. Matthews and Miss M. Studart in checking the references, and that of Miss J. Buchanan for her investigations on my behalf.

I am indebted to Drs W. J. Griffiths, R. R. McSwiney, J. R. Colley and W. W. Holland for Figs 9 and 38.

1958                                                          H. E. de W.

# Contents

# 1

# Structure of the kidney

A kidney contains about 1 000 000 nephrons. Each nephron is a tube approximately 20–50$\mu$ wide and 50 mm long with one end closed and the other opening into a collecting duct. The total length of the tubules in the two kidneys is about 110 km. The blind upper end of each nephron lies in the cortex, invaginated and expanded by a cluster of capillaries (the glomerulus); next to the glomerulus the tube is coiled into a compact mass (the proximal tubule); it then plunges straight towards the hilum of the kidney, some of the tubules reach into the medulla for a variable distance; the tubule then turns back in a tight hairpin bend (the loop of Henle) and once again lies in a coil (the distal tubule) next to its own glomerulus. Finally, it straightens out and together with several other distal tubules joins a collecting duct. Several collecting ducts join together and empty their contents into larger tubes called the papillary ducts which open directly on the surface of the papillae. The proximal tubules of the nephrons which lie in the superficial parts of the cortex are half the length of the proximal tubules of the nephrons which lie more deeply. There are approximately four long nephrons to one short nephron.

Most of the proximal and distal tubules lie in the cortex, while the loops of Henle and the collecting ducts from the bulk of the medulla.

## Glomerular structure

The glomerulus is composed of 4–6 capillary loops which spring from the afferent arteriole and end in the efferent arteriole; they lie within a space whose peripheral wall is known as the glomerular capsule (or Bowman's capsule). This cluster of capillaries shares a central stalk of mesangial cells. The outer part of the stalk is hollowed out to form the lumens of the capillary loop. The total surface area of the glomerular capillaries of two human adult kidneys is about 1.5 square metres. The wall of each capillary loop consists of a sandwich of epithelial cell cytoplasm, basement membrane and endothelial cell cytoplasm. The endothelial cell nuclei can only be distinguished from the mesangial cell nuclei by electron microscopy. The mesangial cell is of mesenchymal origin. In normal circumstances it gives

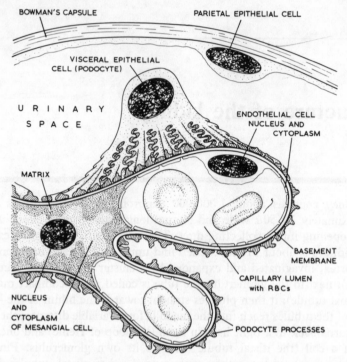

BOWMAN'S CAPSULE

PARIETAL EPITHELIAL CELL

VISCERAL EPITHELIAL
CELL (PODOCYTE)

U R I N A R Y
S P A C E

ENDOTHELIAL CELL
NUCLEUS AND
CYTOPLASM

MATRIX

BASEMENT
MEMBRANE

CAPILLARY LUMEN
with RBCs

NUCLEUS
AND
CYTOPLASM
OF MESANGIAL CELL

PODOCYTE PROCESSES

**Fig. 1.1** Diagram of electron microscopy appearances of glomerular capillary illustrating the disposition of the epithelial, endothelial and mesangial cells. It is to be noted that there is no basement membrane between the lumen and the mesangium.

rise to the endothelial cells. Electron microscopy (Fig. 1.1) reveals that the epithelial cell gives rise to many thin extensions which envelope the surface of the capillary like the tentacles of an octopus. Each extension is ringed by small protrusions called podocytes or foot processes which interdigitate with each other so that they cover the external surface of the basement membrane of the capillaries.

In the slits between the foot processes there are multiple layers of regularly spaced membranes which lie parallel to the basement membrane, the slit pore membranes or the slit diaphragm. The surface area of the pores totals about 2–3% of the surface area of the glomerular capillaries. the disposition of the slit pore membranes resembles that of a zipper in that the membranes arise alternately from each side of the slit and extend to just beyond the mid point of the slit inter-leaving at the centre with it's neighbour. The membranes are covered by negatively charged sieloproteins

The cytoplasm of the endothelial cells, where it forms the inner surface of the capillary loop has round punched out areas approximately 600 Å wide where the thickness of the cytoplasm is also about 70 Å. The basement membrane has a thickness of 800 Å. In man, in contrast to the rat, the basement membrane has a homogenous marzipan like structure, it consists of a fibrillar collagen network, originating from both the epithelial and the endothelial cells, embedded in a carbohydrate and glycoprotein matrix. Within the matrix there are two layers of annionic sites consisting of glycosaminoglycans rich in heparin sulphate in aggregates of 5–10 molecules distributed at regular 60 nm intervals.

On it's passage from the capillary lumen to Bowman's space glomerular filtrate first passes through the highly permeable attenuated cytoplasmic film covering the fenestrae of the endothelial cytoplasm. The first filtration barrier is the inner layer of anionic sites in that portion of the basement membrane adjoining the endothelium. The second barrier, which is the main barrier, is in the middle of the membrane which, because of the highly packed and cross linked collagen molecules, acts as a mechanical filter. The third barrier is formed by the outer layer of anionic site and the slit pore membranes which alter the composition of the filtrate by both ion exchange and mechanical obstruction. The final flow of filtrate is controlled by the epithelial cells adjusting the foot processes and slit pore membranes in a valve like action. Molecular size, shape and charge therefore determine the rate of passage of the various constituents of plasma through the glomerular capillary wall. The fixed anions in the wall hold-up polyanions such as albumin, the collagen network neutral macromolecules, and the slit diaphragms may limit the passage of cationic macromolecules. The mesangial cells have walls which can only be detected by electron microscopy. Between the mesangial cells there lies mesangial matrix which consists of a homogeneous ground substance in which is embedded fine fibres, similar to, but not idential to basement membrane. The matrix appears to be manufactured by the mesangial cells. In normal kidneys there are only small quantities of matrix present. It is also noticeable that there is no basement membrane between the perforated cytoplasm of the endothelium cell and the cytoplasm of the mesangial cell. The lumen of the capillary and the blood that it contains are therefore in contact with the cytoplasm of the mesangial cell. This is why large particles or molecules such as carbon or ferritin appear in the mesangial area within one minute of an intravenous injection. In some diseases the mesangial cells may multiply, large masses of mesangial cell cytoplasm may be formed and the mesangial cells may give rise to fibrocytic cells and collagen. It is possible that such mesangial changes are due to abnormal substances travelling directly from the lumen of the capillary into the mesangial cell cytoplasm. Carbon particles and ferritin molecules are phagocytosed within a few hours and the mesangial area is cleared within a few days.

## Tubular structure

The outer surface of the nephron is covered by a continuous layer of basement membrane. The proximal tubule is composed of irregularly cuboidal cells with coarse granular cytoplasm and ragged inner margins (the brush border). The cells of the descending thin limb of the loops of Henle are extremely thin and flat and have clear cytoplasm, whereas about two-thirds of the ascending limb is composed of cuboidal cells and is known as the thick part of the ascending limb. The length of the loops varies greatly; those that originate from glomeruli near the cortico-medullary junction are the longest and penetrate deeply into the medulla. The cells of the distal tubules are cuboidal but they are smaller than those in the proximal tubules; they have clear cytoplasm and sharp margins.

With the electron microscope the brush border of the proximal tubule cells is seen to consist of multiple projections of cell cytoplasm about 1 $\mu$ long covered by surface membrane. Between these projections there are invaginations of the surface membrane which penetrate into the cell cytoplasm and extend towards the mitochondria (Fig. 1.2). These projections and invaginations increase enormously the area of contact between the tubular fluid and the contents of the cells. The membranes of the lateral and basal surfaces of the proximal tubule cells are also invaginated into a number

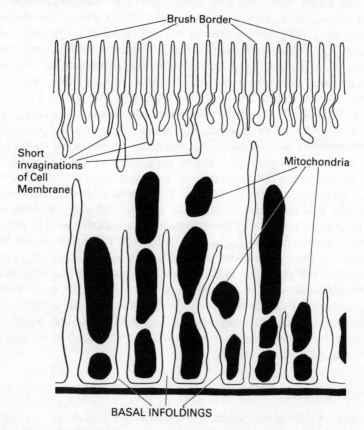

Fig. 1.2 Tubule. Schema of the electron microscopy appearances of a proximal tubule cell; the nucleus has been omitted.

of inlets which lie between the mitochondria. These form an extensive and complex extracellular compartment situated within the cell but in contact with the extracellular fluid space. The proximal tubule cells are seperated from one another by an intercellular space into which empty the many lateral membrane unfoldings. The cells appear to lie free of each other except at the luminal end of the intercellular spaces where the membrances of adjacent cells fuse to form 'tight junctions' of variable permeability. These block off the lumen of the tubule from the intercellular space, the other end of which opens out at the basal end of the cell at the level of the basement membrane. Electron microscopy and micropuncture studies agree that the distal tubule, i.e. that portion of the nephron which extends from the thick ascending limb of the loop of Henle to the cortical collecting duct, is structurally and functionally mainly a continuation of the ascending limb of Henle which extends to the beginning of the collecting duct.

The collecting ducts are an extensive system which have important functions other than that of leading the tubule fluid towards the papilla. They make the final adjustments to some of the contents of the tubule, and thus control the net overall bodily balance of these substances. And the remarkable impermeability of the cortical and outer medullary cortical duct to urea, whereas the inner medullary and papillary segments are freely permeable to urea, play an important part in building up the hypertonicity of the medullary interstitium without which the final urine cannot be made hypertonic (p. 61).

## Interstitial space

The cortex is almost free of connective tissue and in an ordinary histological preparation the peritubular venous capillaries and the tubules are contiguous, which suggests that there is no interstitial space. It is by no means certain however that this is true in life. Sections from kidneys which have been frozen instantaneously, after being excised from living animals, show that there exists a clear area around each tubule, between the tubule and the peritubular capillary. It is also well established that the blood that drains from a kidney which has just been excised from a living animal has a much lower haematocrit than the haematocrit of that animal's arterial or venous blood. It is probable that the extra plasma lies in the clear areas around the tubules. Usually these spaces are not visible, for the plasma they contain escapes with the blood in the capillaries via the cut renal artery and vein. The presence of an interstitial space in the medulla is certain, for the many parallel tubes that it contains are separated by a lagging of connective tissue which is particularly thick towards the apex of the pyramids. The cortical interstitial space contains only a few cells whereas in the medulla they are both numerous and prominent. Morphologically there are three distinct types and their number and appearance are related to sodium metabolism and hypertension. Some of the cells may be involved in the synthesis of prostaglandins. The interstitial cells in the medulla lie in a space filled with an amorphous 'cotton wool' like material.

The flow of lymph in the interstitial spaces of the cortex probably takes place in the capacious peri-arterial spaces. These must form relatively unyielding tunnels within which the pulsations of the arteries intermittently compress the adjoining lymphatics to ensure a flow of lymph. There are no lymph channels in the medulla.

### Juxta-glomerular apparatus

In each nephron the first part of the distal tubule rises from the medulla and comes to lie next to its own glomerulus (Fig. 1.3). At this point the afferent and efferent arterioles of the glomerulus are in close contact with the distal tubule. The area where this contact takes place is called the juxta-glomerular apparatus. At this point the cells of the afferent arteriole contain cytoplasmic secretory granules of renin. The distal tubular cells next to the granular cells of the afferent arteriole are columnar with their nuclei placed near the lumen of the tubule. In the space between these specialised arter-iolar and tubular cells there lies a third type of cell which form a lace-work pattern, known as lacis cells, they also extend into the intercapillary mesangial area of the glomerulus and resemble mesangial cells. The juxta glomerular apparatus is extensively innervated. Electron microscopy studies

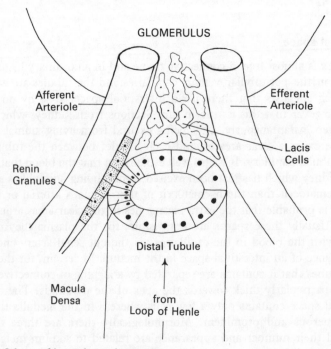

GLOMERULUS

Afferent Arteriole

Efferent Arteriole

Lacis Cells

Renin Granules

Distal Tubule

Macula Densa

from Loop of Henle

**Fig. 1.3** Schema of juxta-glomerular apparatus.

suggest that the granular cells of the arterioles, the lacis cells and the mesangial cells of the glomerulus are related to each other and to smooth muscle. This hypothesis is strengthened by the finding that in cultures of human glomeruli the mesangial cells contract intermittently, and all do so synchronously. Smooth muscle cells in culture do the same. In addition immunofluorescent studies have shown that anti-muscle immunoglobulin adheres to mesangial cells.

Renin is secreted both into the lumen of afferent arteriole and into the interstitial space where it, and angiotension II can be found in high concentrations. The glomerular tubular feed back mechanism by which the rate of flow of sodium to the macula densa causes reciprocal changes in glomerular filtration rate may be due to changes in the concentration of interstitial angiotensin altering the tone of the afferent arteriole.

## Lobules and lobes

The nephrons are arranged in bundles called lobules. Each bundle is not unlike a mushroom. The renal cortex, consisting of glomeruli, proximal and distal tubules are the expanded overlapping head of the mushroom, while the medulla and papilla which contain the loops of Henle and collecting ducts are the stalk. The kidney consists therefore of a collection of mushroom like lobules closely apposed to each other. The 'head' of each lobule lies just under the renal capsule, its sides dipping down away from the capsule. In other words the renal cortex lies not only on the surface of the kidney but at intervals, it also extends a short distance away from the capsule towards the renal pelvis. This is very obvious on a good intravenous pyelogram when the opacified cortex appears as an arcade. The lobules are themselves grouped into multiples called lobes.

## Cortico-medullary junction

At the junction of the cortex with the medulla there is a thick, wide-meshed fibrous net to which the renal pelvis is attached and through which the medulla and pyramids project. The vessels and lymphatic channels; ie outside the lumen of the pelvis and have to travel up to the cortico-medullary junction before they can enter into the renal parenchyma.

## Renal vasculature

About 26% of kidneys have multiple renal arteries, i.e. they have an artery arising from the aorta or the iliac artery in addition to the main renal artery. The renal artery divides into five segmental arteries (Fig. 1.4). It is important to note that, apart from the two poles, separate arteries supply the anterior and posterior surface of the kidney. In an ordinary antero-posterior view therefore angiography will reveal abnormalities of the arterial

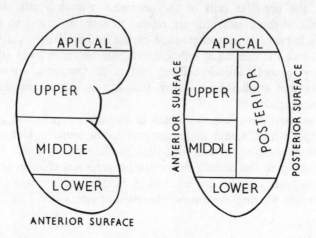

Fig. 1.4 Segmental distribution of renal arterial supply.

supply of the two poles, but isolated lesions of the arteries to the rest of the kidney may be obscured by overlying kidney substance to which the arterial supply is normal. The segmental arteries divide into interlobar arteries which, at the corticomedullary junction, divide into the arcuate arteries. Contrary to original descriptions, these are only linked together by capillary connections (Fig. 1.5). The intralobular arteries branch off at right angles to the arcuate arteries, and penetrate straight into the cortex, where they give rise to short afferent glomerular arterioles, so that even the most distal glomerulus receives its afferent arteriole direct from a relatively large artery. The smooth muscle of the afferent arteriole ceases as the arteriole joins the area of the juxtaglomerular apparatus. Beyond the glomerulus the blood flows into the efferent arteriole and then into a capacious intercommunicating plexus of capillaries situated between the tubules (the peritubular venous capillaries) which empties into the interlobular veins. Though some of the fluid filtered at the glomerulus returns via the distal tubule and the macula densa to influence the glomerulus from whence it came, the blood that flows through a glomerulus spreads far and wide to perfuse the peritubular venous capillaries of several nephrons. The endothelial cytoplasm of the peritubular venous capillaries has the same electronmicroscopic appearance as that of the endothelial cells in the glomerular capillaries. It contains multiple round areas approximately 600 Å wide in which the thickness of the cytoplasm is reduced to 70 Å, an arrangement which must facilitate the transport of substances to and from the blood.

The blood supply to the medulla passes through those glomeruli which are nearest to the medulla; these are sometimes known as juxtamedullary glomeruli. Their blood supply is quite different from other glomeruli. Instead of the blood flowing through an afferent arteriole which enters the

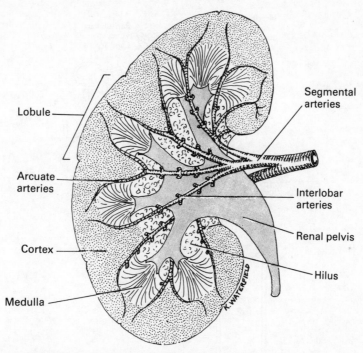

**Fig. 1.5** Renal blood supply related to renal lobes.

glomerulus, breaks up into capillaries and then emerges as an efferent arteriole, the afferent and efferent arteriole form one large continuous vessel which contains smooth muscle throughout and in which there is little evidence of renin secretory activity. The lumen into the glomerular capillaries opens directly on one side of this arteriole in such a way that a proportion of the blood which flows to the medulla does not pass through glomeruli (Fig. 1.6).

The blood to the medulla courses through two distinct systems. One consists of compact bundles of long tubes of capillary thickness which carry the blood down to, and away from, the apex of the pyramids; these are the descending and ascending vasa recta. The other system consists of a thick network of fine capillaries, it is situated in the outer half of the medulla; the same area as that occupied by the thick parts of the ascending limbs of the loop of Henle. The venous blood from the medulla empties into the arcuate veins. The striking feature of the medullary circulation is that the blood in the long bundles of vasa recta is forced to flow in a counter-current fashion. It follows that the vasa recta with their capillary-like walls not only act as conduits for blood, but because the blood within them is in equilibrium with the interstitial fluid, there is imposed upon the environment of the medulla the physical properties of a counter-current system (p. 60).

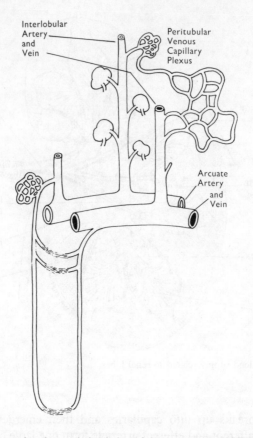

**Fig. 1.6** Schema illustrating the renal circulation of the cortex and medulla.

## Renal nerves

The innervation of the kidneys comes from both the sympathetic and the vagus via the splanchnic nerves. The sympathetic supply is usually from T6 to T12. Within the renal parenchyma there is a widespread distribution of nerves and it is possible to trace nerve fibres until they reach and envelop the tubules as well as the capillaries. There are no ganglia in the kidney. Adenergic nerve fibres are present in relation to interlobar, intralobular, and arcuate arteries, and the afferent arteriole. They are never found in the glomerulus, or the efferent arteriole. Some nerve terminals have been ident- ified in the peritubular basement membrane. These may be directly re- sponsible for changes in sodium reabsorption.

BIBLIOGRAPHY

Boijsen E 1959 Angiographic studies of the anatomy of single and multiple renal arteries. Acta radiol (Stockh): suppl 183

Bowman W 1842 On the structure and use of the Malpighian bodies of the kidney with observations on the circulation through that gland. Phil Trans Roy Soc 132 (i): 57

Brenner B M, Hostetter T H, Humes H D 1978 Molecular basis of proteinuria of glomerular origin. New Eng J Med 298 (15): 826

Gruber C M 1933 The autonomic innervation of the genito-urinary system. Physiol Revs 13: 497

Ishii M, Tobian L 1969 Interstitial cell granules in renal papillaries and the solute composition of renal tissue in rats with Goldblatt hypertension. J Lab Clin Med 74: 47

Jacobsen N O Jorgensen F, Thoen A C 1966 An electron microscopic study of small arteries and arterioles in the normal human kidney. Nephron 3: 17

Kanwar Y S, Linker A, Farquhar M G 1980 Increased permeability of the glomerular basement membrane to ferritin after removal of glycosaminoglycans (Heparan Sulfate) by enzyme digestion. J Cell Biol 86: 688

Latta H, Maunsbach A B 1962 Relations of the centrolobular region of the glomerulus to the juxta-glomerular apparatus. J Ultrastructure Res 6: 547, 562

Mayerson H S 1963 The lymphatic system with particular reference to the kidney. Surg Gynec Obstet 116:

Michael A F, Keane W F, Raij L et al 1980 The glomerular mesangium. Kidney Int 17: 141

Moffat D B, Fourman J 1963 The vascular pattern of the rat kidney. J Anat (Lond) 97: 543

Mueller C B, Mason A D Stout D G 1955 Anatomy of the glomerulus. Amer J Med 18: 267

Page I H, McCubbin J W, 1968 Structure of the juxta-glomerular complex. Renal hypertension. Year Book Medical Publishers, Chicago p 40

Peirce E C 1944 Renal lymphatics. Anat Rec 90: 315

Bennke H G, Venkatachalam M A 1979 Glomerular permeability of macromolecules. Effect of molecular configuration on the fractional clearance of uncharged dextran and neutral horseradish peroxidase in the rat. J Clin Invest 63: 713

Ryan G B, Rodewald R, Karnovsky M J 1975 An ultrastructural study of glomerular slit diaphragm in aminonucleoside nephrosis. J Lab Invest 33: 461

Schurer W, Flevren G J, Hoedemaeker P J et al 1980 A model for the glomerular filter. Renal Physiology 3: 237

Swann H G, Norman R J, 1970 The periarterial spaces of the kidney. Texas Rep Biol Med 28, 3: 317

Swann H G, Valdivia L, Ormsby A A et al 1956 Nature of fluids which functionally distend the kidney. J Exp Med 104: 25

Tisher C C 1976 Anatomy of the kidney. In: Brenner B M, Rector F C Jr (eds) The kidney. Saunders, Philadelphia, p 3

# 2

# Tests of renal structural integrity

The following methods are used to obtain information about the anatomical and histological structure of the kidney. Most of them yeild direct information about renal anatomy, but some, particularly intravenous urography and the radionuclide studies, only provide information on structure via their involvement with function.

Clinical examination of the abdomen
Plain film of the abdomen
Ultrasound examination
Intravenous urography
Renal tomography
Isotope (radionuclide) examination
Retrograde pyelography
Percutaneous (antegrade) pyelography
Cyst puncture
Renal arteriography
Renal venography
Micturating cystogram
Computer tomography
Renal biopsy

## Clinical examination of the abdomen

Obviously this is most helpful in thin patients and may give information about the presence of a tumour, hydronephrosis and polycystic kidneys; if the kidneys are readily palpable it is usually easy to decide whether or not they are much larger than normal. To obtain the best results from this examination it is essential that the patient move his diaphragm well down with each inspiration, while relaxing the anterior abdominal muscles. Some patients seem unable to do this, but may be taught to do so by being told to place their hands, palm downwards, on the surface of their abdomen while they practise. Tenderness in the renal angle or over the kidney anteriorly indicates that there is inflammation which may be due either to infection, infarction or an allergic reaction.

A distended bladder is often an invaluable clue to the presence and cause of renal failure.

## Plain film of the abdomen

Such an X-ray is less revealing than an intravenous pyelogram, but it has certain advantages. It can be performed at short notice and it causes no discomfort. Often it is possible to distinguish the outline of the kidneys so that their size, shape and position can be determined, and it may also be possible to decide whether there are any shadows consistent with the presence of calculi or renal calcification. It is useful to take two films, one in full expiration and another in full inspiration.

## Ultrasound examination

This technique is safe, non-invasive, the patient does not have to be prepared and it does not depend on renal function. But in contrast to most other diagnostic manoeuvres it's value depends strikingly on the trust that is placed on the person who manipulates the probe. Ultrasound can be used repeatedly and is therefore very useful in monitoring the progress of events such as a renal transplantation where it can detect changes in kidney size, ureteric obstruction, and perinephric collections of urine, blood, lymph or pus. As an initial diagnostic tool however, it should be used to complement other methods.

Ultrasound can usually distinguish whether a renal mass, demonstrated by intravenous urography is a cyst or a tumour. It should also be able to determine the size, position and shape of the two kidneys, and the nature of any adjacent structure or mass which may be displacing the kidney. It is particularly useful in the early diagnosis of polycystic kidneys, even in the intrauterine fetus. And it can be used with impunity in pregnancy where irradiation is undesirable. It may be very helpful in revealing the presence of urinary tract obstruction particularly in those difficult occasions when the obstruction is bilateral and causing acute renal failure, but it is particularly dangerous to rely on ultrasound for this purpose, for false negatives can occur.

## Intravenous urography

This is achieved by the rapid intravenous administration of sodium diatrizoate (Hypaque), or a mixture of sodium and methylglucamine diatrizoate (Urografin) or a mixture of sodium and methylglucamine iothalamate (Conray), at a time when the rate of urine flow in minimal. These substances consist of dense molecules containing three radio-opaque atoms which because they are not protein bound are filtered through the glomerulus in large amounts. A very small amount is also secreted into the tubular fluid, by the proximal tubules. When a considerable concentration of these substances has accumulated in the tubular fluid the renal parenchyma becomes faintly visible, while their presence in the urine causes the calyces, pelves and ureters to be densely shadowed. The shadow cast by the paren-chyma is called the nephrogram and that cast by the pelvis and calyces the pyelogram, the older term intravenous pyelogram, or IVP, dates from the days when the value of the nephrogram was not appreciated. On the whole nephrologists are interested in both the nephrogram and the pyelogram, but in that order, whereas urologists tend to be predominantly interested in the pyelogram.

Intestinal gas and faeces and fat may considerably abscure and confuse the results. An aperient should be taken the preceding evening and, if it has failed to act, a small enema should be given. It is best to allow the patient to be up and about for 24 hours before the examination, and a low-residue diet and no medicine containing bismuth or similar radio-opaque substances should be taken for at least two days previously. Intestinal gas can some-times be dispelled by an injection of aqueous vasopressin or neostigmine methyl-sulphate. When renal function is *normal* the rate of urine flow is reduced by fluid deprivation.

The density of the two renal shadows is dependent on the following:
1. The concentration of radio-opaque dye in the blood perfusing the glomeruli.
2. The number of glomeruli and therefore the rate of glomerular filtration.
3. The proportion of water which is removed from the glomerular filtrate as it travels down the tubule, thus concentrating the radio-opaque dye.
4. The antero-posterior depth of urine through which the X-rays have to penetrate.

The optimum concentrations in the blood are obtained with 1 ml/kg body weight of 60% sodium diatrizoate when the glomerular filtration rate is greater than 25 ml/min, and with 2 ml/kg body weight when the glomerular filtration rate is below 25 ml/min. Larger quantities increase the amount in the tubular fluid, but because of the accompanying osmotic diuresis their opaqueness to X-rays may be reduced. Nothing can be done to increase the number of nephrons, but it is probable that noxious stimuli (see below), including perhaps the radio-opaque substances themselves may decrease the function of the nephrons by renal vasoconstriction.

To increase the amount and depth of the urine in the pelves and ureters they are sometimes forcibly distended by partially obstructing the lower ureters by compression of the lower abdomen with an inflatable rubber balloon. This is best done about 5–10 min after the injection of the contrast solution, when its concentration in the pelves has reached a plateau. The final film should be taken after the compression has been released with the patient in the erect position. Failure of most of the contrast medium to empty out of the calyces, pelvis or ureters reveals the presence of obstruction.

The main value of excretion urography is that it demonstrates the size and configuration of the parenchyma, and of the pelvis and calcyes; it is helpful in determining the size, shape and position of the kidneys; it is particularly useful in first suggesting that there may be unilateral parenchymal disease (p. 271). Occasionally distortion of a calyx is best seen on a lateral or oblique view. If the radio-opaque substance is given rapidly and films are taken at 15 sec, 1,2 and 3 min intervals after the injection, additional information can be obtained which is useful in the detection of those occlusions of the renal arteries which are sufficient to cause hypertension; this manoeuvre must be performed without ureteric compression.

Excretion urography give very misleading information about renal function. Small diseased kidneys with little renal function often give dense pyelograms, while absent or faint unilateral or bilateral shadows may be found when the kidneys are normal. Occasionally there may be no shadow during the first urogram, yet a normal shadow is seen a few days later during a second. The reason for these transient anomalies are not always clear. Occasionally they are due to a transient hypotension or ureteric obstruction. It is also possible that the apprehension and discomfort, which are an unavoidable part of intravenous urography, may sometimes be responsible. The patient has to remain in one position on a hard X-ray table for a considerable time and for some of this time he may endure a severe compression of the lower abdomen. Much less stress is known to cause a brisk rise in urine-flow from inhibition of antidiuretic hormone secretion, or an osmotic salt diuresis (p. 71).

*Excretion urography in patients with renal failure. Patients suffering from renal failure must not be dehydrated* for this will make little difference to the concentration of the urine while it may aggravate the renal failure. It is therefore imperative that all those concerned with the urogram be specifically told not to deprive such patients of fluid. The presence of renal failure due to diabetes or myelomatosis however are almost absolute contraindications to excretion urography.

When an excretion urogram is being performed in a patient with renal failure it is sometimes useful, in addition to the usual procedure to continue taking films for some hours, and to include tomography, for in this way the presence of dilated calyces may be revealed which may be due to chronic obstruction. Films are usually taken 20–30 min after the contrast medium has been administered, but it may be necessary to take films intermittently for up to 24 hours to obtain all the available information. The renal outline and the renal substance can nearly always be visualised so that obstruction of the urinary tract is almost invariably demonstrated and excluded, however severe the renal failure, even in patients who are oliguric or anuric. The ability to detect urinary tract obstruction is one of the most useful contributions an intravenous urogram can make in renal failure. The dangers of giving large amounts of contrast media are minimal, if the patient is not deprived of fluid.

### Renal tomography

This technique is most useful when a patient presents with advanced renal failure of unknown cause and when investigating a 'non functioning kidney'. It is also useful in seeing whether calcification is within or simply overlying the kidneys. If an injection of contrast medium is given immediately before taking the tomogram the technique can also help in the differential diagnosis of a renal mass.

### Renal structure shown by radionuclide investigations

Radionuclide studies share with intravenous urography the fact that they can only demonstrate structure if the kidney is functioning, however poorly. Unlike renal ultrasound, or X-ray computer tomography investigations, therefore, which can be performed on a cadaver, renal radionuclide investigations are impossible in the absence of viable renal tissue. Radionuclide tests therefore have unique features.

*Excretion renography with a radioactive substance.* A radio active substance which the kidneys secrete into the urine is injected intravenously, with subsequent serial imaging of the kidneys by means of a gamma camera. (The original renography technique, merely recording time/activity curves over each kidney, gave no structural information and is obsolete.) The usual radio pharmaceutical is Tc DTPA (Technetium Diethylene Triamine Penta Acetic Acid) which is excreted exclusively by glomerular filtration. An alternative is radio-iodinated hippuran which is excreted by both glomeruli and tubules. Though theoretically preferable, the available radioactive forms of iodine have disadvantages. There are two, 131–I which is convenient but gives a greater patient radiation dose than is desirable, and 123–I which is preferable but is not easily available. In contrast, Tc DTPA has a low radiation dose and is readily available.

As might be expected, the excretion renogram using Tc DTPA has some features in common with the intravenous urogram. The earliest images of the kidneys show an 'arteriogram' phase and then, as the radio activity collects in the kidneys, there is 'nephrogram' phase. Subsequent pictures show the function of the outflow tract. As with intravenous X-ray urography, the quality of the study is dependent on the degree of renal function but satisfactory pictures can often be obtained even in extreme renal failure. Unlike the X-ray studies, images obtained from detected radioactivity are not degraded by intestinal gas or gut contents. Computer treatment of the gamma camera images allows quantitation of radioactivity in the two kidneys in the early stages. This closely parallels the relative contribution of each kidney to total renal function and as a measure of total glomerular filtration rate can easily be obtained by some other method, it is possible to obtain an absolute measure of the glomerular filtration rate of each kidney. The excretion renogram is also a valuable aid to the management of renal transplants. It provides information about graft perfusion, size and shape, function, and the outflow tract. The test is atraumatic and can be repeated every other day if necessary. It may be particularly helpful in the anuric post transplantation state when conventional tests of renal function are inappropriate.

*Imaging the kidney with radioactive substances which remain fixed in kidney tissue.* A radio pharmaceutical is used which fixes itself in the cells of the proximal tubules. A number of compounds do this but the most popular currently is Tc DMSA (Technetium Dimercaptosuccinic Acid). As this agent persists in the kidney for some hours, renal images, including lateral and oblique views may be obtained without haste. Accumulation of radio-activity indicates the presence of functioning renal tissue and so it is the technique of choice to search for ectopic renal tissue or to confirm the absence of a kidney. It can demonstrate exagerated foetal lobulation or localised hypertrophy which may distort the renal outline and suggest a space occupying lesion. It is excellent for showing the presence of paren-chymal scars and has been used to monitor growth and progress in reflux nephropathy. It may also demonstrate functioning renal tissue around the periphery of grossly distorted kidneys, as in massive hydronephrosis. Quan-titation of radioactivity on the two sides gives an excellent estimate of the relative contribution of each kidney to total renal function, so long as the kidneys are not displaced.

Radionuclide tests of the kidneys produce pictures with poor detail compaired with most X-ray studies and this may lead to their usefulness being underrated. In fact the detail is perfectly adequate for many purposes and the tests are very simple to perform and should be readily available. The physiological processes which underline the production of these renal images gives them a special significance and can make then uniquely helpful.

## Retrograde pyelography

A radio-opaque solution is introduced directly into the pelvis of the kidney after cystoscopy and ureteric catheterisation. Sodium diatrizoate (25%) or sodium acetrizoate (15%) is injected under condiderable pressure to distend the pelvis and ureter; this is done after the patient has recovered from the anaesthetic so as to avoid overdistension. It is a dangerous procedure when the urinary tract is obstructed for it may cause a severe urinary infection.

The information to be derived from a retrograde pyelogram is obviously confined within the borders of the pelvis, calyx and ureter. The need for retrograde pyelography has considerably diminished since the ureters, pelvis and calyces have been so well demonstrated with the large amounts of contrast media which are now given routinely for intravenous pyelography.

## Percutaneous (antegrade) pyelography

This technique is used, instead of the more dangerous retrograde examin-ation when there is obstruction or dilatation of the upper urinary tract but excretion urography has been inconclusive as to it's cause. Contrast medium is injected directly into the pelvis of the kidney via a needle placed under direct radiological visualisation, with the patient lying on his face. If therapeutically necessary, a catheter can then be threaded through the needle and left in situ to relieve the obstruction and improve renal function until the patient is sufficiently recovered to withstand some more extensive surgical procedure.

## Renal cyst function

When other techniques such as excretion urography and ultrasound have indicated that a renal mass is very probably a cyst a needle is placed into the cyst to first obtain 10–20 ml of fluid for cytological examination and then to inject contrast medium directly into the cyst in order to outline its walls.

## Renal aortography and arteriography

A renal aortogram is obtained by injecting a radio-opaque substance directly into the abdominal aorta at a point just above the origin of the renal arteries; 20–40 ml of 50% sodium diatrizoate are administered via a catheter introduced through a femoral artery; and total volume is administered in 1 to 2 sec. This outlines the abdominal aorta and the origin of the renal arteries where most of the atheromatous obstruction to the renal arteries occurs. It also reveals the presence of accessory renal arteries. Aortography is also of help when the kidney has been injured when it reveals the extent of vascular and parenchymal damage.

A renal arteriogram is performed by injecting the contrast medium directly into the renal artery. Exposures are made at rapid intervals following the injection in order to demonstrate successively the filling of the arteries, veins and tubules (the nephrographic phase). It is a highly specialised technique which gives good pictures of the renal vascular tree. Its greatest use is to identify localised obstructions of the renal artery and its main branches. It can also be useful in defining the existence of localised areas of disease in the renal parenchyma, and distinguishing between tumours and cysts. In principle the tumours being vascular become radio-opaque in contrast to cysts which do not cast a shadow, but there are anomalies. Serious complications after aortography or arteriography are rare, but include acute renal failure, and transient obstruction to the femoral artery.

## Renal venography

One method is to occlude the inferior vena cava momentarily by two rubber balloons, one above the renal veins and the other below. An injection of radio opaque material into this partitioned segment of vena cava may delineate the renal veins and the intrarenal venous system. A more usual technique is to catheterise the renal artery and vein. Contrast material is first placed into the renal artery. With venous thrombosis the passage of the contrast materiial through the kidney is considerably delayed. Collateral venous channels may also become evident. Then nor-adrenaline is injected into the renal artery to cause a transitory fall in renal blood flow and at the same time a retrograde injection of contrast material is made into the renal vein.

## Micturating cystogram

Contrast medium is injected into the bladder via a urethral catheter until the bladder is considerably distended. The patient is then asked to micturate. As he does this, films are taken of bladder, ureters and urethra. This manoeuvre reveals the presence of vesico-ureteric reflux, the principal cause of the scarring of the renal parenchyma which is characteristic of reflux nephropathy (p. 455), and of anatomical abnormalities of the bladder neck and urethra which may be hindering the flow or urine from the bladder.

## Computer tomography (CT scanning)

An expensive X-ray technique with which it is possible to obtain a picture of transverse sections of the body. It's use in nephrology has still to be delineated. At present it's main value appears to be in investigating the retroperitoneal space and the presence and spread of tumours in the pelvis.

## Renal biopsy

A renal biopsy can be performed in two ways. Either the biopsy needle can be inserted through the intact skin. Or the biopsy needle is inserted into the kidney under direct vision through a deep formal surgical approach in the patient's flank. There is little doubt that in centres where renal biopsies are performed infrequently it is probably safer, and a satisfactory sample of renal tissue is more likely to be obtained more frequently, if the biopsy is performed under direct vision. This technique has the additional advantage that haemorrhage into the perirenal tissues can be prevented. On the other hand, in order to perform an open biopsy the patient has to be anaesthetised and he has to suffer the discomforts and possible complications of an abdominal operation.

In most centres, therefore, where renal biopsies are frequently needed it is customary to use the first technique. The biopsy is usually performed with the patient in the prone position. A general anaesthetic is rarely given unless the patient is particularly nervous or very young. A sand-bag is placed under the abdomen, or if the patient is on an operating table, the bridge is raised. A previously performed intravenous urogram, or sometimes only a plain film of the abdomen has demonstrates that the patient has two kidneys and where they are. A fine exploring needle is inserted through the renal angle and the structures down to the kidney infiltrated with local anaesthetic. The fine needle is then withdrawn and the procedure repeated with the biopsy needle when an attempt is then made to bring a fragment of the kidney to the surface. The procedure is more certain if it is performed with the aid of a television screen having given the patient some radio-opaque contrast medium intravenously.

Experience greatly improves performance. Apart from the recurring difficulty of bringing the piece successfully to the surface, there are certain patients who present special difficulties. For instance, those with extensive spinal deformities such as spondylitis deformans or lumbar scoliosis, and those with ascites or pregnancy. There is general agreement that the contraindications to renal biopsy are (1) the presence of only one kidney, (2) a tendency to bleed, and (3) the presence of a hypernephroma, a large renal cyst, a perinephric abscess, or hydro- or pyonephrosis, and (4) an uncooperative patient. Some workers would also include a high blood urea (greater than 100 mg/100 ml), and malignant hypertension, unless the blood pressure is controlled during and for a few hours after the biopsy is performed. If the patient is being treated with an artificial kidney it is usual not to do a biopsy for two days before and one day after a dialysis because of the heparin which is used during the dialysis.

After the biopsy the patient is placed on his back and told to remain in that position uninterruptedly for at least 12–18 hours. This is more likely to produce haemostasis than reliance on a tight abdominal bandage. The patient is also given a large drink of water to induce a diuresis. This not only diminishes the possibility of clot formation if there is haematuria but more quickly demonstrates its presence and extent. The serious complications of biopsy are preponderantly those of haemorrhage either into the renal pelvis or into the retroperitoneal space. Microscopical haematuria always occurs, and direct observation of the retroperitoneal tissues during an open renal biopsy also shows that there is always a perirenal haematoma. It is generally considered, however, that a 'complication' has occurred only when either the haematuria is macroscopic, particularly if there is clot formation, or if the retroperitoneal haemorrhage is sufficiently large to cause pain in the flank and a fall in haemoglobin. Gross haematuria occurs in about 5–10% of cases, and perirenal haematoma in about 2%. Occasionally macroscopical haematuria persists for several days, and there are a few instances of a delayed onset of haematuria. Blood transfusions have been used in about 2% of cases. Other complications include pain during the biopsy which is usually in inverse relationship to the patient's nervousness. A sharp but unimportant pain is produced if the ileoinguinal nerve is transfixed as it emerges from the border of the sacrospinalis, while a dull ache radiating into the iliac fossa indicates that a retroperitoneal haemorrhage is forming. A few patients complain of a transient pain in the back after the biopsy. Comparisons of renal functional capacity before and after the biopsy have demonstrated that unless there is ureteric obstruction from a clot there is no disturbance of function. Serial renal aortograms have been performed in a few patients after renal biopsy. They have revealed a disturbing number of transient intrarenal arterio-venous shunts which may take several months to resolve.

A renal biopsy is clearly the only method of making an exact histological diagnosis during life. The information which has been obtained in this way has been of the greatest value in throwing light upon the natural course of renal disease. And even in the present era of therapeutic helplessness in regard to most renal diseases there are an increasing number of occasions when an exact histological diagnosis is of importance in deciding the patient's future treatment.

BIBLIOGRAPHY

Barrett T M 1975 Renal biopsy. In: Rubin M I, Barrett T M (eds) Pediatric nephrology. Williams & Wilkins, Baltimore
Britton K E 1979 Radionuclides in the investigation of renal disease. In: Black D, Jones N F (eds) Renal disease. Blackwell Scientific, Oxford, p. 270
Davies P, Roberts M B, Roylance J 1975 Acute reactions to urographic contrast media. Brit Med J 2: 434
D'Elia J A, Gleason R E, Alday M et al 1982 Nephrotoxicity from angiographic contrast material. Amer J Med 72: 719
Eisenberg R L, Bank W O, Hedgcock M W 1980 Renal failure after major angiography. Amer J Med 68: 43
Harkomen S, Kjellstrand C M 1977 Exacerbation of diabetic renal failure following intravenous pyelography. Amer J Med 63: 939
Hodson C J 1977 Radiology and the kidney. In: Contributions to nephrology, 5. Karger, Basel
Kincaid O W, Davis G R 1966 Renal angiography. Year Book Medical Publishers, Chicago
Kirkland J A 1959 Massive albuminuria following aortography. Lancet 2: 1144
Maxwell M H, Gonick H G, Witta R et al 1964 Use of rapid-sequence intravenous pyelogram in the diagnosis of renovascular hypertension. New Eng J Med 270: 213
O'Reilly P H, Osborn D E, Testa H J et al 1981 Renal imaging: a comparison of radionuclide, ultrasound and computed tomographic scanning in investigation of renal space-occupying lesions. Brit Med J 282: 943
O'Reilly P H 1979 Nuclear medicine in urology and nephrology. Butterworth, London
Radiology in renal disease. 1972 Brit Med Bull 28, no 3: 189
Rahimi A, Edmondson R P S, Jones N F 1981 Effect of radiocontrast media on kidneys of patients with renal disease. Brit Med J 282: 1194
Seldinger S I 1953 Catheter replacement of the needle in percutaneous arteriography; a new technique. Acta radiol (Stockh) 39: 368
Sherwood T 1971 The physiology of intravenous urography. Scientific basis of medicine annual review: 336
Sherwood T, Trott P A 1975 Needling renal cysts and tumours: cytology and radiology. Brit Med J 3: 755
Wells P N 1977 Ultrasonics in clinical diagnosis, 2nd edn. Churchill Livingstone, Edinburgh
White R H R 1963 Observations on percutaneous renal biopsy in children. Arch Dis Child 38: 260

# 3

# Structural changes (histological) in response to disease and their relation to function

The various ways the glomerulus, tubule or interstitial space may react to disease are limited. And many of the responses can occur in association with more than one renal disease. Structurally, therefore, individual diseases are recognised more often by a pattern of structural disturbance than by any specific change. This explains why to the beginner the histological appearances of most renal diseases all look so much the same. The similarity of the more obvious individual changes is more easily recognised than is the difference between their collective patterns. The analogy with function is relatively close. There are very few abnormalities of function which occur in only one form of renal disease, but patterns of abnormalities can be discerned in certain diseases more often than in others. In the present climate of knowledge it is accepted that functional changes can be studied and discussed separately from the diseases which cause them. The first part of this section attempts to do the same for the structural changes which result from disease. The second part discusses the use of immuno fluorescence, and the third the relation between the histological appearance and renal function.

## Glomerulus

### Epithelial cells

These cells line the inside of Bowman's capsule and the outer surface of the glomerular capillaries. Those lining Bowman's capsule may proliferate and become cuboidal when they then look identical to proximal tubule cells. Occasionally when there are severe focal destructive lesions of the glomerular basement membrane some of the contents of the capillary lumen spill out into Bowman's space. A crescentic collection of fibrin forms in the space which is then invaded by macrophages which lie in parallel crescentic rows. Later this cellular crescent is replaced by basement membrane like material. Crescents are seen most conspicuously but are by no means confined to patients suffering from rapidly progressive glomerular nephritis (p. 390).

The epithelial cells on the outer surface of the capillary loop may swell or lose their foot processes. The swellings are due to the ingestion of large macromolecules and occur with proteinuria. The loss of foot processes is only seen with the electron microscope, it may be focal or general and is also related to proteinuria. Both these changes are most evident but are not limited to patients who have a nephrotic syndrome. Sub-epithelial cell deposits are discussed later.

## Endothelial cells and the capillary lumen

Endothelial cells may proliferate and/or swell. These changes may occlude the lumen of the capillary, a result which may also be produced by intra-luminal aggregation of platelets and leucocytes, or the insinuation of mesangial cytoplasm between the basement membrane and the endothelial cell (see below). The lumen may also be occluded by sub-endothelial deposits. Occlusion of the capillary by endothelial cell swelling and some proliferation occurs in toxaemia of pregnancy, while in acute glomerular nephritis it may be caused by several of the changes described above.

## Mesangium

Mesangial cells are highly phagocytic and their function has been described as one of 'garbage disposal'. Nearly all conditions which affect the glom-erulus are associated with some structural change of the mesangial cells. The most conspicuous is that of proliferation and particularly the formation of deposits of mesangial cell cytoplasm and matrix. Small changes cause what has been described as mesangial stalk 'thickening', a change which is often seen after acute glomerular nephritis. More pronounced changes include either focal nodules of mesangial matrix such as are seen in diabetes, or diffuse masses of matrix which occupy most of the glomerular tuft as in the 'lobular' form of persistent glomerular nephritis. Later the mesangial proliferation disappears while the mass of matrix remains as large acellular areas. These changes can occur without, initially, any involvement of the capillary loop.

In other circumstances the mesangial cells may proliferate and send out cytoplasmic extensions between the endothelial cell and the basement membrane. These may extend peripherally so that the capillary loop is surrounded. The wall of the capillary is then considerably thickened and consists of five layers, the epithelial cell, the basement membrane, the mesangial cytoplasm and matrix, another layer of basement membrane and the endothelial cell (Fig. 3.1). Eosin stains the whole wall a diffuse pink including the mesangial cell cytoplasm and matrix, while PAS and silver selectively stain only the fibrils of the matrix, and the basement membrane. As the mesangial cytoplasm infiltrates itself between the endothelial cells

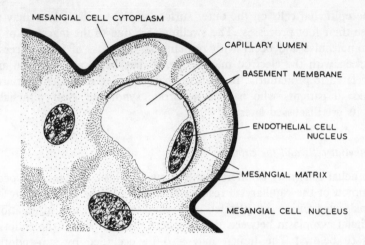

**Fig. 3.1** Diagram of light microscopy appearances in mesangiocapillary glomerular nephritis.

and the basement membrane the fibrils of matrix tend to condense on either side of the cytoplasm. With PAS stain therefore, there is what looks like a split basement membrane surrounding a clear space. The space contains non-PAS staining mesangial cell cytoplasm. This particular abnormality of the mesangium has been called a 'mesangiocapillary' change, a term which is more evocative of what is seen than the older term 'membrano-proliferative'. It is seen in persistent glomerular nephritis, diffuse lupus erytheomatosis and sometimes in diabetes.

*Basement membrane*

Basement membrane surrounds the periphery of a capillary loop, but where the capillary faces the mesangium there is no basement membrane, the lumen of the capillary being in direct contact with the mesangial matrix through the perforations of the endothelial cell cytoplasm (Fig. 1.3). Nevertheless as both basement membrane, and the mesangial cytoplasm and matrix which lie next to the lumen react to disease in much the same way they can be considered together. The basement membrane appears to be altered in all diseases of the kidney, except for that form of glomerular nephritis which is associated with a nephrotic syndrome but in which no histological changes can be detected in the renal biopsy.

The basement membrane and adjoining mesangial matrix may be uniformally thickened, or have focal excrescences, or erosions; they may also be the site of various deposits. Extensive relatively uniform thickening of the basement membrane may occur in diabetes and nephrosclerosis while focal erosions are found in acute glomerular nephritis. Focal excrescences of varying sizes, and various extravagant shapes are found in most prolonged

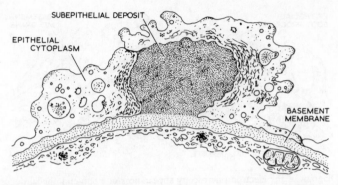

**Fig. 3.2** Diagram of electron microscopy appearance of a hump-like extra-membranous deposit in acute glomerular nephritis.

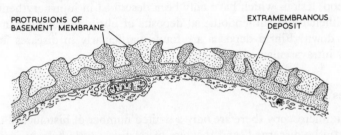

**Fig. 3.3** Diagram of the electron microscopy appearances of the deposits and the basement membrane in extra-membranous glomerular nephritis.

immunological disturbances of the kidney such as chronic glomerular nephritis and lupus erythematosus. The commonest deposits to be found in relation to the basement membrane consist of focal and diffuse masses of material which contain various substances known to be involved in immunological reactions. They may be sub-epithelial or sub-endothelial. Focal sub-epithelial deposits are characteristic of acute glomerular nephritis and are known colloquially as 'humps' (Fig. 3.2). Diffuse sub-epithelial deposits cause those changes which are described under the term extra-membranous glomerular nephritis. In this condition the basement membrane, at first, appears normal but silver stains demonstrate that it extends upwards at relatively regular intervals for a short distance between the deposits (Fig. 3.3). The appearance of the basement membrane is thus like that of a comb with short irregular teeth, the deposits lying between the teeth. Later the deposits increase in size until they become incorporated into a thickened basement membrane which may then totally surround them. Deposits can sometimes be found within the basement membrane, this is particularly characteristic in diffuse lupus erythematosus. Sub-endothelial deposits (Fig. 3.4) occur in a wide variety of conditions including lupus erythematosus, diabetic glomerulosclerosis and pre-

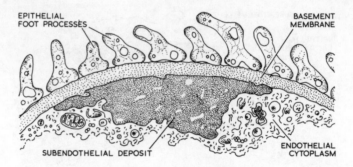

**Fig. 3.4** Diagram of the electron microscopy appearances of a sub-endothelial deposit.

eclampsia. Large focal accumulations may give rise to what have been called 'wire loop' lesions which have only been described in lupus erythematosus. Sub-epithelial and sub-endothelial deposits of fibrin and amyloid may also be laid down. Fibrin deposits are found particularly in diseases in which there is intravascular coagulation.

## Tubules

On light microscopy there are only a limited number of histological changes which can be discerned, and they are of relatively little help in identifying the disease process with which they are associated. Electron microscopy however has revealed that, at the level of the organelle, there are a large number of changes which can be detected.

The so-called hyaline droplet degeneration is seen in a wide variety of renal diseases. It consists of numerous eosinophilic droplets within the cytoplasm of the tubule cell. It is usually due to the tubule cell having absorbed a large quantity of protem from the tubule fiuld. The protein is ingested into lyosomes at a rate greater than the lyosomes can dispose of protein, so that the droplets consist of distended lyosomes filled with proteinaceous material. Pale unstainable vacuolations of the tubule cell are found after the administration of sucrose, manitol and glucose. Again these vacuoles are due to the rapid accumulation of these substances into the cells at a rate greater than the digestive powers of the lyosomes so that they become distended. Hypoxia, hypokalaemia, certain nephrotoxins, partial occlusion of the renal vein and hydronephrosis may cause a sub-lethal injury to the tubule cells leading to an increased number of pale vacuoles which are also due to distended lyosomes. Sometimes these contain fat or necrotic debris such as mitochondria. The vacuoles associated with hypokalaemia are particularly large, and in man are found within the proximal tubules. Tubule cells may also become calcified.

Many disease processes, and some nephrotoxins such as mercury or Amphotericin B may directly inhibit the sodium pump of the tubule cell.

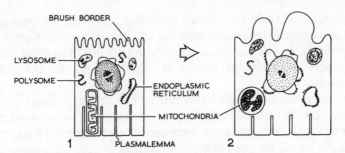

**Fig. 3.5** Diagram of electron microscopy of tubular damage (reproduced from Trump, Tisher & Saladino 1969 In: Bittar E E, Bittar N (eds) The biological basis of medicine. Academic Press, London, vol 6, p 387, with kind permission).

Sodium then accumulates within the cell, water is drawn into the cell and the cell swells. This change has been described as that of 'cloudy swelling' or 'hydro degeneration' (Fig. 3.5). Up to a point this change is compatible with prolonged survival. Prolonged injury may give rise to tubular atrophy, a feature which is seen in all forms of renal disease. The tubule may then appear as a shrivelled mass surrounded by a thick collar of PAS positive basement membrane. Acute necrosis of the tubules may occur from acute ischaemia or nephrotoxic poisons. In those sites in which the necrosis does not involve the basement membrane the flat necrotic tubular epithelium regenerates rapidly.

The nucleus of the tubule cells may swell when the sodium pump is inhibited. Otherwise the nuclearplasm may show inclusion bodies such as virus particles in cytomegalic inclusion disease, or dense accumulations due to poisoning with heavy metals such as bismuth or lead.

### Interstitial space

In most renal diseases the interstitial space shows some abnormality. The most common is a variably distributed widening of the space between the tubules, best known as 'tubular separation' and sometimes referred to as 'oedema of the interstitium'. It is remarkable how often this most obvious and important abnormality is not mentioned in a report on a renal biopsy. Chronic inflammatory cells are usually found in these widened areas of interstitium, scattered thinly and in focal collections. Such collections are often accompanied by degeneration of the adjoining tubules so that it is difficult to make out if the pathological process began in the interstitium or in the tubule. Very occasionally, however, it is easier to decide, as in acute glomerular nephritis in which there may be focal collections of acute and chronic inflammatory cells surrounded by tubules which show necrosis only of the wall next to the collection of inflammatory cells, the whole area looking as if a small inflammatory explosion had occurred in the interstitial space.

Sometimes the whole interstitium is widely separated and packed with chronic and acute inflammatory cells, an appearance known as acute interstitial nephritis. In this condition, which is usually due to an acute immunological process, most of the tubules are also damaged but the glomeruli appear normal.

If the underlying pathological abnormality persists the widened interstitial space fills up with fibrous tissue. In most instances the cause of the change in the interstitial space cannot be discerned. A chronic interstitial nephritis, however, in which the predominent inflammatory cells are plasma cells is probably associated with Sjögen's syndrome. And the associated presence of the characteristic histological changes of glomerular nephritis in the glomeruli, the presence of urate crystals calcium deposits, or bacteria or the appearance of advanced vascular disease may make it easier to speculate about the cause of the interstitial widening and fibrosis. A radiological diagnosis of phenacetin nephropathy, reflux nephropathy (chronic pyelonephritis), obstructive uropathy or medullary cystic disease will also help.

## Vessels

This is a contentious and difficult area. The principal difficulty is that the vascular changes in the ageing kidney are up to a point the same as those which accompany hypertension, and they are also seen in other renal diseases, in the absence of hypertension e.g. gouty nephropathy. The arterial tree in the ageing kidney develops sub-intimal thickening particularly of the arterioles, with elastic reduplication of the media in larger vessels, both changes which tend to narrow the lumen. These changes are accompanied by patchy, sometimes wedge shaped, cortical areas of tubular atrophy with focal areas of tubular separation and scattered inflammatory cells. The glomerular tufts tend to shrink and collections of collagen accumulate on the *inside* of Bowman's capsule, an appearance frequently misnamed *peri*-glomerular fibrosis. If the patient is young these changes are pathological, in an older subject a decision between the normal ageing process and a pathological process is more difficult. More florid changes are unlikely to be due to age. These consist of arteriolar necrosis, arteriolar occlusion with micro thrombi, or complete occlusion of the lumen of larger arteries, particularly of the interlobular arteries, by shredded collagen interspersed by much amorphous material in which are embedded a few nuclei. Necrosis of vessels is often accompanied by focal areas of necrosis in the glomeruli.

## Immunofluorescent staining

The development of this technique has made it possible to detect the presence of certain substances such as antigens and antibodies in the renal parenchyma which are not there normally. The first step in the technique consists of repeatedly injecting an animal with a pure preparation of some intrinsic or extrinsic substance which is antigenic to the animal. In this connection it must be remembered that human immunoglobulin antibodies are antigenic to the experimental animal. Intrinsic substances which have been used include IgG, IgM, IgA, IgE, IgD, $\beta_1$C complement, renin, fibrin, insulin, some nucleoside fractions of DNA and neoplastic antigens. Extrinsic antigens include those obtained from malarial parasites, schisosoma, the leprosy bacillus and the Australia antigen. The animal develops circulating antibodies to the particular antigenic substance which has been injected. The antibodies are then extracted from the blood and labelled with a fluorescent stain. This preparation can now be used to detect the presence of that antigenic substance in a section of kidney from a patient. A renal biopsy is performed and a section is made when it is freshly frozen. A drop of the liquid preparation containing the fluorescent antibody which has been obtained from the experimental animal is then placed on the surface of the frozen section. If the antigen against which the animal formed the antibody is present in the renal biopsy the fluorescent antibody will bind onto it and will adhere to the section. After a suitable interval the section is repeatedly washed to remove any unbound fluorescent antibody. The section is then examined under ultra-violet illumination. The sites in the section which contain the antigenic substance will be fluorescent against a dark background.

In this way it has been possible to demonstrate that in various renal diseases one or more of the various substances listed above are present within the renal parenchyma. It has therefore made it possible to infer which renal diseases are probably associated with a humoral immunological disturbance. And, when deposits of intravascular fibrin have been found, it has led to the conclusion that perhaps some of the structural changes are due to intravascular clotting which may itself cause inflammatory proliferative changes and ischaemia. Conversely the inability to detect any of these substances in various other renal diseases makes it possible that they are due to one or more mechanisms other than a humoral immunological disturbance, or intravascular clotting.

Some characteristic patterns have emerged. They depend not only on which particular substance is present, which should not normally be in the renal parenchyma, but also on the way the substance is distributed. The most characteristic patterns are almost all found in the glomerulus. For instance in membranous glomerular nephritis IgG is nearly always found lying along the glomerular capillary wall as a fine granular deposit, while there is none in the mesangial areas (Fig. 3.6). Whereas in Henoch-Schönlein nephritis IgA is seen predominantly in the mesangial areas. In acute glomerular nephritis IgG is again found lying along the glomerular capillary wall but in a rather lumpy distribution. In Goodpasture's syndrome, or in other syndromes in which the blood contains anti-glomerular basement membrane antibody, IgG is laid down along the capillary wall in smooth

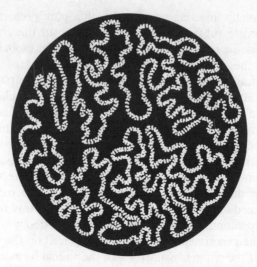

**Fig. 3.6** Diagram of the appearances of the immunofluorescent granular deposits along glomerular capillary walls.

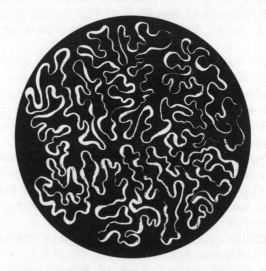

**Fig. 3.7** Diagram of the appearances of immunofluorescent linear diffuse deposits along glomerular capillary walls.

homogeneous lines (Fig. 3.7). Depositions of IgG are also found in renal vein thrombosis, embolic nephritis and in the nephrotic syndrome associated with neoplastic disease.

IgA is seen in focal proliferative glomerular nephritis not associated with a systemic disease, it is then deposited in the mesangial areas and is almost never found in the capillary walls (Fig. 3.8). Similar deposits of IgA are

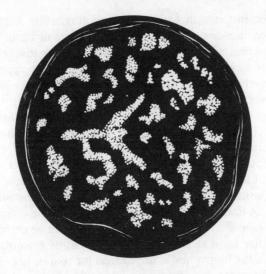

**Fig. 3.8** Diagram of the appearances of immunofluorescent deposits in mesangial areas.

found in long standing liver disease. Granular deposits of IgM lying along the capillary wall occur in transplanted kidneys and in focal sclerosing glomerular nephritis. Large intraluminal deposits of IgM are also seen in macroglobulinaemia. $\beta_1C$ complement is usually found, though less frequently, in association with the immunoglobulins mentioned above. In membranoproliferative glomerular nephritis however $\beta_1C$ is found in nearly all cases laid down in a coarse granular pattern both in the capillary wall and the mesangial areas; often there is no associated fixation of immunoglobulin. Intracapillary fibrin is seen in many conditions, particularly in those in which deterioration of renal function is most rapid such as Goodpasture's syndrome and rapidly progressive glomerular nephritis. In toxaemia of pregnancy fibrin is usually found without any accompanying deposition of immunoglobulins. Deposits of various fractions of DNA and IgG are present in disseminated lupus erythematosus both in the capillary wall and in the mesangial areas. Antigenic fractions of the malarial parasite, schistosomes, and the leprosy bacillus have been found in the glomeruli of patients suffering from infections by these agents when they have had an associated renal disturbance such as proteinuria or a nephrotic syndrome.

In contrast it has not been possible to demonstrate either the presence of immunoglobulin or abnormal antigens in the renal parenchyma of patients suffering from nephrosclerosis, chronic pyelonephritis and phenacetin nephropathy.

*Relation between the structural changes found with light microscopy and electron microscopy, and the findings obtained with immunofluorescence.* Each one of these three techniques has something of individual importance to contribute. For instance in focal sclerosing glomerular nephritis electron microscopy may demonstrate intravascular deposits of fibrin which are too small to be detected with immunofluorescence. Alternatively immunofluorescent deposits have been detected in biopsies which appear normal on both light and electron microscopy. The routine use of a wide variety of immunofluorescent antibodies and the use of special preparations against certain unusual antigens such as those obtained from the malarial parasite and tumour cells has been of immense value in elucidating the probable aetiology of certain renal diseases. At the moment, however, there are many confusing exceptions. For example in a proportion of patients with mesangial proliferation no immunofluorescent staining can be detected, while others only show deposits of $\beta_1 C$. Many patients with focal sclerosing glomerular nephritis have no immunofluorescent deposits. One thing is clear. It is that to examine renal biopsies with light microscopy only can be extremely misleading. On the other hand electron microscopy permits examination of only a small portion of the biopsy and is impractical for routine use. The technique of immunofluorescent staining is more practicable but the findings still demonstrate many unexplained inconsistencies.

### Relation between structural changes and individual nephron function

In individual nephrons from a diseased kidney there is a close relationship between structure and function, but there are wide differences between nephrons. Some nephrons are hypertrophied or hyperplastic and have supernormal single nephron filtration rates, others are atrophic with low glomerular filtration rates. Nevertheless as glomerular filtration rate falls overall tubular function remains remarkably normal. In other words as renal failure develops though the body's content of those substances which depend mainly on filtration for excretion rises (e.g. urea and creatinine), its content of those substances which depend mainly on tubular function remains remarkably normal (e.g. sodium, potassium and water). If follows that overall tubule function adapts to the overall decrease in filtration rate. And precise measurement of proximal tubule reabsorption in individual nephrons indicates that this adaptation takes place to the same extent in all nephrons whatever their structure and glomerular filtration rate. In other words each tubule adjusts its reabsorption according to its filtration rate so that the proportion of filtrate reabsorbed by each proximal tubule is the same. The mechanisms underlying this phenomenon are not obvious. One partial explanation is that tubule function in a diseased kidney may control glomerular filtration rate much more closely than in a normal kidney. If this is true then the adaptive phenomenon in the diseased kidney can be stood on its head, it is the filtration rate that is adapting to the variations in the tubule's structure and function. Theoretically the tubule could do this by altering the luminal pressure in the tubule thus changing the hydrostatic pressure gradient across the glomerular capillary wall.

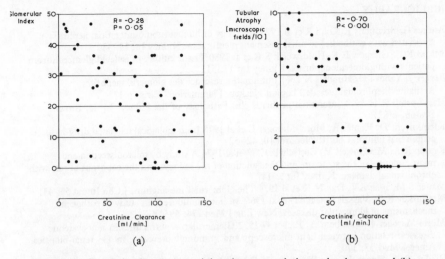

**Fig. 3.9** (a) Correlation between creatinine clearance and glomerular damage and (b) between creatinine clearance and tubular atrophy (reproduced from Risdon, Sloper & de Wardener 1968 Lancet 2: 363, with kind permission).

## Relation between structural changes and overall renal function

Total glomerular filtration rate bears a much closer relation to the extent of tubular damage and interstitial separation than to the extent of glomerular damage (Fig. 3.9). In other words it is not unusual to find patients with relatively unimpaired glomerular filtration rates in whom the renal biopsy demonstrates extensive glomerular damage with large eosinophilous deposits but in which the extent of tubular and interstitial changes are minimal; the reverse can be seen in both acute and chronic renal failure. One explanation is that as mentioned above the abnormality of the tubule (or perhaps the widened oedematous interstitium) impairs the efficiency of tubular reabsorption. This may then lower glomerular filtration rate by raising the intratubular hydrostatic pressure. A similar effect as that which presumably occurs when the tubule lumen is obstructed by a cast or cell debris. On the other hand, it is possible that interstitial abnormalities may also compress the arterioles so that the glomerular filtration rate might fall because of a fall in renal blood flow. It is also possible that, though the substances used to measure glomerular filtration rate do so accurately when the tubules are normal they may not do so when the tubule is damaged. There is certainly evidence in acute renal failure that filtered substances which do not pass through a normal tubule wall may diffuse out of a damaged tubule. In some patients therefore the measured glomerular filtration rate may be much lower than the true filtration rate because the substance used to measure filtration rate (e.g. inulin) has leaked from the tubule lumen into the interstitium and back into the blood.

## BIBLIOGRAPHY

Andres G, Brentjens J, Kohli R et al 1978 Histology of human tubulo-interstitial nephritis associated with antibodies to renal basement membranes. Kidney Int 13: 480

Atkins R C, Glasgow E F, Holdsworth S R et al 1980 Tissue culture of isolated glomeruli from patients with glomerulonephritis. Kidney Int 17: 515

Berger J, Yaneva H, Hinglais N 1971 Immunofluorescence des glomerulonephrites. Actualites nephrologiques de l'hopital Necker. Flammarion, Paris, p 17

Hepstinstall R H 1974 Interstitial nephritis. In: Pathology of the kidney. Little, Brown, Boston, p 821

Kleinknecht D, Kanfer A, Morel-Maroger L et al 1978 Immunological mediated drug-induced acute renal failure. Contrib Nephrol 10: 42–52

Kramp R A, MacDowell M, Gottschalk C W et al 1974 A study by microdissection and micropuncture of the structure and the function of the kidneys and the nephrons of rats with chronic renal damage. Kidney Int 5: 147

Mauer S M, Fish A J, Day N K et al 1974 The glomerular mesangium. J Clin Invest 53: 431

McCluskey R T, Vassali P, Gallo G et al 1966 An immunofluorescent study of pathogenic mechanisms in glomerular diseases. New Eng J Med 274: 695

Morel-Maroger L, Leathem A, Richet G 1972 Glomerular abnormalities in non-systemic diseases: relation between light microscopy and immunofluorescence in 433 renal biopsies. Amer J Med 53: 170

Risdon R A, Sloper J C, de Wardener H E 1968 Relationship between renal function and histological changes found in renal-biopsy specimens from patients with persistent glomerular nephritis. Lancet 2: 363

Trump B F, Tisher C C, Saladino A J 1969 The nephron in health and disease. In: Bittar E E, Bittar N (eds) The biological basis of medicine. Academic Press, London, vol 6, p 387

# 4

# Introduction to renal function and some theoretical considerations concerned in testing its integrity

The function of the kidney is to assist in keeping the volume and composition of the extracellular fluid within normal limits; it is also concerned with the maintenance of a normal blood pressure, erythropoisis, vitamin D metabolism and certain endocrine functions.

The composition and volume of the extracellular fluid is controlled by glomerular filtration, and tubular reabsorption or secretion. In a day approximately 180 litres of almost protein-free fluid is filtered through the glomerular capillaries into the glomerular space, from whence it passes into the tubule. As this filtrate travels down the tubule various substances are either subtracted or added to it, so that eventually only about 1 litre emerges as urine; this is the water and solutes which the body needs to discard. The renal mechanisms involved in regulating the blood pressure and erythropoiesis are obscure; they are discussed in Chapter 16 (p. 260) and Chapter 15 (p. 245).

In normal circumstances every glomerulus is continuously being perfused with blood. The rate of blood flow is adjusted by alterations in the afferent and efferent glomerular arterioles. Such changes must influence the glomerular capillary pressure and in turn the rate of glomerular filtration. Alterations in glomerular filtration rate are, within wide limits, affected by changing the rate of filtration in each glomerulus. There is no evidence that new nephrons are opened up when glomerular filtration rate increases, and complete closure of some glomeruli only occurs when glomerular filtration rate is suddenly reduced below 50%.

Normally approximately 120 ml of filtrate are separated from the 600 ml of plasma that pass through the kidneys each minute. The ratio glomerular filtration rate: renal plasma flow is known as the filtration fraction. It can be seen that in health it is about 0.2. In disease it may vary from 0.1 to 0.3, but it is clear that, as might have been expected, the relationship between the rate of renal plasma flow and the glomerular filtration rate remains relatively close.

Glomerular filtrate contains all the ultrafiltrable substances present in plasma and, ignoring a slight difference caused by the plasma proteins, they are present in the same concentrations. There is also some indirect evidence that the filtrate contains small concentrations of protein, probably less than 300 mg/l; though this is a relatively insignificant concentration, it nevertheless amounts to a filtration of about 50 g of protein in 24 hours.

## Theoretical considerations

The contents of the urine are selected from the plasma by a wide variety of mechanisms. It follows that the methods used to measure the efficiency of these mechanisms also vary. For instance, it will be shown in Section 5 that one of the best methods for testing the kidney's ability to control the sodium content of the extracellular fluid is to place the patient on a salt-free diet, and then to observe whether the kidney is able to diminish the excretion of sodium. Such a method is obviously unsuitable for measuring the kidney's ability to control the extracellular fluid concentration of substances which, regardless of intake, are continuously being manufactured by the body, e.g. urea and creatinine.

It has been found empirically that the most convenient gauge of the kidney's ability to control the extracellular fluid concentration of substances such as urea and creatinine is to calculate the quotient

$$\frac{\text{amount excreted in the urine per min } (\mu\text{mol})}{\text{concentration in the plasma } (\mu\text{mol/ml})} \quad \text{or} \quad \frac{UV}{P}$$

where U = the concentration in the urine ($\mu$mol/100 ml), V = the urine volume per min (ml/min), and P = the plasma concentration ($\mu$mol/100 ml). This quotient can of course be calculated for any substance which is present in the plasma and the urine, but it is of little value if the result is greatly influenced by factors unrelated to renal function (e.g. diet). It is relatively useless, for example, to calculate the quotient for sodium for, in a normal person, it may vary by more than 100% during a single day. The quotients for urea and creatinine, however, are relatively constant, for their urinary excretion throughout the day is far more uniform.

The quotient UV/P is expressed as ml/min, i.e. ($\mu$mol/min)/($\mu$mol/ml) = ml/min, and is conventionally referred to as a 'clearance'. This curious term derives from an extension of the fact that the result of dividing the amount excreted in the urine by the plasma concentration gives the least volume of plasma which could have contained the amount excreted. It follows that the quotient can therefore be considered as representing the volume of plasma which must be completely 'cleared' to provide the amount appearing in the urine. The concept of a clearance is only a particular way of thinking about the quotient UV/P, it is obviously unrelated to what is actually happening in the kidney, for there is no evidence that some of the plasma is stripped of certain of its contents while the remainder emerges unchanged. The disadvantages of the word 'clearance' are the tortuous explanations and frequent misconceptions to which it gives rise.

## Measurement of glomerular filtration rate

The most precise measurement of glomerular filtration rate is obtained with inulin, for after passing freely through the glomerulus it travels down the tubule without any being subtracted or added by the tubule cells. The quantity that is excreted in the urine in one minute is therefore the same as that which is filtered. But it is known from puncture of the glomerular capsule by micropipettes that the fluid in Bowman's space (i.e. the glomerular filtrate) is identical to plasma ultrafiltrate. Therefore the quantity of insulin present in the urine must, as it passed through the glomerulus, have been accompanied by a quantity of water sufficient to keep the inulin concentration in the capsular space the same as in the plasma. This volume is clearly that of the glomerular filtrate; it is estimated by calculating the least volume of water (i.e. plasma) that can have contained the amount of inulin excreted in the urine, i.e. UV/P. The inulin clearance is thus a measure of glomerular filtration rate. For instance, if the plasma concentration of inulin is 10 mg/100 ml, and 10 mg of inulin is excreted in the urine in one minute, it is clear that if inulin is not reabsorbed or secreted by the tubule cells, 100 ml of water is passing through the glomerular filter in one minute.

For similar reasons creatinine clearance is also used as a measure of glomerular filtration rate, but it is not so exact as inulin for a small quantity of creatinine is secreted into the tubular fluid by the tubules.

## Measurement of renal plasma and blood flow

The renal plasma flow (RPF) can theoretically be calculated by the Fick principle using any substance excreted in the urine, provided that the renal arterial (RA), and renal venous (RV) plasma concentrations, the urine flow (V), and the urine concentration (U) of that substance are known:

$$RPF \ (ml/min) = \frac{UV \ (excretion \ per \ minute)}{RA - RV \ (arterio\text{-}venous \ difference)}$$

From this renal blood flow (RBF) can be calculated from the arterial haematocrit (Hct):

$$RBF = \frac{RPF}{1 - (Hct/100)}$$

It will be seen below that this laborious procedure is seldom necessary, but it is feasible by obtaining samples of arterial blood from the femoral artery, while renal venous blood is obtained via a catheter introduced through an antecubital or femoral vein.

Clearly a substance that is almost completely excreted by the kidney and therefore has a large RA – RV difference will give more accurate results than one like sodium which has an insignificant RA – RV difference. An almost ideal substance is para-amino-hippuric acid (PAH) which is infused intravenously until a steady plasma concentration is achieved.

If the plasma PAH level is less than 5 mg/100 ml about 90% of the PAH reaching the kidney is promptly excreted in the urine (except in cases of advanced renal failure). In general, therefore, it is not necessary to catheterise the renal vein to sample the renal venous blood, for it can be assumed that RV is negligible (i.e. RV = o) or:

$$RPF = \frac{UV}{RA}$$

In other words the clearance of PAH is a measure of renal plasma flow.

Furthermore, since the *peripheral* venous plasma concentration of PAH is almost identical to that in the arterial blood, it is also unnecessary to sample arterial blood, and the whole technique is greatly simplified.

In clinical work PAH clearances are hardly ever estimated. There is a relatively rigid relationship between the renal blood flow and the glomerular filtration rate, and it is easier to estimate filtration rate than renal blood flow. The simplest way to perform a PAH clearance is to inject 12 ml 20% PAH mixed with 6 ml 2 per cent xylocaine into the loose subcutaneous tissues of the axilla. The urine collection periods are begun 30–45 min later. Alternatively the use of small quantities of [125]I-Hippuran greatly simplifies the technique.

BIBLIOGRAPHY

Berliner R W 1971 Outline of renal physiology. In: Strauss M B, Welt L G (eds) Diseases of the kidney. Little Brown, Boston, p 31
Goldring W, Chasis H 1944 Hypertension and hypertensive disease. Commonwealth Fund, New York (for inulin and para-amino hippuric acid clearance techniques)
Gutman Y, Gottschalk C W, Lassiter W E 1965 Micropuncture study of inulin absorption in the rat kidney. Science 147: 753
Ram M D, Evans K, Chisholm G D 1967 Measurement of effective renal plasma-flow by the clearance of [125]I-Hippuran. Lancet 2: 645

# 5

# Tests of glomerular functional integrity and proteinuria

The mean hydrostatic pressure in the glomerular capillary in the rat, in which it has been measured directly, is considerable. It is approximately 60 cm $H_2O$. The effective filtration pressure, which is the hydrostatic pressure less the plasma protein osmotic pressure is therefore about 14 cm $H_2O$. The permeability of the glomerular capillary wall is also higher than capillaries elsewhere. This combination of a relatively high capillary hydrostatic pressure and permeability accounts for the high rate of filtration which occurs across the glomerular capillary wall. Though there is mean driving force of approximately 14 cm $H_2O$ at the afferent end of the capillary, the rise in plasma protein osmotic pressure which occurs as fluid is filtered from the plasma across the capillary wall gradually raises the plasma protein osmotic pressure so that at the efferent end of the capillary the net driving force across the wall is 0, a phenomenon known as filtration equilibrium.

It has been mentioned earlier that in man approximately 600 ml of plasma pass through the glomeruli per minute from which are filtered about 120 ml of fluid that is almost free of protein and blood cells. Glomerular integrity can thus be studied by measuring glomerular filtration rate and by examining the urine for the presence of protein, cells and casts.

## GLOMERULAR FILTRATION RATE

The four methods most widely used to obtain an indication of the glomerular filtration rate are, in descending order of accuracy:
1. Inulin clearance
2. $^{51}Cr$ EDTA clearance
3. Creatinine clearance
4. Urea clearance.

Estimations of plasma creatinine and urea are also used to get a rough idea of the glomerular filtration rate, and particularly to follow changes in the filtration rate. In addition Tc DTPA is also used occasionally to get an impression of the overall glomerular filtration rate, but it is most useful in helping to provide an accurate estimate of the glomerular filtration rate of each kidney (p. 16).

## Inulin clearance

An inulin clearance is a protracted procedure, many blood samples are needed and, as urine is collected at short intervals, relatively large errors due to incomplete bladder emptying may occur which can only be avoided with certainty by catheterisation. For these reasons glomerular filtration rate, except for research purposes, is hardly ever determined by inulin clearance. For clinical purposes an inulin clearance can most easily be performed after an intravenous injection of 90 ml of 10% inulin. The urine collections are begun 30 min later.

## $^{51}$Cr EDTA clearance

Ethylenediaminetetracetate (EDTA) is handled by the kidney in almost the same way as inulin. The clearance of EDTA can therefore be used to measure glomerular filtration rate. It has an enormous advantage over inulin, however, for it can be labelled with $^{51}$Cr which is a gamma emitter. $^{15}$Cr EDTA is a stable substance while $^{51}$Cr has a usefully long half life, is relatively innocuous and is rapidly eliminated in the urine. All the advantages of using a gamma emitting isotope can therefore be used to measure glomerular filtration rate. $^{15}$Cr EDTA clearance can either be determined in the usual way from the quotient UV/P during the administration of $^{51}$Cr EDTA by a continuous intravenous infusion, or it can be calculated from the fall in plasma concentration of $^{51}$Cr EDTA 2 hours after a single intravenous injection. The latter, though indirect, avoids the hazards inherent in trying to collect a timed sample of urine.

## Creatinine clearance

This remains by far the most convenient method of obtaining a fairly accurate estimate of glomerular filtration rate. The clearance of pure creatinine however is slightly greater than that of inulin, indicating that some creatinine is actively secreted by the tubules. The amount of creatinine that is actively secreted is related to the level of plasma creatinine. With advancing renal failure therefore the discrepancies between the clearance of creatinine and inulin increases. When the plasma creatinine is about 350 $\mu$mol/l (4 mg/100 ml) the creatinine to inulin clearance ratio is 1.4. At higher levels this effect diminishes so that at plasma creatinine concentrations around 900 $\mu$mol/l (10 mg/100 ml) the ratio has fallen to 1.2. Nevertheless at these plasma levels of creatinine the glomerular filtration rate is so small that such discrepancies are of no moment.

The clearance of creatinine is a much more convenient determination to make than that of inulin, for creatinine is already present in body fluids; its plasma concentration being remarkably steady throughout the 24 hours. Creatinine clearance tests can therefore be performed over long periods without the necessity of continuous intravenous administration; and because the plasma concentration of creatinine, if the patient is on a normal protein intake, is relatively stable, only one sample of blood need be taken during a 24-hour collection of urine. Such long periods minimise inaccuracies caused by incomplete bladder emptying or slipshod timing of the duration of urine collection; they also diminish the effect of transient emotional reactions on renal function.

*Procedure for a 24-hour creatinine clearance*

The basic requirements are a 24-hour collection of urine and one sample of blood preferably taken before lunch. Because an accurately timed collection of urine is so incredibly difficult to obtain (except in a metabolic ward), it is perhaps worth while describing some of the difficulties which are encountered. A 24-hour collection of urine can start at any convenient hour, e.g. 9 a.m.; at this time the patient is asked to empty his bladder and this urine is discarded; for the next 24 hours all the urine that is passed is collected into one container and the collection ended when the patient is asked to empty his bladder for the last time 24 hours after the collection period began, e.g. at 9 a.m., this urine being included in the 24-hour collection. It is clearly of no importance if the actual duration of the collection period is a few hours more or less than 24, so long as it is accurately timed. The volume of the urine is then measured and the rate of urine flow per minute is calculated by dividing this volume by the number of minutes which the collection period has lasted. A convenient slogan is that the urine collection should be 'timed to the nearest minute and measured to the nearest ml'. A screw-topped bottle full of this urine, and the blood sample, are then sent together to the laboratory for creatinine estimation and calculation of the clearance.

This simple manoeuvre may be vitiated by the following accidents: (1) unless the patient has been warned, urine may be passed during defaecation and thrown away; (2) unless urine is placed immediately into a large container it may be lost and not included in the 24-hour collection; (3) occasionally the urine passed at the beginning of the collection period is included in the total collection; though the patient may have four or five hours urine in his bladder; (4) it is not unknown for a 24-hour collection to cease when the container into which it is being collected is full, regardless of the time the collection began; beware, therefore, of a 24-hour collection bottle filled to the brim. Many of these troubles can be avoided by making the patient responsible for his own urine collection.

**Urea clearance**

The clearance of urea used to be the most widely used test of renal function. Its value depends on the fact that urea clearance is directly related to the

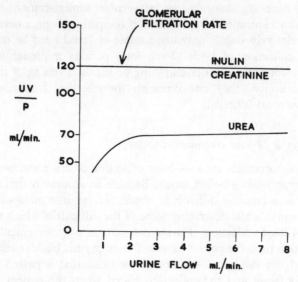

**Fig. 5.1** Schema showing the relationship between the clearances of inulin, creatinine and urea to the urine flow and to each other.

glomerular filtration rate. As a guide to the rate of glomerular filtration, however, it is greatly inferior to the creatinine clearance. Its main disadvantages are: (1) the clearance of urea is considerably less than the rate of glomerular filtration; (2) this discrepancy varies with the rate of urine flow; and (3) the ward procedure involved in a urea clearance makes it very vulnerable to technical inaccuracies.

In normal subjects, when the urine flow is greater than 2 ml/min urea clearance is about three-fifths of the glomerular filtration rate; at lower urine flows it is less. This relationship is illustrated in Figure 5.1. It suggests that though there is every reason to believe that urea is filtered through the glomerulus at the same rate as inulin and creatinine, for urea is a small highly diffusible molecule, a great deal must be reabsorbed as it passes down the tubule. At urine flows above 2 ml/min the amount reabsorbed is constant and is about two-fifths of the quantity which has been filtered, and as the urine flow becomes less so gradually more urea is reabsorbed. In an average man, therefore, the urea clearance at urine flows above 2 ml/min is 3/5 × 120 = 74 ml/min; such a clearance (obtained at urine flows greater than 2 ml/min) is sometimes called the maximum urea clearance.

When the urine flow is less than 2 ml/min urea clearance varies with the rate of urine flow, but in normal subjects if the clearance is then multiplied by the square root of the rate of urine flow, a figure is obtained which approximates to an average of 54 ml/min, regardless of the rate of urine flow. This mathematical jugglery is called a 'standard urea clearance'; it is a manoeuvre which adjusts all the true clearances measured at rates of urine flow below 2 ml/min as if they had been estimated at a standard urine flow of 1 ml/min. This rigmarole probably caused more confusion about the nature of renal function in those not familiar with the subject than any other of the many mathematical obscurities which so often enshroud the kidney. It is obvious that a 'standard urea clearance' is *not* a clearance and that the use of the word 'standard' in this context is misleading. For clinical purposes these complications are best avoided by doing urea clearances at rates of urine flow above 2 ml/min.

*Procedure for a urea clearance test*

It is customary to perform this test over a short period in the morning when the patient is fasting. In order to to raise the urine flow above 2 ml/min two glasses of water are given about half an hour before the beginning of the first period when the bladder is emptied and the urine discarded. An hour later the bladder is emptied again, the urine is saved and a sample of venous blood is taken. Finally the urine is collected once more after a further hour. The volume of the two urine collections is measured and a sample of each collection is then sent, together with blood, to the laboratory for urea estimation and calculation of the clearance. The point of having two collection periods is to enable a comparison to be made between these two clearances so that the accuracy of the urine collection may be gauged.

Serious errors will occur if the bladder cannot be emptied properly or if those concerned with noting the duration of the urine collection period are horologically amoral. Occasionally the test may be influenced by the emotional reactions of the patient to having to empty his bladder at predetermined intervals, or to having to submit to venepuncture.

There is a point in the laboratory technique which sometimes causes confusion. The urea clearance is usually expressed as a 'blood' clearance, i.e. UV/B (as opposed to UV/P). This is possible because urea is freely diffusible into red cells, and the concentration of urea in whole blood is almost identical to its concentration in plasma. If necessary therefore blood urea estimations can be performed on spun red cells, leaving the supernatant plasma available for other estimations.

## Plasma concentrations of urea and creatinine as a guide to the rate of glomerular filtration

Normal plasma urea concentrations vary between 2–6 mmol/l (15–35 mg/100 ml), the lower values tending to be found principally in children, and during pregnancy: normal plasma creatinine concentrations vary between 45–120 $\mu$mol (0.5–1.4 mg/100ml). If the clearance of these substances parallels the rate of glomerular filtration it is clear that when the filtration rate falls their plasma concentration will rise. It would seem simpler therefore, when trying to gauge the state of the glomerular filtration rate, to be guided by an estimation of these plasma concentrations instead of having to perform clearances. Unfortunately the relation between glomerular filtration and plasma concentration is such that these concentrations are only of limited usefulness in this respect. The reasons for this are given below.

The plasma concentrations of urea and creatinine depend on their rate of production and elimination. If their route of elimination is via the glomerular filtrate and their daily production is relatively constant, then a fall in glomerular filtration rate will cause their plasma concentration to rise until a new equilibrium is reached. Conversely, if glomerular filtration rate remains constant and the rate of urea or creatinine production increases, their plasma concentrations will also increase. The connection between glomerular filtration, the production of urea and creatinine, and their plasma concentrations are analogous to the situation that obtains when fluid is being poured into a funnel. The height of the level of the fluid in the funnel depends on the diameter of the funnel's outlet and the rate at which the fluid is being delivered into the funnel. The level rises until it has become sufficiently high above the outlet to force the fluid out as fast as it is being poured in at the top. If the outlet is then partially occluded or the rate of delivery into the funnel is increased the level of fluid in the funnel rises higher until a new equilibrium is reached. The supply of liquid into the funnel represents the production of urea and creatinine; the height of liquid in the funnel their plasma concentrations; and the diameter of the outlet the rate of glomerular filtration. When a new equilibrium is reached the rate of elimination equals the rate of production.

The relationship between the blood concentration of urea and the glomerular filtration rate is illustrated in Figure 5.2. It can be seen that as the glomerular filtration rate diminishes there is at first only a small absolute rise in blood urea so that when the filtration rate is down to half its normal value the blood urea is still only 6–8 mmol/l (35–50 mg/100 ml). Further reductions in filtration rate, however, produce large absolute changes.

The implications behind this relationship are most interesting: (1) plasma concentrations of urea and creatinine show little absolute change until, functionally, the patient has lost one kidney; (2) when the glomerular filtration rate is low a small additional reduction in filtration rate will produce large changes in plasma concentration. The latter is particularly striking in a patient with a moderate degree of renal failure and a blood urea of 8–10 mmol/l (50–60 mg/100 ml) who develops cardiac failure, or who has a haemorrhage; the blood urea may then rise to 25–33 mmol/l (150–200 mg/100 ml) due to a superimposed decrease in glomerular filtration rate of only 10–20 ml/min.

It is clear that if the blood urea concentration is greater than 10 mmol/l (60 mg/100 ml), or the plasma creatinine above 200 $\mu$mol/l (2 mg/100 ml), there is probably severe depression of glomerular filtration rate; but these are indifferent indications of glomerular function (Fig. 5.3). This is not only

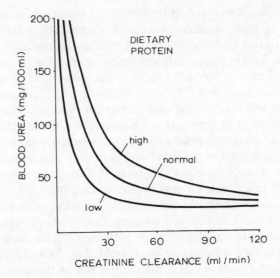

**Fig. 5.2** Schema of the relationship between glomerular filtration rate (creatinine clearance) and the blood urea at varying levels of protein intake (conversion: traditional to SI units — urea 10 mg/100ml = 1.7 mmol/l).

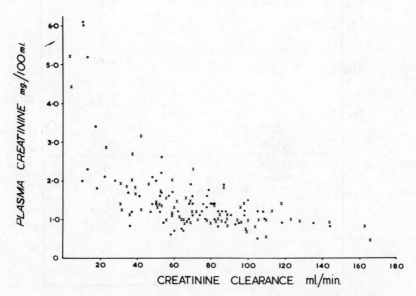

**Fig. 5.3** The relationship between plasma creatinine concentration and the creatinine clearance in 140 patients. It can be seen that at any one clearance the plasma creatinine concentrations are widely scattered. For instance, there are several clearances below 50 ml/min with normal creatinine concentrations (conversion: traditional to SI units — creatinine 1 mg/100 ml = 88 μmol/l).

because at these lower concentrations large disturbances of glomerular filtration cause small absolute changes in plasma concentrations, but also because such small changes may be due to other factors than alterations in filtration rate. This is particularly applicable to urea, for (1) its rate of elimination in the urine is not only related to the glomerular filtration rate but also to the urine flow, and (2) its rate of production is profoundly affected by dietary protein content and endogenous protein catabolism. Figure 5.2 illustrates the effect of high and low protein diets on the relation between blood urea and glomerular filtration rate in normal subjects. It shows that with low protein intakes the level of blood urea may remain within the normal range though there is a substantial fall in glomerular filtration rate (the impaired production of urea in liver disease may also cause a similar effect). Figure 5.5 illustrates this point in a patient with advanced renal failure (creatinine clearance of 5 ml/min). Conversely, a high protein diet (Fig. 5.4), will raise the blood urea to pathological levels though the glomerular filtration rate is normal or unchanged. Paradoxically starvation may also be associated with a raised blood urea due to the associated acceleration of endogenous protein catabolism. These factors also influence the plasma concentrations of creatinine but to a much smaller extent (Fig. 5.4) for the rate of creatinine production is mainly a function of the size of the

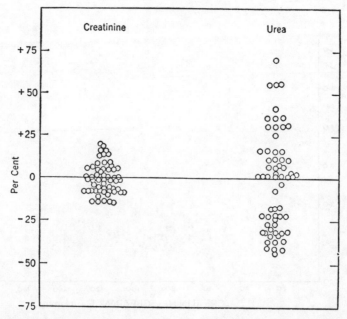

**Fig. 5.4** Serum concentration of creatinine and urea. The percentage variation from the average serum concentrations of creatinine and urea in normal men on diets containing 0.5 to 2.5 g of protein per kg body weight. It is apparent that the creatinine concentrations vary less than those of urea (reproduced from Addis 1949 Glomerular nephritis, Macmillan, New York, with kind permission). See also Fig. 5.5.

muscle mass. On the other hand when patients with small muscle masses develop renal failure they may have plasma creatinines which are misleadingly low, e.g. plasma creatinine of 200 μmol/l (2.0 mg/100 ml) with a glomerular filtration rate of 12 ml/min.

Finally, plasma concentrations of both urea and creatinine are often misleading because they lag behind changes in glomerular filtration rate. This is most obvious during the first few days of acute renal failure when there may be a gross reduction in glomerular filtration rate with initially a relatively small rise in blood urea or creatinine.

*Conclusion*

In a patient in whom renal disease is suspected the finding of a substantial rise in blood urea or creatinine is nearly always good evidence of a severe reduction in glomerular filtration rate. If the patient has been on a low protein diet however, an estimation of the plasma concentration of urea may be grossly misleading (e.g. blood urea of 10 mmol/l (60 mg/100 ml) with a glomerular filtration rate of 10 ml/min; in these circumstances the creatinine concentration permits a much more accurate assessment of the filtration rate. With plasma concentrations in or near the normal range it is necessary

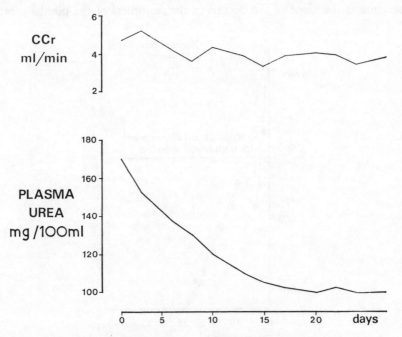

**Fig. 5.5** The effect of a 20 g protein diet on the blood urea and creatinine clearance in a patient suffering from advanced renal failure. There is a profound fall in blood urea though there has been a fall in creatinine clearance (Conversion: traditional to SI units — urea 100 mg/100 ml = 17 mmol/l).

to estimate a 24-hour creatinine clearance or preferably a $^{51}$Cr EDTA clearance before it can be decided whether there is any impairment of filtration rate.

The only advantage of a urea clearance is that when the glomerular filtration rate is below approximately 10 ml/min, then an accurate urea clearance estimated over a short collection period is close to the inulin clearance regardless of the rate of urine flow. In addition, an abnormally low urea/$^{51}$Cr EDTA clearance ratio indicates an increased back diffusion of urea through damaged tubules.

Once it has been established that the patient is suffering from renal failure further progress is followed by repeated measurements of plasma urea and creatinine. Plasma urea gives information about protein metabolism and glomerular filtration rate, while plasma creatinine mainly gives information about glomerular filtration rate. If both are measured it is therefore possible to follow what is happening to protein metabolism and renal function separately. This is particularly important when eventually the patient is placed on a low protein diet. The blood urea may then stay around 30 mmol/l (180 mg/100 ml) obscuring the fact that renal function continues to deteriorate.

*The reciprocal of the plasma creatinine.* The slope of a steady decline in glomerular filtration rate, which is not unusual in glomerular nephritis, is the same as the slope of the decline in the reciprocal of the plasma creati-

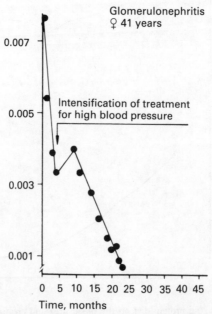

**Fig. 5.6** Plot of the reciprocal of the plasma creatinine against time in a patient with glomerular nephritis (reproduced from Oksa, Pasternak, Luomala et al 1983 Nephron 35: 31, with kind permission).

nine. In the absence of frequent measurements of glomerular filtration rates, therefore, scrutiny of the reciprocal of the plasma creatinine gives a much closer feel for what is happening to the filtration rate than looking at the exponential rise in the concentration of creatinine in the plasma. Furthermore, as the slope of the rate of decline in renal functions is often a straight line, it is usually reasonable to extrapolate the slope of the reciprocal of the plasma creatinine to the point where it will cross the time axis, i.e. when renal function will be zero (Fig. 5.6). This gives a relatively good indication of when the patient will need to be dialysed. Computer manipulation and presentation of numerical data in graphic form makes the use of the reciprocal of the plasma creatinine in the day to day clinical management of the patient an instantaneous procedure.

## PROTEINURIA

Glomerular filtrate contains up to 5 mg of plasma proteins per 100 ml. A normal person therefore filters approximately 7 g of protein per day, but in that time only $80 \pm 25$ mg of protein is excreted in the urine. It is clear that most of the filtered protein is reabsorbed by the tubule. The amount of a protein that will pass through the glomerular capillaries is determined by the glomerular filtration rate and the permeability of the capillary wall to the protein. And this in turn is determined by the protein's size, shape, plasma concentration and charge. The most important is its size. Anionic proteins such as albumin are held up, in part, by the fixed anionic composition of the basement membrane (p. 3) while the slit diaphragms between the podocytes probably prevent the passage of larger cationic molecules. The proximal tubule reabsorbs most if not all of the filtered protein by a process of endocytosis followed by intracellular 'digestion'. The maximum reabsorptive capacity of the tubule for albumin appears to be close to the amount which is normally filtered, whereas it's capacity to absorb lower molecular weight proteins may considerably exceed the amount that is filtered.

Electrophoretic or immunoprecipitin methods of separating urinary proteins demonstrate that, of the plasma proteins, albumin is excreted in the largest quantity (up to 35 mg/day) and $\beta_2$ microglobulin in the smallest (0 to 0.14 mg/day). Nevertheless though the urinary excretion of the smallest molecular weight protein is much less than that of the larger proteins, their urinary clearance

$$\frac{\text{(urinary concentration of the protein} \times \text{urine volume)}}{\text{plasma concentration of the protein}}$$

is considerably greater. When proteinuria is present ($>100$ mg/day) the ratio of the clearances of the larger proteins to the smaller proteins is sometimes used to provide an index of the selectivity of the glomerular permeability to plasma proteins (p. 166).

In addition to plasma proteins the urine contains about 50 mg/day of a protein (known as Tam-Horsfall protein) which is secreted into the tubule lumen by the ascending thick limb of Henle, the distal tubule and the collecting duct. Tam-Horsfall protein may contribute to the remarkable impermeability of this area of the tubule to water. It is certainly responsible for hyaline casts and it forms the binding material for cellular casts.

Children excrete proportionally less protein than adults, and in normal man urinary protein excretion is less in the standing than in the lying position. In the diseased kidney proteinuria may either fall or rise on standing. There are three principal mechanisms responsible for proteinuria.

### Overflow proteinuria

This is due to the presence in the plasma of an excess concentration of a protein, usually of small molecular size which is filtered through normal glomeruli in amounts which saturate the tubule's capacity for reabsorption, e.g. immunoglobulin light chains (Bence Jones proteins) in myelomatosis, or lyzozymes in leukaemia.

### Glomerular proteinuria

An abnormal increase in glomerular permeability allows such an excess of normal plasma proteins, present in the plasma in normal concentrations, to pass through into the tubule that its capacity for reabsorption is exceeded, e.g. most renal diseases.

### Tubular proteinuria

Failure of the tubule to reabsorb normal plasma proteins, present in the plasma in normal amounts, which have been filtered through a normal glomerulus. In this form of proteinuria the amount of albumin in the urine is normal but the quantity of smaller molecular weight proteins such as $B_2$ microglobulin are present in excess. The condition is most easily recognised when there are discreet lesions of the tubules e.g. with exogenous tubular poisons such as cadmium or lead or in selective congenital lesions of the tubule (Fanconi syndrome) (p. 360).

For routine clinical purposes it is best to test for proteinuria by precipitation either by boiling or by the addition of salicyl sulphonic acid. 'Stick' tests such as Albustix and Multistix do not detect Bence Jones proteins (p. 516) and should therefore not be used in a ward. The use of 'stick' tests for the detection of proteinuria is fraught with other hazards particularly if the test is used infrequently. The bottle containing the sticks must be tightly closed and stored at below 90°F, though not in a refrigerator, and the sticks should be used before the expiry date! In artificial light the small colour changes may be difficult to detect so it is useful to use a control stick which has been dipped in water for comparison. Alkalis and detergents can some-times give false positives.

The normal low protein concentration of the urine is not apparent with these tests; otherwise they are relatively delicate and with 25% salicyl sulphonic acid a protein concentration of 0.2 g/l is evident as a 'trace', and 5.0 g/l will give a heavy flocculent precipitate. For clinical purposes it is traditional to comment on the proteinuria in a semiquantitative manner, a barely percep-tible precipitate being called a 'trace' and a heavy precipitate + + + +, with + to + + + in between. This is more useful if the concentration (i.e. specific gravity) of the urine is measured at the same time, for usually the rate of protein excretion is relatively constant throughout the 24 hours and is related to the glomerular filtration rate, whereas the concentration of protein fluctuates with urine flow. In other words, the finding of + of protein in a dilute urine indicates a much greater rate of protein loss than a similar finding in a concentrated urine. The only accurate way to measure the extent of proteinuria is to measure the amount of protein excreted in 24 hours.

In general persistent proteinuria does not occur with disease of the lower urinary tract; neoplasms of the urinary tract, however, will sometimes give rise to intermittent or persistent proteinuria; and with severe exudative or haemorrhagic lesions there may be protein +, but this will only occur when the pus and blood are visible macroscopically. It is essential to realise that it is the presence of protein in the urine which is the important abnormality; and that the rate of protein excretion is of secondary importance. Advanced renal failure may be associated with only a trace of protein in the urine. Proteinuria is almost always present when there is disease of the renal parenchyma, and though there are many transient and unimportant causes of proteinuria, such as fever or exercise, it should not be dismissed, particu-larly if it is persistent. In women a trace of protein may be caused by con-tamination with vaginal discharge.

## URINARY DEPOSIT

Red and white cells and hyaline casts are found in normal urine. In order to determine accurately the extent of white and red cell excretion it is necessary to measure their rate of excretion per unit time.

The subject empties his bladder as completely as possible, the time is carefully noted, and the urine discarded. Three to four hours later, the bladder is emptied once more, the time again noted and the urine kept. In women it is necessary to avoid including cells from the urethra and introitus. In men it is necessary to avoid preputial contamination. The urine from one voiding is therefore collected in two containers. The concentration of cells is measured only in the urine that is excreted into the second container; the rate of excretion is then calculated by multiplying this concentration by the total volume, i.e. the volume of urine in both containers. Within the two subsequent hours the specimen is thoroughly shaken, precipitated phosphates dissolved by adding a few drops of glacial acetic acid, and 10 ml is measured into a graduated centrifuge tube. After spinning at 2000 r.p.m. for 5 min, 9 ml of the supernatant is discarded and the remaining 1 ml thoroughly mixed with a Pasteur pipette. The cells in a drop of this fluid are then counted in 2 mm$^3$ of the ruled area of a Fuchs-Rosenthal counting chamber under 1/6 objective. Only unequivocal polymorphs in which the lobes of the nuclei can be distinguished are counted, disrupted and degenerated cells are not included. The results are calculated as follows, and expressed either as the number of red cells or the number of leucocytes cells excreted per hour:

$$N = \frac{500 \times C \times V}{10\ T} = \frac{50\ CV}{T}$$

where C = actual number of cells counted, V = volume of specimen in millilitres, T = time in hours over which the specimen was formed, and 500 = the factor to convert 2 mm$^3$ to 1 ml. The cells are more easily recognised if the urine is not too concentrated; it is useful therefore, to see that the patient passes about 200–400 ml of urine in the three to four hours of the collection period.

With this technique an excretion of white cells greater than 200 000 per hour is abnormal; the average normal excretion is about 50 000 per hour with a range of 0 to 200 000/hr though occasionally normal subjects have rates between 200 000 and 400 000/hr. The rate of excretion of red cells is approximately the same. This is a relatively laborious technique which again suffers from those recurrent difficulties which are associated with trying to obtain a timed sample of urine. It has been found, however, that a close approximation to the red or white cell excretion rate can be obtained by simply measuring the *concentration* of red or white cells in a drop of fresh uncentrifuged urine (Fig. 5.7). Again a counting chamber is used but it is not necessary to time the urine collection or to spin the urine. When there are more than 10 white or red cells per mm$^3$ the white or red cell excretion rate is abnormally high, whereas if there are less than three per mm$^3$ it is normal; when the result lies between 3 and 10 per mm$^3$ it is best to repeat the test. These criteria apply to children and adults; in infants less than 10 white cells per mm$^3$ is considered to be normal.

There are two other ways in which the white cell content of the urine has been gauged in the past. One consisted of anecdotal remarks such as 'scanty white cells', 'a moderate number of white cells' and the now famous 'white cells seen'. This technique is only of use when the white cells are very numerous. In the other method a sample of urine is spun for 10 min, a drop of the deposit is then placed on a plain glass slide and covered by a cover slip. The numbers of cells seen per high power field (usually with a 1/6 objective) is then reported. Figure 5.8 compares the number of white cells seen per high power field in each of 155 urines against the white cell

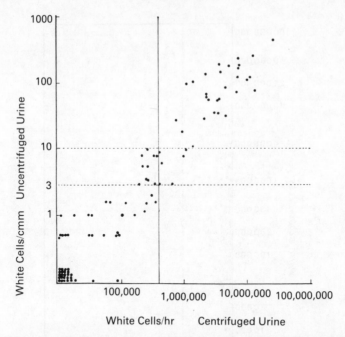

**Fig. 5.7** Comparison of the white cell concentration measured in uncentrifuged urine (white cells per mm³) with the white cell excretion rate calculated from counts made on centrifuged urine (white cells per hour). The vertical line is at 400 000 cells per hour. The horizontal lines at 3 and 10 cells per mm³ (reproduced from Little 1964 Brit J Urol 36: 360, with kind permission).

excretion rate. It is clear that this technique is only useful when there are more than five cells seen per high power field when it can be safely assumed that there is a high urinary excretion of white cells. When there are less than five cells per high power field the excretion rate may be normal or raised. As this technique is more complicated and less reliable than the one in which a drop of unspun urine is examined in a counting chamber there is no good reason why it should linger.

It is important to note that there is a misleading relationship between the colour of the urine and the concentration of red cells it contains. For instance, frank haematuria, i.e. the macroscopic appearance of red cells in the urine sufficient to cause an acid urine to be brown or an alkaline urine to be red is, produced by only 0.2 ml of blood in 500 ml of urine. When blood in the urine comes from the renal parenchyma the red cells tend to look damaged and have odd shapes in contrast to red cells originating from the lower urinary tract.

Many different types of casts may be seen — blood, granular, hyaline waxy, and broad — the most important diagnostically being granular and blood casts. All are basically formed by the precipitation of Tam-Horsfall

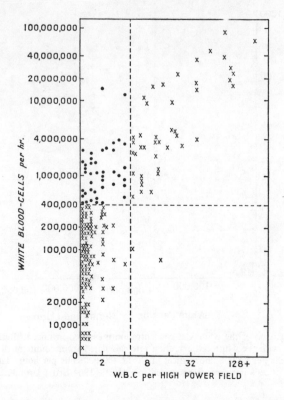

**Fig. 5.8** Urinary white cell excretion rate compared with the number of cells seen per 'high power field' examination of the same urines. The horizontal line is at 400 000 cells per hour; the vertical line is at five cells per 'high power field'. O = urine with high w.b.c. excretion but with less than five cells seen per 'high power field' (reproduced from Little 1962 Lancet 1: 1149, with kind permission).

protein secreted by the tubule into which are imbedded either the red cells that are leaking through the diseased glomeruli, or the degenerated tubule cells that are flaking off the walls of the nephron. Hyaline casts are transparent, without any cells attached to their surfaces; they are of no importance clinically. Blood casts are characterised by a diffuse orange-yellow colour which is the haemoglobin from haemolysed red cells; these casts tend to break into short, stumpy, ragged, rectangular masses which are easily overlooked. Granular casts contain either relatively intact red cells or desquamated tubular cells. The highly significant fact about blood and red cell granular casts is their indication, beyond any shadow of doubt, that the haemoglobin and red cells they contain must have originated from the renal parenchyma and not from the lower urinary tract.

BIBLIOGRAPHY

Braude H, Forfar J O, Gould J C et al 1967 Cell and bacterial counts in the urine of normal infants and children. Brit Med J 4: 697

Brenner B M, Deen W M, Robertson C R 1976 Glomerular filtration. In: Brenner B M, Rector F C (eds) The kidney. Saunders, Philadelphia, p 251

Brenner B M, Hostetter T H, Humes H D 1978 Molecular basis of proteinuria of glomerular origin. New Eng J Med 298: 826

Chantler C, Garnett E S, Parsons V et al 1969 Glomerular filtration rate measurement in man by single injection method using $^{51}$Cr EDTA. Clin Sci 37: 169

Donath A 1971 The simultaneous determination in children of glomerular filtration rate and effective renal plasma flow by the single injection clearance technique. Acta Paediat Scand 60: 512

Farquhar M G 1975 The primary glomerular filtration barrier — basement membrane or epithelial slits. Kidney Int 8: 197

Francois B, Pozet N, Rattanachane B et al 1971 L'estimation de la filtration glomerulaire par l'EDTA $^{51}$Cr. Nephron 8: 147

Goldring W, Chasis H 1944 Hypertension and hypertensive disease. Commonwealth Fund, New York (for inulin and para-amino-hippuric acid clearance techniques)

Heath D A, Knapp M S, Walker W H C 1968 Comparison between inulin and $^{51}$Cr labelled EDTA for the measurement of glomerular filtration rate. Lancet 2: 1110

Hilton P J, Roth Z, Lavender S et al 1969 Creatinine clearance in patients with proteinuria. Lancet 2: 1215

Kumar R, Steen P, McGeown M G 1972 Chronic renal failure or simple starvation. Lancet 2: 1005

Lavender S, Hilton P J, Jones N F 1969 The measurement of glomerular filtration rate in renal disease. Lancet 2: 1216

Little P J 1964 A comparison of the urinary white cell concentration with the white cell excretion rate. Brit J Urol 36: 360

Little P J 1965 Diagnostic criteria of pyelonephritis. J Clin Path 18: 556

McQueen E G 1966 Composition of urinary casts. Lancet 1: 397

Richards P, Brown C L 1975 Urea metabolism in an azotaemic woman with normal renal function. Lancet 2: 207

Robinson R R 1980 Isolated proteinuria in asymptomatic patients. Kidney Int 18: 395

Shannon J A 1935 The renal excretion of creatinine in man. J Clin Invest 14: 403

Shannon J A, Smith H W 1935 The excretion of inulin, xylose and urea by normal and phlorizinised man. J Clin Invest 14: 393

Symposium on proteinuria and renal protein catabolism 1979 Kidney Int 16, No 3: 247

# 6

# Tubular function and tests of tubular functional integrity

The functions of the tubule are to reabsorb, or prevent the reabsorption of the contents of the tubular fluid, and to secrete into the tubular lumen substances which are either circulating in the peritubular venous capillaries or which are formed by the tubule cell. These processes are under the control of many hormones, some plasma and intracellular electrolyte concentrations, and the hydrostatic, plasma protein, and gas pressures in the peritubular capillaries.

The principal function of the proximal tubule is to reabsorb about 80% of the total solids and water from the glomerular filtrate. The solids are reabsorbed in unequal proportions so that while proteins and glucose, for instance, appear to be almost completely reabsorbed (Fig. 6.1), sodium

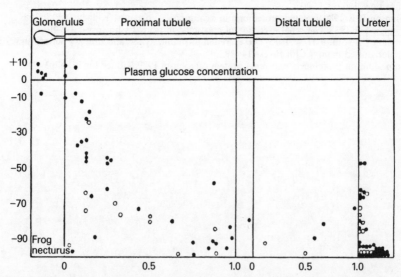

**Fig. 6.1** Site of glucose reabsorption. Difference in glucose concentration between plasma and fluid collected with a micropipette from various levels of the renal tubules of normal Necturi and frogs. Zero on the ordinate represents plasma, figures above and below zero represent percentage differences from plasma. (reproduced from Walker & Judson 1937 Amer J Physiol 118: 130, with kind permission).

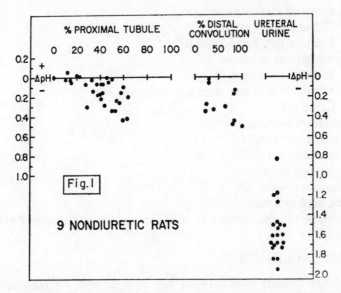

**Fig. 6.2** Localisation of urine acidification in the rat kidney. The points show the difference in pH of the tubular fluid obtained in various parts of the nephron and the ureter, from that of arterial blood. Points below the horizontal line = pH below that of plasma. Note that the fluid begins to be acidified in the proximal tubule but that the main increase in acidity occurs between the distal tubule and the ureteric urine, i.e. in the collecting tubule (reproduced from Gottschalk, Lassiter & Mylle 1960 Amer J Physiol 198: 581, with kind permission).

chloride and urea are only partly reabsorbed, and there is no reabsorption of creatinine. Reabsorption from the proximal tubule takes place in such a way that the fluid in the proximal tubule always remains isosmotic to arterial blood. The pH of the fluid, however, may change, and when the urine is acid the process of acidification begins in the proximal tubule (Fig. 6.2). The main function of the loop of Henle is to make the interstitial fluid in the medulla *hypertonic* and the tubular fluid that emerges from it, into the distal tubule, *hypotonic*; these changes permit the concentration of the final urine to be modified over a wide range. The hypotonic tubular fluid which flows into the distal tubule contains considerable quantities of sodium chloride and waste products and has a pH which is much the same as that in the fluid emerging from the proximal tubule. The principal functions of the distal and collecting tubules are to adjust the pH, osmolality and electrolyte content of this fluid and to prevent or impede the reabsorption of the waste products.

The following tubular functions will be discussed:
1. Water excretion
    *a.* Urine concentration
    *b.* Urine dilution and water elimination

2. Sodium and chloride excretion
   a. Tubular reabsorption
   b. Relation to volume control
3. Hydrogen ion excretion
   a. Bicarbonate excretion
   b. Titratable acid and ammonia excretion
   c. Urine pH
4. Potassium excretion
5. Calcium excretion
6. Magnesium excretion
7. Phosphate excretion
8. Amino-acid excretion
9. Uric acid excretion
10. Maximal tubular capacity to reabsorb glucose and secrete PAH.

## WATER EXCRETION

The kidney's ability to modify the rate of urine flow is largely responsible for the constancy of the volume and osmolality of body fluids; and the rate of urine flow is mainly determined by the tubule's ability to control the concentration of the urine. The terms *hypertonic, isotonic* and *hypotonic* refer respectively to osmolalities which are greater than, equal to, and less than those of plasma. Osmolality can be defined as the concentration of particles in a solution. The highest urine concentration attainable is about 1300 mosmol/kg/$H_2O$ (SG 1.040) which is about four times greater than the concentration of plasma, approximately 300 mosmol/kg/$H_2O$ (SG 1.008), while the lowest concentration is about 50 mosmol/kg/$H_2O$ (SG 1.001).

The osmolality of the urine is mainly dependent on four interlocking factors: (1) the functional integrity of the loop of Henle, (2) the counter current flow of blood through the vasa rectae, (3) the concentration of circulating anti-diuretic hormone (ADH), and (4) the functional integrity of the collecting duct. The loop of Henle produces a hypotonic tubular fluid (Fig. 6.3) and initiates the mechanism responsible for producing a hypertonic interstitial environment (Fig. 6.4). The vasa rectae magnify and safeguard this hypertonicity, and ADH controls the movement of water and urea across the wall of the collecting duct, and the flow of blood through the vasa rectae.

The vasa rectae perform their role by their ability to act as counter current multipliers and exchangers. Their counter current multiplying function is due to the downward flow of plasma in the descending vasa recta. The increase in medullary hypertonicity occurs in the following manner. As the isotonic plasma in the descending vasa recta travels down it comes into equilibrium with an area of interstitium into which the water impermeable thick ascending limb of Henle in the outer medulla is actively pumping chloride (accompanied by a passive movement of sodium). This raises the

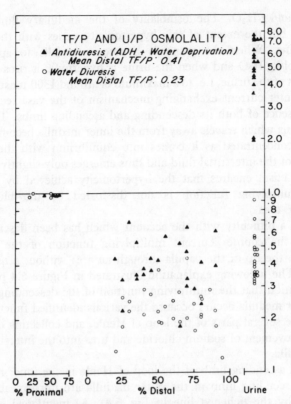

**Fig. 6.3** Site of dilution and concentration of the urine in the dog. Each triangle or circle represents the results obtained in a sample of tubular fluid removed by micropuncture. The site of each micropuncture is represented along the horizontal axis as a percentage of the length of the proximal or distal tubule. The tubular fluid or urine/plasma osmolal ratio is indicated along the vertical axis. At the horizontal line 1.0 the tubule fluid is isosmotic with the plasma; above this line the urine is hypertonic, and below the line the fluid or urine is hypotonic. ▲ = results in dehydrated dogs; ○ = results in dogs having a water diuresis. It can be seen that the tubular fluid in the proximal tubule is always isosmotic whereas in the distal tubule it is always hypotonic whether the urine is hyper- or hypotonic. In the dehydrated animal the osmolality of the distal fluid is about 150 mosmol/kg (plasma = 300 mosmol/kg/$H_2O$), whereas in the dogs having a water diuresis it is approx 75 mosmol/kg/$H_2O$(reproduced from Clapp & Robinson 1966 J Clin Invest 45: 1847, with kind permission).

osmolality of the plasma in the vasa recta by a certain amount. The now slightly hypertonic plasma travels further down and has a further quantity of sodium added to it by the same mechanism so that there is a further rise in its concentration. In this way the osmolality of the plasma is raised by a succession of graduated steps until it reaches the lower border of the thick ascending limb. At this point it travels down into the inner medulla where no active transport of solute has been identified. Nevertheless the counter multiplying function of the descending vasa rectae continues to the tip of the papilla (see below). The highest osmolality reached is about

1300 mosmol/kg/$H_2O$. The osmolality of the medullary fluid is always hypertonic but the extent of this hypertonicity varies with the osmolality of the urine. When the urine is hypotonic it falls to approximately 400 mosmol/kg/$H_2O$ and when the urine is hypertonic it rises to the same level as that of the urine, i.e. to a maximum of around 1300 mosmol/kg/$H_2O$.

The counter current exchanging mechanism of the vasa rectae depends on the presence of both its descending and ascending limbs. The hyperosmolar plasma which travels away from the inner medulla becomes progressively less concentrated as it comes into equilibrium with the decreasing osmolality of the interstitial fluid and thus emerges only slightly hypertonic. This mechanism ensures that the hypertonicity achieved by the counter current multiplying function is not dissipated by the blood flowing through the area.

There is a difficulty with the account which has been described above. It is that the counter current multiplying function of the vasa rectae continue to the tip of the papilla through an area without *active* transport of solute. The following explanation illustrated in Figure 6.4 puts forward the proposition that the multiplying function of the descending vasa recta, in the inner medulla occurs because the various identified functional differences of the several parts of the loop of Henle, and collecting duct, induce a *passive* movement of sodium chloride and urea into the interstitium of the inner medulla.

The thin ascending limb of the loop of Henle in the inner medulla and the thick ascending limb in the outer medulla are impermeable to water (indicated by the tichened line in Fig. 6.4). As mentioned above active ($\rightarrow$ in Fig. 6.4) chloride reabsorption in the thick portion of the ascending limb is accompanied by a passive ($--\rightarrow$ in Fig. 6.4) movement of sodium This process is indicated by the notation ① in Figure 6.4. It causes the tubule fluid to become dilute and the adjoining medullary interstitium to become hypertonic. In the last part of the distal tubule, and the collecting tubules, which are both water permeable and urea impermeable, water is reabsorbed passively ($--\rightarrow$) down its osmotic gradient ② in Figure 6.4 thus increasing the concentration of urea that remains in the tubule fluid. In the inner medulla both water and urea are reabsorbed from the water and urea permeable collecting duct ③ in Figure 6.4, and some urea thus goes back into the medullary interstitium and re-enters the urea permeable part of the loop of Henle (Fig. 6.5). This medullary recycling of urea causes urea to accumulate in large quantities in the medullary interstitium where it excretes a powerful osmotic force which extracts water passively from the sodium chloride impermeable descending limb of the loop of Henle, ④ in Figure 6.4, thus concentrating the sodium chloride of the tubule fluid in the descending limb. When this fluid which now contains a raised concentration of sodium chloride comes around the bend of the loop of Henle and enters the sodium chloride permeable (but water impermeable) thin ascending limb, sodium chloride moves down its concentration gradient out of the tubule

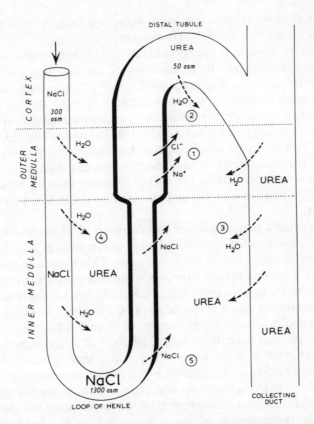

**Fig. 6.4** Mechanism involved in the concentration of the urine as proposed by Koko, Rector and Stephenson (modified and reproduced from Jamison 1981. In: Brenner, B M, Rector F C (eds) The kidney. Saunders, Philadelphia, p. 495, with kind permission).

lumen making the tubule fluid relatively hypo-osmotic to the adjoining interstitium⑤in Figure 6.4.

When the plasma ADH concentration is low, following a drink of water or disease of the neurohypophysis, the urine is hypotonic and is excreted in large volumes, and when the ADH concentration is raised following dehydration the urine is hypertonic and only small amounts are excreted. ADH alters the concentration of the urine by changing the permeability of the distal and collecting tubule to water; the presence of ADH causing the permeability to increase. In this way when ADH is absent the impermeability of the collecting tubules is intact, the hypotonic fluid which continuously emerges from the loop of Henle then remains hypotonic as it travels down, and hypotonic urine is excreted. This phenomenon is aided by the simultaneous fall in the osmolality of the interstitial fluid in the medulla, which occurs when the concentration of circulating ADH is low for ADH directly increases the permeability of the collecting duct to urea (see below) and indirectly restricts blood flow through the vasa recta. A rise in medullary blood flow lowers interstitial fluid osmolality.

When ADH is present, the permeability of the distal tubule to water is relatively unaffected, but the permeability of the collecting duct to water is much increased. The hypotonic fluid which emerges from the loop of Henle therefore remains hypotonic as it travels through most of the distal tubule, though its volume is reduced. As it enters the final part of the distal tubule its osmolality is approximately 180–200 mosmol/kg/$H_2O$. In the collecting duct where the adjoining interstitial fluid of the medulla is hypertonic this reduced volume of moderately hypotonic fluid from the distal tubule becomes hypertonic by the passage of water from the tubule lumen into the interstitial space so that an even smaller volume of hypertonic urine is excreted.

It is clear that a part of the total concentration of solutes which build up the hyperosmolality of the interstitial space of the medulla is accounted for by sodium chloride. Most of the rest is urea. This is because the permeability of the collecting tubules to urea is controlled by ADH. In the absence of ADH when the urine is hypotonic, the reabsorption of urea is at its lowest and the excretion of urea is at its highest; in the presence of ADH, however, when the urine is hypertonic, the movement of urea out of the tubular fluid into the hypertonic medullary interstitial fluid is at its highest, and the excretion of urea is at its lowest. The initial step in achieving a high concentration of urea in the medulla is the passive movement of urea from the medullary collecting ducts. As with sodium chloride the counter current of fluid within the vasa rectae then traps the urea within the medulla and increases its concentration so that it is greatest at the tip of the papilla (Fig. 6.4). It follows that the final urine osmolality, when the urine is concentrated, is approximately equal to the sum of the osmolalities of the sodium chloride and urea in the interstitial space. Therefore one of the factors responsible for the kidney's well known increased capacity to concentrate the urine on a high protein diet is the increased excretion of urea that then occurs.

In addition to its effect on the tubule's permeability to water and urea ADH has also been shown to increase the rate of active sodium transport in isolated membranes such as frog skin. If ADH has the same effect on the ascending limb of the loop of Henle it is possible that the increase in the hypertonicity of the medulla, which occurs when there is a rise in the concentration of circulating ADH, is due not only to its effect on the tubule's permeability to urea but also to an increased delivery of chloride and sodium into the medullary interstitial fluid.

It is intuitively understandable that the counter-current exchanger phenomenon of the vasa recta is likely to be more efficient at relatively low rates of blood flow. It is interesting therefore that when ADH is present and there is a need for as high a medullary interstitial fluid osmolality as possible, the flow of blood through the vasa recta is reduced. This is probably due to the constricting effect on the vasa recta of the rise in the interstitial fluid osmolality.

## Methods used to measure the concentration of the urine

It is customary to measure the concentration of the urine by its specific gravity, which is an indication of the weight of the solutes in solution. The kidney's capacity to concentrate however, is related to the concentration of particles in solution (i.e. the osmolality*) and not to their weight. This fact is most easily demonstrated by measuring the specific gravity of urine following an intravenous pyelogram when values of SG 1.060 may be found. Such values are much greater than any obtained following dehydration and are due to the excretion of large heavy molecules of radio-opaque substance; the particle concentration of such urine is within normal limits.

The concentration of particles, i.e. the osmolality of a solution, may be calculated from a determination of its freezing point or vapour pressure. These techniques are laboratory procedures, and it is fortunate that when urine contains only normal constituents, the correlation between specific gravity and osmolality is sufficiently close for specific gravity to be used as a clinical guide to the osmolality of the urine. This relationship is illustrated in Figure 6.5 which also shows that if urine contains much glucose the specific gravity will be greater at a fixed osmolality, than in normal urine; and, conversely, if the urine contains much urea (a less dense molecule) the specific gravity will be lower.

Clinical hydrometers are convenient but relatively coarse instruments with which to measure specific gravity; it is important therefore that they should be used with care. In order to check incorrect graduations clinical hydrometers should always be tested in water each time they are used; and, to avoid surface tension errors on the stem, the hydrometer should be spun and plunged well into the urine. Detergents should not be used for cleaning urine bottles or specimen glasses, for these lower surface tension and increase the measured specific gravity. And the specific gravity should never be measured in freshly passed warm urine, for hydrometers are standardised at a temperature of 16°C; for every 3°C above this temperature the specific gravity will appear to be 0.001 less than its true value, i.e. if a hydrometer is placed in urine at 37°C and shows a reading of 1.013 the true specific

---

* The osmolality of a solution is an index of the number of particles it contains in 1 kg of water, whereas the osmolarity of a solution is an index of the number of particles contained in one litre of the solution. In biological fluids the two are very similar. Determinations of freezing point and vapour pressure measure osmolality, i.e. $mosmol/kg/H_2O$. Some years ago some of us failed to appreciate these facts and the term osmolarity was used when osmolality was measured. This explains why some of the diagrams in these pages, which have been taken from earlier papers mention osmolarity and mosmol/l instead of osmolality and $mosmol/kg/H_2O$. It should be noted that in this context the symbol $H_2O$ is often omitted, and osmolality described as mosmol/kg.

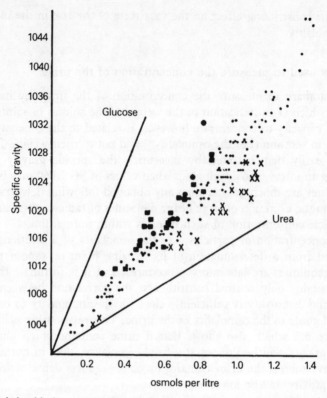

**Fig. 6.5** Relationship between specific gravity and osmolality of urine. Different urines are shown as follows: with no sugar or protein (○), with +++ sugar (●), with +++ protein (■), after 25 g urea by mouth (×). Lines are also given showing the relationship between specific gravity and osmolality of glucose and urea solutions (reproduced from Miles, Paton & de Wardener 1954 Brit Med J 2: 901, with kind permission).

gravity is 1.020. An adjustment is also necessary when there is gross proteinuria; 0.001 is subtracted for every 5 g/l of protein.

## Procedure used to test the tubule's ability to concentrate urine

This test can be performed by depriving the patient of fluid or preferably by giving one dose of diamino, 8-D-arginine vasopressin (Desmopressin) DDAVP, a synthetic analogue of arginine vasopressin which is a powerful antidiuretic agent with negligible vasoactive properties. Before doing either, however, the specific gravity of a sample of urine passed on waking should be measured, for if such a random sample is greater than 1.018 it is most unlikely that the maximum concentration achieved by fluid deprivation of DDAYP administration will be below normal.

*Fluid deprivation.* Fluid deprivation results in a rise of plasma osmolality and a shrinkage of the extracellular volume, both changes which are known

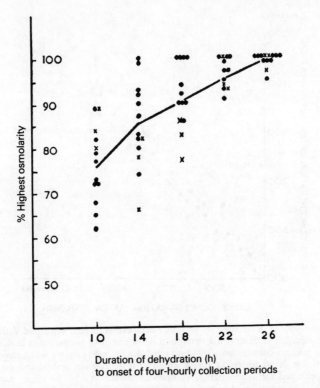

**Fig. 6.6** The effect of progressive water deprivation on the urine osmolarity in thirteen subjects. The osmolarity is expressed as a percentage of the highest osmolarity reached in each subject during thirty hours fluid deprivation. Urines were collected between 8 a.m. and 4 a.m. in cases marked with a dot, and between 8 p.m. and 4 p.m. in those marked with a cross (reproduced from Miles, Paton & de Wardener 1954 Brit Med J 2: 901, with kind permission).

to increase antidiuretic hormone production. The urine become concentrated but often does not approach its maximal value for 24–36 hours (Fig. 6.6). This is rather a long time to dehydrate patients and a convenient clinical compromise is to do the test over a period of 24 hours as follows. The period starts at 8 a.m. when the intake of all fluid, including ice creams, soups and fruit, ceases until 8 a.m. of the following day. The concentration of all urine samples passed during the last 12 hours of this period is estimated, and one of these should equal or be greater than SG 1.022. The normal range of urine concentration obtained with this procedure varies from SG 1.022 to SG 1.040. The highest figures are rarely seen in persons over the age of 20. Occasionally an apparent inability to concentrate is due to the test being performed during a diuresis caused by the spontaneous (and sometimes induced) excretion of oedema fluid.

Fluid deprivation is nearly always unpleasant for the patient, and occasionally, if a severe negative fluid balance develops because of an

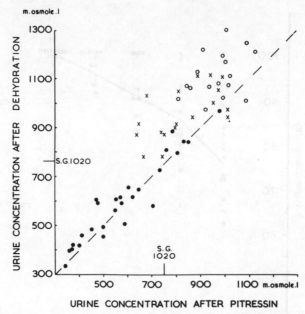

**Fig. 6.7** Osmolarity of urine after 36–48 hours deprivation of fluid compared with that following an injection of vasopressin tannate in oil in sixty-two persons: (○) healthy persons, (×) patients convalescent from non-renal disease, (●) patients with renal disease. The diagonal line shows where the points would lie if deprivation of fluid and vasopressin tannate concentrated the urine equally. Vasopressin tannate in oil is no longer manufactured for it was an awkward material to use, painful intramuscularly, and which occasionally could cause hypersensitivity reactions and angina in susceptible persons. It has been superceded by DDAVP. It is probable, however, that the results depicted here would be similar, if instead, repeated doses of DDAVP were used over a period of 36 to 48 hours (reproduced from de Wardener 1956 Lancet 1: 1037, with kind permission).

inability to concentrate, the test may even be dangerous. The test should always be terminated if the loss of body weight exceeds 4%. For these reasons the test is hardly ever repeated, which greatly lowers its value. The test may also be vitiated by the patient's emotional reactions to having his kidneys 'tested' for it may induce him to have an emotional diuresis.

*DDAVP.* If the information required is only to find out the kidney's capacity to concentrate the urine, fluid deprivation and its discomforts and disadvantages can be avoided by giving instead either 20 μg IM, 40 μg IV or 20 μg into each nostril of DDAVP. If, however, the information required is to find out if the patient can secrete ADH then it is necessary to perform a fluid deprivation test. Theoretically one might expect the concentration of the urine to rise to the same extent whether fluid deprivation or DDAVP is used but in practice the concentration of the urine is slightly less following vasopressin than after fluid deprivation (Fig. 6.7).

The kidney's ability to concentrate can be adequately tested by combining DDAVP and a short period of fluid deprivation beginning at 6 p.m. At

8 p.m. the DDAVP is given and the bladder is emptied at 10 p.m. The concentration of the first urine passed in the morning is measured. An even simpler test is to give DDAVP in the morning (e.g. at 9 a.m.) and to measure the urine concentration of the two subsequent urine specimens passed. The mean osmolality of the second specimen — that is of the urine passed 5 to 9 hr after the administration of the DDAVP is only slightly less than when the test is performed with a period of overnight dehydration. Nevertheless it is advisable to advise the patient to drink only small amounts during the daytime test. With these methods the highest specific gravity obtained should be 1.020 or above. The effect of DDAVP only lasts about 12 hr so that the test can be repeated at fairly frequent intervals to confirm earlier results and to follow the course of the disease.

### Interpretation of the urine concentration test

In order to understand the result of a concentration test it is necessary to keep in mind the three factors which are directly concerned in concentrating the urine; they are:
1. The concentration of circulating antidiuretic hormone (ADH)
2. The ability of the tubules to respond to the antidiuretic hormone
3. The rate of solute output.

*The concentration of circulating ADH* is regulated by both the amount of ADH produced by the neurohypophysis and the rate at which it is being destroyed at the periphery, particularly in the liver and kidney. An abnormal rate of destruction is rare though there are occasional reports of the spontaneous appearance of an antibody to endogenous ADH. In general, therefore, changes in the circulating level of ADH are due to alterations in its production by the neurohypophysis. A wide variety of factors influences neurohypophyseal function including the osmolality of a extracellular fluid, the blood volume and certain disease processes involving the hypothalamus or the posterior pituitary.

*The ability of the tubules to respond to ADH* depends on the integrity of the loop of Henle, the collecting tubule and the flow of blood through the vasa recta. The response may be impaired because of a congenital defect or an acquired disturbance; the latter may be reversible. The acquired disturbances which may be reversible initially include fever, urinary tract obstruction (Fig. 6.8), potassium deficiency, hypercalcuria, water intoxication, hypoadrenalism, and occasionally certain acute phases of some generalised allergic diseases. In many of these conditions the urine may be persistently hypotonic even during dehydration or the administration of vasopressin; this is particularly characteristic of hypercalcaemia and potassium deficiency. Reflux nephropathy (chronic pyelonephritis) is also occasionally responsible for a state of fixed hypotonicity particularly when the urine is infected.

*The rate of solute output in a normal kidney.* If a person is dehydrated for a considerable time so that the level of circulating ADH, and the concentration

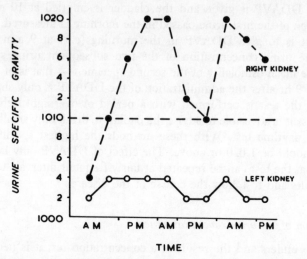

**Fig. 6.8** The effect of a raised intrapelvic pressure on the ability to concentrate. The observations were made on a patient with a left-sided hydronephrosis due to a recent obstruction of the left ureter. The urine from the left kidney was obtained through a nephrostomy tube, and from the right kidney in the usual way. The hydronephrotic kidney continually excreted a very hypotonic urine, though the high concentrations of the urine from the right kidney indicated that there were adequate concentrations of antidiuretic substances in the circulating blood.

of the urine are high, and if at this time some substance is then administered which is promptly excreted by the kidney, there is not only a prompt increase in solute output, but also a rise in urine flow and *a decrease in urine concentration*. This phenomenon is called an osmotic diuresis and is illustrated by the curve A in Figure 6.9. It can be seen that in these conditions of maximal ADH activity an osmotic diuresis is associated with a fall in urine concentration towards that of plasma, but that the urine concentration remains greater than plasma.

If on another occasion an osmotic diuresis is induced when the level of circulating ADH is less than during the experiment just described (in a patient with diabetes insipidus) similar changes in urine flow and concentration will take place, but the curve will be at a lower level; i.e. line B in Figure 6.10. The lower the concentration of circulating ADH therefore, the lower the curve until, when there is no ADH in the circulation, an osmotic diuresis increases the urine flow but there is little or no associated change in the urine concentration, for it is already at its lowest (line C).

The increase in the rate of urine flow and fall in urine concentration during an osmotic diuresis are due to several factors. As the proximal tubule wall cannot sustain an osmotic gradient the fluid in the lumen of the proximal tubule is always isosmotic, therefore water can only be absorbed from the proximal tubule when solutes are reabsorbed. It follows that if a solute is not reabsorbed (e.g. glucose because of hyperglycaemia) less water will

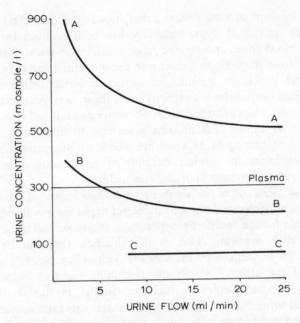

**Fig. 6.9** Osmotic diuresis in the normal kidney during an IV infusion of mannitol: A was obtained in a normal subject during severe dehydration; B in a patient with diabetes insipidus during the infusion of minimal quantities of vasopressin and C in the same patient when no vasopressin was being given (reproduced from de Wardener & del Greco 1955 Clin Sci 14: 715, with kind permission).

be reabsorbed. But the presence of this excess water in the lumen of the proximal tubule reduces the intraluminal concentration of sodium, thus increasing the concentration gradient across the tubule wall so that sodium reabsorption is impaired. The unabsorbed sodium then further reduces water reabsorption from the proximal tubule. Consequently the flow of tubular fluid from the proximal tubule into the descending limb of Henle is increased and it contains an increased quantity of sodium chloride. As this limb is freely permeable to water but relatively impermeable to sodium chloride (and urea) and it is surrounded by a hyperosmolar interstitium some of the excess fluid diffuses into the interstitial space. But the fall in the osmolality of the interstitium increase medullary blood flow (see above) which greatly reduces the hyperosmolality of the interstitial space. Therefore much of the large volumes of fluid and all the excess sodium that travel into the descending limb of Henle pass on into the impermeable ascending limb of Henle. The main function of this part of the nephron is to reabsorb chloride and sodium and to prevent reabsorption of water. But during an osmotic diuresis the reabsorption of chloride (and consequently of sodium) is impaired for reasons which are not at all clear. Much of the water and sodium chloride that enter into the ascending limb of Henle therefore travels on into the distal tubule and collecting duct as a large flow of hypotonic fluid. In the collecting duct, the urine does not become concentrated, however much ADH is present, because the interstitial hyperosmolality has been reduced by the raised medullary blood flow, and by the large amounts of water that are being transferred from the collecting duct into the interstitial space. In addition it appears that the large amounts of sodium chloride delivered into the collecting duct overwhelm it's capacity for reabsorption. An osmotic diuresis therefore causes a loss of large amounts of water and salt and thus a depletion of extracellular fluid. This in turn gives rise to hypotension and large quantities of circulating ADH which are unable to concentrate the urine.

The most important clinical example of an osmotic diuresis is that associated with the glycosuria of diabetes mellitus.

*The rate of solute output per nephron in a diseased kidney.* If the total solute output remains unchanged but the number of nephrons is reduced, the solute excretion rate for the remaining nephrons in increased and osmotic diuresis occurs in each nephron. This is the situation that can be produced experimentally in animals by excising one kidney completely and about 50 per cent of the other. Though the remaining piece of kidney contains presumably normal nephrons such an animal is unable to produce concentrated urine. It is likely that similar conditions exist in many forms of renal disease associated with much parenchymatous destruction. If the patient is eating normally the total solute excretion rate must remain relatively unchanged, yet these solutes are being excreted through a considerably reduced number of nephrons. In such circumstances a diminished capacity to concentrate is probably due in part to the osmotic diuresis *per nephron* which must be taking place, rather than any particular inability of the tubules to respond to circulating ADH.

### Procedure to test the tubule's ability to produce a dilute urine and eliminate a water load

The test is started early in the morning and is performed in the fasting state. After emptying the bladder the patient is asked to drink 20 ml of water per kg body weight in about 10–20 min. It is inadvisable to ask the patient to drink this amount more rapidly, for in some cases this will induce nausea and vomiting with the release of large quantities of ADH; it is also advisable to sweeten the water with fruit juice. Urine is collected at hourly intervals for four hours and the concentration of each specimen and the cumulative total are measured. During these four hours a normal person should excrete 75% or more of the amount ingested, and the concentration of at least one specimen should be below S.G. 1.004.

Apart from the risks of nausea and vomiting, this test is subject to other causes of inaccuracy. For instance, smoking may inhibit a water diuresis; or emotional reactions may cause either (1) an exuberantly high rate of urine flow unrelated to the patient's normal response to a water load; or (2) an almost complete inhibition of the expected diuresis; an example of both of these occurring in the same patient is illustrated in Figure 6.10

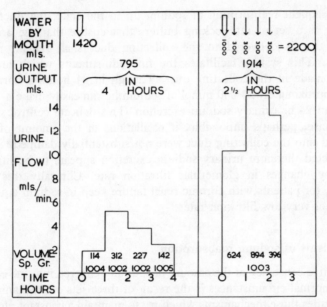

**Fig. 6.10** The effect of a water load in an emotional subject. On the first occasion only 50% of the amount ingested was excreted in the subsequent four hours, but the next time nearly 100 per cent was passed in only two and a half hours.

In addition to renal disease a persistent impairment in the ability to excrete a water load can be caused by many other disturbances including hypoadrenalism, or an inverted diurnal rhythm.

## SODIUM EXCRETION

Sodium is the principal solid constituent of the extracellular fluid, the volume and osmolality of which are closely related to the amount of sodium it contains. In one hour a pair of normal adult kidneys filter and reabsorb rather more than 1000 mmol of sodium. Or in other words 6 litres of physiological saline. Whereas less than 1% of this amount, about six to eight mmol, is excreted in the urine.

The rotation of these large quantities of sodium in and out of the tubule is the inevitable accompaniment of the high glomerular filtration rates needed to dispose of those materials that can only be excreted in the urine by filtration. One of the most important functions of the kidney therefore, as regards the control of sodium excretion, is to ensure that the bulk of these enormous quantities of sodium are reabsorbed. This takes place in the proximal tubule and the loop of Henle. A second function is then to adjust the small amounts of sodium that are excreted in the urine in such a way that sodium balance is maintained. This occurs in the collecting duct. One unifying view of these mechanisms, which are responsible for the filtration and subsequent reabsorption of sodium up to the collecting duct, is that they act as a set of interlocking buffers that ensure that the amount of sodium that is delivered to the collecting duct shall remain relatively constant. This system facilitates the fine adjustments which are subsequently made in the collecting duct. Though in 24 hours a normal man filters approximately 24 000 mmol of sodium he can easily make a 10 mmol change in 24 hr urinary sodium excretion. This delicate control would be less precise, perhaps impossible, if oscillations in the amount of sodium delivered into the collecting duct were not substantially damped. As might be expected therefore urinary sodium excretion appears to be little influenced by changes in glomerular filtration rate. Clinically this is very obvious, for patients with chronic renal failure keep in sodium equilibrium in spite of very low filtration rates.

## Mechanisms of sodium reabsorption

The relative constancy of the amount of sodium delivered into the collecting duct in normal circumstances is the result of three sets of mechanism. The first includes those mechanisms which try to maintain a constant glomerular filtration rate, or in other words a constant load of sodium into the proximal tubule. The second are those mechanisms which adjust sodium reabsorption in the proximal tubule on the one hand and the ascending limb of Henle and early distal tubule on the other. And the third are those factors which control the reabsorption of sodium in the collecting duct.

The relative constancy of glomerular filtration rate is ensured by circulatory autoregulation to changes in hydrostatic pressure (p. 77) and haematocrit, and the distal tubule to glomerulus feed-back mechanism. The latter, probably working via the juxtaglomerular apparatus reduces filtration rate when a sudden surge of tubular fluid emerges out of the ascending limb of Henle into the first part of the distal tubule (Fig. 6.11).

### Proximal tubule

Two thirds of the filtered sodium (and water) is reabsorbed in the proximal tubule though the tubule fluid in the proximal tubule always remains isosmotic to plasma, i.e. there is no gradient for sodium across the proximal tubular epithelium. Nevertheless in certain experimental conditions it can be shown that sodium reabsorption can occur against a steep electrochemical gradient, which provides direct proof that sodium is actively pumped out of the proximal tubule. Additional evidence that sodium transport is an active process comes from the finding of a linear relationship between renal oxygen consumption and sodium reabsorption. Even so it is not immediately obvious how large quantities of water move from one isotonic fluid in the lumen of the proximal tubule across the wall of the proximal tubule into another isotonic area on the outside of the tubule in which lie the tubular capillaries.

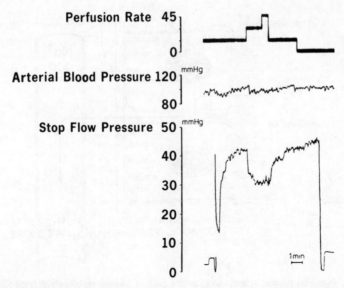

**Fig. 6.11** Tubuloglomerular feedback. Effect on stop flow pressure in early proximal tubule of changing the rate of microperfusion of loop of Henle with modified Ringer solution (reproduced from Schnerman, Hermle, Schmidmeier et al 1975 Pflügers Archives 358: 325, with kind permission).

The following hypothesis to explain the movement of water has been put foward. It is based on the ultrastructural finding that the tubule cells are associated with two groups of long narrow channels (Fig. 6.12). One group consists of channels between the cells (the intercellular channels). These are partially blocked at their luminal end while the other end opens directly into the interstitial space on the basal and capillary side of the cell. The other groups of channels consist of deep infoldings at the base of the cell (Fig. 1.4). Lining the intercellular channels and the basal infoldings there is a layer of adenosine triphosphatase, an enzyme which is closely connected with sodium transport. It has been proposed that sodium is actively transported from the inside of the cell into the intercellular channels and basal infoldings. This makes the fluid within them hypertonic. Water consequently flows across the walls of the channels down the osmotic gradient and into their lumen so that the sodium and the water in the channels are then swept towards their open end at the base of the cell towards the capillary. In this way there is a continuous movement of sodium and water, from the tubule lumen to the interstitial space in contact with the peritubular venous capillaries, through the intercellular channels and basal infoldings. Or, in other words, an isotonic solution passes from one isotonic solution in the tubule lumen to another isotonic solution in the interstitial space via a standing osmotic gradient built-up deep in the intercellular channels and basal infoldings.

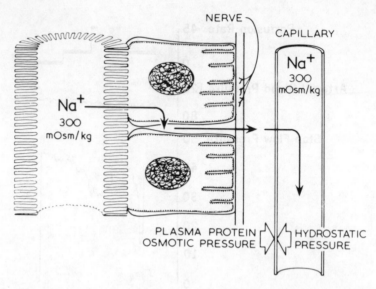

**Fig. 6.12** Proximal tubule: schema to illustrate path of sodium reabsorption (reproduced from de Wardener 1978 In: Dickinson C J, Marks J (eds) Developments in cardiovascular medicine. MTP Press, London, p. 179, with kind permission).

There is also evidence that about one third of filtered sodium is reabsorbed *passively* across the tight juction of the proximal tubules. In the earlier parts of the proximal tubule this is due to the avid reabsorption of glucose, amino acids and bicarbonate, and as the proximal tubule cannot sustain an osmotic gradient water follows the reabsorption of these substances. This in turn raises the intraluminal sodium concentration and sodium therefore leaks out passively through the tight junction into the capillaries via the intracellular channels. Further along the proximal tubule, the epithelium of the proximal tubule is more permeable to chloride, a lumen-positive electrical potential therefore develops which generates a driving force for passive net sodium efflux from the lumen.

Some sodium ions also travel across the cell from the lumen to the interstitial space by means of a co-transport mechanism whereby certain sugars and amino acids form carrier complexes with sodium which move down electrical and chemical gradients for sodium, which have been established by other means. This mechanism appears quantitively more important for the transport of glucose and amino acids, which it accelerates markedly, than for the bulk transport of sodium.

*Factors which influence the reabsorption of sodium in the proximal tubule.* The constancy of the amount of sodium that emerges from the distal end of the proximal tubule and which is thus delivered into the loop of Henle is ensured by a mechanism known as glomerulotubular balance. This phenomenon becomes evident when there are spontaneous changes in filtra-

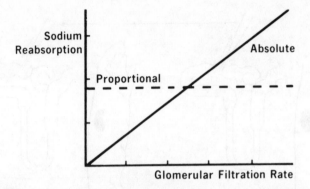

**Fig. 6.13** Proximal tubule: relation of sodium reabsorption to sodium delivered into the tubule with spontaneous changes in glomerular filtration rate (reproduced from de Wardener 1978 In: Dickinson C J, Marks J (eds) Developments in cardiovascular medicine. MTP Press, London, p. 179, with kind permission).

tion rate and therefore of sodium delivered into the proximal tubule. There is then a parallel change in sodium reabsorption. This phenomenon is illustrated in Figure 6.13 where it can be seen that changes in glomerular filtration rate are accompanied by parallel changes in absolute reabsorption but the proportion reabsorbed remains the same. It was believed at one time that this was due to parallel changes in the plasma protein concentration in the peritubular capillaries. It was proposed that a rise in glomerular filtration rate unaccompanied by a rise in plasma flow would raise the plasma protein concentration of the plasma flowing from the glomerulus to the peritubular capillaries, and that such a rise would produce a compensatory increase in proximal tubule reabsorption. It is now known that though changes in plasma protein concentration in the peritubular capillaries may have a small effect on sodium reabsorption from the proximal tubule such changes cannot account for glomerulotubular balance. It appears more probable that the rate of proximal tubule reasbsorption is so perfectly related to the rate of glomerular filtration rate because glomerular filtrate contains substances which stimulate it's own reabsorption. The evidence in support of this hypothesis comes from experiments Häbeler in which a proximal tubule is perfused with proximal tubule fluid harvested from another proximal tubule (Fig. 6.14). It can then be demonstrated that changes in perfusion rate with harvested fluid are accompanied by parallel changes in reabsorption (Fig. 6.15b). The control experiment is to perfuse the tubule with Ringer's solution when changes in perfusion produce little or no change in reabsorption (Fig. 6.15a). Thus the parallel change in sodium reabsorption which accompanies changes in filtration rate or perfusion with harvested fluid are not due simply to a change in the rate of delivery of fluid into the proximal tubule but due to some special property of the fluid.

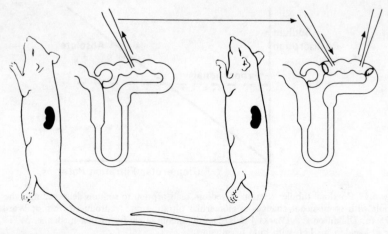

**Fig. 6.14** Proximal tubule: technique of perfusing a proximal tubule with fluid obtained from another proximal tubule (Häberle's experiment: Häberle D A, Shiigai T T, Maier G et al 1981 Dependency of proximal tubular fluid transport on the load of glomerular filtrate. Kidney Int 20: 18). See Fig. 6.15.

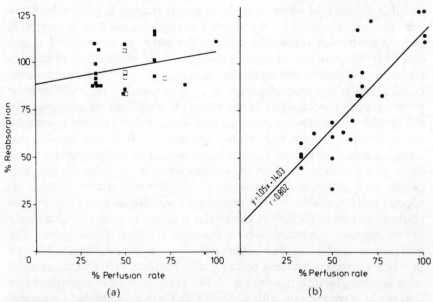

(a)  (b)

**Fig. 6.15** (a) Microperfusion of the lumen of the proximal tubule with Ringer's solution. (b) Microperfusion of the lumen of the proximal tubule with proximal tubule fluid harvested from late proximal tubules. In each experiment the tubule was perfused at two rates of flow, one between 10 and 20 nl/min and the other between 20 and 30 nl/min. The perfusion rates are expressed as a percentage of the highest perfusion rate used in each experiment. Reabsorption is expressed as a percentage of the reabsorption at the highest perfusion rate in that experiment. Each re-puncture value is corrected for differences in the length of the tubule perfused (Häberle's experiment) (reproduced from de Wardener 1978 In: Dickinson C J, Marks J (eds) Developments in cardiovascular medicine. MTP Press, London, p. 179, with kind permission).

Other factors which may influence sodium reabsorption from the proximal tubule include, the hydrostatic pressure in the peritubular venous capillaries, locally produced angiotensin, an osmotic diuresis, renal nerves and the permeability of the brush border. It appears that sodium entry across the brush border is the rate limiting step of transcellular sodium transport. Active sodium extrusion at the other side of the cell into the intercellular channels and basolateral membranes is not saturated under normal conditions.

It is also important to note the effect that changes in sodium reabsorption has on the reabsorption of many other substances. For instance an increased back pressure due to a decrease in proximal tubule fluid reabsorption due to diminished sodium reabsorption enhances the leakiness of the tight junctions. The reabsorption of other substances is then made that much more difficult. In addition, as the luminal concentration of a substance which is being reabsorbed tends to fall there is back leak of the substance down the concentration gradient from the interstitial space back into the lumen. These are the probable mechanisms which explain why a diminution of sodium reabsorption which occurs in extracellular volume expansion is associated with an increased excretion of chloride, calcium, phosphate, amino acids, glucose and particularly bicarbonate.

## Loop of Henle

The loop of Henle, including the early part of the distal tubule, can also be shown to have a form of 'glomerulotubular' balance in that reabsorption again adjusts itself to the delivery of sodium. The outstanding difference between the proximal tubule and the loop of Henle and early distal tubule, however, is that in the loop and distal tubule absolute reabsorption *is* directly related to the rate of sodium delivery, whether the sodium delivered is contained in a normal tubule fluid delivered in the natural way from the end of the proximal tubule, or whether the sodium is contained in Ringer's solution delivered by microperfusion. The parallelism between the rate of delivery of sodium from the proximal tubule and reabsorption from the loop and the distal tubule cannot, as in the glomerulotubular balance of the proximal tubule, therefore, be due to the tubule fluid containing any substance which controls active sodium reabsorption. There are two other relevant important differences between the proximal tubule, and the loop of Henle and early distal tubule; one is that movement of sodium in the ascending limb of Henle is secondary to the reabsorption of chloride, and the other is that as the wall of the ascending limb of Henle and early distal tubule are relatively impermeable to water, the tubular fluid they contain is hypotonic and the interstitial fluid is hypertonic. Consequently there is a steep ionic gradient across the tubule wall of the ascending limb of Henle where back-diffusion must be greater than in the proximal tubule. This likelihood is accentuated by the fact that the intercellular tight junctions in

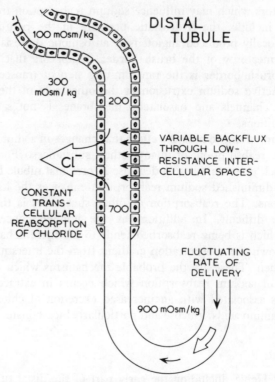

**Fig. 6.16** Ascending limb of Henle and early distal tubule. Schema of possible explanation for parallelism between sodium delivered and sodium reabsorption (reproduced from de Wardener 1978 In: Dickinson C J, Marks J (eds) Developments in cardiovascular medicine. MTP Press, London, p. 179, with kind permission).

the ascending limb of are particularly leaky. The extent of the ionic gradient and the decreased resistance to back diffusion are probably responsible for the paralellism between sodium delivery into, and reabsorption out of, the ascending limb of Henle and early part of the distal tubule. For example, assuming an unchanging active reabsorption of chloride, a greater delivery of chloride into the loop of Henle from the proximal tubule will cause the concentration of chloride in the tubule to rise. This will reduce the concentration gradient across the tubule wall so that back diffusion of chloride from the interstial space into the lumen will be less. Therefore without a change in active reabsorption, a higher delivery of chloride and sodium into the loop of Henle causes an increased net reabsorption of chloride and therefore of sodium.

*Collecting duct*

The pattern of sodium reabsorption in the collecting duct is totally different from those parts of the nephron which precede it. There is no parallelism between the amount of sodium that is delivered into the early distal tubule and the collecting duct, and the amount that is reabsorbed. For instance the natriuresis of chronic sodium loading, or of an acutely administered *small* amount of intravenous saline is not accompanied by any changes in proximal tubule sodium reabsorption. Presumably in both of these instances there is little change in sodium delivery into the collecting duct and yet the amount of sodium leaving the collecting duct increases. It would appear therefore that changes in glomerular filtration rate, or of sodium reabsorption in the proximal tubule or in the loop of Henle and early distal tubule with the exception of what takes place during an osmotic diuresis are usually irrelevant to the changes that occur in urinary sodium excretion. Changes in the urinary excretion of sodium are the result of changes in reabsorption in the collecting duct.

The collecting duct's behaviour as regards sodium handling is mainly determined by the need to maintain sodium and volume balance. In order to understand the control of urinary sodium excretion therefore it is necessary to find out what controls sodium handling in the collecting duct. Unfortunately this is the site which is the most difficult to get at experimentally and has thus been the least investigated. There are certain intrarenally-produced substances such as dopamine, bradykinin, prostaglandin and angiotensin all which are known to alter urinary sodium excretion. Some of these probably do so by acting on the collecting duct but it must be pointed out that the release of these substances is usually subservient to extrarenal influences.

The extrarenal factors which influence the collecting duct in response to changes in sodium and volume balance are aldosterone, the natriuretic hormone and the arterial pressure. The long term effects of angiotensin and the renal nerves, the action of both of which can be antinatriuretic, is not clear. The antinatriuretic effect of aldosterone is due to it's capacity to increase the permeability of the luminal border of the distal tubule and collecting duct to sodium. The resultant increase in sodium entry into the cell is compensated for by an increase in $Na^+-K^+$-ATPase activity along the walls of the basal infoldings and intercellular channels which actively pump the sodium out of the cell into the interstitial space. There is some evidence that the natriuretic hormone may inhibit sodium reabsorption along the whole length of the nephron but particularly the collecting duct. Acute changes in arterial pressure effect sodium reabsorption in the collecting duct. Persistent changes in arterial pressure, however, unless they are very great, do not seem to have much effect on sodium excretion.

There is a hypothesis that urinary sodium excretion is controlled in part by changes in regional perfusion. It stems from the observation that when sodium excretion is low the blood flow to the nephrons with glomeruli near the medulla is also low, and vice versa. It is not at all certain whether this phenomenon is one of cause or effect.

### The natriuretic hormone and circulating sodium transport inhibitor

The initial experiments on the natriuretic hormone demonstrated that the plasma of a volume expanded animal was natriuretic (Fig. 6.17). It was then shown that normal plasma has the capacity to inhibit sodium transport in frog skin, toad bladder and other types of intact cells. And it was also shown that this inhibitory capacity was greatest in plasma obtained from a volume expanded animal. It is now apparent that the sodium transport inhibitory capacity of plasma is due to at least in part to its ability to inhibit $Na^+$-$K^+$-ATPase (Fig. 6.18). As a first approximation many have assumed that the natriuretic capacity of plasma obtained from a volume expanded animal, and its increased capacity to inhibit $Na^+$-$K^+$-ATPase are due to a change in the concentration of the same substance but it is very possible that they are due to at least two substances.

There is evidence that the site of production of the substances responsible for the natriuresis and inhibition of $Na^+$-$K^+$-ATPase may be the hypothalamus. On the other hand highly potent peptides (1000 times more active than frusemide) have been isolated from the cardiac atria. These substances do not inhibit $Na^+$-$K^+$-ATPase and at the time of writing it is not known whether they are present in plasma.

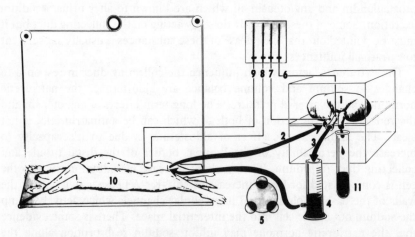

**Fig. 6.17** Diagram of the isolated kidney preparation which demonstrates the presence of a natriuretic substance in plasma. The isolated kidney (1) is placed in a constant temperature-humidity chamber where it is perfused with blood from the femoral artery (2) of a second dog (10). Renal venous blood (3)flows by gravity into a reservoir (4) from which it is pumped (5) to the femoral vein of the perfusion animal. The perfusion animal (10) rests on an adjustable platform and by raising or lowering the platform with respect to the isolated kidney, renal arterial pressure in the isolated kidney can be regulated. Pressure in the femoral artery (9) and vein (8) and renal artery (7) and vein (6) are monitored with pressure transducers. Urine (11) is collected from a catheter secured in the ureter. When the blood volume of the dog was expanded with equilibrated blood from the reservoir the isolated kidney had a natriuresis (reproduced from Kaloyanides & Azer 1971 J Clin Invest 50: 1603 by copyright permission of The American Society for Clinical Investigation).

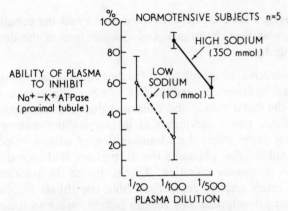

**Fig. 6.18** Inhibition of ouabain sensitive Na$^+$-K$^+$-ATPase in proximal tubules of guinea pig kidney by dilutions of plasma from 5 healthy subjects each on a high (●———) and on a low sodium diet (0, -----) The plasma from the subjects when they were on a high sodium diet had a greater capacity to inhibit Na-K ATPase. (reproduced from de Wardener, MacGregor, Clarkson et al 1981 Lancet 1: 411 with kind permission).

The afferent mechanism which controls the secretion of natriuretic hormone may monitor changes in intrathoracic blood volume. Immersion of a man up the neck in water, or acute elevation of the left auricular pressure in an animal increases the intrathoracic blood volume and causes a sustained increase in urinary sodium excretion, despite a gradual decrease in total blood volume. The cause of the natriuresis is not clear. It is unrelated to the aldosterone angiotensin system or the renal nerves and it is abolished by vagotomy. There is some fragmentary evidence that it may be due to the natriuretic hormone. It is possible therefore that normally the changes in extracellular volume and blood volume which produce changes in intrathoracic blood volume affect vagal afferents which in turn influence the secretion of the natriuretic hormone by the hypothalamus (Fig. 6.19).

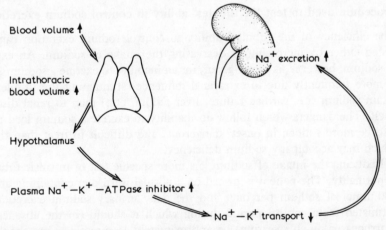

**Fig. 6.19** Possible afferent system for controlling the secretion of natriuretic hormone.

### The relationship between sodium reabsorption and the tubular handling of potassium, hydrogen, and calcium ions in the distal tubule and collecting duct

Sodium reabsorption in the distal and collecting duct is closely related to potassium and hydrogen excretion. For instance the greater delivery of sodium into the distal tubule and collecting duct the higher the excretion of potassium. Or under conditions of intense sodium reabsorption (e.g. during sodium deprivation) the administration of sodium sulphate causes a precipitate fall in urine pH and a rise in tritatable acid excretion, together with a rise in potassium excretion. This is due to the positively charged sodium ions being actively reabsorbed from the tubule lumen while the negatively charged sulphate ions remain behind owing to their poor penetrative qualities. The electrical gradient which results is then responsible for a passive movement of hydrogen and potassium ions from the tubule cells into the tubule lumen. Such an intravenous infusion of sodium sulphate during sodium deprivation is a highly abnormal situation, but the urinary changes which it induces probably reflects the normal pattern of events, i.e. active sodium reabsorption from the tubule lumen into the tubule cells sets up a potential gradient along which chloride ions travel into the cell while hydrogen and potassium ions move in the opposite direction from the cell into the tubule fluid.

A close and parallel relationship between the urinary excretion of sodium and calcium ions can be demonstrated in acute experiments when the urinary excretion of one of them is acutely changed. It seems therefore that the mechanism of reabsorption for these two ions are related. Nevertheless in chronic situations the urinary excretion of the two ions is not related. For instance a person on a low calcium diet who is excreting small amounts of calcium does not become oedematous.

### Procedure used to test the tubules' ability to control sodium excretion

The efficiency of the tubules' ability to control sodium excretion can be tested either by increasing or decreasing the intake of sodium. An excess of sodium, however, is rarely given, for an inability to excrete a sodium load is more frequently due to extrarenal influences stimulating the tubules to retain sodium (i.e. cardiac failure, liver failure, etc.) than to renal disease itself. The dangers which follow an inability to excrete a sodium load may also be more sudden in onset, dangerous, and difficult to treat than those which may accompany sodium deficiency.

Reducing the intake of sodium is a more specific test of intrinsic tubular abnormality. The patient is placed on a normal ward diet containing about 100 mmol of sodium per day, and the daily urinary sodium excretion is estimated for a control period during which it should (in the absence of diarrhoea or much sweating) be approximately 15 mmol/day less than the intake (to allow for loss in sweat and faeces). The dietary intake of salt is then reduced to about 10 mmol/day, which is the content of the average hospital 'salt-free' diet. Within 7–10 days urinary sodium excretion should also be down to 10 mEq per day.

The kidney's response to a low salt diet depends not only on tubular function but also on the many mechanisms which influence the tubule to retain salt. A more direct test of tubular ability to control salt excretion is obtained by keeping the patient on a normal diet and giving 2 mg of 9-$\alpha$-fluoro-hydrocortisone twice a day for two or three days when the urinary excretion of sodium should fall below 10 mmol/day.

Apart from Addison's disease and severe glycosuria, an inability to conserve sodium is seen occasionally in chronic renal failure; it also occurs sometimes during the diuretic phase of acute renal failure, and very rarely as a result of a primary disturbance of tubular function (renal tubular acidosis, p. 362). In contrast, in chronic renal failure there may sometimes be an impaired ability to excrete a high intake of sodium.

## CONTROL OF ACID-BASE BALANCE AND URINE ACIDITY

Plama hydrogen-ion concentration is maintained close to pH 7.4 by a variety of mechanisms. The most important are the buffering capacity of the cells and the skeleton, and the control of the $B.HCO_3/H.HCO_3$ buffer system in the plasma (where B = metallic cations, i.e. sodium, potassium and calcium). In this system the level of carbonic acid is regulated by the excretion of $CO_2$ by the lungs, and the concentration of bicarbonate (mainly in the form of sodium bicarbonate) by the kidney's ability to control bicarbonate and hydrogen ion secretion, and to generate bicarbonate.

On a normal diet and with a normal ventilation the pH of the blood can only remain constant if about 40–60 mmol of hydrogen ions are excreted in the urine each day. This represents the net load which remains to be disposed of, when metabolism is normal. The kidney's ability to excrete hydrogen ions depends on the tubule's capacity to secrete both hydrogen and ammonia ions into the tubular fluid. In the urine the hydrogen ions are either (1) free, or potentially free in association with a buffer, or (2) combined with ammonia in the form of ammonium.

The amount of alkali that must be added to acid urine to return the pH to that of plasma is a measure of the net quantity of free and potentially free hydrogen ions in the urine and is known as the titratable acid. The sum of the urinary titratable acidity and ammonium is a measure of the kidney's excretion of hydrogen ions, i.e. its contribution towards preventing the internal environment from becoming acid.

### Tubular control of hydrogen ion secretion and bicarbonate reabsorption

The tubular fluid pH is consistently acid along the length of the tubule indicating that bicarbonate is reabsorbed by a process which involves hydrogen ion secretion. Direct reabsorption of bicarbonate would not be associated with these low pH values. The secretion of hydrogen ions into the tubular fluid permits the excretion of free hydrogen ions which is necessary for the reabsorption of sodium bicarbonate, it is also responsible for generating fresh bicarbonate.

Hydrogen ion secretion from the tubule cell and bicarbonate reabsorption from the tubule lumen occur in both the proximal and distal tubule and are dependent on the intracellular production of free hydrogen ions. Throughout the nephron, both in the cells and tubular fluid, this is due primarily to the formation of carbonic acid from the hydration of carbon dioxide. Some of the carbonic acid then dissociates into hydrogen and bicarbonate ions, i.e.

$$CO_2 + H_2O \rightleftharpoons H_2CO_3 \rightleftharpoons H^+HCO_3^-$$

In the cells, therefore, hydrogen and bicarbonate ions are continuously being generated. The hydrogen ions are transferred into the tubular fluid in exchange for the sodium ions which are being actively and independently transported from the tubule lumen into the cell. The positively charged hydrogen ions diffuse into the tubule lumen not only because of their higher intracellular concentration (consequent upon their continuous intracellular production) but also because of the electrical gradient caused by the simultaneous active transport of the positively charged sodium ions from the tubule lumen.

Most of the hydrogen ions which enter the tubular fluid combine with bicarbonate to form carbonic acid most of which (Fig. 6.20) is then dehydrated in the tubule lumen to carbon dioxide and water, when the carbon dioxide then diffuses back into the cell. Once in the cell the carbonic acid or carbon dioxide are then reutilised or diffuse into the blood. The hydrogen ions which remain in the tubule fluid are finally excreted in the urine, either as free ions or in association with a buffer, particularly phosphate (Fig. 6.20), or they are combined with ammonia. The transfer of hydrogen ions from the tubule cell into the tubule fluid in the distal tubule can continue in the face of a steep rise in the concentration of hydrogen ions in the tubular fluid; the highest concentration which can be sustained is about pH 4.3 At this point the further transfer of hydrogen ions depends on the supply of buffer or ammonia.

The bicarbonate that is generated in the cells by the hydration of carbon dioxide joins the reabsorbed sodium that is passing through the cell and thus it is sodium bicarbonate that diffuses into the peritubular capillaries. It is to be noted therefore that strictly speaking bicarbonate is not reabsorbed from the tubule fluid. The bicarbonate that accompanies the sodium out of the cell into the blood is fresh bicarbonate generated in the cell, while the bicarbonate in the tubule fluid is destroyed. In this exchange equilibrium is maintained, there is no gain to the body of acid or alkali. The formation of titratable acid follows the same principle. Hydrogen ions formed in the re-

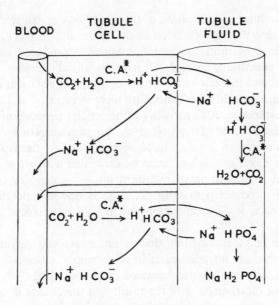

* C.A.= CARBONIC ANHYDRASE.

**Fig. 6.20** Secretion of hydrogen ions in the distal tubule, and bicarbonate reabsorption and generation. Note that the excretion of titratable acid is chiefly in the form of acid phosphate, and that the formation of this salt is accompanied by the generation of fresh bicarbonate ions.

nal tubule cells are again exchanged for sodium in the tubule fluid. If bicarbonate is scarce in the tubule fluid the hydrogen ions join the phosphate ion $HPO_4$ and convert it to $H_2PO^-_4$ i.e.:

$$Na_2\ HPO_4 + H^+ \rightarrow Na\ H_2PO_4 + Na^+$$

During this process however, there is a net loss of acid from the body. And in addition the sodium ion as it passes through the cell picks up a bicarbonate ion generated in the tubule cell so that there is a net gain of bicarbonate to the body. This regeneration of bicarbonate stores also occurs when hydrogen ions generated in the cells are trapped in the tubule lumen by ammonia.

The intracellular formation and concentration of hydrogen ions in the tubule cells and their secretion into the tubule lumen is dependent on a variety of factors. In the proximal tubule it appears to be dependent on the ambient carbon dioxide tension. In the distal tubule it is also dependent on the carbon dioxide tension but it is also related to the intracellular content of carbonic anhydrase which accelerates the hydration of carbon dioxide. In addition, in the distal tubule, sodium reabsorption from the lumen of the tubule into the cell can cause potassium ions to move from the cell into the tubule lumen as well as, or instead of, hydrogen ions. The relative intracellular concentration of these two ions probably determines in what proportions they are excreted in the urine. For instance, the increase in intracellular potassium concentration which is produced by the administration of potassium chloride diminishes distal tubular secretion of hydrogen ions and increases the urinary excretion of potassium. As a result less bicarbonate is reabsorbed, therefore more is excreted and there is a fall in plasma bicarbonate. Alternatively, if the cellular production of hydrogen ions in the distal tubule is inhibited by the administration of a carbonic anhydrase inhibitor such as acetazoleamide (Diamox) the reabsorption of sodium in the distal tubule will again be associated with a rise in potassium excretion and a diminution of hydrogen ion excretion. On this occasion, however, the increased potassium excretion is due to a decrease of intracellular hydrogen ion concentration and not to an increase in potassium concentration.

Bicarbonate reabsorption, like that of phosphate and sodium, is closely related to glomerular filtration rate. In other words, changes in glomerular filtration of bicarbonate are accompanied by almost equal change in tubular reabsorption of bicarbonate with the result that the change in filtration produces little if any change in bicarbonate excretion. It is important that this phenomenon be remembered when studying the effect of various stimuli on tubular reabsorption, if such stimuli also produce changes in glomerular filtration rate. It is for this reason that in such studies changes in bicarbonate (and phosphate) reabsorption are related to a constant glomerular filtration.

*Other mechanisms involved in the control of bicarbonate excretion*

It is clear from the above that one of the main factors which influences bicarbonate excretion is the secretion of hydrogen ions into the tubule lumen. And this in turn appears to be a direct function of the plasma $pCo_2$. When a sufficient quantity of hydrogen ions are secreted into the tubule lumen all the filtered bicarbonate can be reabsorbed — if less hydrogen ions are secreted some of the filtered bicarbonate will bot be reabsorbed and will therefore be excreted. It has been pointed out that the intracellular potassium concentration can also influence the secretion of hydrogen ions.

Aside from $pCo_2$ and intracellular potassium, the secretion of hydrogen ions and therefore the reabsorption and excretion of bicarbonate are also influenced by:
1. Expansion and contraction of body fluids
2. Adrenal cortical hormones
3. Parathyroid hormone
4. Plasma calcium
5. Plasma chloride
6. The integrity of the counter-current system in the medulla.

Changes in the volume of the extracellular fluid can profoundly influence bicarbonate reabsorption. At one time it was considered that the tubule had a limited capacity to reabsorb bicarbonate, i.e. a Tm $HCO_3$ (see p. 110). This conclusion was based on experiments which were performed by raising the plasma bicarbonate progressively by the intravenous infusion of large volumes of sodium bicarbonate solutions. It has now been demonstrated that this apparent limitation of bicarbonate reabsorbed is an artefact produced by expanding the extracellular fluid volume with the bicarbonate solution. If the experiment is repeated in such a way that the rise in plasma bicarbonate is produced with a minimal expansion of body fluid there is no discernible limit to the tubule's capacity to reabsorb bicarbonate (Fig. 6.21).

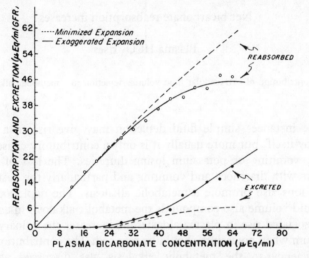

**Fig. 6.21** The effect of extracellular fluid volume expansion on bicarbonate reabsorption in the rat. Bicarbonate reabsorption is depressed by extracellular fluid volume expansion (reproduced from Pukerson, Lubowitz, White et al 1969 J Clin Invest 48: 1754, by copyright permission of The American Society for Clinical Investigation).

The effect of changes in extracellular fluid volume on bicarbonate reabsorption is due to their effect on the tight junctions of the intracellular channels, a phenomenon described earlier when discussing the control of sodium excretion. The greater the extracellular fluid volume, the less tight the junctions and therefore the greater the diffusion of many substances including bicarbonate from the interstitial fluid back into the tubule lumen, i.e. the bigger the extracellular fluid volume the lower the net bicarbonate reabsorption, the greater the urinary excretion of bicarbonate and the lower the plasma bicarbonate. Conversely, and clinically much more important, extracellular fluid volume depletion due to salt depletion gives rise to an increased net bicarbonate reabsorption a diminished excretion of bicarbonate, and a rise in plasma bicarbonate (Fig. 6.22).

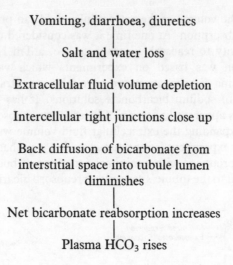

Vomiting, diarrhoea, diuretics
|
Salt and water loss
|
Extracellular fluid volume depletion
|
Intercellular tight junctions close up
|
Back diffusion of bicarbonate from
interstitial space into tubule lumen
diminishes
|
Net bicarbonate reabsorption increases
|
Plasma HCO₃ rises

Fig. 6.22 Contribution of extracellular fluid volume depletion to a metabolic alkalosis.

In some instances simple fluid depletion may give rise to a metabolic alkalosis by itself, but more usually it is only a contributory cause e.g. with diarrhoea, vomiting or potassium losing diuretics. The loss of potassium that occurs with diarrhoea and vomiting and particularly the gastric loss of hydrogen ions also promote a metabolic alkalosis. The depletion of extracellular fluid volume also compounds the metabolic alkalosis in another way for the associated rise in plasma aldosterone increases the urinary excretion of potassium when potassium should be retained. The contribution of potassium deficiency to the metabolic alkalosis was discussed above. The decrease in the potassium content of the tubule cells increases hydrogen ion secretion from the cells into the tubular fluid thus increasing bicarbonate reabsorption.

Insufficiency of adrenal cortical hormones leads to a metabolic acidosis and an excess to a metabolic alkalosis because of the changes in volume and potassium metabolism discussed in the preceding paragraph. Parathyroid hormone increases bicarbonate excretion so that in primary hyperparathyroidism there is an initial metabolic acidosis and in hypoparathyroidism an initial metabolic alkalosis. Hypercalcaemia has an opposite effect to that of parathyroid hormone in that it causes a rise in urinary hydrogen excretion and thus a diminition of bicarbonate excretion probably by stimulating carbonic anhydrase activity. If the hypercalcaemia is so severe that it causes vomiting then the viscious circle of circumstances which will aggravate the metabolic alkalosis is formidable. In addition to the effect of the hypercalcaemia itself on the tubule's ability to secrete hydrogen ions there is the gastric loss of hydrogen ions, sodium, and potassium and water. The lowered ability to concentrate the urine which is associated with hypercalciuria and hyperkalaemia will enhance the effect of the fall in extracellular fluid volume on not only bicarbonate reabsorption but also on calcium reabsorption, and the latter will perpetuate the hypercalcaemia.

Plasma chloride concentration affects the secretion of hydrogen ions and therefore bicarbonate excretion in the following way. Let us assume that the plasma chloride concentration is low but that of plasma sodium is normal, and that the tubule attempts to reabsorb nearly all the sodium in the normal way. It has been pointed out earlier that the reabsorption of the positively charged sodium ions from the tubule lumen causes a rise in the electrical potential difference between the cell and the lumen of the tubule; the cell tending to become increasingly positive and the lumen increasingly negative. This potential gradient causes the negatively charged chloride ions to diffuse from the tubule lumen into the cell and the positively charged hydrogen ions to diffuse from the cell into the lumen. If the supply of chloride ions to the tubule lumen falls because of a fall in plasma chloride and if at the same time sodium reabsorption remains normal, it is clear that even if all the chloride ions diffuse back into tubule cell, the steepness of the potential gradient will remain higher than when the supply of chloride is normal. Then the passive flux of hydrogen ions from the tubule cell into the tubule lumen will increase and enhance bicarbonate reabsorption.

The $P_{CO_2}$ of an alkaline urine excreted by a normal person may be around 100 mmHg. The kidney's ability to excrete a urine with such a high $P_{CO_2}$ is due to counter-current systems in the medulla which traps the carbon dioxide (p. 58). This phenomenon permits the presence in the urine of very high concentrations of bicarbonate and thus increases the kidney's capacity to excrete large amounts of bicarbonate.

## Procedures used to detect the presence of an abnormal handling of bicarbonate by the kidneys

The plasma bicarbonate tends to be low when the ability to reabsorb bicarbonate is reduced and raised when the ability to reabsorb bicarbonate is raised.

One method used to detect the presence of an abnormal handling of bicarbonate by the kidney is to estimate the tubules 'maximal' capacity to reabsorb bicarbonate (Tm $HCO_3$, see p. 110). Though this is a spurious Tm, and is only apparent because of the way in which the plasma bicarbonate is increased (see above) it is sufficiently reproducible to be used as a test of bicarbonate handling by the kidney. A low Tm $HCO_3$ is evidence of bicarbonate wastage due to diminished bicarbonate reabsorption in the proximal tubule. The patient should not be taking diuretics and should be emotionally at rest to avoid hyperventilation. A large intravenous infusion of sodium bicarbonate is given so as to raise the plasma bicarbonate to approximately 28–30 mmol/l. As bicarbonate reabsorption is related to glomerular filtration the maximal rate of bicarbonate reabsorption is then adjusted to a standard quantity of glomerular filtrate; it is usually adjusted to one litre of filtrate.

The normal maximal rate of bicarbonate reabsorption under these conditions is 26 to 29 mmol/1 of glomerular filtrate. It is lowered in chronic renal failure, and it is reduced in many diseases in particular, those associated with hyperglobulinaemia when it is almost invariably associated with many selective disturbances of distal tubule function (p. 362). Tm $HCO_3$ is also low in some patients with essential hypertension without overt evidence of other renal functional abnormalities, it is also lowered when hyperventilation lowers $Pco_2$; on the other hand, it is raised in respiratory failure with a raised $Pco_2$, in vomiting with hydrochloric acid loss, in potassium deficiency and hyperadrenalism.

In chronic renal failure the leak of bicarbonate into the urine may be an important contributory cause of metabolic acidosis. The easiest way to spot a bicarbonate leak in chronic renal failure is to find bicarbonate in the urine when the plasma bicarbonate is 20 mmol/1 or lower. Sometimes with a plasma bicarbonate which is much lower, e.g. 10 mmol/1, the urine may be free of bicarbonate. If, however, the plasma bicarbonate is increased by the intravenous administration of bicarbonate, bicarbonate is then observed to appear in the urine at a plasma bicarbonate of between 15 and 20 mmol/l. This leak of bicarbonate is partly due to an insufficient secretion of hydrogen ions by the reduced number of nephrons (see below) and to the raised concentration of plasma parathyroid hormone which inhibits bicarbonate reabsorption. If the patient is acidotic it can be presumed that the kidneys are at all times under maximal stimulation to reabsorb bicarbonate. It is for this reason that a good approximation of a Tm $HCO_3$ can be obtained simply by measuring the urine bicarbonate and then calculating the reabsorption of bicarbonate from a concomitant creatinine clearance.

### Acidosis

In chronic *respiratory acidosis* (e.g. chronic obstructive airways disease) the rise in $Pco_2$ causes an increase in the concentration of hydrogen ions both in the plasma and the cells, including the tubule cells. This in turn increases the tubular secretion of hydrogen ions from the cells into the tubule lumen and thus causes a rise in both the urinary excretion of hydrogen ions and an increased intracellular generation of bicarbonate. The increased secretion of hydrogen ions into the tubule lumen ensures that all the filtered bicarbonate is reabsrobed, in addition, however some of the extra bicarbonate generated in the tubule cell also diffuses into the blood. The combination of total bicarbonate reabsorption, intracellular bicarbonate generation with diffusion into the plasma, and increased urinary hydrogen ion excretion causes a rise in plasma bicarbonate. The ability to reabsorb all the filtered bicarbonate increases in parallel with rise in $Pco_2$ and remains complete with $Pco_2$ tensions of 80 mmHg and above (Fig. 6.23). The generation of extra

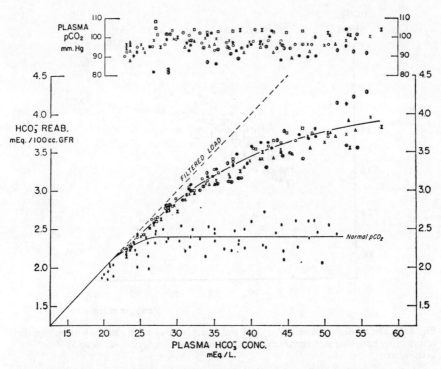

**Fig. 6.23** Bicarbonate reabsorption in the dog. The effect of acute increases in $P_{CO_2}$ during the progressive elevation of plasma bicarbonate by the intravenous infusion of $NaHCO_3$ in large volumes of water. The lower line = values obtained at normal $P_{CO_2}$ between 35 and 45 mmHg. The upper curved line = values obtained when the $P_{CO_2}$ was between 80 and 110 mmHg. It can be seen that the bicarbonate reabsorption is greater when the $P_{CO_2}$ is raised. It is clear that at both concentrations of $P_{CO_2}$ the capacity to reabsorb bicarbonate flattens out, but at different values. This flattening is due to the effect of the large expansion in body fluids caused by the sodium bicarbonate infusion which inhibits bicarbonate reabsorption (reproduced from Schwartz, Falbriard & Lemieux 1959 J Clin Invest 38: 939, by copyright permission of The American Society for Clinical Investigation).

bicarbonate and urinary excretion of hydrogen ions, however, are only sufficient to compensate for a rise of $P_{CO_2}$ up to 60 mmHg. This can be seen in Figure 6.24 where up to a rise in $P_{CO_2}$ of 60 mmHg the accompanying rise in bicarbonate is sufficient to prevent a major change in plasma pH. Above a $P_{CO_2}$ of 60 mmHg the urine remains free of bicarbonate but the rise in plasma bicarbonate is minimal and there is a sharp fall in plasma pH. The inadequacy of urinary hydrogen ion excretion is particularly striking and is due to an impaired production of ammonia. It is probable that this impairment is due directly to the poisonous effect of the rise in $P_{CO_2}$ on the tubule cell's capacity to form ammonia (in metabolic acidosis the ammonia production is much higher). The sustained rise in bicarbonate reabsorption is associated with a sustained diminution in chloride reabsorption. It results in a severe chloride loss and a low plasma chloride.

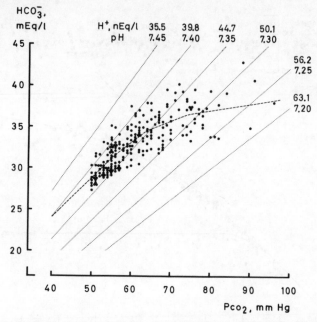

**Fig. 6.24** The relation of arterial $P_{CO_2}$, pH and bicarbonate in δ-210 patients with pulmonary insufficiency breathing air (reproduced from Refsum 1964, Clin Sci 27: 407, with kind permission).

*Metabolic acidosis* is due either to the retention of acids other than carbonic acid or to loss of bicarbonate. Acids consist of a combination of an anion and a hydrogen ion. A metabolic acidosis due to the retention of acids other than carbonic acid can therefore be inferred from a calculation of the plasma 'anion gap'. The anion gap is calculated by subtracting the sum of the concentrations of plasma chloride and total $CO_2$ from the plasma sodium concentration, i.e.

$$[Na^+] - ([Cl^-] + [T_{co2}]) = 143 - (102 + 28)$$
$$= 12 \text{ mmol/l anion gap}$$

The anion gap varies between 10 and 16 mmol/l. It is raised above 16 in (a) diabetic ketoacidosis with retention of acetoacetic acid and β-hydroxy butyric acid, (b) lactic acidosis due to severe anorexia increasing glycolysis, (c) chronic renal failure due in part to retention of sulphate, phosphate and other anions, (d) the ingestion of various poisons such as salicylates, methanol and glycol which give rise to formic and oxalic acids respectively. It is of course the simultaneous retention of the accompanying hydrogen ions which is responsible for the acidosis.

Obviously when metabolic acidosis is simply due to bicarbonate loss, the reduction of plasma bicarbonate tends to *reduce* the anion gap to below 12 mmol/l. There is at the same time a compensatory conservation of chloride by the kidney so that the plasma chloride rises to 106 mmol/l or more. The condition is therefore often referred to as hyperchloraemic acidosis. This occurs with (a) severe diarrhoea due to loss of bicarbonate in the stools, (b) ureterosigmoid transplant when the urinary chloride is reabsorbed by the bowel in exchange for bicarbonate (p. 342) (c) renal tubular acidosis due in part to an impaired ability of the kidney to secrete hydrogen ions and therefore to reabsorb bicarbonate (p. 362), (d) rupture of bladder or ureter with consequent reabsorption of urinary chloride from the peritoneum, (e) the administration of acetozolamide (Diamox) which inhibits the reabsorption of bicarbonate by the tubule. Amonium chloride administration also causes hyperchloraemic acidosis but not because of loss of bicarbonate (see below).

In a metabolic acidosis the increased concentration of hydrogen ions in the plasma cause hyperventilation so that the carbon dioxide tension in the plasma is *reduced*, (Fig. 6.25). Nevertheless the tubules again increase the secretion of hydrogen ions and the reabsorption of bicarbonate. It appears therefore that in a metabolic acidosis the inhibitory effect of the reduced carbon dioxide tension on the intracellular production of hydrogen ions is swamped by the persistent rise in extracellular fluid hydrogen ion concentration which presumably causes a rise in intracellular hydrogen ion concentration. In normal man when the plasma bicarbonate concentration falls below 25 mmol/1 the urinary excretion of bicarbonate rapidly diminishes. In the metabolic acidosis associated with renal disease, however, this compensatory mechanism may not occur and in some patients bicarbonate

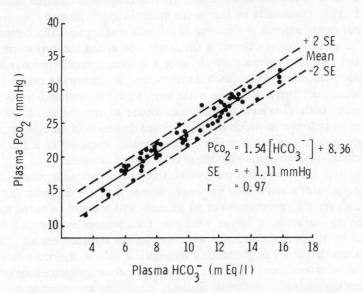

$$Pco_2 = 1.54 \left[ HCO_3^- \right] + 8.36$$
$$SE = \pm 1.11 \text{ mmHg}$$
$$r = 0.97$$

**Fig. 6.25** Respiratory response induced by metabolic acidosis. SE, standard error (reproduced from Albert, Dell & Winters 1967 Ann Intern Med 66: 312, with kind permission).

excretion may continue down to plasma bicarbonate levels of about 20 mmol/1 (see above). The maximum acidity which the tubule can sustain is approximately pH 4.6, which limits the kidney's ability to excrete large quantities of hydrogen ions unless the urinary content of phosphate buffer is raised or there are large volumes of urine, as in diabetic ketosis.

## Alkalosis

When there is a *respiratory alkalosis* (e.g. voluntary hyperventilation, left heart failure, or excessive artificial ventilation) there is a fall both in plasma hydrogen ion concentration and carbon dioxide tension. Both these factors will decrease the availability of the hydrogen ions in the tubule cell so that less hydrogen ions are excreted and bicarbonate reabsorption is decreased; both of which will tend to reduce the alkalinity of the plasma. In an *acute* respiratory alkalosis there is a simultaneous increase in the excretion of sodium and potassium. The rise in sodium excretion is due to a cardiovascular reflex, the afferent limb of which is probably a change in venous pressure in the left side of the heart. The rise in potassium excretion is due to a sudden rise in intracellular potassium concentration consequent upon the alkalosis.

*Metabolic alkalosis* can be caused by:

*Extrarenal loss of hydrogen ions or chloride.* Extrarenal loss of hydrogen ions can be due to vomiting of gastric secretion and is relatively common (p. 339). Extrarenal loss of chloride is very rare. It may be lost in the stools with a villous adenoma of the colon, or with congenital chloride diarrhoea. And it may occasionally be lost in the sweat in cystic fibrosis.

*Renal loss of chloride or excessive bicarbonate reabsorption* The commonest cause of a renal loss of chloride is the careless or willful use of powerful loop diuretics such as frusemide which cause a disproportionally greater loss of chloride than bicarbonate. Such diuretics may also cause an excess loss of potassium (and therefore cause potassium depletion) and sodium (volume depletion) both of which will also contribute to the metabolic alkalosis. Bartter's syndrome in which there is volume depletion of unknown cause is thought (when it is not secondary to surreptious vomiting or secret use of diuretics and purgatives) to be due to renal loss of chloride.

Excessive tubular reabsorption of bicarbonate occurs with volume depletion (see above) when it may not be recognised that it is the main factor responsible for the perpetuation of an alkalosis which could be cured by simply giving intravenous saline. Excessive bicarbonate reabsorption is also caused by potassium deficiency by a mechanism outlined earlier. Though potassium deficiency may induce a metabolic alkalosis unaided e.g. in primary aldosteronism and Cushing's disease it usually accompanies one or more concomitant causes of metabolic alkalosis (e.g. diuretics, vomiting).

*Massive ingestion of bicarbonate.* The only remaining example of this condition is the vanishing 'milk-alkali' syndrome in which a person who has been tortured by dyspepsia for many years finally resorts to the ingestion of extraordinary amounts of milk and indigestion powders (containing sodium bicarbonate and calcium carbonate).

In a metabolic alkalosis there is a fall in hydrogen ion concentration but, because of the accompanying hypoventilation, there is a rise in the carbon dioxide tension. The rise in carbon dioxide tension does cause a slight increase in bicarbonate reabsorption but, when the plasma bicarbonate concentration rises above 27 mmol/1 bicarbonate reabsorption does not increase further and unless there is volume depletion or potassium deficiency, bicarbonate excretion then equals the increasing quantities which are filtered. If the glomerular filtration rate is normal this spill over prevents the concentration of plasma bicarbonate from rising steeply. With volume depletion or potassium deficiency this balance is struck at a much higher concentration of plasma bicarbonate. In contrast to metabolic acidosis therefore, which is controlled entirely by tubular mechanisms, the ability of the kidneys to control a metabolic alkalosis is mainly related to the glomerular filtration rate. But tubular function is also involved for very large quantities of bicarbonate can only be excreted if the counter-current system in the medulla is sufficiently intact to maintain a high $P_{CO_2}$ (p. 58).

### Ammonia excretion

Ammonia ($NH_3$) is formed in the tubule cells throughout the whole length of the nephron, with the exception of the thin part of the loop of Henle (Fig. 6.26). Ammonia is a base with no electrical charge which is highly soluble in lipids, for this reason it diffuses easily across cell membranes. When ammonia combines with a hydrogen ion, however, and becomes ammonium ($NH_4^+$) it is charged, has a low lipid solubility and only diffuses across cell membranes with some difficulty. The ammonia formed within the tubule cells diffuses passively from the cells into the tubular lumen on one side of the cell and the peritubular venous capillaries on the other. When the ammonia in the tubule fluid combines with a hydrogen ion and forms an ammonium ion it is trapped within the lumen and most of it remains there to be excreted in the urine, a most important mechanism for getting rid of excess hydrogen ions, particularly in chronic acidosis. The formation of ammonium in the tubule lumen diminishes the intraluminal concentration of ammonia so that the diffusion of ammonia from the cell to the tubule lumen down a concentration gradient continues. On the other hand, if the secretion of hydrogen ions from the cell into the tubule lumen is diminished the formation of ammonium will be less and the intraluminal concentration of ammonia will rise; this in turn will reduce the rate of diffusion of ammonia from the cell to the lumen.

Ammonia is formed within tubule cells mainly from the action of glutaminase on glutamine, though other amino acids are also involved. This process is depressed by accumulation of intracellular ammonia and accel-

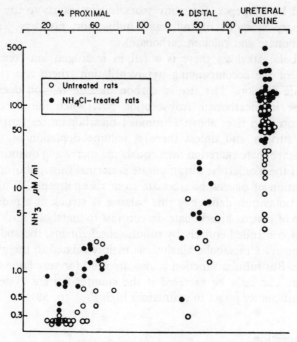

**Fig. 6.26** Site ot ammonia production in the rat nephron (reproduced from Glabman, Klose & Giebisch 1963 Amer J Physiol 205: 127, with kind permission).

erated when the concentration falls; conversely, it is accelerated in potassium deficiency, perhaps because of the intracellular acidosis that then occurs which probably reduces the concentration of free ammonia. It is important to remember that free ammonia diffuses both into the tubule lumen and into the peritubular venous capillaries and that the amount that diffuses into the blood is therefore inversely proportional to that which is secreted into the urine. Clinically this is particular relevant in patients with liver failure who develop oliguria or anuria in whom there is thus a shift in the direction of ammonia secretion into the blood.

Urinary ammonium excretion is inversely related to the pH of the urine and almost ceases when the urine becomes alkaline. The increase in ammonium excretion, which occurs as the urine pH falls, is due in part to the increased formation of ammonia in the tubule cell mentioned above and due to the depletion of intracellular ammonia. But if the urine continues to be acid the amount of ammonium excreted continues to rise after the pH has reached its minimum. This adaptive mechanism in chronic acidosis is not yet understood. It may be due to a circulating substance of unknown structure.

In normal circumstances the daily excretion of ammonium and free hydrogen ions is approximately the same (i.e. 20–30 mmol of each). When there is a need for an increased excretion of both (as in diabetic ketosis) the increase in ammonium greatly exceeds that of free hydrogen ions. Ammonium excretion may reach 400 mmol/day whereas the simultaneous excretion of free hydrogen ions will only be 70–100 mmol/day. These are very high excretion rates and are rarely seen except in prolonged diabetic ketosis. The response of a normal person to large quantities of ammonium chloride is illustrated in Figure 6.27. It can be seen that after a delay of five days the ammonium excretion is about three times greater than that of free hydrogen ions.

## Procedure used to estimate the tubule's ability to excrete an acid urine and to excrete hydrogen ions and ammonia

The tubule's capacity to excrete hydrogen ions and ammonia is estimated by measuring its response to the oral administration of ammonium chloride. The ammonium chloride molecule is metabolised to urea and HC1. The addition of these hydrogen ions into the extracellular fluid tends to make it acidotic, and in order to compensate for this tendency the kidney excretes increased quantities of hydrogen ions both as titratable acid and as ammonium, and the urine becomes more acid. Ammonium chloride is given either as a single dose in the morning, the urine being studied within the next eight hours; or it is administered in divided doses each day for five days when each daily collection of urine is studied, particularly that obtained on the fifth day. If the patients plasma bicarbonate is below 20 mmol/1 the administration of ammonium chloride is unnecessary and may be dangerous.

*The short test.* After two control collections of urine of about 1–2 hours duration the patient is given 0.1 g (1.9 mmol) of ammonium chloride per kg body weight orally at about 10 a.m.; in a patient of average size this is about 7 g. In order to avoid gastric irritation this amount is given over an hour, in gelatin capsules of 0.5 to 1.0 g together with a litre of water (enteric coated tablets are not used for they often appear intact in the stools). Venous blood is taken before and 2–4 hours after the administration of ammonium chloride. The urine may be collected at hourly intervals, but as the changes are maximal and relatively constant after the fifth hour a single urine collection taken between 3 and 5 p.m. will usually suffice. The urine pH should fall below 5.3, and hydrogen ion excretion (i.e. combined titratable acidity and ammonium) should rise above 60 $\mu$mol/min; the titratable acid excretion should be greater than 25 $\mu$mol/min and ammonium excretion greater than 35 $\mu$mol/min.

*The long test.* Following two to three days control observations 7.5 g (140 mmol) of ammonium chloride is given by mouth in divided doses each day for five days. The maximum titratable acidity is reached in three to four days, whereas ammonium excretion takes four to five days to reach its peak. The chloride ions of the ammonium chloride are also eliminated through the kidney; at first these are excreted with almost equal quantities of

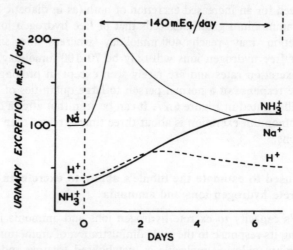

**Fig. 6.27** The effect of 140 mEq/day of ammonium chloride by mouth on the urinary excretion of sodium, hydrogen and ammonium in a normal subject.

sodium, but after two to three days the initial increase in sodium excretion subsides (Fig. 6.27). At the end of four to five days the urine pH should have fallen below 5.0 and the daily combined excretion of ammonium and titrable acid should rise above control values by about 120 mmol/day. If the renal response is normal, plasma bicarbonate and chloride concentrations should not alter by more than 6 mmol/1.

The ability to reduce the pH of the urine is always impaired in renal tubular acidosis (p. 362) and potassium deficiency (p. 324), it is sometimes impaired in hypercalcuria, while it appears normal in the chronic renal failure which accompanies loss of nephrons (p. 187). The ability to excrete titratable acid normally is depressed in renal tubular acidosis; potassium deficiency, hypercalcuria and chronic renal failure. As ammonium excretion is related to the pH of the urine the value obtained in these tests must be considered in relation to the pH of the urine. The normal relationship is illustrated in Figure 6.28. It can only be claimed that the capacity to excrete ammonium is depressed if it is lower than a normal person's capabilities at the same urine pH. According to these criteria ammonia excretion is depressed in chronic renal failure and in some cases of hypercalcuria, it is normal in most cases of renal tubular acidosis and some cases of potassium deficiency; and it is raised in most cases of potassium deficiency and some cases of renal tubular acidosis.

## POTASSIUM EXCRETION

Potassium is the principal intracellular cation.

The potassium that is filtered at the glomerulus is nearly all reabsorbed in the proximal tubule, while the potassium that appears in the urine is

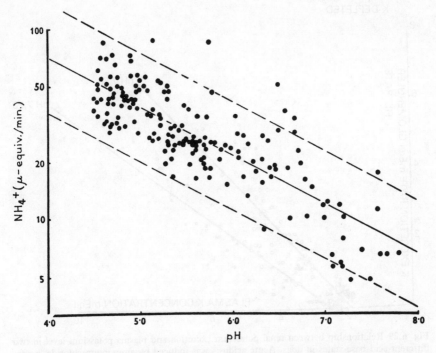

**Fig. 6.28** Relation between the excretion of ammonium and urinary pH in normal subjects a few hours after the oral ingestion of a single dose of ammonium chloride ('short test'). The calculated regression line and 95% range of observations are shown (reproduced from Wrong & Davies 1959 Quart J Med 28: 259, with kind permission).

secreted by the distal nephron, particularly the collecting duct. As with sodium, therefore, though for different reasons, glomerular filtration rate is unrelated to potassium excretion. This is a point of the greatest importance to patients suffering from most forms of chronic renal disease who, though glomerular filtration may be reduced to less than 5 ml/min, usually remain in potassium balance with a normal plasma potassium.

The secretion of potassium by the distal nephron (i.e. the urinary excretion of potassium) is controlled by the concentration of plasma aldosterone, the dietary content of potassium, plasma pH and the rate of flow of the fluid entering the distal nephron, and it's sodium concentration. Aldosterone increases the secretion of potassium by the distal tubule, and the secretion of aldosterone is in turn directly related to the concentration of plasma potassium. On the other hand it is unlikely that though the dietary intake of potassium directly effects plasma potassium that the effect of dietary potassium on tubular secretion of potassium is entirely due to parallel changes in plasma aldosterone. The effect of plasma pH on the urinary excretion of potassium has been mentioned earlier. It is illustrated in Figure 6.29.

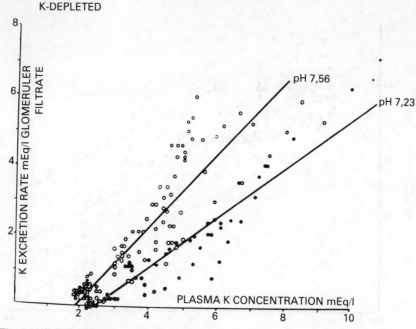

**Fig. 6.29** Relationship between renal potassium excretion and plasma potassium level in two different acid base states in dogs. Acute acidosis was induced by ammonium-chloride, acute alkalosis by bicarbonate infusion. The urinary excretion of potassium is greater the higher the urine pH (reproduced from Toussaint & Vereerstraaeten 1962 Amer J Physiol 202: 768, with kind permission).

Diffusion of potassium from the tubule cell into the tubule lumen is passive. It is dependent in part on the cell's ability to maintain the potassium concentration gradient between the lumen and the cell but more importantly on the electronegativity of the tubule lumen, which is a consequence of active sodium reabsorption. There is no evidence that the potassium that is secreted is in any way exchanged for sodium that is reabsorbed. For instance during the intravenous infusion of sodium sulphate the impermeant negatively charged sulphate ions are not reabsorbed. A small amount of sodium reabsorption therefore causes the electronegativity of the tubule lumen to become very great. This then increases back diffusion of sodium from the cell into the lumen so that effective sodium reabsorption from the lumen is small. Nevertheless there is a simultaneous maximal secretion rate of potassium ions from the cells to the tubule lumen. There is also evidence that the diffusion of potassium into the lumen proceeds at such a rate that the same potassium concentration gradient is achieved however high the rate of flow of the tubule fluid. In other words the more fluid delivered into the distal tubule the greater the urinary excretion of potassium, even if distal tubule sodium reabsorption remains unchanged. (Fig. 6.30). There is also evidence that the net movement of

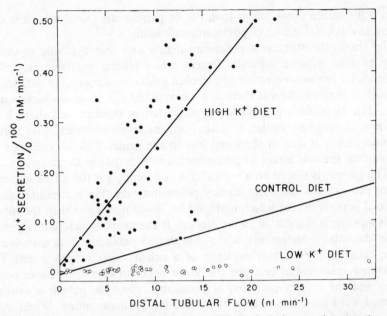

**Fig. 6.30** Plot of absolute rates of normalized (0–100%) distal tubular potassium secretion as function of distal tubular volume flow rate. The latter had been varied by loading with saline or saline-urea solutions given at progressively higher rates intravenously. Data are from rats kept on a low, normal and high dietary potassium intake (reproduced from Khuri Wiederholt 1975 Amer J Physiol 228: 1249, with kind permission).

potassium into the tubule lumen is dependent on the concentration of sodium in the tubular fluid, the permeability of the cell membrane on the luminal side of the cell and on the presence of a potassium pump which moves potassium back from the lumen into the cell. Though there is a certain reciprococity between potassium and hydrogen ion secretion there is again no evidence that there is a direct 'pump-related' relationship between potassium and hydrogen secretion. It is more probable that the apparent reciprocity is due to changes in intracellular potassium and hydrogen ion concentration. For instance when $PCO_2$ rises there is a rise in intracellular hydrogen ion concentration and a fall in the intracellular potassium concentration. These changes are accompanied by a rise in urinary hydrogen secretion and a fall in potassium excretion.

## Procedure used to test the tubules ability to control potassium excretion

Unlike sodium, where the serum concentration tends to remain unchanged or *fall* with sodium retention, serum potassium *rises* with potassium retention. This makes the testing of the kidney's ability to deal with an increased potassium load a potentially dangerous procedure, and it is therefore never attempted. Urinary excretion is the main route of potassium elimination, and if the serum potassium is found to be persistently raised it is clear that there is a tubular defect of potassium excretion.

To show that there is a potassium deficit and that it is due to excess urinary loss is more difficult. Except when plasma potassium is below 3 mmol/1 a low concentration is uncertain evidence of potassium deficiency; though it is more likely if there is a concomitant rise in serum bicarbonate (p. 325). If potassium depletion is suspected or evident, and there is no obvious diminished intake, or leak from the intestinal tract, it is almost certain that it is due to abnormal loss in the urine. This is confirmed by measuring the oral intake of potassium and its output in the urine.

The patient is placed on a normal diet containing 80–100 mmol of potassium per day and the daily urinary potassium excretion is measured for a control period, during which it should be 10–20 mmol less than the intake (this amount is eliminated in the faeces). If the urinary excretion is greater than the intake particularly when the plasma potassium concentration is low, there is unequivocal evidence of a urinary leak of potassium. The following relationship between the lower concentrations of plasma potassium and the urinary excretion of potassium, when the patient is eating a normal ward diet, is a reliable substitute for a balance study. When there is a renal leak of potassium and the plasma concentration of potassium has fallen to 3 mmol/1 or lower, the urinary excretion of potassium is greater than 20 mmol/24 hours; whereas if the potassium deficiency is due to some other cause (such as diarrhoea) the urinary excretion of potassium at these low plasma potassium concentrations will be less than 20 mmol/24 hours. This distinction will usually persist even when potassium deficiency has caused severe renal functional impairment. After some years, however, the potassium deficiency itself may affect the kidney's ability to retain potassium.

If the findings on a normal diet are within normal limits and yet a urinary leak of potassium seems very likely, the patient is placed on a low potassium diet, since in some instances the tubular abnormality may only become apparent when the potassium intake is reduced. On a diet containing 25–30 mmol/day of potassium the urinary excretion of potassium should fall to 25–30 mmol/day within four to seven days.

Potassium excretion may be excessive in hyperaldosteronism, and Cushing's disease, following the use of diuretics, and in certain tubular disorders, particularly those associated with renal tubular acidosis. In all of these there may be hypokalaemia. Potassium excretion may be abnormally low in hypoaldosternism (Addison's disease), acute renal failure and in terminal chronic renal failure.

## CALCIUM EXCRETION

Calcium reabsorption along the nephron is similar to that of sodium in that about half of the filtered calcium is reabsorbed in the proximal tubule, about a third in the loop of Henle and less than 10% in the collecting duct. And in the same manner as sodium it would appear that the urinary content of calcium is mainly determined by changes in calcium absorption in the collecting duct.

Acute volume expansion which produces an acute natriuresis is accompanied by acute parallel changes in calcium excretion, but in the steady state urinary calcium excretion is largely independent of sodium excretion.

Under normal circumstances urinary calcium excretion is mainly under the control of parathyroid hormone. Parathyroid hormone increases calcium reabsorption and thus decreases calcium clearance. But with excess parathyroid hormone the increase in calcium liberated from the bone and the increased calcium absorption from the gut (via the associated stimulation of 1,25 $(OH)_2$ Vit $D_3$) raise the plasma calcium and thus tend to increase calcium excretion in spite of the increased tubular reabsorption of calcium.

In addition to excess parathyroid hormone, hypercalcuria also occurs with exess 1,25 $(OH)_2$ vitamin D, (iatrogenic or pathological) excess ingestion of calcium, excess glucocorticoids, metabolic acidosis and loop diuretics such as frusemide. Renal tubular acidosis is the only primarily tubular lesion which may give rise to hypercalcuria, but it is difficult to distinguish whether this may not be secondary to the accompanying metabolic acidosis. The initial functional disturbances associated with hypercalcuria are an impairment in the ability to concentrate and to acidify the urine. The commonest clinical conditions in which hypercalcuria produces renal failure are mentioned on page 331.

Apart from changes in plasma calcium, hypocalcuria is mainly due to chronic renal failure and thiazide diuretics. It is interesting that if glomerular filtration rate is sufficiently depressed hypercalcaemia may not cause hypercalcuria.

## Procedure used to determine the presence of hypercalcuria

The upper limit of normal calcium excretion at any time of the year is about 400 mg (10 mmol) per day. Urinary calcium is considerably greater in the summer than in the winter. More precisely hypercalcuria can be defined as the daily excretion of more than 200 mg (5 mmol) of calcium when the diet contains less than 150 mg (3.8 mmol). A simple way to perform such a balance study is to place the patient on a rice diet. The diet is cooked in distilled water, but salt can be added in normal amounts, and jams, sugar and fruit are allowed; drinking water must also be distilled. Such a diet contains about 90–130 mg (2.3–3.3 mmol) of calcium a day. The urine calcium excretion is estimated on the fourth day when it should contain less than 200 mg (5 mmol). In children the upper level of urinary calcium excretion is 7 mg/kg/24 hr (175 $\mu$mol), the usual rate is about 3–4 mg/kg/24 hr (75–100 $\mu$mol).

## MAGNESIUM EXCRETION

The average daily intake of magnesium is approximately 250 mg (10 mmol) with a urinary excretion of 100 mg (4 mmol) per day. The filtration of magnesium at the glomerulus and its reabsorption from the tubule parallel that of calcium. In the same way the control of urinary magnesium excretion appears to be almost identical to that of calcium in that it is raised by a rise in the concentration of circulating parathormone, etc. It is probable that calcium and magnesium share a common intratubular transport mechanism. Nevertheless magnesium metabolism is less disturbed than calcium metabolism in renal disease. Paradoxically in acute renal failure, though the urinary excretion of both calcium and magnesium cease there is a fall in plasma calcium and a rise in plasma magnesium.

In chronic renal failure plasma magnesium tends to remain normal. It is usual for the intake of magnesium to fall and for there to be an accompanying reduction in magnesium absorption and urinary magnesium excretion; magnesium balance remains undisturbed (Fig. 6.31). Very rarely a renal lesion may be caused by some exogenous therapeutic nephrotoxic poison such as gentamycin, cis-platinum or methotrexate, when the excessive loss of urinary magnesium rapidly gives rise to the acute symptoms of hypomagnasaemia.

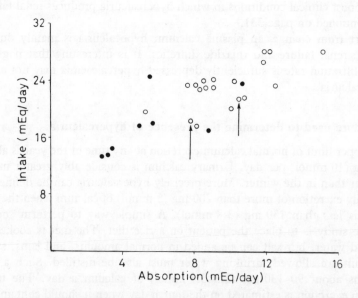

**Fig. 6.31** Relationship between intake and alimentary absorption of magnesium in eight patients with chronic renal failure (●) and nineteen normal subjects (○) (reproduced from Clarkson, McDonald, de Wardener et al 1965 Clin Sci 28: 107, with kind permission).

**Procedure used to detect a renal leak of magnesium**

No special procedure is necessary. Normally renal conservation of magnesium is extremely efficient. If a normal man is deprived of dietary magnesium, urinary magnesium falls within a few days to around 1 mmol/day, although the concentration of plasma magnesium is only slightly below normal. Therefore if a patient is found to have a low plasma magnesium and the urinary content of magnesium is greater than 1–2 mmol/l there is a urinary leak of magnesium.

## PHOSPHATE EXCRETION

Normally all the phosphate in the plasma is filtrable. Approximately 80% of the filtered phosphate is reabsorbed in the proximal tubule and relatively little is reabsorbed in the loop of Henle. The amount that is reabsorbed by the collecting duct controls the urinary content of phosphate. Phosphate reabsorption (like that of sodium and bicarbonate) is directly related to glomerular filtration in that changes in filtered sodium are paralleled by compensatory changes in phosphate reabsorption. Nevertheless changes in plasma phosphate are much more obviously reflected by parallel changes in urinary phosphate excretion than is the urinary excretion of sodium by changes in the concentration of plasma sodium, presumably because the percentage changes in plasma phosphate are so much greater. There are very pronounced diurnal swings of plasma phosphate, a point of some importance when studying the control of urinary phosphate excretion.

Phosphate reabsorption is under the control of parathyroid hormone, calcitonin and the extracellular fluid volume, a rise in any of which will diminish reabsorption, increase urinary phosphate excretion and tend to lower plasma phosphate. It is probable that in addition there are other as yet unidentified factors which control tubular phosphate reabsorption for, experimentally, thyroparathyroidectomised animals can alter phosphate excretion to match changing intake without large changes in plasma phosphate. Certain inherited or acquired lesions of the tubule's reabsorption of phosphate cause hyperphosphaturia and hypophosphataemia (p. 350). In contrast vitamin D, growth hormone, and possibly thyroxin increase tubular phosphate reabsorption.

**Procedure used to detect the presence of an abnormal handling of phosphate by the kidney**

The only reliable and reproducible method is to estimate the maximal capacity of the tubules to reabsorb phosphate (Tm $PO_4$, p. 106). This is achieved by raising the plasma phosphate concentration by an intravenous infusion of about 200 ml of buffered phosphate over three hours

until the plasma phosphate rises to a level greater than 5 mg/100 ml
(1.6 mmol/l). Conditions both before and during this test have to be rigorously controlled; a high phosphate diet before the test must be avoided;
because of the diurnal rhythm of phosphate the test should always be done
at the same time of day; as glucose is absorbed along the same pathways
as phosphate the patient should be fasting; other substances such as PAH
which may compete for tubular transport mechanisms should be avoided;
and the test should not be prolonged for otherwise it may induce endocrine
changes which will alter the result. And when all these precautions have
been taken the normal range is still wide. Figure 6.32 shows the results in
normal subjects. The maximal capacity to reabsorb phosphate (Tm PO$_4$) is
$38 \pm 5$ mg/l of glomerular filtrate. It is necessary to relate the maximal rate
of phosphate reabsorption to a fixed volume of glomerular filtrate because
changes in filtration rate are accompanied by automatic and parallel changes
in phosphate reabsorption.

When patients are grouped according to their Tm PO$_4$ per litre of glomerular filtrate, the groups will polarize according to their diseases. It is then
possible to discriminate groups of patients with hyper-and hypoparathyroidism, thyrotoxicosis, and over production of growth hormone, from
healthy persons. Tm PO$_4$ unrelated to filtration rate does not discriminate

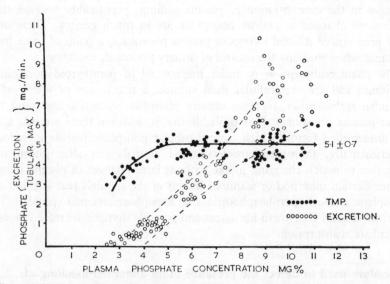

**Fig. 6.32** Single estimation of Tm PO$_4$ and phosphate excretion corrected for filtration rate,
plotted against phosphate concentrations in normal subjects ('phosphate tubular max' =
phosphate reabsorbed). Phosphate reabsorption reaches a maximum of about 5.0 mg/min
and then levels out. The value at which it does so is the Tm PO$_4$, or maximum capacity of
the tubule to reabsorb phosphate. In this figure the reabsorption and excretion have been
adjusted to a glomerular filtration rate of 131 ml/min; it is now more usual to relate these to
1 litre of filtrate (see text) (reproduced from Anderson & Parsons 1963 Clin Sci 25: 431,
with kind permission).

patients. There is a close correlation between Tm $PO_4$ per litre of glomerular filtration rate and the fasting plasma phosphate so that when the capacity to reabsorb is diminished the plasma phosphate falls, and when the capacity to reabsorb is increased the plasma phosphate rises.

Tm $PO_4$ per litre of glomerular filtration rate (Tm $PO_4/l$ GFR) is a time consuming performance subject to many technical pitfalls. It has been found however that in the fasting state it is possible to predict Tm $PO_4/l$ GFR from the relation of urinary phosphate excretion ($U_{PO_4} \times V$/GFR) to the plasma phosphate. A prediction made in this way is even simpler to make than it at first appears for $U_{PO_4} \times V$/GFR is

$$U_{PO_4} \times V \bigg/ \frac{U \text{ creatinine} \times V}{P \text{ creatinine}}$$

which becomes

$$\frac{U_{PO_4} \times P \text{ creatinine}}{U \text{ creatinine}}$$

Thus a prediction of Tm $PO_4/l$ GFR can be made from a measurement of the concentration of phosphate and creatinine in the plasma and in an untimed (as V has been eliminated) but simultaneous sample of urine. The error of the prediction is too large to be of value in single determinations, but the prediction is much improved by repeat determinations. Moreover the use of the prediction makes it practicable to make successive observations when following the clinical progress of a patient.

Other methods used to detect the presence of an abnormal handling of phosphate by the kidneys include estimates of the clearance of phosphate alone, or the phosphate to creatinine clearance ratio. The first is valueless and the second is only of value if the duration of the clearance period is twenty four hours, the dietary intake of phosphate is constant from day to day and the plasma phosphate sample is always taken 4–5 hours after the last meal (e.g. at midday). As the phosphate to creatinine clearance ratio rises as the plasma phosphate concentration increases the results obtained must therefore be compared with those obtained over a wide range of plasma phosphate concentrations in normal subjects.

## AMINO ACID EXCRETION

Amino acids are filtered, and actively reabsorbed in the proximal tubule by four main transport mechanisms, each of which deals with one of the following groups of amino acids:
1. The monoamino-monocarboxylic amino acids such as alanine, valine, tryptophan and cysteine
2. The dibasic amino acids; lysine, arginine, ornithine and cystine
3. The dicarboxylic amino acids: glutamic and aspartic acids
4. The imino-acid and glycine group: proline, hydroxyproline and glycine.

Amino-aciduria or excessive excretion of amino acids is classified into 'overflow' or 'renal' types. Overflow amino-aciduria is due to disorders of metabolism in which there is a rise in the circulating concentration of certain amino acids. The amount of these amino acids which is then filtered exceeds the tubules' capacity for reabsorption and the quantity which is not reabsorbed 'overflows' into the urine. The inability to deaminate amino acids in severe liver failure causes an overflow of all groups of amino acids, while phenylketonuria which is due to an impaired ability to metabolise phenylanaline is an example of a single amino acid overflow amino-aciduria.

In renal amino-aciduria the primary defect is either an absence or deficiency of one group of active transport mechanisms. This can arise either as a hereditary anomaly of amino acid transport without other evidence of abnormal tubular function, e.g. cystinuria; or as one of several tubular abnormalities all of them caused by damage to the proximal tubules. Such damage may develop acutely as in cadmium and uranium poisoning or more chronically with copper in Wilson's disease, or galactose in infantile galactosaemia.

## URATE EXCRETION

98% of the filtered urate is reabsorbed by the proximal tubule, while 80% of the urate in the urine is secreted by the distal tubule. Reabsorption of urate (like sodium and bicarbonate) is in part controlled by the state of extracellular fluid volume. An infusion of saline greatly increases urate excretion but more familiarly the state of mild chronic volume depletion associated with prolonged diuretic therapy diminishes the back leak of urate from the interstitial space to the tubule lumen thus increasing net reabsorption and diminishing urate excretion so that there is a rise in plasma urate. Plasma urate is also raised by a diminution in tubular urate secretion by competitive inhibitors such as lactic acid (e.g. toxaemia of pregnancy and alcohol) and by acetic acid and B hydroxybutyric acid (e.g. starvation and diabetes). The hyperuricaemia of one form of familial gout is also due to an impaired ability of the tubule to secrete urate which appears to be a primary disturbance of the tubule. An increased production of urate of unknown cause in another form of familial gout can also cause hyperuricaemia. Sometimes, however, an increase in urate production is due to an easily identifiable cause such as a high cellular turn-over as in leukaemia, or when a tumour is rapidly destroyed e.g. radiotherapy to a large retroperitoneal lymphosarcoma. In renal failure the ability to secrete urate per nephron increases as the number of surviving nephrons diminish. The mechanism of this compensatory increase is not known.

The concentrations of urate found in the urine are such that the urate is in a supersaturated state. The liability to precipitation is obviously greatest when the urine is acid. The solubility of free uric acid and urates in urine is only 8 mg/100 ml (0.48 mmol/l) at pH 5.0, 22 mg/100 ml (1.3 mmol/l) at pH 6.0, and 158 mg/100 ml (9.4 mmol/l) at pH 7.0. In addition precipitation of sodium urate in the urine and in the medulla is probably enhanced by the high concentrations of sodium in the medulla and urine when concentrated urine is being formed.

## Procedures used to test the ability of the tubules to secrete uric acid; and to detect the presence of an increased urate production

Plasma urate may be raised because of a diminished tubular secretion of urate, an increased endogenous production of urate, or a high protein intake.

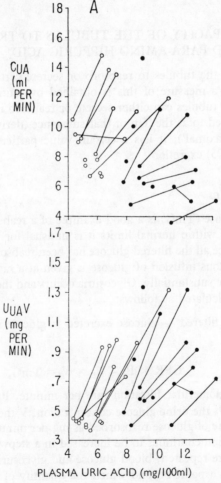

**Fig. 6.33** The effect of the ingestion of large amounts of ribonucleic acid for three days on plasma urate concentration and the clearance of uric acid ($C_{UA}$) and the urinary excretion of uric acid ($U_{UA}V$) in patients with gout ●; and in individuals without gout ○. The patients with gout have an impaired ability to excrete uric acid (conversion: traditional to SI units — urate 1 mg/100 ml = 0.06 mmol/l) (reproduced from Nugent, MacDiarmid & Tyler 1964 Arch Int Med 113: 115, with kind permission).

In order to assess the capacity of the kidneys to excrete urate, large amounts of RNA are given per day to progressively raise plasma urate and urinary urate excretion. An impairment in the ability to secrete urate is evident from the slope of the rise in the urinary output of urate in relation to the change in plasma uric acid. A normal subject excretes much more urate at each plasma urate level than a person who has an impaired ability to excrete urate (Fig. 6.33). An excess endogenous production can be discerned by placing the patients on a purine free diet consisting of milk, bread, fats and eggs for seven days. Twenty-four hour urine collections are made on the last two days when the daily urate excretion should be less than 600 mg (3.6 mmol).

## MAXIMAL CAPACITY OF THE TUBULES TO TRANSPORT GLUCOSE AND PARA-AMINO HIPPURIC ACID

The capacity of the tubules to reabsorb or secrete certain substances may be limited, and a measure of this is obtained by estimating the maximal amount that the tubules can either secrete or reabsorb in one minute. This amount is referred to as the Tm of that substance (derived from the words 'tubule' and 'maximal'); it has a certain value particularly in relation to phosphate (p. 105) excretion.

### Reabsorption Tm

The Tm of glucose (TmG) is a good example of a reabsorptive Tm. When blood glucose is within normal limits it is unusual for there to be glucose in the urine, since all the filtered glucose has been reabsorbed. To determine $Tm_g$ an intravenous infusion of glucose is given at a rate sufficient to raise the blood glucose substantially. Glycosuria occurs and the amount of glucose reabsorbed is calculated as follows:

glucose filtered — glucose excreted = glucose reabsorbed

or

$$GFR \times P_g - U_g \times V = TmG,$$

where GFR is glomerular filtration rate per minute, $P_g$ is plasma glucose concentration, $U_g$ the urine glucose concentration, V the rate of urine flow, and TmG the rate of glucose reabsorbed as mg per minute. The rate of glucose administration continues to be increased in a stepwise manner and the measurements are repeated; blood glucose and glycosuria increase steadily, but there comes a point beyond which the quantity of glucose reabsorbed remains constant; this is the TmG, and in normal man is $323 \pm 64$ mg/min.

The plasma glucose concentration at which glucose first appears in the urine is sometimes referred to as the renal threshold for glucose. This level is roughly correlated with TmG but is a less constant value, for it is influenced by alterations in glomerular filtration rate. At the renal threshold for glucose the quantity of glucose being presented to the tubules by the glomerular filtrate is only just sufficient to exceed the tubule's ability to reabsorb all the glucose passing through; if plasma glucose remains unchanged but there is a fall in filtration rate, no glucose will appear in the urine and the renal threshold will have altered. But when estimating TmG the blood glucose concentration is raised to such high values that, so long as a nephron has some filtration, the amount of glucose being presented to the tubule for reabsorption is far in excess of its maximum reabsorbing capacity; in this way alterations in glomerular filtration rate cannot influence the amount reabsorbed.

The main value of a TmG is that it gives a quantitative expression of the total mass of functioning tubular cells but it is rarely estimated.

The Tm of bicarbonate and phosphate reabsorption have been discussed earlier (p. 87, 105). The reabsorption of these ions is influenced by changes in the extracellular fluid volume. For instance it has been pointed out (p. 87) that there appears to be no limit to the tubule's capacity to reabsorb bicarbonate if the plasma bicarbonate is raised in such a way that the rise in the extracellular fluid volume is minimal. And it has also been demonstrated (p. 89) that even when the technique of raising the plasma bicarbonate includes a substantial expansion of the extracellular fluid volume Tm $HCO_3$ can still be altered by altering $P_{CO_2}$.

The influence of extracellular fluid volume expansion on Tm $PO_4$ is not nearly so profound but can be easily demonstrated. Tm $PO_4$ is also influenced by parathormone. It is clear therefore that for Tm $PO_4$ and Tm $HCO_3$ to be of any value they must be measured during rigorously standardised conditions. In addition, unlike $Tm_g$ which is uninfluenced by changes in glomerular filtration, tubular reabsorption of bicarbonate and phosphate varies directly with changes in glomerular filtration rate, so that for purposes of comparison Tm $HCO_3$ and Tm $PO_4$ have to be related to a standard glomerular filtration rate (p. 106).

## Secretion Tm

In this context a substance is considered to be secreted by the tubules only if the amount excreted in the urine is greater than that which has been filtered. This is, of course, a convenient but grossly arbitrary definition, for some substances which are actively secreted by the tubules (e.g. potassium) have a total urinary excretion which is usually less than that which has been filtered. To measure the true amount secreted, therefore, it would be necessary to know the amount which has been reabsorbed, and in ordinary circumstances this is not possible.

Those substances which have the greatest rate of tubular secretion according to the definition given above are those which are not normally present in body fluids, and include diodone, phenol red, penicillin and para-amino-hippuric acid (PAH). Because of its ease of estimation and its high rate of active secretion PAH is the substance which has been most often used to obtain a secretory Tm. The procedure is similar to that used for estimating glucose Tm. Intravenous PAH is administered at a rate sufficient to maintain plasma PAH level at about 20 mg per 100 ml at which level the tubules are being presented with PAH at a rate much greater than their ability to secrete it into the tubule lumen; Tm PAH is then calculated as follows:

$$PAH \; excreted - PAH \; filtered = PAH \; actively \; secreted,$$

or

$$U_{PAH} \times V - GFR \times P_{PAH} = Tm \; PAH.$$

In normal man Tm PAH is $68 \pm 11$ mg/min. Again, it is rarely estimated. It is of great interest that the secretion Tm of PAH, in line with the reabsorption Tm of $HCO_3$ and $PO_4$, is also depressed by expansion of the extracellular fluid volume. This is probably due in part to the effect of the rise in the plasm's ability to inhibit $Na^+$-$K^+$-ATPase which occurs with volume expansion, for PAH transport is closely related to $Na^+$-$K^+$-ATPase activity.

## Limitations of existing renal function tests

There is as yet no test which will give information about the number of functioning nephrons. This is a serious disadvantage. The kidney's capacity to hypertrophy is very great and it has been repeatedly shown that the removal of one kidney produces little or no permanent change in overall function. Similarly there is much histological evidence that in those chronic renal diseases in which nephrons are destroyed, the surviving nephrons hypertrophy, and it must be assumed that the function of the surviving nephrons increase with their size. It is therefore theoretically possible for a renal disease to destroy about half the nephron population and yet produce little or no change in renal function, and it follows that an unchanging renal function is not proof that a disease is quiescent. Conversely, when renal function is persistently reduced to half its normal value it is almost certain that a great deal more than half of the original renal parenchyma must have been destroyed. These speculations would be unnecessary if, during life it were possible to obtain an estimate of the number of surviving nephrons.

BIBLIOGRAPHY

Aber G M, Bishop J M 1965 Serial changes in renal function, arterial gas tensions, and the acid-base state in patients with chronic bronchitis and oedema. Clin Sci 28: 511
Anderson J, Parsons V 1963 The tubular maximal resorptive rate for inorganic phosphate in normal subjects. Clin Sci 25: 431

Ardaillou R, Fillastre J P, Milhaud G et al 1969 Renal excretion of phosphate, calcium and sodium during and after a prolonged thyrocalcitonin infusion in man. Proc Soc Exp Biol Med 131: 56

Barker E S 1960 Physiologic and clinical aspects of magnesium metabolism. J Chron Dis 11: 278

Beck N, Kim K S, Wolak M et al 1975 Inhibition of carbonic anhydrase by parathyroid hormone and cyclic AMP in rat renal cortex in vitro. J Clin Invest 55: 149

Brazy P C, McKeown J W, Harris R H et al 1980 Comparative effect of dietary phosphate, unilateral nephrectomy and PTH on phosphate transport by the rat proximal tubule. Kidney Int 17: 788

Clapp J R, Robinson R R 1966 Osmolality of distal tubular fluid in the dog. J Clin Invest 45: 1847

Denis G, Preuss H, Pitts R 1964 The $pNH_3$ of renal tubular cells. J Clin Invest 43: 571

Dunn M J, Walser M 1966 Magnesium depletion in normal man. Metabolism 15: 884

Giebisch G 1978 The proximal tubule. In: Andreoli T E, Hoffman J F, Fanesti D (eds) Physiology of membrane disorders. Plenum Press, London, p 629

Giebisch G 1978 Renal potassium transport. In: Giebisch G, Tosteson D C, Ussing H H, (eds) Membrane transport in biology. Springer Verlag, Berlin, 5, p 216

Gutman A B, Yu T F, Berger L 1959 Tubular secretion of urate in man. J. Clin Invest 38: 1778

Häberle D A, Shiigai T T, Maier G et al 1981 Dependency of proximal tubular fluid transport on the load of glomerular filtrate. Kidney Int 20: 18

Jamison R, Robertson C R 1979 Recent formulations of the urinary concentrating mechanism; a status report. Kidney Int 16: 537

Jacobson H R 1981 Functional segmentation of the mammalian nephron. Amer J Physiol 241: F203

Kangawa K, Matsuo H 1984 Purification and complete amino acid sequence of α-human atrial matriuretic polypeptide (p-hAMP). Biochem Biophys Res Com 1118 No 1:131

Kassirer J P, Schwartz W B 1966 The response of normal man to selective depletion of hydrochloric acid. Amer J Med 40: 10

Kinne R, Schwartz I L 1978 Isolated membrane vesicles in the evaluation of the nature, localization and regulation of renal transport processes. Kidney Int 14: 547

Koko J P, Rector F C 1972 Counter current multiplication system without active transport in inner medulla. Kidney Int 2: 214

Kwong T F, Bennett C M 1974 Relationship between glomerular filtration rate and maximum tubular reabsorptive rate of glucose. Kidney Int 5: 23

Lang F, Greger R, Knox F G et al 1981 Factors modulating renal handling of phosphate. Renal Physiol 4: 1

Lemann J, Lennon E J, Goodman A D et al 1965 The net balance of acid in subjects given large loads of acid or alkali. J Clin Invest 44: 507

Malnic G, Giebisch G 1978 Cellular aspects of renal tubular acidification. In: Giebisch G, Tosteson D C, Ussing H H (eds) Membrane transport in biology. Springer Verlag, Berlin, 6, p 300

Manitius A, Epstein F 1963 Some observations on the influence of a magnesium deficient diet on rats with special reference to renal concentrating ability. J Clin Invest 42: 208

Maesaka J K, Levitt M F, Abramson R G 1973 Effect of saline infusion on phosphate transport in intact and thyroparathyroidectomized rats. Amer J Physiol 225: 1421

Massry S G, Coburn J W, Kleeman C R 1969 Renal handling of magnesium in the dog. Amer J Physiol 216: 1460

Miles B E, Paton A, de Wardener H E 1954 Maximum urine concentration. Brit Med J 2: 901

Milne M D 1964 Disorders of amino-acid transport. Brit Med J 1: 327

Monclair T, Mathisen Ø, Kiil F 1980 Renal bicarbonate reabsorption during bicarbonate loading. Kidney Int 17: 577

Neumann K H, Rector F C 1976 Mechanism of NaCl water reabsorption in the proximal convoluted tubule of rat kidney. J Clin Invest 58: 1110

Pak Poy R K, Wrong O 1960 The urinary $pCO_2$ in renal disease. Clin Sci 19: 631

Pitts R F 1964 Renal production and excretion of ammonia. Amer J Med 36: 720

Quamme G A, Wong N L M, Dirks J H et al 1978 Magnesium handling in the dog kidney: A micropuncture study. Pfleuger's Arch 377: 95

Rabinowitz L 1979/80 Aldosterone and renal potassium excretion. Renal Physiol 2: 229

Relman A S 1968 The acidosis of renal disease. Amer J Med 44: 706

Ross B, Leaf A, Silva P et al 1974 Na-K-ATPase in sodium transport by the perfused rat kidney. Amer J Physiol 226: 624

Sajo I M, Goldstein M B, Sonnenberg H et al 1981 Site of ammonia addition to tubular fluid in rats with chronic metabolic acidosis. Kidney Int 20: 353

Schafer J A, Barfuss D W 1980 Membrane mechanisms for transepithelial amino acid absorption and secretion. Amer J Physiol 238: F335

Schnermann J, Persson A E G, Agerup B 1973 Tubulo-glomerular feed-back. Non linear relation between glomerular hydrostatic pressure and loop of Henle perfusion rate. J Clinc Invest 52: 862

Schrier R W 1976 Water metabolism Kidney Int 10: 1

Smith H W, Goldring W, Chasis H 1938 The measurement of the tubular excretory mass, effective blood flow and filtration rate in the normal human kidney. J Clin Invest 17: 263

Stanbury S W 1958 Some aspects of disordered renal tubular function. (Phosphaturia) Advan, Intern Med 9: 231

Stephenson J L 1965 Ability of counterflow systems to concentrate. Nature 206: 1215

Struyvenberg A, de Graeff J, Lameijer L D F 1965 The role of chloride in hypokalaemic alkalosis in the rat. J Clin Invest 44: 326

Suki W N 1979 Calcium transport in the nephron. Amer J Physiol 237: F.1

Thibault G, Garcia R, Seidah N G et al 1983 Purification of three atrial matriuretic factors and their amino acid composition. FEBS 1041, 164 no 2:288

Tröhler U, Bonjour J-P, Fleisch H 1976 Inorganic phosphate homeostasis. Renal adaptation to the dietary intake in intact and thyroparathyroidectomised rats. J Clin Invest 57: 264

Verney E B 1946 Absorption and excretion of water. The antidiuretic hormone. Lancet 2: 739 and 781

Walker A M, Hudson C L 1937 The reabsorption of glucose from the renal tubule in amphibia and the action of phlorizin upon it. Amer J Physiol 118: 130

Wardener de H E 1973 The control of sodium excretion. In: Orloff J, Berliner R W (eds) Handbook of physiology — renal physiology. Amer Phys Soc (Washington DC), ch 21

Wardener de H E 1977 The natriuretic hormone. Clin Sci Mol Med 53: 1

Wardener de H E, Clarkson E M 1982 Editorial review on the natriuretic hormone: recent developments. Clin Sci 63: 415

Wardener de H E, del Greco F 1955 The influence of solute excretion rate on the production of a hypotonic urine in man. Clin Sci 14: 715

Warren Y, Luke R G, Kashgarian M et al 1970 Micropuncture studies of chloride and bicarbonate absorption in the proximal renal tubule of the rat in respiratory acidosis and in chloride depletion. Clin Sci 38: 375

Weinman E J, Eknoyan G, Suki W N 1975 The influence of extracellular fluid volume on the tubular reabsorption of uric acid. J Clin Invest 55: 283

Whang R, Welt L G 1963 Observations in experimental magnesium depletion. J Clin Invest 42: 305

Wilcox C S, Cemerikic D A, Giebisch G 1982 Differential effects of acute mineralo-and glucocortico-steroid administration on renal acid elimination. Kidney Int 21: 546

Wolgast M, Larson M, Nygren K 1981 Functional characteristics of the renal interstitium. Amer J Physiol 241: 105

Wrong O, Davies H E F 1959 The excretion of acid in renal disease. Quart J Med NS 28: 259

# 7

# Renal circulation

At rest about one-fifth of the cardiac output flows through the kidney, though the oxygen consumption of the kidney does not amount to more than 8–10% of the oxygen consumption of the whole body. The normal renal blood flow is approximately 1100 ml/min. It is a greater irrigation per unit weight of tissue than any other organ. This extraordinary phenomenon is confined to the cortex which has a blood flow of about 5 ml/g/min. On the other hand the medulla which receives only 6% of the total renal blood flow has a blood flow of about 0.3 ml/g/min which is considerably *less* than any other tissue in the body. The reason for the high cortical perfusion is not understood for, though experimentally a substantial and sustained reduction in renal blood flow is always associated with some fall in glomerular filtration rate, renal function in all other measurable respects may remain perfectly normal. In the following discussion it is to be remembered that changes in renal blood flow are generally accompanied by similar changes in the glomerular filtration rate, though frequently the degree of change may be different.

## SOME FACTORS WHICH CAUSE A REDUCTION IN RENAL BLOOD FLOW

The normal renal blood flow is very great, consequently if a change does occur, the flow is nearly always reduced. The upright posture, undernutrition, exercise, pain, heat, adrenaline and advancing years are some of the physiological factors associated with such a reduction. The pathological causes are discussed below.

### Circulatory insufficiency

Clinically the most frequent cause of a fall in renal blood flow is circulatory insufficiency. Contraction of the blood volume and cardiac failure both cause renal vasoconstriction and a fall in renal blood flow, whether or not there is a concomitant decrease in blood pressure.

115

*Contraction of the blood volume* may be secondary to traumatic, surgical or spontaneous bleeding, acute haemolysis, severe diarrhoea and vomiting, barbiturate poisoning, burns, or negative protein balance. Sudden changes in blood volume produce the most marked changes in the renal circulation, but there is a delay between the time of the haemorrhage and the onset of renal vasoconstriction. A haemorrhage which is severe enough to induce peripheral vasoconstriction, with pallor and coldness of the hands, feet and face, may not cause a fall in renal blood flow within the next one to two hours. If, however, the blood volume remains reduced for four to seven hours there is severe renal vasoconstriction, which, in association with other factors, may be sufficient to cause necrosis of the renal cortex. The cause of this vasoconstriction is nervous and humoral. Therapeutically the delay is sometimes an advantage, for early transfusion may prevent the onset of severe renal ischaemia; but conversely once ischaemia has developed, transfusion is only associated with a slow recovery; the ischaemia continuing for several hours after the blood volume is normal.

*Cardiac failure* induces renal vasoconstriction both when the cardiac output is low (when the fall in renal blood flow is proportionately greater than the fall in cardiac output) and when the output is high as in cor pulmonale and thyrotoxicosis. In the latter the cardiac output may be doubled and yet the renal blood flow may fall to 20% of its normal value. The cause of this vasoconstriction is uncertain, but the inability of a high spinal anaesthetic to alter the renal blood flow in established cardiac failure suggests that it may be humoral. This is supported by the finding that some increase in renal blood flow occurs following the administration of adrenergic antagonists and (propranolol) angiotensin converting enzyme inhibitors (captopril). Large increases in renal venous pressure have been found to produce transient reductions in renal blood flow. But this is not the cause of the fall in renal blood flow in cardiac failure, for the renal venous pressures usually encountered are not in this high range, and in chronic heart failure the venous pressure and renal blood flow may vary independently.

A teleological explanation for the renal vasoconstriction which occurs with circulatory distress is that it maintains the arterial pressure and switches the available cardiac output to organs which are less able than the kidney to function with a reduced blood flow.

## Acute uterine catastrophies

There is a close association between the incidence of abortion, accidental haemorrhage, and eclampsia on the one hand and severe renal ischaemia on the other. Abortion used to be the most frequent cause of acute renal failure.

In many of these conditions haemorrhage must be partly responsible for the renal ischaemia, but it is probable that other mechanisms are also involved. The intravascular laying down of fibrin in the glomerular capillaries in accidental haemorrhage is one mechanism, and endothelial capillary swelling in eclampsia is another. In experimental animals an acute rise in intra-uterine pressure causes a marked fall in renal blood flow; if such a mechanism is present in man it may be an important contributory factor in the causation of renal ischaemia in some of the conditious mentioned above (e.g. concealed accidental haemorrhage).

## Electrolyte and endocrine abnormalities

Many forms of electrolyte abnormalities cause a reduction in renal blood flow. With simple water depletion, or with combined salt and water depletion, this reduction is caused by the contraction of the blood volume. But with water intoxication due to salt loss, or excess water intake, the mechanism is obscure. Potassium deficiency and hypercalcaemia also cause a fall in renal blood flow. Initially these circulatory changes are quickly and completely reversible; if, however, they are prolonged and are associated with the development of structural changes, recovery will be incomplete.

The renal blood flow is also reduced in hyper- and hypo-adrenalsim, hypopituitarism and myxoedema.

## Vasoconstrictors other than those produced by the endocrine glands

These consist mainly of exogenous substances and include a variety of cytotoxic poisons such as carbon tetrachloride, corrosive sublimate (mercuric chloride), propylene glycol, etc. Frequently tubular necrosis follows, both from direct action of the poison on the cells and from intense renal ischaemia (p. 139).

Some infections such as Weil's disease and scrub typhus are also associated with severe reductions in renal blood flow.

## Disorders of the renal vasculature

Atheroma of the large intrarenal arteries may occasionally lead to wedge-shaped loss of renal parenchyma and a substantial fall in renal blood flow; while hypertension (particularly the malignant form), polyarteritis nodosa, eclampsia, diabetes and amyloidosis frequently produce such obliterative changes in the arterioles and glomerular capillaries that severe fatal renal ischaemia may result. Changes in the renal vessels in diffuse lupus erythematosus and scleroderma may also lead to renal failure. The acute glomerular capillaritis of acute glomerular nephritis, though it causes a fall in glomerular filtration rate, does not usually effect renal blood flow. If acute glomerular nephritis, however, is associated with severe interstitial oedema there is severe, but potentially reversible renal ischaemia, and a profound fall in glomerular filtration rate.

**Gradual destruction of the renal parenchyma as a cause of a decrease in renal blood flow**

Loss of nephrons is at first compensated for by an increased flow of blood through the remaining hypertrophied nephrons, e.g. the changes which occur following unilateral nephrectomy. Eventually, however, with further loss of nephrons the renal blood flow inevitably diminishes. Among the conditions which have not yet been considered and which produce a graudal destruction of the renal parenchyma there are: persistent glomerular nephritis, reflux nephropathy polycystic disease, congenital tubular disorders, renal tuberculosis and urinary tract obstruction.

## SOME FACTORS WHICH CAUSE RENAL HYPERAEMIA

These include cold, large protein intake, hyperpyrexia, sudden increase in blood volume, emotion, aminophylline derivatives, magnesium sulphate, polycythaemia, pregnancy, and growth hormone. In general, transient increases in renal blood flow are of no clinical importance, though occasionally aminophylline is used to raise the renal blood flow and glomerular filtration rate when trying to obtain an adequate diuresis with diuretics (p. 176). It is possible, however, that a permanent increase in renal blood flow produces glomerulosclerosis which may eventually destroy the glomerulus.

## ADJUSTMENT OF THE RENAL CIRCULATION TO CHANGES IN HAEMATOCRIT

In the normal kidney the fall in haematocrit which occurs in anaemia is associated with a substantial decrease in renal blood flow, a small reduction in plasma flow and an almost unchanged glomerular filtration rate; when the haematocrit falls below approximately 20, however, the renal ischaemia becomes much more pronounced and there is a marked reduction in plasma flow and glomerular filtration (Fig. 7.1). These changes are more pronounced when the anaemia causes salt and water retention ('cardiac failure').

Conversely the rise in haematocrit which occurs in polycythaemia is associated with a substantial *increase* in renal blood flow, but again there is only a small reduction in plasma flow and an almost unchanged rate of glomerular filtration; at haematocrits above approximately 75, however, both the renal plasma flow and glomerular filtration rate tend to be sharply depressed.

These changes suggest that the kidney is mainly concerned with the maintenance of a constant renal plasma flow and glomerular filtration, and not with the total renal blood flow. The mechanisms responsible for these adjustments are not known, but they appear to be local in origin and unrelated to changes in cardiac output.

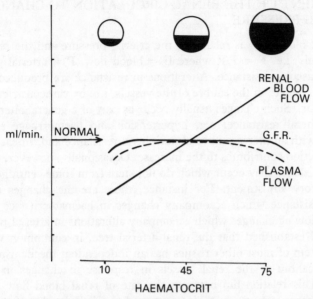

**Fig. 7.1** Schema of the changes in renal blood flow, plasma flow and glomerular filtration rate which occur in the normal kidney in response to changes in haematocrit. The three circles illustrate what is presumably taking place in the renal vessels, i.e. the renal plasma flow remains constant because the diameter of the renal vessels varies directly with the changing fraction of red cells.

Clinically the important point is that such adjustments may take some days to complete, and that in diseased kidneys they take place even more slowly or not at all. The result is that a perfectly justifiable transfusion for anaemia in chronic renal failure may be followed by a rapid deterioration in renal function. The explanation is as follows. It has been pointed out earlier that a reduction in glomerular filtration rate to 50% of normal produces little absolute change in the blood concentrations of waste products, but with further reductions in filtration rate these concentrations rise steeply. If, therefore, owing to renal parenchymal destruction the glomerular filtration rate is low, it is clear that a further small decrease in filtration will produce a large increase in blood concentrations of waste products. Such a decrease in filtration may follow the rise in haematocrit which accompanies a ʳransfusion; it is due to the failure of the renal vessels to dilate sufficiently quickly to accommodate the rising fraction or red cells; the renal plasma flow and filtration rate are automatically reduced and the patient may die of acute anuria. If it is considered necessary to treat the chronic anaemia of chronic renal failure with transfusions, it is best to give small amounts of packed cells and not to try and raise the PCV above 25. It is best to give packed red cells in order to minimise the risk of causing heart failure which is the other hazard of transfusing patients with renal failure. An estimate of glomerular function should be obtained between each transfusion.

## ADJUSTMENT OF THE RENAL CIRCULATION TO CHANGES IN ARTERIAL PRESSURE

The rate of blood flow is related to the arterial pressure and the resistance of the vessels, i.e. $F = P/R$ where $F$ = blood flow, $P$ = arterial pressure and $R$ = vascular resistance. Alterations in resistance are produced almost entirely by changes in the calibre of the vessels, i.e. by vasoconstriction and vasodilatation. Such changes usually occur as part of a general alteration in total peripheral resistance, e.g. hypertension and haemorrhage are both associated with an increase in total peripheral resistance and, in each, renal vasoconstriction contributes to the increase. Occasionally, however, changes in renal resistance may occur which do not stem from some central demand for circulatory adjustment. For instance, there are the changes in renal vascular resistance which accompany changes in haematocrit (see above), and the following changes which accompany alterations in arterial pressure.

It is well established that the renal arterial tree, in commmon with the arterial system of most other tissues has an independent mechanism which alters the calibre of the renal vessels in response to changes in arterial pressure. This relationship between the rate of renal blood flow and the arterial pressure is most easily demonstrated in the isolated perfused dog's kidney, and is illustrated in Figure 7.2. It can be seen that over a pressure range of about 0 to 90 mmHg the blood flow rises with the pressure; from 90 to 200 mmHg the flow remains relatively unaltered; and after 200 mmHg the flow rises once again. The alterations in vascular lumen mainly occur in the arteries on the afferent side of the glomerulus, for the glomerular

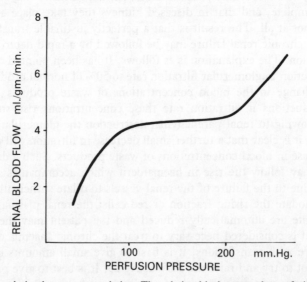

**Fig. 7.2** Renal circulatory autoregulation. The relationship between the perfusion pressure (i.e. renal artery pressure) and the renal blood flow in a dog's kidney, showing the relative constancy of the blood flow when the perfusion pressure is between 100 and 200 mmHg.

filtration rate parallels the changes in the renal blood flow. The changes in the diameter of the arterial lumen are due to the innate property of the smooth muscle in the arterial walls to respond to a stretching force by a contraction, and a diminution of tension by a relaxation; a property which can be demonstrated in the arteries of many other organs and the umbilical artery. It is probable, for instance, that this phenomenon is responsible for the dilatation of an artery that occurs distal to the site of an obstruction. The constancy of the renal blood flow during alterations in blood pressure is known as circulatory autoregulation. It is particularly well developed in the kidney where it influences the 94% of the total renal blood flow that flows through the cortex. Circulatory autoregulation does not occur in the medulla.

It has been suggested that renal circulatory autoregulation might be due to the tubulo-glomerular feed-back mechanism (p. 73) implying that in the kidney circulatory autoregulation is due to a completely different mechanism than elsewhere in the body. The proposal is that changes in perfusion pressure cause an initial change in renal blood flow and glomerular filtration rate which causes a change in the sodium concentration delivered to the macula densa of the distal tubule, that this in turn induces a change in the rate of renin production by the granular cells in that part of the afferent arteriole near to the macula densa and that this causes the afferent arteriole to change the size of its lumen in the direction which will correct this sequence. There are many serious objections to this hypothesis. One is that renal circulatory autoregulation can be demonstrated in a kidney in which the tubules have been blocked by an inert oil. Perhaps one of the potent objections is that it cannot explain the rapid oscillations of renal blood flow which take place in the first few seconds after the renal perfusion pressure is suddenly altered (Fig. 7.3).

Indirect evidence for the presence of a similar stabilising mechanism in the renal vasculature of man has been obtained on several occasions, though the exact range over which it occurs is not known. It must almost certainly be over a lower range than in the dog, for the mean blood pressure in man is lower than that in the dog. There is some evidence that renal circulatory autoregulation in man is present down to a mean arterial pressure of about 60 mmHg. Such observations are difficult to obtain, for in most circumstances changes in arterial pressure produce a central demand for compensatory alterations in the peripheral resistance which have priority over purely local circulatory reflexes; the latter are best observed following small changes in arterial pressure produced by changes in cardiac output.

Teleologically this intrinsic pressure-flow relationship is difficult to understand. One suggestion is that it protects the glomerular filtration rate from the normal fluctuations in pressure, so that the tubules are presented with a continuous steady quantity of materials. As many of the factors which influence tubular function are slow to change the extent of their activity, a stability of this nature may be of value.

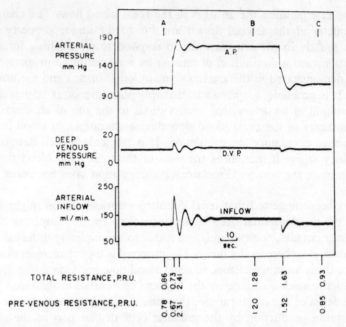

**Fig. 7.3** Circulatory autoregulation. The effect on renal arterial blood flow to an isolated kidney of increasing the arterial pressure. There are several rapid oscillations of blood flow before the renal blood flow stabilises at a level slightly greater than before the rise in pressure. Such oscillations could not be a function of a reflex from the distal tubule to the afferent arteriole. See text (reproduced from Waugh 1964 Circ Res Suppl I, 14–15: 1–157, with kind permission).

Clinically there are two aspects of this local pressure-flow relationship which are of interest. The first is purely speculative; does this mechanism, which responds to a rise in arterial pressure by vasoconstriction ever become so disordered in disease that it becomes set at a higher or lower plateau than normal. If the whole arterial tree were set at a higher level it could theoretically cause hypertension. This aspect is related to the treatment of hypertension with hypotensive drugs. When renal function is substantially normal the renal blood flow and glomerular filtration rate remain unchanged as the blood pressure falls. But if there is evidence of renal damage (reduced glomerular filtration, etc.) before the administration of the hypotensive agent the normal pressure-flow relationship may either fail, or only become manifest after a long interval. In these circumstances glomerular filtration rate will fall, the blood urea rise steeply, and the patient may die of acute upon chronic renal failure. It is always wise therefore to induce a fall in blood pressure gradually in such patients, and to repeat estimations of glomerular function at frequent intervals.

In renal artery stenosis there may be a profound fall in perfusion pressure and consequently a persistent autoregulatory vasodilatation of the afferent arteriole beyond the obstruction. When there is a substantial fall in perfusion pressure beyond the obstruction however glomerular filtration rate is maintained by efferent arteriolar constriction due to a high local concentration of inactive angiotensin I converted to the active angiotensin II. This mechanism is revealed when captopril is administered to control the hypertension of renal artery stenosis. Captopril inhibits the conversion of the inactive angiotensin I to angiotensin II there is thus a fall in the local concentration of angiotensin II, a drop in glomerular filtration rate and a rise in plasma creatinine and urea, which sometimes may be sufficiently severe to cause alarm.

## ADJUSTMENTS OF REGIONAL DISTRIBUTION OF RENAL BLOOD FLOW AND THE URINARY EXCRETION OF SODIUM

It has been established both in man and animals that when the urinary excretion of sodium is low the blood flow to the outer cortex of the kidney is often reduced, and that to the medulla is increased, and vice versa. It was, at first, assumed that these changes were accompanied by parallel changes in glomerular filtration rate. And it was therefore proposed that the low urinary sodium excretion was due to a greater proportion of glomerular filtrate passing through the deep juxta medullary nephrons. It was proposed that these nephrons reabsorbed sodium more avidly because they have long loops of Henle. None of these assumptions seem to be warranted. It has been found that redistribution of glomerular filtration does not occur with changes in urinary sodium excretion. And it has been pointed out that though the juxta medullary nephrons do have longer loops of Henle they also have a much higher rate of filtration. Thus any overall redistribution, if it did occur, might not have any effect on sodium reabsorption. It is possible therefore that the redistribution of blood flow that occurs with changes in sodium excretion may be the consequence, rather than the cause, of the changes in sodium excretion. This conclusion is re-enforced by the observation that the rise in urinary sodium excretion produced by frusemide and ethacrynic acid are also associated with a redistribution of regional blood flow.

## SHUNTS

There is no convincing evidence that true shunting of blood ever takes place in the kidney. Nevertheless, there are two renal circulatory phenomena which have sometimes had the word shunt applied to them. One is the kidney's capacity for intense vasoconstriction, and the other is the way in which it separates plasma from red cells.

### 'Shunting' of whole blood

It has been claimed that in some circumstances, the cortex may become ischaemic because the blood which should have travelled to the cortex is shunted through the medulla. This conclusion was first reached from observations made on experimental animals subjected to the following stimuli: prolonged application of tourniquets to the hind limbs, bleeding, stimulation of the sciatic nerves and the administration of certain substances such as adrenaline, in large quantities. During and immediately after stimulation the renal circulation was studied by means of angiographs, injections of methylene blue, and histological sections. These techniques give an indication of the *distribution* of blood within the kidney at any one time, but are not measures of the *rate* of blood flow in any one place. It was found that these noxious stimuli were associated with the following change in the distribution of blood; the cortex contained less and the medulla more, that is, the cortex on section was pale and the medulla was dark. Mainly from this evidence it was suggested that the ischaemia of the cortex was due to the hyperaemia of the medulla; the blood intended for the cortex having been by-passed, diverted, or shunted through the medulla.

This assumption was unwarranted, for to demonstrate that ischaemia is due to the opening of a shunt it is necessary to show that the decrease in flow in the ischaemic area is of the same order as the increase in flow in the shunt, i.e. if a large diversion of the normal cortical blood flow takes place it should be possible to demonstrate cortical ischaemia without significicant reduction in renal blood flow. But when renal blood flow is measured, the cortex becomes pale and the medulla dark only when the total renal blood flow is greatly reduced. It is clear therefore, that the ischaemic pallor of the cortex cannot be due only to an increase in medullary flow, whether or not a small increase does occur. That such an increase is unlikely has been demonstrated with temperature measuring needles simultaneously recording from medulla and cortex; for when the total renal blood flow is markedly reduced by nor-adrenaline, adrenaline and stimulation of the renal nerves, the changes in temperature which take place (and which presumably reflect changes in blood flow) are the same in the two sites. It has even been suggested that when there is pallor of the cortex and congestion of the medulla it is probable that there is no blood flowing through the medulla, for it has been found that indian ink injected intravenously may sometimes fail to appear in the medulla.

The importance of the observations which led to the renal shunt hypothesis is that they showed that in certain circumstances the cortex of the kidney has a disconcerting tendency to shut off its blood supply almost completely. It is probable that in most instances of intense renal vasoconstriction the blood flow through the cortex virtually ceases while medullary blood flow may continue at a very reduced rate.

### 'Shunting' of plasma from red cells

The haematocrit of the blood in the renal cortex is about 50% of that in the large blood vessels, and in the medulla it is only 30% This high proportion of plasma in the cortex is partly due to (1) its predominantly capillary bore circulation, for there is a tendency for red cells in small vessels to travel quickly down the centre in a narrow stream, while plasma passes more slowly in a wide peripheral cuff; and (2) there is some evidence that some plasma probably lies in the interstitial space (p. 5).

The even higher proportion of plasma in the medulla indicates that the blood flow through the medulla is mainly plasma. The most reasonable hypothesis for this phenomenon is that the plasma is 'stripped' from the red cells at the point where the afferent arterioles supplying the juxtamedullary glomeruli leave the interlobular arteries. It has been shown on models that when blood flows through a tube whose branches come off at right angles (as they do from the interlobular arteries) the sleeve of plasma in the main tube passes selectively into the branches with little admixture of red cells. The functional importance of this manoeuvre is obscure. It is possible that it contributes to a low intramedullary $pO_2$ (see below).

## SIGNIFICANCE OF THE COUNTER-CURRENT CIRCULATION IN THE MEDULLA

It has been pointed out (p. 58) that the blood supply to the medulla flows through long looped vessels (the vasa recta) which, though they are relatively wide, have walls of capillary thickness throughout their entire course. And that the blood within them is obliged to flow in a counter-current fashion, first down towards the tip of the papilla and then upwards to the corticomedullary junction. As the walls of the vasa recta are of capillary thickness the blood they contain is in nearly all respects in equilibrium with medullary interstitial fluid, and therefore with the fluid flowing through the thin capillary like descending limbs of Henle. In addition it is very likely that at all times the fluid in the collecting ducts must also be in equilibrium with the $pO_2$ and $Pco_2$ of the medullary interstitial fluid, and there is evidence that under the influence of ADH the fluid in the collecting ducts is also in equilibrium with respect to its osmolality, urea concentration and probably hydrogen ion concentration.

The importance to the medullary interstitial fluid of a counter-current flow in the vasa recta is two-fold: (1) it magnifies the *rise* in concentration which follows the transfer of any solute or gas from the tubules into the medullary interstitial fluid; (2) it magnifies the *fall* in concentration of any solute or gas which is removed from the medullary interstitial fluid. Both are clinically important.

An example of the first consequence of the counter-current circulation was detailed on page 58 where it was shown how it contributes to the high medullary concentrations of sodium chloride and urea, which in turn make it possible for the urine to become hypertonic. It is probable that it is also responsible for the high $Pco_2$ of alkaline urine and the low pH of acid urine.

The high osmolality of the medulla is one reason why the medulla is so susceptible to infection, for it inhibits the action of complement and the mobilisation and phagocytic properties of polymorphonuclear leucocytes. The most clear-cut example of the second consequence is the fact that the $pO_2$ of urine is lower than that of renal venous blood. This is because the initially high $pO_2$ of the arterial blood in the descending limb of the vasa recta is in equilibrium with the low $pO_2$ of the venous blood in the ascending limb; it follows that the $pO_2$ of the supposedly arterial blood reaching the tip of the papilla, and which is in equilibrium with the urine emerging from the collecting tubule, is lower than normal arterial blood. This hypoxic effect of the counter-current circulation is accentuated by the low red cell content of medullary blood, the medulla's poor renal blood flow, and it's inability to adjust blood flow to changes in perfusion pressure. To compensate for this hypoxia the medulla has a greater capacity for anaerobic metabolism. Clinically it is probable that medullary hypoxia is a factor in the characteristic localisation renal tuberculosis to the tip of the papilla, and in the aetiology of papilliary necrosis in diabetes, sickle cell anaemia and phenacetin nephropathy.

BIBLIOGRAPHY

Barger A C 1966 Renal hemodynamic factors in congestive heart failure. Ann N Y Acad Sci 139: 276 (regional redistribution of blood flows)

Bradley S E, Bradley G P 1947 Renal function during chronic anaemia in man. Blood 2: 192

Earley L E, Schrier R W 1973 Intrarenal control of sodium excretion by hemodynamic and physical factors. In: Orloff J, Berliner R W (eds) Handbook of physiology, section 8, Renal physiology. Am Phys Soc, Washington DC, ch 8

Eichna L W, Farber S J, Berger A R et al 1953 Cardio-vascular dynamics in heart failure. Circulation 7: 674

Emery E W, Gowenlock A H, Riddell A G et al 1959 Intrarenal variations in haematocrit. Clin Sci 18: 205

Epstein F H, Post R S, MacDowell M 1953 The effect of an arteriovenous fistula on renal haemodynamics and electrolyte excretion. J Clin Invest 32: 233

Fishman A P, Maxwell M H, Crowder C H et al 1951 Kidney function in cor pulmonale. Circulation 3: 703

Fourman J, Moffat D B 1971 The blood vessels of the kidney. Blackwell Scientific, Oxford

Guyton A C, Langston J B, Navar G 1964 Theory for renal autoregulation by feedback of the juxta-glomerular apparatus. Circ Res 15: Suppl. 1–187

Hollenberg N K 1979 The physiology of the renal circulation. In: Black D A K, Jones N F (eds) Renal Disease. Blackwell Scientific, Oxford, ch 2

Ladefoged J, Munk O 1971 Distribution of blood flow in the kidney. In: Fisher J W (ed) Kidney hormones. Academic Press, London, p 31

Lauson H D, Bradley S E, Cournand A 1944 Renal circulation in shock. J Clin Invest 23: 381

Phillips R A, Dole V P, Hamilton P B et al D D 1946 Effects of acute haemorrhagic and traumatic shock on renal function of dogs. Amer J Physiol 145: 314

Rennie D W, Reeves R B, Pappenheimer J R 1958 Oxygen pressure in urine and its relation to intrarenal blood flow. Amer J Physiol 195: 120

Scher A M 1951 Focal blood flow measurements in cortex and medulla of kidney. Amer J Physiol 167: 539

Selkurt E E, Elpers M J 1963 The influence of hemorrhagic shock on renal hemodynamics and osmolar clearance in the dog. Amer J Physiol 205: 147

Semple S J G, de Wardener H E 1959 The effect of increased renal venous pressure on circulatory autoregulation of isolated dog kidneys. Circ Res 7: 643

Stein J H, Boonjarern S, Wilson C B 1973 Alterations in intrarenal blood flow distribution. Methods of measurement and relationship to sodium balance. Circ Res 32 Suppl: 1–61

Symposium on autoregulation of blood flow 1964 Circ Res 15: Suppl 1

Thurau K 1964 Renal hemodynamics. Amer J Med 36: 698

Wardener de H E, McSwiney R R, Miles B E 1951 Renal haemodynamics in primary polycythaemia. Lancet 2: 204

Waugh W H 1958 Myogenic nature of autoregulation of renal flow in the absence of blood corpuscles. Circ Res 6: 363

Wirz H, Dixic R 1973 Urinary concentration and dilution. In: Berliner R W, Orloff J (eds) Handbook of physiology, section 8, Renal physiology. Amer Phys Soc, Washington DC, ch 13

# 8

# Renal function in relation to age

## RENAL FUNCTION IN THE FETUS

The outstanding fact is that fetal urine is hypotonic to its own plasma.

## RENAL FUNCTION IN INFANCY

In contrast to adults the intake of food and the rate of growth are more important than the kidney in keeping the biochemical environment of the infant stable. In addition, though the infant's kidney is perfectly adequate for normal purposes it is less adaptable than that of an adult in an emergency. The normal daily rhythms of urinary excretion are not present at birth. They only gradually become established over a period of years, though some difference between 'day' and 'night' excretory rates manifest themselves at an early stage. Failure to develop a normal diurnal rhythm may occasionally be the cause of nocturnal enuresis after infancy.

*Glomerular filtration rate*, calculated on a surface area basis, is proportionately less than in an adult and yet the concentration of urea in the blood is lower. This is due to the relatively larger quantities of nitrogen that are being retained at this time of life, and in normal circumstances the lower glomerular filtration rate is perfectly adequate to dispose of the small amount of waste products of protein catabolism. The hazards of this situation are evident when the child becomes ill and ceases to store nitrogen. A sharp increase in protein catabolism is then liable to produce a rise in blood urea and, if protein administration is continued the blood urea may rise even more rapidly though there has been no alteration in the glomerular filtration rate.

*Tubular function.* The ability to dilute and concentrate the urine to adult levels does not take place until approximately the fourteenth day and the third month respectively. The ability to excrete a water load does not reach adult proportions until the end of the first month. The inability to concentrate the urine is due initially to (1) an inability to respond to ADH because the renal medulla has not developed sufficiently, and (2) the small amounts of urea passing down the tubule consequent upon the retention of nitrogen needed for growth. After a few weeks the kidney has matured sufficiently to enable it to respond to ADH but the ability to concentrate remains low because of the small amounts of urea that are sequested in the medulla. At this point, however, if an infant is given suitable quantities of urea by mouth the ability to concentrate rises to adult levels within a few hours, the increase in osmolality being equal to the increased concentration of urea in the urine. Consequently, during the first few months an inadequate intake of water or an attack of diarrhoea may lead to severe dehydration; or an excessive administration of water may cause overhydration.

The control of sodium excretion is even less elastic than that of water and an excess infusion of normal saline may produce a hypertonic oedema because of the greater difficulty in getting rid of sodium. In infants five to seven months of age retention of sodium occurs when the intake is greater than 50 mEq/day. Alternatively, urinary sodium excretion may continue though there is a negative balance of sodium from diarrhoea or vomiting.

The other tubular functions which have been found to be relatively less efficient than in an adult are the ability to excrete a highly acid urine, and both TmPAH and TmG. All functions become comparable to those of an adult by the end of the first year. Ammonia excretion, however, is within normal limits in the first few days.

Titratable acid excretion is remarkably low for the first year of life. This is due in part to a poor ability to secrete hydrogen ions against a gradient and also to the low phosphate content of the urine. The low urinary phosphate content is due to the infant's retention of phosphate for the formation of bone and muscle. If phosphate is administered titratable acid excretion rises and the usually low plasma bicarbonate values rise to adult levels. The infant's renal threshold for bicarbonate is 21.5 to 22.5 mmol/l which is much lower than the 24 to 26 mmol/l found in the adult. It appears therefore that the infant's normal state of mild metabolic acidosis is secondary to a combination of inadequate kidneys and insufficient urinary buffer. This explains the infant's liability to develop severe acidosis if given large quantities of dietary protein.

Proteinuria and glycosuria occur in about a quarter of normal premature infants, and infants up to the third day, when the urine then becomes free of protein and glucose.

## RENAL FUNCTION DURING SENESCENCE

After the age of 30 there is a gradual reduction in renal functional capacity. This is due principally to involution and is independent of renal vascular occlusion though it can be accelerated by arteriosclerosis. The functions which have been studied include glomerular filtration, renal blood flow, secretion Tm, urea clearance, and the ability to concentrate.

By the age of 90 each of these functions has decreased to approximately half its value at the age of 30. It is important to note however that though

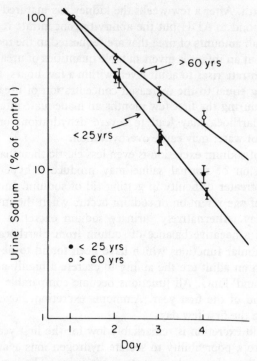

**Fig. 8.1** Changes in urinary sodium excretion in response to a sudden restriction in sodium intake in two groups of normal men, one under 25 years and the other over 60 years. The rate at which urinary sodium excretion fell in the younger group was significantly faster than in the older group (reproduced from Epstein 1979 Fed Proc 38: 170, with kind permission).

the creatinine clearance may be halved, the plasma creatinine is normal. This is because the production of creatinine by the reduced muscle mass of the elderly is smaller than normal. It must not be assumed, therefore, if the plasma creatinine of an elderly person is normal, then his glomerular filtration rate is the same as that of a younger person with the same plasma creatinine. This is extremely relevant when administering digitalis and certain antibiotics which, if the dose is not adjusted to the depressed glomerular filtration rate, may accumulate and cause toxic symptoms. Histological appearances show that there is a gradual loss of nephrons so that it is highly probable that every function is involved. It is also very noticeable that elderly patients are not able to concentrate their urine to the same extent as adolescents and that they are also much slower in responding to a dietary reduction of sodium, a combination which makes their already impaired renal function very vulnerable (Fig. 8.1).

BIBLIOGRAPHY

Alexander P, Nixon D A 1961 The foetal kidney. Brit Med Bull 17: 112

Boss J M H, Dlouka H, Kraus M et al 1964 The structure of the kidney in relation to age and diet in white rats during the weaning period. J Physiol 168: 196

Cutler R E, Orme B M 1969 J Amer Med Ass 209: 539

Edelman C M, Barnett H L, Troupkou V 1960 Renal concentrating mechanisms in newborn infants. Effects of dietary protein and water content, role of urea, and responsiveness to antidiuretic hormone. J Clin Invest 39: 1062

Edelman C M, Soriano J R, Boichis H et al 1967 Renal bicarbonate reabsorption and hydrogen ion excretion in normal infants. J Clin Invest 46: 1309

Krecek J, Heller J 1962 Neurohypophysis and the regulation of water and electrolyte metabolism in infants and mammals. Proc Internat Union of Phys Sci, 22nd Congress 1: 53

McCance R A, Hatemi N 1961 Control of acid-base stability in the newly born. Lancet 1: 293

McCance R A, Widdowson E M 1956 Metabolism and renal function in the first two days of life. Modern views on the secretion of urine. Churchill, London, p 217

Miller J H, Shock N W 1953 Age differences in the renal response to antidiuretic hormone. J Gerontol 8: 446

Rhodes P G, Hammel C L, Berman L B 1962 Urinary constituents of the new born infant. J Paediat 60: 18

Sakai T, Leumann E P, Holliday M A 1969 Single injection clearance in children. Pediatrics 44: 905

Shock N W 1946 Kidney function tests in aged males. Geriatrics 1: 232

Shock N W, Davies D F 1950 Age changes in glomerular filtration rate, effective renal plasma flow, and tubular excretory capacity in adult males. J Clin Invest 29: 496

Spitzer A 1971 Renal physiology impact of recent developments on clinical nephrology. Pediatrics clinic of North America 18: 377

Vernier R L, Birch Anderson A 1962 Studies of the human foetal kidney. J Paediat 60: 754

Watkin M, Shock M H 1955 J Clin Invest 34: 969

# 9

# Diurnal rhythm

The urinary excretion of water and most electrolytes is normally greater during the day than at night, a fortunate phenomenon which ensures that sleep shall be undisturbed. This pattern is not only due to the fact that fluid and food are usually ingested during the day; it will persist even if identical quantities of food and water are ingested at regular intervals throughout the 24 hours. As the evening approaches and during the night, the excretion of sodium, potassium, bicarbonate and chloride ions gradually diminishes, while the pH of the urine falls, and its concentration rises; the process is reversed in the morning (Fig. 9.1).

The mechanism responsible for this rhythm is unknown; it has been shown that there is a small nocturnal fall in glomerular filtration rate, but this cannot explain all the changes that occur; for instance, the excretion of phosphate *increases* at night and diminishes during the day. It is possible that the changes in water excretion, and particularly the changes in urine concentration, follow a diurnal alteration in antidiuretic hormone secretion. There is no doubt that an antidiuretic mechanism is present, for at night a large drink of water only produces a small increase in urine flow. The changes in electrolyte excretion are preceded, by a few hours, by similar fluctuations in steroid excretion. It is probable that this is only coincidental, for it fails to explain why the changes in sodium and potassium excretion should be parallel; it has also been reported that under certain conditions the excretion of steroid will rise gradually throughout the day and night, and yet the diurnal rhythm of electrolyte and water excretion continues uninterruptedly.

A normal diurnal rhythm persists during undernutrition, water deprivation; salt deprivation, the sustained action of pitressin and a temporary disturbance of sleep rhythm. For instance, a person going from east to west on a ship across the Atlantic will show a peak of electrolyte excretion one hour (ship time) earlier each day. But the clock 'gains' an hour each day so that in fact the diurnal rhythm remains unchanged in relation to European time. Reversal or abolition of the diurnal rhythm occurs commonly in the four most frequent causes of generalised oedema, i.e. cardiac failure, liver failure, the nephrotic syndrome and malnutrition (e.g. anorexia

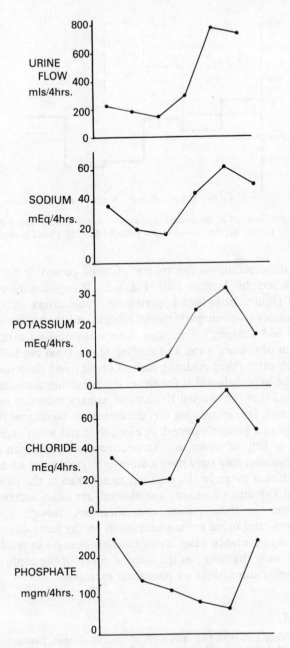

**Fig. 9.1** Diurnal rhythm of urinary excretion of water, sodium, potassium, chloride and phosphate in a normal subject.

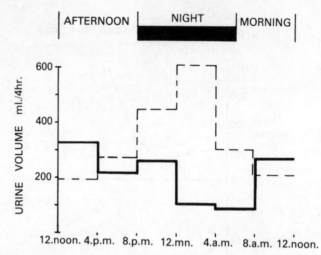

**Fig. 9.2** Pathological reversal of the diurnal rhythm (‒ ‒ ‒ ‒ ‒) of urinary excretion of water compared with the normal rhythm (——————) in a patient following a head injury.

nervosa). In these conditons the volume of urine passed at night may be equal to or exceed the daytime total (Fig. 9.2). It may also be reversed in chronic renal failure, malignant hypertension, renal artery stenosis, small bowel insufficiency (e.g. idiopathic steatorrhoea), Addison's disease, hyper-aldosteronism and Cushing's Syndrome. Very occasionally a reversal of the diurnal rhythm of urinary water and electrolyte excretion can follow a head injury. In such cases other evidence such as obesity and sleep disturbances suggest that the hypothalamus is the site of the persisting abnormality. This in turn suggests that the diurnal rhythms of urinary excretion originate in the hypothalamus. It is interesting that the foetus has no diurnal rhythm.

A knowledge of a patient's pattern of electrolyte and water excretion may sometimes be of help in treatment. An oedematous person with a reversed rhythm, for instance, may only have a diuresis following the administration of a diuretic, if it is given in the evening, rather than in the morning.

The diurnal rhythms of urinary constituents are often accompanied by diurnal rhythms in their plasma concentrations, though synchronous changes in blood and urine are not necessarily in the same direction. This is of the utmost importance when trying to assess changes in renal function. Inattention to these rhythms was the cause of much of the confusion which surrounded earlier discussions on phosphate excretion.

BIBLIOGRAPHY

Borst J G G, de Vries L A 1950 The three types of 'natural' diuresis. Lancet 2: 1
Dunger D B, Wolf O H, Leonard J V et al 1980 Effect of naloxone in a previously undescribed hypothalamic syndrome. A disorder of the endogenous opioid peptide system? Lancet 1: 1277

Finkenstaedt J T, Dingman J F, Jenkins D et al 1954 The effect of intravenous hydrocortisone and corticosterone on the diurnal rhythm in renal function, and electrolyte equilibria in normal and Addisonian subjects. J Clin Invest 33: 933

Flear C I G, Cooke W T, Quinton A 1959 Water diuresis and steatorrhoea. Clin Sci 18: 137

Fourman P, Reifenstein E C, Kepler E J et al Effect of desoxycorticosterone acetate on electrolyte metabolism in normal man. Metabolism 1: 242

Goldman R 1951 Studies in diurnal variation of water and electrolyte excretion: nocturnal diuresis of water and sodium in congestive cardiac failure and cirrhosis of the liver. J Clin Invest 30: 1191

Kleitman N 1949 Biological rhythms and cycles. Physiol Rev 29: 1

Lewis P R, Lobban M C 1956 Patterns of electrolyte excretion in human subjects during a prolonged period of life on a 22-hour day. J Physiol (Lond) 133: 670

Papper S, Rosenbaum J D 1952 Diurnal variation in the diuretic response to ingested water. J Clin Invest 31: 401

Payne R W, de Wardener H E 1958 Reversal of urinary diurnal rhythm following head injury. Lancet 1: 1098

Rosenbaum J D, Ferguson B C, Davis R K et al 1952 The influence of cortisone upon the diurnal rhythm of renal excretory function. J Clin Invest 31: 507.

Stanbury S W, Thomson A E 1951 Diurnal variations in electrolyte excretion. Clin Sci 10: 267

Thomas J P, Coles G A, El-Shaboury A H 1970 Nocturia in patients on long term steroid therapy. Clin Sci 38: 415

Thomas S 1959 Effects of change of posture on the diurnal renal excretory rhythm. J Physiol 148: 489

Wesson L G 1964 Electrolyte excretion in relation to diurnal cycles of renal function. Medicine 43: 547

Wesson L G, Lauler D P 1961 Diurnal cycle of glomerular filtration rate and sodium and chloride excretion during responses to altered salt and water balance in man. J Clin Invest 40: 1967

# 10

# Orthostatic proteinuria

This benign condition is also called postural proteinuria. It consists of the excretion of protein in the urine only when the patient is in certain positions.

### Aetiology

Proteinuria can be produced in 75% of youths if they are placed in extreme lordosis. With increasing age the proportion gradually dwindles and, of men over 50, only 10% will have proteinuria in this position.

It has been demonstrated that in the lordotic position the liver in these persons rotates forwards and downwards thus kinking the inferior vena cava. As a result there is a rise in the pressure within the inferior vena cava and renal veins, and protein appears in the urine.

If, however, the patients stands in the lordotic position but the liver is prevented from sliding forward by firm digital restraint under the right costal margin, the inferior vena caval pressure does not rise and there is no proteinuria. In bed, the lordosis of the upright position disappears and again there is no proteinuria, though it can be made to reappear by purposely assuming the lordotic position. Conversely, proteinuria will not appear in the upright posture if the patient remains bent forward.

### Renal function

Excluding the proteinuria renal function is normal.

### Clinical features

Orthostatic proteinuria occurs most frequently in children, adolescents and young adults. It has been reported in 12–40% of children aged 10–16 years; and it is claimed that this proportion is greater if the urine is examined at frequent intervals. Orthostatic proteinuria occurs in about 5% of young adults.

The presence of protein in the urine is usually detected during a routine examination on going to school or university, or on entering the services. Occasionally it is noted as an incidental finding during an illness which is unrelated to the kidney. If many urine samples are tested it is found that protein is present throughout the day, except in the first sample passed in the morning. The concentration of protein rarely exceeds + + and is usually + or less; the daily excretion is seldom more than 2–3 g. It is not unusual to find protein on some days and not on others. Orthostatic proteinuria is of no importance; it does not influence the patient's health or the functional capacity of his kidneys. The majority of patients lose their proteinuria as they become older though it may continue for 10–30 years.

For routine purposes orthostatic proteinuria is distinguished from persistent proteinuria by asking the patient to empty his bladder just before going to bed, and to keep for examination the urine he passes next morning immediately he gets up. This test can be combined with a 16- to 24-hour fluid deprivation test, when the ability to concentrate can be tested simultaneously.

## Differential diagnosis

If proteinuria can be made to disappear with a change in posture it is almost certain that there is no renal disease. Nevertheless it is also characteristic of the proteinuria of renal disease that it is greater when the patient is up and about, and diminishes upon lying down. On very rare occasions the proteinuria of renal disease may be altogether absent from the urine formed during the night, when it is then indistinguishable from benign orthostatic proteinuria. These confusing cases usually declare themselves eventually; sometimes they can be differentiated earlier by an examination of the urinary deposit, or a renal biopsy. It is a paradox that orthostatic proteinuria like that which occurs with fever and exercise demonstrates a pattern of unselective glomerular permeability (p. 166) though the glomeruli show no histological changes. Orthostatic proteinuria should not be dismissed too lightly when it occurs in a patient over 30 years old.

## Treatment

No treatment is necessary.

## PROTEINURIA FROM NON-GONOCOCCAL URETHRITIS

Superficially, this appears to be a variant of orthostatic proteinuria, but in fact it has no direct relation to posture. It is an important diagnostic trap. The proteinuria is present in the *morning* and disappears during the course of the day. The condition is most commonly seen in young men. Urethral massage in the morning, before any urine has been excreted, and examination of the contents of the urethra establishes the diagnosis. The two glass test is also a useful screening test.

## BIBLIOGRAPHY

Bull G M 1948–49 Postural proteinuria. Clin Sci 7: 77
King S E 1955 Patterns of protein excretion by the kidneys. Ann Intern Med 42: 296
King S E 1957 Postural adjustments and protein excretion by the kidney in renal disease. Ann Intern Med 46: 360
Lowgren E 1955 Studies on benign proteinuria (with special reference to the renal lymphatic system). Acta Med Scand suppl 300
Lyall A 1941 Classification of cases of albuminuria. Brit Med J 2: 113

# 11

# Acute renal failure

Acute renal failure can be arbitrarily defined as any condition in which the daily volume or urine passed into the bladder is suddenly reduced below 400 ml*. This definition inevitably includes severe but physiological oliguria, which is sometimes called 'acute renal insufficiency'. Acute renal failure can be divided into four main categories.
1. Severe functional changes without structural damage
2. Severe functional changes with acute structural damage
3. Functional changes of perhaps moderate severity but occuring in a patient with chronic structural damage
4. Acute urinary tract obstruction.

## Severe functional changes without structural damage ('pre-renal azotaemia')

The most important of these changes is severe but initially reversible renal vasoconstriction, the causes of which have been discussed on page 115; they are predominantly those which cause acute circulatory insufficiency. Typical examples are the sudden reductions in blood volume which may accompany acute diarrhoea and vomiting, burns and haemorrhage. The reduced renal blood flow which results is associated with a reduced renal blood flow and glomerular filtration rate and thus a decreased excretion of solutes. Usually there is a simultaneous stimulation of the supra-optico-hypophyseal system and an increase in the level of circulating antidiuretic hormone. The oliguria which results is thus associated with a urine which at first is highly concentrated. Some of the most severe but rapidly reversible oliguric episodes may occur in the first two days after operation when the 24-hour urine volume may be 150 ml.

* This excludes a transient form of acute renal failure in which the glomerular filtration rate falls and the blood urea rises, but the urine flow remains normal. The condition has been described in association with the administration of aminoglycosides, burns and after open heart surgery, it has a good prognosis.

## Severe functional changes with acute structural damage

A wide variety of conditions may give rise to acute structural changes severe enough to cause acute renal failure; they are illustrated in Figure 11.1. They include severe forms of certain renal diseases which usually present in a less acute form, i.e. acute nephritis, acute pyelonephritis with acute necrotising papillitis, malignant hypertension, polyarteritis nodosa and eclampsia. Acute renal failure may also be caused by an acute interstitial nephritis due to a drug sensitivity (e.g. phenindione). Numerically these are not important causes of acute renal failure. The most common form of structural damage is acute tubular necrosis. In the past this condition has been called 'lower nephron nephrosis', 'shock kidney' and 'crush syndrome'.

Tubular necrosis may follow directly from the action of nephrotoxic poisons or severe prolonged renal vasoconstriction. Poisons act directly by causing the death of those tubular cells which transport the substance from the blood into the lumen of the tubule; they also cause intense renal vaso-constriction and irregularly distributed focal patches of renal ischaemia, which in turn becomes the sites of ischaemic tubular necrosis. Mercury, arsenic, lead, bismuth, carbon tetrachloride, potassium chlorate, propylene glycol, sulphonamides, cephaloridine and amino glycosides are some of the substances which have been known to cause acute tubular necrosis. Some endogenous substances such as porphyrins and bilirubin are also liable to produce acute tubular necrosis if present in excess quantities in the plasma.

The causes of renal vasoconstriction which may produce tubular necrosis are the same as those which have been discussed above and in Chapter 7. In addition to these hypovolaemic causes of ischaemia most patients who develop acute renal failure initially pass through a phase of disseminated intravascular coagulation with microemboli which intensifies the vasocon-striction. Necrosis is due to the intensity and duration of renal ischaemia, i.e. it must be present for a matter of hours, a point of immense importance in trying to prevent the condition. Abortion, multiple wounds and extensive surgery with inadequate blood replacement and bacteraemia are the most frequent causes of tubular necrosis. Though it is possible that renal vaso-constriction without a concomitant fall in blood pressure may occasionally be sufficiently intense to cause necrosis, it is clear that necrosis is more likely if there is a combination of vasoconstriction and hypotension. It is not always appreciated that (1) renal vasoconstriction abolishes circulatory autoregulation so that a fall in pressure is now accompanied by a further reduction in renal blood flow and (2) that the more intense the vasocon-striction the higher the minimal arterial pressure necessary to keep the vessels open. These conditions are important clinically, for when there is severe renal vasoconstriction, minor falls in blood pressure may be sufficient to cause a complete ischaemia.

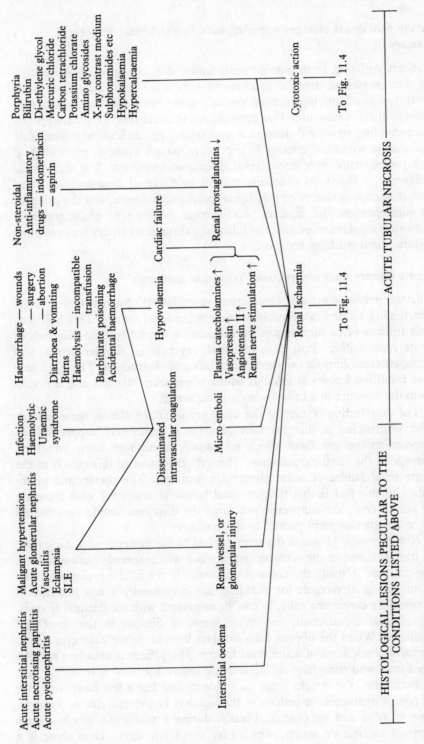

**Fig. 11.1** Initiating causes and mechanisms in acute renal failure.

## Acute functional changes superimposed upon chronic structural damage

Patients suffering from chronic renal failure due to a gradual obliteration of their nephrons may be precipitated into acute renal failure by some disturbance which, in a normal person, would cause only an insignificant change in renal function. This combination of acute functional changes and long-standing structural damage is sometimes very difficult to differentiate from acute structural damage in previously normal kidneys, particularly if the pre-existence of chronic renal disease is unknown. The differential diagnosis is based on obtaining clinical evidence of long-standing renal failure such as a history of polydipsia, polyuria, lassitude, and the presence of pigmentation and anaemia. Radiological evidence of phalangeal sub-periosteal erosions or evidence of bilaterally shrunken kidneys are even more helpful distinguishing features.

## Acute urinary tract obstruction ('post-renal azotaemia')

Bilateral pelvic or ureteric obstruction, or unilateral obstruction to a single functioning kidney can obviously cause acute renal failure. This indisputable truth is often forgotten when considering the differential diagnosis of acute renal failure. Pus, clots of blood, crystalluria, tubular debris, and retroperitoneal fibrosis can cause acute bilateral obstruction. There is also a rare condition known as calculus anuria when acute bilateral anuria results from the presence of a calculus in only one ureter.

The outstanding feature of the acute renal failure due to acute urinary tract obstruction is that the flow of urine is completely suppressed, as opposed to the low flows which are usually found with acute structural damage to the renal parenchyma. The only exception to this rule is in the acute renal failure of acute glomerular nephritis. The therapeutic implication of this fact is that if acute renal failure is associated with complete or almost complete suppression of urine the diagnosis should be assumed to be obstruction until proved to the contrary.

*Retroperitoneal fibrosis* is the term applied to the presence of a thick mass of fibrous tissue in the retroperitoneal space which spreads outwards from the mid-line. Usually the cause is unknown. It can follow prolonged treatment with methysergide for migraine; and occasionally it is a response to invasion by carcinoma cells. It may be associated with mediastinal fibrosis, oesophageal constriction, and other forms of fibrosis in the chest and abdomen. When the fibrous mass involves both ureters it may give rise to a characteristic form of acute renal failure. The patient is usually a middle-aged man who complains of increasingly severe bouts of unremitting pain in both loins, the attacks come on suddenly and last a few hours or a day or two. A hydrocoele or oedema of the legs may be present, due to compression of veins and lymphatics. Finally, during a prolonged attack of pain there is oliguria or anuria, which may last a few days. Then there is a profuse polyuria, perhaps only for a few hours, followed by a return of complete anuria. The concentration of blood urea fluctuates wildly with the changes in urine flow, and the urine is free of protein, a most revealing point which excludes a disturbance of the renal parenchyma as the cause of the anuria. Surprisingly ureteric catheters often pass up the ureters without difficulty and urine flows down the lumen of the catheters, but when they are removed, the anuria persists. Radiographic studies may show that the ureters have been pulled inwards towards the mid-line or that they are deformed in a zig-zag pattern along part of their course. The ureteric abnormalities are best seen by filling the ureters with hypaque from below using a bulb type of ureteric catheter. Treatment consists in freeing the ureters and placing them laterally beyond the fibrous mass. The idiopathic form of the disease is thought to be self-limiting.

## TUBULAR NECROSIS

The following sections describe the pathological findings, clinical features, treatment and prognosis in acute tubular necrosis. The clinical features and treatment of acute renal failure due to other causes have many points in common.

### Pathology of acute tubular necrosis

Macroscopically the kidneys do not look greatly disturbed and may often be passed as normal. When the kidney is incised there is a tendency for the cortex to bulge and to look slightly pale. The only unmistakable macroscopical appearances are those associated with extensive necrosis such as are found with eclampsia and accidental haemorrhage (p. 499) when the condition is called acute cortical necrosis.

Microscopically the lesions are most clearly displayed in nephrons which have been microdissected. By this technique is has been possible to show that there are two distinct lesions; one is due to ischaemia and occurs in a random distribution throughout all nephrons and in any part of the nephron down to the collecting tubule; the other, which is due to nephrotoxins, affects all nephrons equally, and is confined to the same part of each *proximal* tubule. Each ischaemic lesion involves only a relatively short length of the nephron and consists of complete necrosis of the tubule cells and the basement membrane, thus exposing the lumen of the tubule to the renal interstitial space (Fig. 11.2). The nephrotoxic lesion involves a considerable segment of each proximal tubule and consists of necrosis of tubule cells only, without involvement of basement membrane (Fig. 11.3). Nephrotoxins, however, not only cause the death of those tubule cells which transport them, but in additon their presence in high concentrations causes intense renal vasoconstriction. In acute tubular necrosis from nephrotoxins, therefore, both ischaemic and cytotoxic lesions are found.

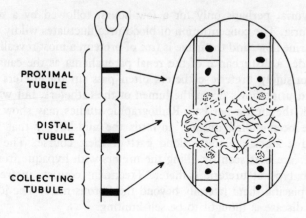

Fig. 11.2 Ischaemic lesion of tubular necrosis.

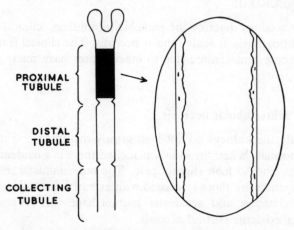

Fig. 11.3 Nephrotoxic lesion of tubular necrosis.

Ordinary histological sections of the kidney at autopsy show that the glomeruli appear to escape injury. The even distribution of the nephrotoxic tubular lesions are easily recognised but the ischaemic lesions are much more widely spaced and more difficult to identify. There are a few foci of round cell infiltration and many of the tubules are surrounded by interstitial oedema. Numerous haemcasts are seen in those instances in which acute renal failure follows an incompatible blood transfusion or widespread muscle injury.

The most striking light microscopy change in renal biopsies obtained from patients in whom acute renal failure was not due to a nephrotoxic poison, nor to one of the well recognised parenchymatous diseases, is how little there is to see. The few histological changes present are quite out of proportion to the severe reduction in renal function. The glomeruli and proximal tubules appear normal unless the patient has been treated with mannitol or dextran, when the tubules are found to be grossly vacuolated. The distal tubules however, show many focal dilatations often in the shape of a fat U which contains pigmented casts. Occasionally the very localised necrotic areas are situated at the site of a cast.

With the electron microscope the extent of the tubular lesions is found to be much greater than with light microscopy, and if the biopsy has been obtained near the onset of the illness marked depositions of fibrin and platelets can be found in the lumen of the glomerular capillaries consistent with intraglomerular capillary thrombosis.

### Aetiological mechanism (Fig. 11.4)

Acute tubular necrosis appears to be initiated by a tansient ischaemic insult which sets in train a set of longer lasting abnormalities in the tubules. The renal ischaemia is due to the raised plasma content of many vasoconstrictors including angiotensin II, catecholamines and vasopressin; and there is also intense renal nerve vasoconstricting activity. In addition there is the powerful local vasoconstricting effect associated with the breakdown of the intravascular thrombi which were formed, initially, as a result of disseminated vascular coagulation. The marked reduction in renal blood flow is accompanied by an even more marked fall in apparent glomerular filtration rate.

If the ischaemia persists beyond a certain critical time or is particularly intense the consequential anoxia causes a reduction in membrane $Na^+$-$K^+$-ATPase activity, mitochondrial respiration and intracellular pH. The former leads to a rise in intracellular sodium and calcium and a fall in intracellular potassium. The rise in the concentration of free calcium and the intracellular acidosis damage the tubule cells. These changes having been set in motion by the ischaemic then continue through the renal blood flow returns to near normal values. The anoxic damage to the tubule cells, however, prevents a parallel rise in glomerular filtration. The persistent reduction in GFR is due to obstruction of the tubule lumina with the debris of proximal cell tubule brush border, cellular oedema, back leak of glomerular filtrate through the walls of the damaged tubules, and a diminution in glomerular permeability. There is also evidence to suggest that persisting obstruction to the lumen of a tubule causes the afferent arteriole of its own glomerulus to constrict, perhaps by preventing the usual flow of prostaglandins along the tubule lumen from the loop of Henle in the medulla (where they are manufactured) to the renal cortex.

It is remarkable that acute renal failure cannot be produced experimentally in animals by a prolonged period of hypovolaemic hypotension (haemorrhagic shock). Possibly it is necessary for there to be the additional vasoconstrictive effect of disseminated intravascular coagulation (which occurs clinically) for the vasoconstriction to be sufficiently intense to

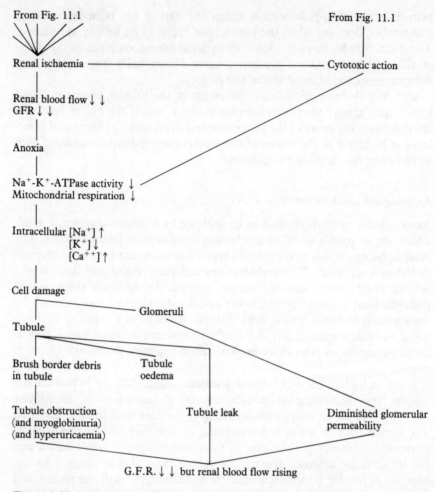

From Fig. 11.1

Renal ischaemia ———————————————————— Cytotoxic action

Renal blood flow ↓ ↓
GFR ↓ ↓

Anoxia

Na⁺-K⁺-ATPase activity ↓
Mitochondrial respiration ↓

Intracellular [Na⁺] ↑
[K⁺] ↓
[Ca⁺⁺] ↑

Cell damage

Glomeruli

Tubule

Brush border debris    Tubule
in tubule              oedema

Tubule obstruction          Tubule leak          Diminished glomerular
(and myoglobinuria)                               permeability
(and hyperuricaemia)

G.F.R. ↓ ↓ but renal blood flow rising

**Fig. 11.4** Mechanisms responsible for persistent functional abnormalities in acute renal failure after initiating insult.

produce irreversible tubular damage. Ischaemic acute renal failure can only be produced experimentally by clamping the renal artery, by an intrarenal infusion of noradrenaline, or by an intramuscular injection of glycerol. Nevertheless even the acute renal failure induced by these Herculean methods, or by the administration of nephrotoxins, can either be prevented or its severity considerably diminished by ensuring that, just before they are used, there is a high solute output by simultaneously giving IV saline or mannitol, or by the administration of frusemide. The exact mechanism whereby a high solute output protects the kidney is not clear. It would certainly sustain the glomerular filtration rate by increasing renal blood flow which together with the high solute output would make the formation of casts more difficult. Very recently a protective effect has been obtained with the use of calcium channel blockers such as verapamil and nifedipine, again if given just before the experimental insult.

## Clinical and biochemical features of acute tubular necrosis

Following the particular episode which has precipitated tubular necrosis and which may be defined at the onset, the natural history of the disorder can be divided into three phases:
1. The oliguric
2. The diuretic
3. The postdiuretic.

### Oliguric phase

The early part of the oliguric phase is frequently unrecognised, for it often begins during a surgical or medical emergency.

A typical example is that of a young patient referred for a nephrological opinion late on a friday afternoon having been admitted several days before suffering from multiple injuries from a car accident. He has been anaesthetised several times for multiple surgical operations. One wound is infected. There may be some evidence of shock lung, and collapse of lung. He has been given, for one or more days, normal quantities of one or more nephrotoxic antibiotics. After the initial attempts to replace blood loss, the amount of plasma and blood which has been administered has been insufficient to cover further losses, whereas the administration of 5% glucose or saline has been too liberal. The patient looks very ill, his face is puffy, pale and moist, perhaps he is cyanosed and he is breathing rapidly and shallowly. He is feverish, has a tachycardia greater than 120/min and a blood pressure around 100/50 mm Hg. His nose and hands are cold. He is hypovolaemic, hyponatraemic, hyperkalaemic, acidotic, anoxic and the blood urea and creatinine are considerably raised because he has acute renal failure and is in a highly catabolic state.

The first clinical indication of incipient renal failure is the onset of oliguria. Anuria does not occur with tubular necrosis. At least 50–100 ml of urine is excreted daily; it is often dark and discoloured by breakdown products of blood, and at first may be thickened by the debris of necrosed tubular cells, yet the specific gravity of this small volume of 'concentrated'-looking urine is nearly always around 1.010, a paradox which confirms the diagnosis. Proteinuria is always present.

The severe reduction in apparent glomerular filtration rate and the tubular damage cause urea, creatinine, potassium, phosphate, sulphate and a considerable quantity of unidentifiable anions (which have been aptly called, for want of a better name, 'anuric anions') to accumulate in the blood and extracellular fluid. There is also an accumulation of hydrogen ions with a fall in plasma pH and bicarbonate. The increase in the concentrations of potassium, phosphate and urea are due to their release from the breakdown of muscle protein. The rate of this release, which is greatest during the first few days of the oliguric phase, largely determines the course of the illness. The rise in plasma potassium is aggravated by the retention of the hydrogen ions, for these tend to be sequestered intracellularly in exchange for potassium ions which are then released into the extracellular fluid. In addition, a fall in arterial oxygen tension (e.g. with a chest infection) may also cause a rapid shift of intracellular potassium into the extracellular fluid and plasma. The immediate danger to life is that the rising concentration of plasma potassium may cause cardiac arrest. This threat is accentuated by the rise in phosphate which lowers the plasma ionised calcium, and, as potassium and calcium ions have opposing actions on heart muscle, the lowered calcium and the raised plasma potassium summate in their ill effects on cardiac function. There is also a rise in plasma magnesium which potentiates the harmful effects of the rise in plasma potassium. The rate of protein catabolism is greatest following injury to muscle, haemorrhage and trauma in the young and healthy; elderly or debilitated patients break down protein at a slower rate. Infection causes a brisk increase in protein catabolism. In most patients protein catabolism is greatest in the first two or three days. On a diet containing about 100 g of carbohydrate per day, and endogenous fat constituting the main source of energy, the average total (endogenous + exogenous) calorie consumption is approximately 2500.

The other major electrolyte disturbance which occurs in the oliguric phase is a decrease in the serum concentration of sodium and chloride. In the past this hypotonicity or overhydration was usually due to an attempt to relieve the oliguria by the administration of large quantities of water; an intuitive therapy based on the naive principle that 'what goes in must come out'. This is a particularly easy trap to fall into for these patients are often extremely thirsty. It has been shown, however, that plasma osmolality gradually falls even if the water intake is limited to an amount which is normally lost by insensible means. At first there was thought to be a shift of sodium into the cells, but it now appears that the most important factor is an increase in the extracellular water. This is derived both from the intake, for the insensible loss of water is below average in these patients, and from 'metabolic water' formed by the endogenous breakdown of protein and fat; a quantity which may amount to 300 ml a day. It is important to recognise the origin of this hypotonicity, for its prevention and correction depends on restricting the intake of water, and trying to diminish the endogenous breakdown of protein and fat, *not* in administering large quantities of normal or concentrated saline intravenously; this only expands the extracellular fluid space and may lead to cardiac failure.

The hypocalcaemia mentioned above is also due to a precipitous fall in plasma $1,25(OH)_2$Vit $D_3$ and a resistance of the bones to the calcium mobilising effect of parathyroid hormone. The low plasma $1,25(OH)_2$Vit $D_3$ certainly causes (1) a diminution in calcium absorption, and it probably causes (2) the resistance of the bones to the calcium mobilising properties of parathyroid hormone and (3) stimulates the parathyroid glands to raise the plasma concentration of parathyroid hormone.

Other changes evident in the blood are the development of anaemia and a leucocytosis. The anaemia develops rapidly, fails to progress beyond a certain severity though the oliguria may continue, and often becomes more pronounced when the blood urea concentration is beginning to fall. The cause of the anaemia appears to be a combination of bone marrow depression and haemolysis.

These many changes in the internal environment can only be diagnosed with certainty by laboratory estimations: they are associated with the following rather vague clinical signs. The fall in plasma pH results in deep regular sighing respirations which are easily recognised. The other electrolyte changes produce signs which are singularly non-specific, even when they are of sufficient severity to threaten the patient's life. Overhydration causes mental dullness and headache, nausea, vomiting and convulsions. It has also been said to cause psychosis and fever. Expansion of the extracellular fluid space is recognised by a rise in jugular venous pressure, oedema, tachypnoea and pulmonary crepitations. The rise in plasma potassium and the fall in plasma calcium concentrations are stated to be responsible for anxiety, restlessness, paraesthesiae and hypotension; these are particularly unreliable signs. Plasma potassium should therefore be measured frequently. Sometimes serial electrocardiograms may be valuable in pre-empting dysrhythmias related to hyperkalaemia. They may be valuable in revealing a rise in plasma potassium. Initially there is 'tenting' of T waves with ST segment depression, flattening of the P wave, and a lengthening of the QRS complex so that it resembles bundle branch block. At higher concentrations of potassium the ECG takes on the appearance of an untidy sine wave and there may be periods of standstill and irregular rhythm. Death occurs from cardiac standstill and ventricular fibrillation. In traumatic cases, particularly those with extensive injury to muscle, the rate of rise of plasma potassium to a lethal concentration may be extremely rapid: a concentration of 6–7 mmol/l rising to 10 mmol/l overnight. The rise in plasma magnesium probably produces some drowsiness and weakness.

Gastro-intestinal disturbances including hiccoughs are frequent during the oliguric phase; their cause is unknown, but they become more severe as the blood urea rises; both vomiting and diarrhoea may occur and they are usually made worse by oral feeding. Occasionally there is haematemesis and melaena. As the oliguric phase lengthens there is a gradual clouding of consciousness, nausea and lassitude, fading into a twitching coma. These features seem to be directly due to the retention of some unidentifiable waste products, for they can be relieved by dialysis even if the concentration of blood urea and identifiable electrolytes are left uncorrected.

A rise in blood pressure is infrequent.

Delayed wound healing and haemorrhage often occur in surgical cases.

Finally, it is important to be aware that these patients are very liable to develop infections which are a common cause of death.

### Diuretic phase

This phase begins when the 24-hour urine volume reaches 1000 ml. Together with the onset of diuresis, the renal blood flow and glomerular filtration rate gradually increase. Sometimes, however, the diuresis begins without any marked changed occurring in either. At first the urine appears to be pure plasma filtrate, for the total concentration of the urine, and of each of its constituents, is identical with that of plasma. As the urine volume increases, the tubules recover some ability to reabsorb salt and concentrate urea so that the urine now contains less salt and more urea than plasma, but the total osmolar concentration still remains about the same as that of plasma. The delay in the return of the ability to concentrate is paralleled by a similar delay in the ability to acidify the urine.

During the first few days of the diuretic phase the patient's general condition changes markedly. There is an increased awareness. Nausea and vomiting cease, and appetite returns. The overall improvement is such that when blood urea estimations are found to be either unchanged or even a little higher than before the onset of diuresis, there is often an atmosphere of disbelief in the accuracy of the estimations. Nevertheless, this is the recurrent pattern of recovery and is another indication that the symptoms of renal failure are not due to the high concentrations of blood urea. The diuretic phase may be a week old before the blood urea begins to fall.

At the height of the diuresis the daily urine volume may be very great (e.g. 6 litre), so that whereas a few days before the patient's life was threatened by an excess of water, salt and potassium, it now appears to be exposed to the perils of dehydration, salt loss and potassium lack. The cause of this extensive diuresis appears to be a combination of three mechanisms: (1) An osmotic diuresis due to the high blood urea; (2) tubular functional inadequacy; and (3) the release of an accumulated surplus of fluid and electrolytes. Obviously if (1) and (2) are responsible for the large diuresis, dangerous electrolyte and water deficiencies may occur, whereas if it is due to (3) it is to the patient's advantage. The urine volume rises to a peak and then falls to normal values.

In some patients, particularly those whose renal failure is due to myoglobinuria the diuretic phase is associated with a transient but sometimes severe hypercalcaemia (Fig. 11.5). This is due to brisk rise in plasma $1,25(OH)_2$Vit $D_3$ before the plasma PTH had returned to normal (Fig. 11.5). The recovering tubule's ability to manufacture $1,25(OH)_2$Vit $D_3$ is stimulated to excess by the raised plasma parathyroid hormone so that there is a sudden brisk risk in calcium absorption from the gut. At the same time the rise in plasma $1,25(OH)_2$Vit $D_3$ lowers the resistance of the bone to parathyroid hormone so that the raised level of plasma parathyroid hormone

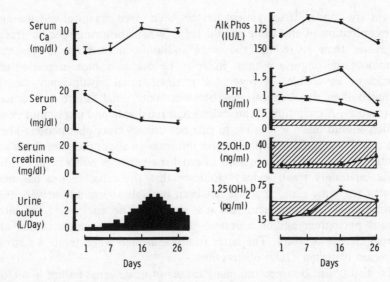

**Fig. 11.5** Graphic representation of biochemical values in six patients at admission and during the oliguric, early polyuric, and late polyuric phases of acute renal failure. PTH estimations, • = carboxy terminal fragment, ▲ = amino terminal fragments. Conversion: traditional to SI units — calcium 10 mg/dl = 2.5 mmol/l: phosphorus 10 mg/dl = 3.2 mmol/l: creatinine 10 mg/100 ml = 880 nmol/l: 25 OH Vit D 20 ng/ml = 50 nmol/l: 1,25(OH)₂Vit D 30 pg/ml = 70 pmol/l. Reproduced from Llach, Felsenfeld, Haussler 1981 New Eng J Med 305: 117, with kind permission.

now mobilizes bone calcium at an unusually rapid rate. The cause of the delayed fall in plasma parathyroid hormone is not clear.

*Postdiuretic phase*

This stage develops imperceptibly from the diuretic phase and is characterised by a normal output of urine although there continues to be some impairment of renal function. Gradually renal blood flow and glomerular filtration rate increase, and the ability to concentrate the urine, and other tubular functions, return towards normal over a period of about one year. Nevertheless, follow-up studies have shown that although renal function is perfectly adequate, full recovery is unusual.

**Differential diagnosis**

A diagnosis of acute intrinsic renal failure is confirmed by trying to make certain that the oliguria and rise in blood urea and creatinine are not due to volume depletion (pre-renal azotaemia) or urinary obstruction (post renal azotaemia). Reversible renal functional insufficiency due to volume depletion may be suspected if the attendant circumstances e.g. diarrhoea, vomiting, a biliary or intestinal fistulae and the patient's recent changes in weight are known. If the patient has not been given mannitol or frusemide an examination of the urine should help. When the urine specific gravity is greater than 1.016 and the urine sodium concentration is less than 20 mmol/l the oliguria is most likely to be due to volume depletion and should be reversible. If reversible intrinsic renal insufficiency can be excluded then the diagnosis lies between acute renal failure and urinary obstruction. A plain film of the abdomen, a renal scan and ultrasound examination should make it possible to rule out urinary tract obstruction. These non invasive techniques will also give information about the size, shape and position of the kidneys. Inequality of renal size suggests reflux nephropathy, while bilaterally small kidneys indicate that the renal failure has been present for some time. If it has not been possible to exclude urinary tract obstruction with these techniques it is sometimes necessary to do an intravenous pyelogram and/or a cystoscopy with ureteric catheterization and retrograde pyelography. The latter is also indicated when there is a strong suspicion of urinary tract obstruction.

To distinguish between the many causes of acute renal failure it is often necessary to do a renal biopsy. It is important not to delay this investigation for in some conditions such as vasculitis or SLE the earlier aggressive treatment with steroids and other agents is begun the better.

Acute renal failure often occurs in a confused clinical setting, as was illustrated by the fictitious case described earlier. There is often more than one possible cause and it may not be possible to decide which is the most relevant. Rhabdomyolysis with myoglobinuria should be suspected from the attendant circumstances e.g. crush injury, prolonged unconsciousness from barbiturate overdose or alcohol, heat stroke etc. At the onset a presumptive diagnosis can sometimes be made if the urine still contains myoglobin. A urinary 'dip stick' will indicate the presence of 'haemoglobin'. If however, the urine is not hypotonic (below a specific gravity of 1.010 or an osmolality below 250 mosmol/kg/$H_2O$) and contains no red cells, and if the colour of the serum is normal while its content of creatinine phosphokinase is raised the diagnosis of myoglobinuria is fairly certain.

If acute renal failure occurs out of the blue in a previously healthy person it is very likely to be due to either to a primary renal disease, or a nephrotoxic poison, often ingested as a suicidal gesture. If on the other hand acute renal failure is preceded by illness it may be due to the use of a some-therapeutic nephrotoxic agent such as an aminoglycoside antibiotics, a non steroidal inflammatory drug or a radiological contrast medium. Acute renal failure from the use of contrast medium is mainly seen in elderly dehydrated diabetics with some pre-existing deterioration of renal function or in dehydrated patients with myelomatosis. Many non nephrotoxic drugs can cause acute renal failure by causing a hypersensitivity reaction in the interstitium of the kidney. This should be suspected from the nature of the drug (e.g. methicillin) and the presence of fever, maculopapular rash, eosinophilia and the presence in the urine of many leucocytes and eosinophils.

## Treatment

The following account is particularly relevant to the treatment of acute tubular necrosis but much of it is applicable to most forms of acute renal failure.

### Treatment of the onset

During the onset of acute renal failure, when there is severe renal ischaemia, but before tubular necrosis has occurred, it should be possible (except in the case of poisons) to prevent necrosis by prompt transfusion, or electrolyte and water replacement, whichever is appropriate. It is imperative that transfusions should not be withheld on the grounds that, as the patient is already suffering from acute renal failure, he should not be exposed to the risks of a mismatched transfusion. It would be as logical to refrain from throwing a lifebelt to drowning man for fear it might hit him on the head. Ideally the patient should never be allowed to become oligaemic long enough for severe renal ischaemia to develop. If acute renal failute does supervene it is essential that its time of onset should be determined as accurately as possible, for though rapid intravenous therapy may be life-saving in the first few hours, 24–48 hours later it may only precipitate pulmonary oedema, cardiac failure and death. It is wise to try and decide by examining a blood film whether the loss of blood has occurred in an already anaemic person, for if such a patient is transfused so that the haematocrit rises above its usual level, renal failure may be aggravated (p. 118), particularly if there is already some degreee of chronic renal structural damage.

When acute renal failure follows diarrhoea and vomiting, pyloric stenosis, etc., electrolyte and water losses should be replaced even though the presence of oliguria makes the dangers of overadministration more likely. In order to find out whether the oliguria is reversible, a litre of saline is given intravenously in one hour; if the urine flow rises to 20–30 ml/hr or more it is reasonable to assume that the oliguria is reversible and to continue the saline administration. In any case it is reasonable to continue to give saline, so long as the jugular venous pressure is closely observed, or preferably if the central venous pressure is measured with a catheter in the superior vena cava. The central venous pressure should not rise above 5–10 cm $H_2O$. The central venous pressure of patients on ventilators, particularly when they are being haemodialysed, should be interpreted with some care.

If volume repletion does not induce an increase in urine flow and there is reason to believe that the oliguria is of recent onset 50 ml of a 25 per cent solution of mannitol can be given intravenously in 5 min, and repeated 30 min later if the urine volume has not risen to 40 ml/hr. If the urine flow does rise repeat boluses of mannitol are given to maintain the diuresis until it is self sustained. Recently it has been claimed that the intravenous administration of dopamine (a powerful renal vasodilator) 1–2 $\mu$g/kg/min for 12 hours can sometimes increase urine flow when oliguria persists after adequate volume repletion (central venous pressure up to 5 to 10 cm of $H_2O$). Frusemide is sometimes used, particularly by the inexperienced but there is no evidence that it is effective, moreover there is something worrying about using a substance to treat acute renal failure which is known to enhance the nephrotoxicity of many of the antibiotics used to treat such patients, and which may cause acute interstitial nephritis on it's own account.

Once it has been decided that the oliguria is irreversible any urinary catheter should be removed from the bladder. From then on the patient's progress is best observed, and clinical decisions are best made, from an inspection of the patient and his plasma biochemical changes, not forgetting his weight which should be measured 4 to 6 times a day (much to the bewilderment of the staff of some intensive care wards). Now that there are commecially available bed weighing machines that are both reliable and small, it is preferable to monitor the patient's weight continuously. It must be stressed that obsessional attention to the urine flow diverts attention away from the patient. In addition the persistent presence of a catheter in a bladder almost invariably causes a urinary infection. If the urine volume is around 300 ml per day or above there will usually be spontaneous bladder voiding at least once a day, if it is below this it is insufficient to influence decisions about treatment.

*Treatment of the oliguric phase*

The aim of treatment during the oliguric phase is to keep the internal environmental normal until the kidneys recover. It is clear that this aim is limited by two factors: (I) the rate at which the internal environment changes, which is mainly dependent on (*a*) the rate of catabolism, and (*b*) the efficacy of treatment; and (2) the duration of the oliguria. If the internal environmental changes relatively slowly, and the oliguria does not last more than two to three weeks, conservative treatment may be sufficient. But if the internal changes are rapid or the oliguria prolonged then it may be imperative to supplement conservative treatment with dialysis. In practice it is the rate of change that is most liable to vary, and this in turn is largely determined by the extent of the associated trauma and infection. When there is no trauma, e.g. following abortion and poisoning, the rise in blood urea and potassium are often so gradual that conservative treatment is adequate. But with extensive trauma, e.g. gunshot wounds and road accidents, deterioration is so rapid that dialysis is usually necessary. This dissimilarity is not only due to probable differences in the rate of catabolism but also to the fact that traumatic cases, and particularly war casualties, are liable to have large quantities of intracellular products released from non-viable muscles which have been overlooked during débridement.

Whatever means are employed to treat acute renal failure, plasma electrolytes, urea and glucose should be estimated at least once a day; the daily urine volume should be measured and its content of electrolytes and glucose estimated. If the patient is being treated by dietary means and not being dialysed he should lose 0.2–0.5 kg per day, for this is approximately the weight of endogenous solids which are metabolised each day.

## Conservative treatment

This form of treatment is mainly for patients in whom the duration of the acute renal failure is likely to be short, the catabolic rate is not raised, and appetite is relatively good e.g. in obstetric cases and non oliguric acute renal failure.

*Control of water intake.* As soon as it is considered that the patient is not deficient in water, the intake of water is limited to 500 ml a day, plus a quantity equal to the amount of urine passed in the previous 24 hours. The total amount is increased in very hot weather and if there is much sweating. The amount of water required is best gauged by the patient's weight and the effective plasma osmolality (i.e. total osmolality less the osmolality due to the urea content); if it is not possible to estimate the plasma osmolality plasma sodium is a less exact but useful substitute. The weight should fall gently while the plasma osmolality or sodium concentration should not change. Unfortunately, the patient's persistent thirst is no guide to his needs.

*Control of electrolyte intake.* Following any initial replacement that may be necessary the further ingestion or administration of electrolytes (except for calcium) must be prevented.

The plasma concentration of potassium should be kept below 6 mmol/l. Some authorities have suggested that this can be done by the intravenous administration of calcium gluconate and insulin (50 units per day) throughout the 24 hours. The latter, in association with a high glucose intake (see below), tends to draw the potassium into the cells and so lower plasma potassium. This is certainly true on a short-term basis, but it is impractical over a prolonged period. Resins in the sodium phase or preferably in the calcium phase are used to lower plasma potassium; the dose is 15 g two to four times a day orally, or 60 g as a retention enema. The most satisfactory way to lower plasma potassium temporarily in an emergency is to give 200 ml of molar sodium lactate intravenously in three hours. The rise in extracellular pH induces a compensating shift of hydrogen ions from the intracellular compartment and this in turn causes potassium to pass from the extracellular space *into* the cells.

The fall in plasma sodium and chloride should be treated by limiting the fluid intake for, unless there is a very clear indication of sodium and chloride loss before the onset of renal failure, its administration in order to correct plasma concentrations is potentially dangerous. This also applies to any attempt to correct the acidosis by giving sodium bicarbonate or sodium lactate, for the dangers of expanding the extracellular fluid volume and causing cardiac failure are greater than any benefit gained by altering the pH. In any case, if such electrolyte cosmetics are thought to be desirable, they are usually better carried out by dialysing the patient.

*Control of protein, carbohydrate and fat intake.* With conservative treatment protein intake should be controlled. Nevertheless a protein-free diet is repugnant and the patient often needs the nitrogen. In addition, it has been shown that if the carbohydrate intake can be maintained at a high level (around 200 g per day) 20–40 g of protein per day will not influence the rate of rise of blood urea; and the patient feels much better. The additional potassium intake which this involves can be controlled with resins.

Carbohydrates should be free of electrolytes. They are given to slow the rate of endogenous protein breakdown and minimise the rise in plasma potassium concentration (see above). 100 g of carbohydrate per day will reduce endogenous protein breakdown by 50%. Additional amounts up to 400 g per day will further reduce protein breakdown. The use of Hycal (Beecham) which contains 400 calories of carbohydrate as disaccharides and dextrose in 180 ml of water is of help, and most patients find this palatable. Caloreen, a soluble glucose polymer, is a useful alternative for patients who find Hycal unpalatable. Anabolic steroids (Nilevar, 16-Ethyl-19-*nor* testosterone or Durabolin, 19-*nor* testosterone-17β phenyl propionate)are sometimes used to delay protein breakdown particularly in obstetric cases.

*Control of Infection.* The likelihood of infection is so great that some centres now treat all patients with acute renal failure in isolation. Antibiotics are not given unless an infection develops, It must be remembered that with many antibiotics the dose has to be adjusted.

*Therapeutic measures to avoid.* The frustration of seeing a patient gradually dying from acute renal failure, who may have been recently saved from death by an emergency operation, has in the past prompted the use of certain useless and dangerous measures. They are enumerated here, so that the lessons of the past shall not be forgotten.

1. The intravenous administration of large volumes of osmotic diuretics or the attempt to force a diuresis by overexpansion of the extracellular fluid space with large quantities of intravenous saline used to cause cardiac failure.

2. Encouraging the patient to drink large quantities of water while giving 5% glucose intravenously caused water intoxication and pulmonary congestion.

3. Renal decapsulation and paravertebral block; the trauma of the first procedure hastened the rise in blood urea, while the second caused hypotension.

None of these measures were beneficial; some were lethal.

*Dialysis*

If the patient is unable to, or won't, eat, or there is a blood urea which is rising rapidly, paralytic ileus, recent abdominal surgery, severe hypo-albuminaemia, or acute or chronic respiratory failure he should be dialysed. There is no question but that this is best done with haemodialysis by an experienced group, and that the ideal method is for the patient to be fed entirely parenentally and be dialysed each day. In this way it is possible to give the large amounts of calories necessary to control protein breakdown, and to attempt to replace the nitrogen losses. With this technique wound healing is quicker and deaths are fewer.

Haemodialysis must start before the blood urea is greater than 30–35 mmol/l (180–210 mg/100 ml) to reduce the risk of subsequent fatal haemorrhages into the gastrointestinal tract or into the pericardium. Daily dialysis not only controls the plasma concentration of urea, potassium etc. but also, by removing fluid by ultrafiltration, reduces the extracellular fluid volume and thus creates a 'space' into which the large intravenous volumes necessary for total parenteral nutrition can be placed without overloading the patient's circulation. Accordingly it is possible via a venous catheter placed centrally to give around 3500 calories per day in 2400 ml of fluid containing 9.4 g of nitrogen (Table 11.1). When protein loss is severe it may be necessary to give up to 8000 calories and 18 g of nitrogen per day.

**Table 11.1** Specimen average daily requirement for a patient with acute renal failure being fed entirely parenterally.

|  | ml | Calories |
| --- | --- | --- |
| 900 ml of 50% Dextrose | 900 | 1800 |
| 500 ml of 20% Intralipid | 500 | 1000 |
| 1000 ml of 'Vamin' glucose | 1000 | 650 |
| Total | 2400 | 3450 |

The blood sugar is controlled by giving 1 to 5 units of soluble insulin hourly by a constant infusion pump intravenously according to blood sugar levels which are measured frequently by a bedside technique. The high glucose intake and the associated insulin will lower the protein catabolic rate from around 300 g/day to 130 g/day which then makes it easier to keep up with the loss of nitrogen. The amino acid infusion (Vamin glucose) is given after a dialysis. Otherwise the amino acids tend to be lost into the dialysis fluid. It is also best to give the intralipid soon after a dialysis. In this way there is at least 12–16 hours before the morning specimen of blood when it can be observed whether the fat has been removed from the circulation. If it hasn't, the daily amount of intralipid should be lowered. Plasma protein fraction (PPF) or plasma is given during dialysis to raise serum albumin and to compensate for the obligatory loss of amino acids across the dialysis membrane.

Daily dialysis and parenteral feeding make it necessary to supply water soluble vitamins, particularly folic acid, the body stores of which are rapidly depleted. In the absence of gastrointestinal loss a dialysate concentration of 1 mmol of magnesium is sufficient to maintain a normal plasma magnesium. If there are gastrointestinal losses of magnesium they are replaced by additions of magnesium sulphate into the Vamin glucose solution (10 ml of 10% magnesium sulphate contains 4 mmol of magnesium) Phosphate depletion may also occur but on the whole is prevented by the 15 mmol of phosphate contained in the 1 litre of 20% intralipid. If plasma phosphate falls below normal a mixed phosphate infusion can be given.

It is important, when starting haemodialysis in a patient with a very high blood urea, not to try and lower it too quickly. This may cause severe headaches, vomiting, fits and unconsciousness. This is due to the fact that during the dialysis the changes in the content of urea and bicarbonate in the brain lag behind those in the blood. This causes two cerebral disturbances. The first is due to the content of urea in the brain falling move slowly than in the blood. This causes an osmotic gradient. Water diffuses into the brain and there is cerebral oedema. The second is due to the brain bicarbonate rising more slowly than the blood bicarbonate. The rise in blood bicarbonate is associated with a reduction in ventilation and a rise in blood $P_{CO_2}$ towards normal. As $CO_2$ is readily diffusible, $P_{CO_2}$ in the cerebrospinal fluid rises at the same rate as in the blood. In the cerebrospinal fluid, however, there is now a relatively unchanged low bicarbonate but a rising $P_{CO_2}$ with the result that the already low pH falls to even lower levels (Fig. 11.6).

For most patients suffering from acute renal failure who are in need of dialysis peritoneal dialysis is a poor substitute for haemodialysis. In many adult patients it is totally inadequate. For children however, peritoneal dialysis is the method of choice. The trouble with peritoneal dialysis, in contrast to haemodialysis, is that though it looks easy it is full of risks. These include peritonitis, pain, leakage around the abdominal catheter, incomplete drainage of the dialysate out of the peritoneal cavity so that the patient becomes overloaded. Dissection of the abdominal wall, wound dehiscence and perforation of a viscus may also occur. In addition pulmonary collapse of the bases and lung infection are quite common. And it is unusual for the patient to have a good appetite so that there is a tendency to try and give the large amounts of calories and protein needed by stomach tube.

*Treatment of the diuretic phase*

With conservative treatment it is vital that the strict regimen of the oliguric phase should be continued until the blood urea begins to fall. Frequently a partial recovery with a daily urine volume of about 700 ml may progress no further for several days; it is imperative that during this time treatment should not be relaxed.

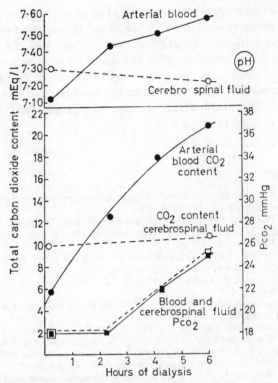

**Fig. 11.6** Changes in pH, total $CO_2$ content of arterial blood and cerebro-spinal fluid brought about by haemodialysis (reproduced from Lambie, Anderton & Robson, 1964 Blackwell Scientific, Oxford with kind permission).

Once the diuretic phase begins the dangers to look out for and correct are water depletion, salt loss and potassium loss. It has become clear that often much of the polyuria which these patients experience is only the evacuation of excess extracellular fluid. And attempts to replace it only prolong the diuretic phase and may lead to overhydration. An exact replacement should not, therefore, be attempted unless there is evidence of need. It is more important to be guided by the patient's general condition, pulse rate, blood pressure, thirst and plasma electrolyte content than by the urine volume and its content. Intravenous therapy and dialysis are stopped unless there is nausea, vomiting, confusion or coma. The patient is encouraged to eat a high potassium, high salt diet, and given easy access to large amounts of water.

## Prognosis

The prognosis of acute renal failure depends on the initiating cause and its associated circumstances (e.g. multiple injuries), the severity of the renal lesion and the efficiency of treatment. It is fair to say, however, that whereas there was a mortality of about 90% before the introduction of conservative treatment and artificial dialysis, it is now nearing 40%. In obstetric and medical cases the mortality is rather less than 15% whereas in surgical cases it is usually greater than 50%. In some of the most advanced centres, however, the mortality in surgical cases has been brought down to between 10 and 30%. 20% of all deaths are due to infection, and it contributes significantly in another 60%.

BIBLIOGRAPHY

Bank N, Mutz B F, Aynedjian H S 1967 The role of leakage of tubular fluid in anuria due to mercury poisoning. J Clin Invest 46: 695

Boen S T 1964 Peritoneal dialysis in clinical medicine. Thomas, Springfield

Brown C B, Ogg C S, Cameron J S 1981 High dose frusemide in acute renal failure: a controlled trial. Clin Nephrol 15: 90

Burke T J, Cronin R E, Duchin K L et al 1980 Ischaemia and tubule obstruction during acute renal failure in dogs: mannitol in protection. Amer J Physiol 238: F305

Cattell W R, McIntosh C S, Moseley I F et al 1973 Excretion urography in acute renal failure. Brit Med J 2: 575

Clarkson A R, MacDonald M K, Fuster V et al 1970 Glomerular coagulation in acute ischaemic renal failure. Quart J Med 39: 585

Counahan R, Cameron J S, Ogg C S et al 1977 Presentation, management, complications and outcome of acute renal failure in childhood: five years experience. Brit Med J 1: 599

Cowie J, Lambie A T, Robson J S 1962 The influence of extracorporeal dialysis on the acid-base composition of blood and cerebrospinal fluid. Clin Sci 23: 397

Cronin R E, de Torrente A, Miller P. D. et al 1978 Pathogenic mechanisms in early norepinephrine — induced acute renal failure: Functional and histological correlates of protection. Kidney Int 14: 115

Donohoe J F, Venkatachalam M A, Bernard D B et al 1978 Tubular leakage and obstruction after renal ischaemia: structural — functional correlations. Kidney Int 13:208

Farber J L 1981 The role of calcium in cell death. Life Sciences 29: 1289

Jackson R C 1970 Exercise-induced renal failure and muscle damage. Proceedings of the Royal Society of Medicine 63: 566

Kaplan S A, Fomon S J 1953 Function recovery pattern in acute renal failure following ingestion of mercuric chloride. Amer J Dis Child 85: 633

Kew M C, Abrahams C, Levin N W et al 1967 The effects of heatstroke on the function and structure of the kideny. Quart J Med XXXVI: 277

Kumar R, Hill C M, McGeown M G 1973 Acute renal failure in in the elderly. Lancet i: 90

Llach F, Felsenfeld A J, Haussler M R 1981 The pathophysiology of altered calcium metabolism in rhabdomyolysis — induced acute renal failure. New Eng J Med 305: 117

Lowe K G 1952 The late prognosis in acute tubular necrosis. Lancet i: 1086

Mason J, Beck, F, Dorge A et al 1981 Intracellular electrolyte composition following renal ischaemia. Kidney Int 20: 61

Mason J, Kain H, Shiigai T et al 1979 The early phase of experimental acute renal failure. V The influence of suppressing the renin-angiotensin system. Pfluger's Arch 380: 233

Myers B D, Hilberman M, Spencer R J et al 1982 Glomerular and tubular function in non-oliguric acute renal failure. Amer J Med 72: 642

Oken D E 1981 On the differential diagnosis of acute renal failure. Amer J Med 71: 916

Oken D E 1975 Role of prostaglandins in the pathogenesis of acute renal failure. Lancet i: 1319

Oliver J 1953 Correlations of structure and function and mechanisms of recovery in acute tubular necrosis. Amer J Med 15: 535

Oliver J, MacDowell M, Tracy A 1951 The pathogenesis of acute renal failure associated with traumatic and toxic injury: renal ischaemia, nephrotoxic damage, and the ischaemuric episode. J clin Invest 30: 1305

Rainford D J 1981 Nutritional management of acute renal failure. Proceedings of the 2nd European Congress of Parenteral and Enteral nutrition. Acta Chirugica Scandinavia Suppl 507: p 327

Richman A V, Narayan J L, Hirschfield J S 1981 Acute interstitial nephritis and acute renal failure associated with cimetidine therapy. Amer J Med 70: 1272

Roxe D M 1980 Toxic nephropathy from diagnostic and therapeutic agents. Amer J Med 69: 759

Sevitt L H, Evans D J, Wrong O M 1971 Acute oliguric renal failure due to accelerated (malignant) hypertension. Quart J Med 40: 127

Saxton H M, Kilpatrick F R, Kinder C H et al 1969 Retroperitoneal fibrosis. A radiological and follow-up study of 14 cases. Quart J Med 38: 159

Sheehan H L, Moore H C 1953 Renal cortical necrosis and the kidney of concealed accidental haemorrhage. Blackwell Scientific Pubs, Oxford

Shubin H, Weil M H 1965 The mechanism of shock following suicidal doses of barbiturates, narcotics and tranquillizer drugs, with observations on the effects of treatment. Amer J Med 38: 853

Stein J H, Lifschitz M D, Barnes L D, 1978 Current concepts on the pathophysiology of acute renal failure. Amer J Phys 234(3): F171

Swann R C, Merrrill J P 1953 The clinical course of acute renal failure. Medicine 32: 215

Thiel G, McDonald F D, Oken D E 1970 Micropuncture studies of the basis for protection of renin depleted rats from glycerol induced acute renal failure. Nephron i: 67

Wardener de H E 1955 The intrarenal pressure in experimental tubular necrosis. Lancet i: 580

Wardle E N 1976 The functional role of intravascular coagulation renal disease. Scottish Med J 21: 83

Wilson D M, Turner D R, Cameron J S et al 1976 value of renal biopsy in acute intrinsic renal failure. Brit Med J 2: 459

# 12

# The nephrotic syndrome

A nephrotic* syndrome is a clinical state in which there is a combination of oedema, proteinuria and hypoproteinaemia, irrespective of aetiology or any other clinical features. This definition stresses the occasional clinical similarities of many unrelated diseases, for the nephrotic syndrome may occur in any of the following conditions: glomerular nephritis, anaphylactoid purpura, disseminated lupus, polyarteritis nodosa, malaria, amyloid disease, diabetes, renal vein thrombosis, cardiac failure, the administration of certain drugs such as troxidone (Tridione) and mercurial compounds (teething powders), it may also occur as a congenital condition.

## STRUCTURAL CHANGES

The changes depend in part upon the aetiology of the nephrotic syndrome. Biopsy studies with the light microscope have shown that the nephrotic syndrome can occur without any changes in the glomerulus. Observations with the electron microscope, however, have shown that even in those biopsies in which there are no changes to be seen with the light microscope there are unequivocal alterations in the cytoplasmic extensions of the epithelial cells (p. 23), and in the basement membrane.

The tubule changes vary widely; they are most marked in the proximal tubules. Some are dilated and lined with flattened pale cells with poorly staining nuclei, while others appear to be occluded by large swollen tubule cells containing vacuoles and much fatty material. Often there are no changes apparent on light microscopy.

---

* The term 'nephrotic syndrome' is blessed by usage and though opinions differ on its exact definition it is clinically useful. Perhaps in time it may be replaced by some more rational substitute such as 'proteinuric hypoproteinaemia' or 'protein losing kidney'. The term 'nephrosis' however, particularly 'lipoid nephrosis', has little justification. Jean Oliver's well-known broadside against the use of the work 'nephrosis' begins '. . . that etymologically absurd and conceptually obfuscatory term nephrosis'. He continues: 'This curious barbarism was introduced by the clinician Friedrich Muller, apparently because to his ear *osis* had the proper antithetical ring to *itis* and so seemed appropriate as a sort of counter-term to nephritis. The suffix *osis* had at the time an accepted meaning, to be full of, as in lipoidosis or carcinomatosis, so that by all the custom and usage of medical nomenclature nephrosis means full of kidney

## FUNCTIONAL CHANGES

In addition to oedema, proteinuria and hypoproteinaemia, the blood lipids are usually raised and the serum calcium reduced. There may also be changes in renal function.

*Oedema* is due to the kidney excreting less sodium in the urine than is being ingested by mouth. And this in turn is due to increased sodium reabsorption in the distal part of the nephron by some unknown intrarenal mechanism, presumably related to the pathological process responsible for the proteinuria (p. 287). There is little evidence that even when the proteinuria is so severe that it leads to a fall in plasma and blood volume and a consequential rise in plasma renin activity and aldosterone that these extrarenal salt retaining influences have any additional salt retaining effect. Hypoproteinaemia per se is of trivial importance in causing generalised oedema. This is well illustrated in patients with hereditary analbuminaemia who have no oedema and in some young patients whose plasma albumin is less than 10 g/l who, nevertheless, have little or no oedema. Presumably in such patients the increased capillary filtration which should accompany the fall in plasma protein osmotic pressure is prevented by some peripheral vascular adjustment which causes a fall in hydrostatic capillary pressure, or the lymphatic system rapidly drains away the increased formation of interstitial fluid.

### Plasma volume

Renal retention of sodium increases the extra vascular volume and at first there is an increase in plasma volume and blood volume with a fall in plasma renin activity and aldosterone. As the proteinuria and hypoproteinaemia become more pronounced however, the plasma volume returns to normal or falls below normal, in spite of a continuously expanding extra-cellular fluid volume. The use of diuretics in such patients, particularly if they cause a rapid daily loss of more than 2–3 kg per day may precipitate such a fall in blood volume that the patient develops severe postural hypotension with all its sequelae such as fits and cardiac arrest.

The blood volume in the nephrotic syndrome shows another interesting phenomenon. It is that upon standing the blood volume may shrink in an exaggerated manner. A fall of blood volume of up to 1000 ml has been recorded. It is possible therefore that for a large part of the day the blood volume of a patient with a nephrotic syndrome is well below the volume measured with the patient lying in bed. It is not surprising therefore that such patients, even when they are not being given diuretics, tend to suffer from mild postural hypotension and faint easily.

Normally there is a continuous leak of albumin molecules through all capillaries which are returned to the plasma via the lymphatics. The dynamic equilibrium of this movement is such that the total quantity of the relatively dilute albumin in the extracellular fluid is approximately the same as the total quantity of the more concentrated albumin in the plasma. The fall in plasma oncotic pressure which accompanies hypoproteinaemia increases capillary filtration, and the resultant increase in flow of plasma filtrate into the intestitial space stimulates lymphatic peristalsis and lymph flow. Paradoxically, however, hypoproteinaemia diminishes capillary permeability to albumin. Thus in hypoproteinaemia less albumin leaks out of the capillaries but what does get through is returned to the plasma more quickly. The net result is that hypoproteinaemia causes a significant amount of albumin to be mobilised from the extracellular fluid into the plasma with a fall in the ratio of extracellular fluid total content of albumin to the plasma's total content of albumin. A useful compensatory mechanism.

## Protein metabolism

Hypoproteinaemia is due to a fall in the albumin fraction of the total plasma proteins, and albumin concentrations below 10 g per litre are sometimes seen. The concentrations of the globulins, however, are liable to increase (except for the smaller globulins) so that if total proteins only are estimated the severity of the decrease in albumin concentration may be disguised. Nevertheless, because globulin molecules are larger and heavier than those of albumin the plasma protein osmotic pressure falls. There is a rough correlation between the appearance of oedema and the plasma albumin concentration, the dividing line being about 25–30 g/l. Today urinary excretion rate of albumin and globulins is usually above 5 g/day, and is often as much as 10–15 g/day. In addition there is a urinary loss of amino acids, the nitrogen content of which may be half the total amount of nitrogen lost as protein. The relation between urinary excretion of protein and plasma albumin concentration is shown in Figure 12.1.

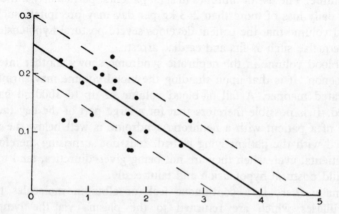

**Fig. 12.1** Relation between reduced serum albumin concentration (abscissae g/100 ml) and daily albumin losses in urine (ordinates g/kg body weight) (reproduced from Squire, Blainey and Hardwicke 1957 Brit Med Bull with kind permission).

The excess nitrogen lost in the urine causes a negative nitrogen balance which, clinically becomes evident as muscle wasting. There is a paradox, however, that the amount of albumin excreted in the urine is usually much less than the maximum which can be synthetised (up to approximately 26 g/day/70 kg man), and yet the total quantity of albumin contained in the plasma and extracellular fluid is considerably reduced, before there is much loss of muscle protein. For instance a plasma albumin concentration of below 10 g/litre can occur in patients only excreting 6–8 g albumin/day. In other words hypoproteinaemia is due, at least in part, to some mechanism, other than the nitrogen loss in the urine. There must be either an increased breakdown or a loss of albumin at some other site. Faecal loss of albumin is not raised. There is therefore an increased breakdown of albumin. The site of this destruction appears to be the proximal tubule. 'Early' proximal tubule fluid in the dog contains about 5 g/l of albumin. Assuming the same concentration in man and a total 24 hr glomerular filtration rate of 180 litres there is normally a tubular reabsorption of around 9 g/day of protein. This is achieved by endocytosis and lyosomal digestion of the albumin and globulins to polypeptides and amino acids. These then diffuse out of the cell, some into the urine and the bulk into the blood in the peritubular capillaries. When glomerular permeability is increased, because of glomerular disease, the increased delivery of protein into the proximal tubule causes a marked increase in the amount of protein being reabsorbed and destroyed. In this way large quantities of albumin can be destroyed without loss of nitrogen.

The pattern of plasma protein concentration in the nephrotic syndrome reflects the preferential passage of lower molecular weight proteins through the diseased glomeruli, and compensatory synthesis. In addition to the low plasma albumin the concentration of other low molecular weight proteins is also reduced, e.g. Vitamin D binding proteins, antithrombin III, transferrin, ceruloplasmin and thyroxin-binding globulin. On the other hand the plasma concentration of large globulins such as alpha-2 macroglobulin, and beta globulin is increased as is that of fibrinogen. None of these appear in the urine and their synthesis is increased perhaps as a side effect of the increase in albumin synthesis. The fall in plasma concentration of gamma globulins and complement proteins are probably responsible for the well-known liability of the nephrotic patient to infection, and the reason why immunisation procedures for polyomyelitis, influenza, tetanus and diphtheria often do not produce satisfactory levels of antibody.

*Proteinuria*. The proteins that appear in the urine are qualitatively the same as those in the circulating blood and in oedema fluid. Proteinuria usually exceeds 5 g/day and characteristically fluctuates widely from day to day, being particularly sensitive to posture and exercise; daily excretions of up to 60 g/day are sometimes seen but the usual rate is 10–15 g/day; it is largely independent of the rate of urine flow. The daily urine volume obviously depends on whether oedema is forming, remaining unchanged or being evacuated. The large quantities of protein being reabsorbed through the proximal tubule cells cause the structural changes in the tubules and these in turn are responsible for the urinary excretion of fatty casts and doubly refractile lipid bodies. It is probable that the changes in the proximal tubules are the cause of the glycosuria which so often accompanies a nephrotic syndrome.

If an immunological technique for the estimation of the albumin in the urine is available, it is possible to dispense with the frustration inherent in trying to collect all the urine passed in a 24-hour period in order to get an index of the extent of the proteinuria. Instead, the albumin to creatinine ratio of a random sample of urine is estimated. In healthy subjects the ratio is well below one whereas in patients with the nephrotic syndrome it is well above one. This boundary is sometimes used to delineate the point at which a relapse or a remission has occurred. With this technique the progress of the proteinuria is easily and accurately followed with a sensitivity which is difficult to achieve in any other way.

*Selective permeability.* The quantity of protein that is excreted, if expressed in terms of its clearance (i. e. the amount of protein excreted per minute divided by its plasma concentration) correlates well with its molecular weight; the smaller the molecular weight, the greater the clearance. In some patients the clearance of large molecular proteins, when compared to the simultaneous clearance of small molecular proteins is greater than in others. Those in whom the clearance of large molecular proteins is high have been defined as having a non-selective proteinuria. The semantics are unfortunate, for clearly the proteinuria cannot select anything. Selective permeability of the kidneys would be more comprehensible way to express the phenomenon.

Selective permeability is measured by comparing the clearance of a large molecule with that of a small one. One way of doing this is to compare the clearances of IgG (CIgG) and albumin (Calb) measuring both these substances with immunological techniques. Thus

$$\frac{CIgG}{Calb} = \frac{UIgG \times V}{PIgG} \bigg/ \frac{Ualb \times V}{Palb}$$

where C = clearance, U = urine, P = plasma, and V=urine flow, and this formula resolves so that V is eliminated and

$$\frac{CIgG}{Calb} = \frac{UIgG}{PIgG} \bigg/ \frac{Ualb}{Palb} \times 100$$

This is most convenient (see p. 43), for a timed collection of urine is not necessary, and selective permeability can then be estimated on any random sample of urine. The ratio CIgG/Calb is the selective permeability and if this is multiplied by 100 it can be expressed as a percentage. In practice the following sub-divisions are useful. Highly selective permeability lies below 15%, moderate selective permeability between 15 and 30%, and poorly selective permeability is greater than 30%.

The quantitative pattern of the proteinuria, i.e. the selective permeability of the kidneys, must derive from the disease process in the kidney. It is hardly surprising, therefore, to find that there is some correlation between the selective permeability of the kidneys and the biopsy findings. As might be expected patients whose kidneys have insignificant histological changes tend to have highly selective permeability and those in whom there are unequivocal histological abnormalities usually have non-selective permeability. The selectivity of the permeability is unrelated to the total amount of protein excreted per day, it remains unchanged during wide fluctuations in protein excretion, and it does not change as the disease progresses. It is interesting that selective permeability remains unchanged even in those patients in whom the proteinuria is reduced by administration of steroids. This suggests that the proteinuria is not due to a simple enlargement of the pores in the basement membrane for if that were the case a diminution of proteinuria would be accompanied by a shrinkage of these pores and a progressive return of selective permeability towards normal.

### Hyperlipidaemia

Total plasma fat, cholesterol, tri-glycerides, and phospholipids are all raised in the nephrotic syndrome. Plasma free fatty acids concentration remains normal. The concentration of total fat in the plasma may reach 20 g/1, with cholesterol concentrations of 26.0 mmol/1 (1000 mg/100 ml). These rises are inversely related to the change in plasma albumin concentration, more specifically to changes in plasma oncotic pressure. A rise in plasma albumin to normal therefore is usually associated with a reciprocal fall in plasma cholesterol whether the rise in plasma albumin is due to a spontaneous remission, treatment with prednisone or the onset of chronic renal failure. Occasionally, however, the plasma cholesterol level may remain elevated for some months after the concentration of plasma albumin has returned to normal. The normal daily urinary excretion of fats is less than 10 mg. In the nephrotic syndrome it may rise to 1000 mg. It appears to be mainly due to the hyperlipidaemia. The cystallisation of cholesterol esters gives rise to the classical birefringent urinary crystals.

The mechanisms responsible for the hyperlipidaemia are obscure. In an experimentally induced nephrotic syndrome in the rat there is an increased synthesis of liporotein by the liver, This overproduction may be due to the increase in albumin synthesis, for the two processes share a common metabolic pathway. The urinary loss of protein lipid-clearing factors may also be important.

### Calcium metabolism

In a nephrotic syndrome unaccompanied by renal failure there is profound hypocalcuria and such a fall in intestinal calcium absorption that often the content of calcium in the faeces is greater than that contained in the diet. There is also a fall in plasma calcium which is principally due to the fall in plasma proteins, but there is also a fall in ionised calcium. Children may develop tetany. These abnormalities are the same as those which take place in chronic renal failure without a nephrotic syndrome. The impairment in calcium absorption from the gut is probably due to the diminished plasma $1,25(OH)_2Vit\ D_3$ but whereas in chronic renal failure the fall in plasma $1,25(OH)_2Vit\ D_3$ is due to a loss of nephrons, in the nephrotic syndrome it is more likely to be due to the digestion and passage of large quantities of protein through the proximal tubule cells, the site of $1,25(OH)_2Vit\ D_3$ production. Hypocalcaemia is due, in part at least, to the malabsorption of calcium, but it is mainly due to the lack of $1,25(OH)_2Vit\ D_3$ at the bone which impairs the calcium mobilising powers of parathyroid hormone.

In contrast to chronic renal failure however, the concentration of plasma $25OHVitD_3$ is low because of the loss of Vit D binding globulin (see above). The fall in plasma $25OHVitD_3$, if prolonged can cause osteomalacia, but this is a rare complication presumably because the usual duration of a nephrotic syndrome is relatively short.

## Potassium metabolism

Many patients have some degree of potassium deficiency and hypokalaemia. It is due to (a) the use of diuretics, resins and steroids, (b) anorexia (c) and in approximately half the patients a raised plasma aldosterone.

## Coagulation

The raised plasma levels of lipoproteins, cholesterol and fibrinogen, and the low antithrombin III levels favour the likelihood of intravascular clotting. In addition the platelet count may be elevated and they may show an increased predisposition to aggregate. These changes probably account for the increased incidence of venous thrombosis which occurs in the nephrotic syndrome, particularly in the renal veins. An increased thrombotic effect in the arteries as evidenced by intermittent claudication, angina and coronary artery deaths however, is more contentious. The excess incidence of these complications, if it exists, seems to be marginal.

## Renal function

All degrees of renal functional efficiency or impairment are seen with the nephrotic syndrome. Some patients, particularly children, have a raised renal blood flow and glomerular filtration rate, while others have varying degrees of renal failure. Because of the negative nitrogen balance the concentration of urea in the blood may be much lower than is expected from the rate of glomerular filtration; this can be very misleading if renal function is being judged only by estimations of the blood urea. On the other hand, it is important to remember that some patients have particularly high creatinine to inulin clearance ratios, and that in such patients a creatinine clearance may be more than double the true glomerular filtration rate. In those patients who have a supernormal filtration rate, very low concentrations of blood urea 1.5 to 2.5 mmol/l (10–15 mg per 100 ml) are seen. If the deterioration of renal function is gradual, proteinuria sometimes diminishes and the oedema recedes. This is presumably because the rate of protein excretion is proportional to the filtration rate, and if this falls sufficiently the negative protein ceases. Often, however, as renal failure advances proteinuria and oedema remain unchanged.

## CLINICAL PICTURE

The incidence of the nephrotic syndrome in relation to age and sex depends largely on its aetiology. The cases can be divided into those in whom the renal lesion is primary, and those in whom it is only a feature in a more generalised disease. The primary lesions are more common in children and men under the age of 60; whereas when the lesion is a feature in a generalised disease the patients are mainly adults and the disease is equally distributed between the sexes.

Whatever the cause of the nephrotic syndrome the onset of oedema is usually gradual and fluctuating. At first there is occasional swelling of the ankles in the evening, or of the face in the morning. There may be transient attacks of more obvious oedema which rapidly disappears.

Eventually, after an interval of weeks or months, oedema persists and recovery from each exacerbation is less complete. When the condition is advanced the accumulation of fluid appears to be controlled only by the skin's limited ability to stretch. The legs and arms are unsightly lobulated balloons, shiny and pale; the abdomen protrudes both with oedema of the subcutaneous tissues and ascites; the face is spherical, bloated and disfigured particularly by circumorbital oedema, the eyes becoming pink pustular horizontal slits between distended eyelids. Pleural effusions are present, and oedema of the scrotum or vulva may produce huge swellings. The oedema is always soft and pits easily with little pressure.

As the oedema accumulates there is an increasing feeling of lethargy and weakness: And when there are pleural effusions there is dyspnoea. Headache is common and, for reasons which are not understood, patients with the nephrotic syndrome frequently have recurrent 'colds' which, though they rarely mature beyond a sore throat and transient nasal obstruction, are often associated with an acute exacerbation of oedema and proteinuria. Bacterial infections also occur frequently and affect principally the skin, the lungs and the peritoneum. When ascites is present there may be sudden attacks of abdominal pain simulating bacterial peritonitis, but laparotomy shows only a few strands of fibrin and sterile fluid; the pain settles gradually after operation. Anorexia and diarrhoea frequently occur and, although oedema of the stomach and intestinal mucosa may be partly responsible for both, it is clear that eventually the anorexia is also due to the state of advanced malnutrition. The latter is probably also the cause of (1) the lowered basal metabolic rate, for the thyroid gland function has been found to be normal, and (2) the occasional presence of anaemia in the absence of renal failure.

The combination of anorexia, increased secretion of aldosterone, treatment with adrenal steroids, and the use of diuretics (particularly chlorothiazide) may sometimes cause severe potassium deficiency with depression of glomerular filtration rate and functional distrubances of the tubule (p. 361).

### Diagnosis

The fact that a patient is suffering from a nephrotic syndrome is easy to observe; its cause is usually more difficult to ascertain. It is suspected from the attendant circumstances and some help can be obtained from renal biopsy. Sometimes the correct diagnosis is only obtained in retrospect or at autopsy. Congenital nephrotic syndrome appears within a few days of birth and is fatal in early childhood. Heterozygotes can be identified during pregnancy in families who have previously had an affected child. The amniotic fluid and maternal serum alpha-fetoprotein is raised.

### Prognosis

The course of the nephrotic syndrome largely depends on its cause; it varies from complete recovery to death from renal failure; it may last only a few weeks or, with remissions and relapses, up to 20 years. In general, the prognosis is better in women than it is in men, and in the young rather than the elderly. Remissions of oedema may occur at any time and may last several months, with persistent proteinuria as the only continuing evidence of disease. Sometimes such a remission may appear complete, with no protein in the urine and yet relapse takes place several years later. Renal failure, hypertensive cardiac failure with malignant hypertension, and intercurrent infections are the usual causes of death. There may be periods of transient hypertension and microscopical haematuria, but these signs, unless they are persistent or severe, do not necessarily imply advancing destruction of the renal parenchyma. Conversely, gradual structural obliteration often takes place without proteinuria diminishing. Renal biopsy may establish the diagnosis. It is of some limited value in prognosis. For instance if the glomeruli appear normal the prognosis is excellent whereas if there are many crescents death occurs within a year.

## Treatment of the initiating condition

This is rarely successful. Cessation of troxidone administration, the surgical removal of a septic focus, which is giving rise to renal amyloidosis, and the treatment of an infection such as syphilis and malaria are some of the exceptions. In addition there is the successful treatment of Hodgkins disease or the removal of a malignant tumor. Unfortunately, however, the cause of the nephrotic syndrome is seldom amenable to treatment, and usually therapy has to be aimed at a lower or more symptomatic level. Such symptomatic treatment, however, is ocassionally followed by a long-lasting remission or even complete recovery.

## Treatment of the proteinuria and salt retention with prednisone

The administration of adrenal steroids to some patients causes a rapid diminution in proteinuria, and there is a large diuresis and loss of oedema. Presumably the diminution in proteinuria is due to some alteration in glomerular permeability. The following account of the use of prednisone is mainly applicable to patients suffering from a nephrotic syndrome due to glomerular nephritis. It is now established that the only form of the nephrotic syndrome in this disease which will consistently respond to prednisone is that in which the renal biopsy shows that the glomeruli are normal on light microscopy (see later). But it must be pointed out that in this group of patients the natural incidence of fairly rapid spontaneous remissions is about 65%. Nevertheless it is usually worthwhile, in children particularly, to try to cut short the dangers of hypovolaemia, protein depletion and oedema. In adults however the complications of prednisone therapy tend to outweigh its advantages.

### Adrenal steroid therapy in children

It is claimed, but not substantiated, that the best response is obtained with large doses. The aim is not only to get rid of the oedema but also to make the urine free of protein. No treatment is given for one week period unless a coincident infection has to be controlled with an antibiotic. Very occasionally, within that time, there is a spontaneous diuresis and proteinuria may disappear or diminish greatly. If proteinuria is then less than 1 g/day no treatment is required but careful supervision should continue, for severe proteinuria usually recurs within two years. Treatment with steroid is divided into two stages: (1) treatment of the first attack, (2) treatment of the relapse.

*Treatment of the first attack* is planned to last 4–8 weeks. As large doses of steroids are administered it is advisable to keep the child in hospital. Care should be taken, however, to keep him away from others with septic conditions such as eczema and tonsillitis. Treatment starts with a high dose of prednisone. The exact amount recommended appears to be falling with the years. At one time a dose of 6–8 mg/kg/day was used. In the continual absence of any controlled trials to ascertain the correct dosage the amount given appears to be decided by personal idiosyncrasy tempered by an inchoate feeling that the very large doses that were given in the past were unnecessarily dangerous and no more effective. Now 1–3 mg/kg/day is recommended, given in three equally divided doses throughout the day until the urine is free of protein or until the end of the fourth week. The same dose is then given on alternate days or half the dose is given each day for a further three weeks. In the following the dose is tailed off and stopped. Up to 97% of children with minimal change glomerular nephritis will respond to this regime. If there has been no response to this course it is probable that the evaluation of the renal biopsy was wrong, and that it does contain some glomerular abnormalities which have been missed. This usually becomes obvious later on a subsequent biopsy. If there has been no response to an eight week course of prednisone it is best to discontinue its use. The possible side effects include hypertension, oedema, cardiac failure, a rising blood urea, infection, potassium depletion, or mental changes. These are rare, and more common in adults but nevertheless the blood pressure, weight, and jugular venous pressure should be observed each day and periodic electrolyte estimations should be made. It is also evident that the contraindications to steroid therapy are cardiac failure, severe hypertension and advanced renal failure; dyspnoea from large pleural effusions is another contraindication. Even when treatment is eventually successful there may be little change in the first seven days except for fluid retention. There is then a gradually increasing diuresis and a marked fall in proteinuria (Fig. 12.2); in the most successful cases there is also a rise in glomerular filtration rate. Prophylactic oral antibiotics (penicillin V) are sometimes given throughout the period of heavy dosage together with potassium supplements (potassium chloride 1–3 g/day), a small amount of calcium and vitamin D, and as much protein as the child will eat. No added salt is allowed. If there is a diuresis it is usually followed by an increase in weight and a phenomenal increase in appetite.

*Treatment of a relapse.* 50 to 80% of those in whom the first course of prednisone produces a remission will have a relapse subsequently. This may occur within days or after several years. If the relapses are so frequent that steroids cannot be stopped it may be possible to control the disease with the continuous administrations of a small dose daily, or on alternate days (e.g. 5 mg). If the amount of steroids which has to be given becomes unacceptable to the patient, parent or the doctor the administration of cyclophosphamide should be considered (see below). Supplements of calcium and potassium are always given during the administration of prednisone.

Nephrotic children frequently have a remission of oedema following an accidental attack of measles. For this reason children were sometimes exposed to measles deliberately. The results were probably due to an increased endogenous secretion of adrenal steroids but they did not seem

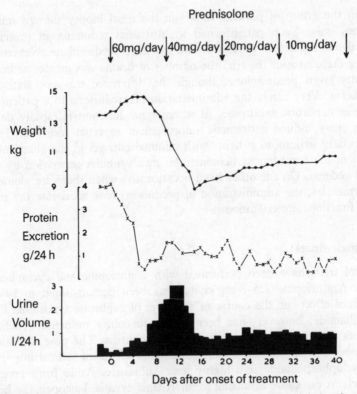

**Fig. 12.2** Treatment of nephrotic syndrome with very large amount of prednisolone in a child with minimal glomerular nephritis. Note the loss of weight early during the administration of prednisolone, preceded in this patient by a profound fall in proteinuria.

any better than after the administration of exogenous adrenal steroids; and measles is certainly far less pleasant for the child.

### Adrenal steroids in adults

In adults deterioration of renal function, and hypertensive side effects of prednisone administration are more common than in children. In addition, large doses may cause acute perforation or haemorrhage from a peptic ulcer, acute psychosis, or reactivation of an old tuberculous lesion. Therefore the amount of prednisolone given to adults with a nephrotic syndrome are considerably less than those given to children.

In a Medical Research Council trial on the use of prednisolone in adults with primary glomerular nephritis 20–30 mg/day of prednisolone was used for at least two months. In patients with unequivocal abnormalities in the glomeruli the course of the disease, and in particular the diminution in proteinuria was the same as in the control patients who did not receive prednisolone. The only advantage gained by the administration of prednisolone was in the group of patients in whom the renal biopsy showed minimal changes only. Such patients had a substantial reduction in proteinuria several months before those who did not have prednisolone. Nevertheless during the course of the trial the number of deaths was greater among the patients given prednisolone, though the difference was not statistically significant. Very rarely the administration of prednisone to a patient with a severe nephrotic syndrome, in whom renal function is rapidly deteriorating, may induce a dramatic improvement in renal function. This is particularly striking in patients with minimal changes in the glomeruli but in whom the renal biopsy demonstrates much tubular seperation by interstitial oedema. On the other hand occasionally, when there are glomerular abnormalities, the administration of prednisone may accelerate the rate of renal functional deterioration.

## Cytotoxic drugs

Control trials have been performed with azathriopine and cyclophosphamide. Azathriopine 2.5–3 mg/kg/day has been demonstrated to have no beneficial effects on the course of any form of nephrotic syndrome. Cyclophosphamide, however, has been shown to confer immense benefits on patients with minimal change glomerular nephritis. The dose, duration of treatment and the timing of its introduction are all of critical importance for cyclophosphamide is a highly toxic substance. Aside from reversible alopecia, it can cause agonising haemorrhagic cystitis, leucopenia, a heightened susceptibility to common viruses (e.g. varicella and measles) and gonadal changes which can be irreversible. There is also the possibility that it may induce leukaemia or a lymphoma.

For these reasons cyclophosphamide is only considered when it has been demonstrated previously that either steroids are ineffective, or more usually, that they have to be given so often and at such high concentrations that they may cause, or have caused, undesirable side effects such as a cushionoid appearance with stunting of growth, hypertension, osteoporosis etc. Cyclophosphamide is then introduced, preferably at the height of a prednisone induced remission and its administration is continued thereafter at a moderate dose until the cyclophosphamide is stopped. 2.5–3 mg/kg/day of cyclophosphamide is given in three divided doses throughout the day for eight weeks. At this dose alopecia is uncommon but with the use of a wig both the patient and the parents accept this temporary unsightliness with equaminity. Photographs of recently bald patients who now have a healthy head of hair also help. The white count should be monitored but at this dose leucopenia is uncommon. Long term assessment of gonadal function in men over the age of 18 years who had received cyclophosphamide during childhood has shown that they now had low ejaculate volumes and sperm densities with an abnormally high percentage of immobile and abnormal forms, but that these abnormalities were never so severe as to suggest infertility. Gonadotrophic hormones were normal.

60% of those treated with such a course of cyclophosphamide will not relapse during the next five years. Earlier relapses may be treated with another course of cyclophosphamide preferably after a one year interval. It is interesting that the 40% of individuals who relapse early after a course of cyclophosphamide have a higher incidence of HLA–B$_{12}$. They also have a high incidence of atopy.

### Treatment of the negative protein balance

The necessity for a high protein diet cannot be overemphasised, for it is imperative that the negative protein balance should be corrected.

The only limit to positive nitrogen balance that can be achieved by these patients is their own capacity for protein ingestion. It has been demonstrated that the rate of proteinuria is not affected by high intakes of protein and there is no evidence that renal function suffers in any way, though in patients with an initially depressed glomerular filtration rate it is important to watch the blood urea. A rising blood urea in these circumstances is, of course, no evidence of a further depression in filtration rate.

Adults should, and can, eat 150–200 g of protein a day, which is not difficult if protein concentrates are used, and salt restriction is not too severe (see below). In the early stages of a nephrotic syndrome anorexia may be severe, but it can often be abolished by prednisone, even if a short course fails to produce any other immediate benefit. It has been shown that a high protein diet, continued for several months, and accompanied by a large accumulating nitrogen balance may at first produce no change in plasma protein concentration or oedema, although the plasma volume is gradually increasing.

### Treatment of low blood volume

It has been mentioned earlier that the blood volume is reduced in only half the patients who present with a nephrotic syndrome. And that even in this group the compensatory increase in the circulating concentration of angiotensin and aldosterone does not contribute to the sodium retention and oedema. Nevertheless when in such a patient the blood volume is further reduced rapidly with powerful diuretics the hypovolaemia may now become so pronounced that it induces a rapid deterioration of renal function. Conversely, correcting a state of hypovolaemia may sometimes make the action of a diuretic more effective. The intravenous administration of albumin is the best way to increase the blood volume. The amount given is empirical e.g. for an adult 200 ml of a 20% solution each day for several days. Packed red cells which, as a blood volume expander should also be useful, are seldom given because of the nephrotic patient's liability to allergic reactions, unless the cells are washed with 5% glucose. For the same reason it is unwise to use infusions of whole blood.

## Treatment of the renal tubule's increased salt reabsorption

Salt and water retention can be minimised by decreasing the salt intake, or increasing the excretion of faecal sodium by giving cation exchange resins; or it may be directly countered by increasing the urinary excretion of sodium with diuretics.

*Dietary salt content.* The amount of salt in the diet should be related to the severity of the oedema and the ease with which it can be controlled with diuretics. In many long-standing cases of the nephrotic syndrome, in whom proteinuria and oedema fluctuate slowly over a period of months, the dietary salt can be adjusted according to the weight chart. When oedema is increasing rapidly it may be imperative to give a 'salt-free' diet. Otherwise the ideal is to give as much salt as the patient can easily excrete; it is often an unnecessary burden to give less, and it increases the difficulties of maintaining a high protein diet. One of the great advantages of the wide range of potent oral diuretics now available is that the dietary control of sodium intake need not be nearly as rigid as it used to be. If renal failure supervenes and the oedema clears it may be important to remember to tell the patient to increase his intake of salt, otherwise he may develop salt deficiency which will aggravate the renal failure.

The difficulties of giving a diet low in salt and yet high in protein can be overcome to a certain extent by the administration of low-sodium concentrated protein preparations such as Casilan, and the use of diuretics or ion exchange resins.

*Diuretics.* The guiding principle to follow is to use that amount of diuretic which will cause a diuresis that is not too precipitous and which preferably does not cause a negative balance of potassium. Failure to produce a diuresis with one diuretic is an indication to add a second. In order to minimise the urinary loss of potassium, treatment is begun with spironalactone and triampterene. Chlorothiazide can be added later and frusemide or bumethanide later still. The dose of oral frusemide is doubled each day until a diuresis is provoked or until the dose has reached 1000 mg per day. If a diuresis has not occurred by this time (which is very exceptional) the large amounts of frusemide are continued (some of it intravenously), while at the same time the blood volume is expanded. A simultaneous intravenous infusion of manitol at this moment gives the *coup de grâce* to any so-called 'diuretic resistant oedema' At the onset of treatment body weight must be measured each day; it is a far better guide to water balance than an 'input-output' chart. Plasma potassium should also be measured every other day.

Once the oedema has disappeared the diuretics should be rapidly cut back in the reverse order in which they were given so that if it is found necessary to continue with diuretics the patient is discharged on spironolactone and/or triampterene. Spironolactone should be avoided, however, in patients with renal failure for they are apt to develop hyperkalaemia. Chlorothiazide and its derivatives and frusemide are dangerous drugs to use in the treatment of patients suffering from a nephrotic syndrome once they are out of hospital. If diuretics are given, potassium supplements must continue to be supplied, but there is no certainty that such supplements will be either ingested or adequate. Plasma potassium concentrations must therefore be measured from time to time. Patients out of hospital are best given chlorothiazide or frusemide intermittently, e.g. on two days a week or an alternate days. On occasion the loss of oedema is associated with diminution or disappearance of proteinuria, a rise in glomerular filtration rate, and a return of plasma proteins to normal.

*Resins.* These are mainly used when there is hyperkalaemia (which is unusual) and a need for the rapid removal of potassium as well as sodium. A cation resin (Katonium, BDH) 75% in the ammonium phase and 25% in the potassium phase, is given orally 15 g four times a day, for an adult. In the small intestine the ammonium and potassium on the resin are exchanged for an equivalent amount of the patient's sodium; but much of this sodium is again exchanged for potassium in the large bowel. The net result is a negative balance of sodium and potassium, and the production of an acidosis from the absorption of ammonium (p. 97). The kidney should be able to prevent the tendency to develop an acidosis by increasing the excretion of ammonia and free hydrogen ions (p. 98). If it is not able to do this adequately an increasing acidosis develops. Cation resins in the calcium phase can also be used. They avoid the acidosis, deplete the body of potassium and sodium, and also contribute some calcium to the patient. They are particularly useful when the patient is suffering from renal failure. Their prolonged use however, may cause hypercalcaemia.

*Dangers of removing oedema fluid too rapidly.* The danger resides in the immense potency of modern diuretics and the variable susceptibility of patients to their effect. It must be remembered that for some patients a dose of 40 mg of frusemide may produce a massive diuresis, a profound loss of weight and symptomatic hypovolaemia with nausea and dizziness due to postural hypotension. This, at best will only cause a reversible deterioration of renal function which admittedly may sometimes take the form of acute oliguric renal failure. At worst however the combination of hypovolaemia and potassium deficiency may be lethal. If the patient faints, the sudden fall in blood pressure releases large quantities of catecholamines into the blood, which in the presence of hypokalaemia can cause ventricular fibrillation, a functional arrest of the heart and death.

### Treatment of the increased capillary filtration and local oedema

The increase in capillary filtration which takes place at all capillary surfaces as a result of the decreased plasma protein osmotic pressure can be minimised below the knees by wearing elastic stockings. In some subjects, particularly young women who have a relatively well-controlled nephrotic syndrome, such a measure may enable them to go out in the evening without looking too conspicuous.

### Treatment of the infections

Though the use of antibiotics does not counteract a specific link in the aetiology of nephrotic oedema, their introduction in recent years has nevertheless been the main factor responsible for the longer survival of patients suffering from the nephrotic syndrome. Such patients seem particularly liable to develop infections, and in turn the infections seem to be more severe and are nearly always associated with an acute exacerbation of the nephrotic syndrome. In order to avoid infections oral penicillin is sometimes given daily as a prophylactic; alternatively the patient is given a short course of a wide-spectrum antibiotic (e.g. cephalexin, or trimethoprim/ sulphamethoxazole (Septrin)) to take home, to be used at the first sign of an infection.

### Synopsis of treatment

Treatment is started with a low salt, high protein diet. Prednisone is given to children in whom the renal biopsy shows the glomeruli to be normal. The administration of prednisone to adults, whatever the renal histology, is hardly justifiable. When prednisone is given, a remission of the proteinuria should occur within two months. If this does not take place within that time prednisone should be discontinued.

Diuretics are given in sufficient amounts to cause a diuresis. If this is unsuccessful, a plasma expander such as 1 l of 10% Dextran or 5% albumin can be given during the administration of the diuretics. Potassium depletion and hypokalaemia frequently occur with nausea, thirst and faintness are useful premonitory symptoms. Supplements of potassium should be used. Antibiotics should be given at the first sign of infection. They can also be given prophylactically.

A high protein diet must be used with some caution when there is renal failure.

In order to be aware of the progress of events it is useful to insist on the following being measured and recorded once a day: (1) body weight; (2) blood pressure *lying and standing*; (3) fluid intake and output, excluding food and faeces. When there are rapid changes in weight, the haematocrit should be measured every day, and at this time plasma potassium and sodium should be measured on alternate days, with plasma urea and creatinine at least twice a week. When the patient is stabilised these estimations can be made less and less frequently. Urinary protein excretion should be measured once a week until the patient is stabilised. Plasma albumin concentration should be measured at least once in two weeks; it is probably the best guide to progress.

## Long term results of treatment

There seems little doubt that the duration of survival is now longer than it was and that in adults this change is due to the use of antibiotics and a high protein diet and the availability of more powerful diuretics. In children, it is still uncertain whether the beneficial effects of prednisone have contributed to the improved survival. There has not yet been a controlled trial of the use of steroids in children.

BIBLIOGRAPHY

Ahlinder S, Birke G, Liljedahl S T O et al 1964 Protein losses studied with double isotope technique. Physiology and patho-physiology of plasma protein metabolism. Proceedings of the 3rd Symposium at Grindelwald, Switzerland. Huber, Bern
Barragry J M, Carter N D, Beer M et al 1977 Vitamin-D metabolism in nephrotic syndrome. Lancet 2: 629
Barratt T M, Bercowsky A, Osofsky S G et al 1975 Cyclophosphamide treatment in steroid-sensitive nephrotic syndrome of childhood. Lancet 1: 55
Barrait T M, McLaine P N, Soothill J F 1970 Albumin excretion as a measure of glomerular dysfunction in children. Arch Dis Child 45: 496
Black D A K, Rose G, Brewer D B 1970 Controlled trial of prednisone in adult patients with the nephrotic syndrome. Brit Med J: 421
Blainey J D 1954 High protein diets in the treatment of the nephrotic syndrome Clin Sci 13: 567
Blainey J D, Brewer D B, Hardwicke J 1979 Proteinuria and the nephrotic syndrome. In: Black D, Jones N F (ed) Renal disease. Blackwell Scientific Publishers, Oxford, p 383
Bourdeau J E, Carone F A 1974 Protein handling by the renal tubule. Nephron 13: 22
Brenner B M, Hosteller T H, Humes H D 1978 Molecular basis of proteinuria of glomerular origin. New Eng J Med 298: 826
Brown, E A, Markandu N D, Roulston J E et al 1982 Is the renin-angiotensin-aldosterone system involved in the sodium retention in the nephrotic syndrome? Nephron 32: 102
Cameron J S, White R H R 1965 Selectivity of proteinuria in children with the nephrotic syndrome. Lancet 1: 463
Chamberlain M J, Pringle A, Wrong O M 1966 Oliguric renal failure in the nephrotic syndrome. Quart J Med 35: 215
Chopra J S, Mallick N P, Stone M C 1971 Hyperlipoproteinaemias in the nephrotic syndrome. Lancet 1: 317
Dirks J H, Clapp J R, Berliner R W 1964 The protein concentration in the proximal tubule of the dog J Clin Invest 43: 916
Earley L E, Forland M 1979 The nephrotic syndrome. In: Earley L E, Gottschalk C W (eds) Strauss and Welt's diseases of the kidney, 3rd edn. Little Brown, Boston, p 765
Eisenberg S 1963 Postural changes in plasma volume in hypoalbuminaemia. Arch Int Med 112: 544
Fawcett I W, Hilton P J, Jones N F et al 1971 Nephrotic syndrome in the elderly. Brit Med J 2: 387

Garnett E S, Webber C E 1967. Changes in blood-volume produced by treatment in the nephrotic syndrome. Lancet 2: 798

Gitlin D 1957 Some concepts of plasma protein metabolism. A.D. 1956 Pediatrics 19: 657

Ichikawa I, Rennke H G, Hoyer J R et al 1983 Role for intrarenol mechanisms in the impaired salt excretion of experimental nephrotic syndrome. J C Invest 71: 91–103

International study of kidney disease in children. Primary nephrotic syndrome in children: Clinical significance of histopathologic variants of minimal change and of diffuse mesangial hypercellularity. Kidney Int 20: 765

Jensen H 1969 Plasma protein metabolism in the nephrotic syndrome, vol 1. Munksgard, Copenhagen

Kaitz A L 1959 Albumin metabolism in nephrotic adults. J Lab Clin Med 53: 186

Kauffmann R H, Veltkamp J J, van Tilburg, N H et al 1978 Acquired antithrombin III deficiency and thrombosis in the nephrotic syndrome. Am J Med 65: 607

Lim P, Jacob E, Tock E P et al 1977 Calcium and phosphorus metabolism in nephrotic syndrome. Quart J Med 46: 327

Mallick N P, Short C D 1981 The nephrotic syndrome and ischaemic heart disease. Nephron 27: 54

Malluche H H, Goldstein D A, Massry S G 1979 Osteomalacia and hyperparathyroid bone disease in patients with nephrotic syndrome. J Clin Invest 63: 494

Seppala M, Rapola J, Huttunen N P et al Congenital nephrotic syndrome: prenatal diagnosis and genetic counselling by estimation of amniotic-fluid and maternal serum alpha-fetoprotein. Lancet 2: 123

Stanbury S W, Macaulay D 1957 Defects of renal tubular function in the nephrotic syndrome. Quart J Med N S 26: 7

Strober W, Waldmann T A 1974 The role of the kidney in the metabolism of plasma proteins. Nephron 13: 35

Thomson C, Forbes C D, Prentice C R M et al 1974 Changes in blood coagulation and fibrinolysis in the nephrotic syndrome. Quart J Med 43: 399

Trompeter R S, Evans P R, Barratt T M 1981 Gonadal function in boys with steroid-responsive nephrotic syndrome treated with cyclophosphamide for short periods. Lancet 1: 1177

Wass V, Cameron J S 1981 Cardiovascular disease and the nephrotic syndrome: the other side of the coin. Nephron 27: 58

Yamauehi H, Hopper J 1964 Hypovolaemic shock of hypotension as a complication in the nephrotic syndrome. Report of ten cases. Am Intern Med 60: 242

# 13

# Chronic renal failure

Chronic renal failure consists of a persistent impairment of both glomerular and tubular function of gradual onset and of such severity that the kidneys are no longer able to keep the internal environment normal. This definition includes mild asymptomatic functional impairment, which is sometimes called 'chronic renal impairment'.

Chronic renal failure follows a great number of conditions which devastate the kidney. Its clinical features, however, are remarkably uniform, for usually renal failure is simply due to a deficiency of nephrons, and a fairly fixed combination of disturbances is inevitable. It is in fact the exceptions to this recurring pattern which cause curiosity, for example, when the blood pressure does not rise and yet at autopsy the kidneys are found to be small and fibrous.

## Vicious cycle mechanisms in renal failure

There is increasing evidence that loss of nephrons, from whatever cause, begets further destruction of nephrons. This may explain the inexorable progress of renal failure in so many patients, and why in patients with progressive renal failure from glomerular nephritis, it is often difficult to find evidence of any continuing active immunological disturbance. This vicious cycle of events appears to be due to several mechanisms.

*Adaptative changes in glomerular haemodynamics* Removal of five-sixths of a rat's renal mass results in proteinuria, hypertension, progressive renal failure and advanced glomerulosclerosis in the remnant kidney. In the early stages, before the onset of systemic hypertension there is a fall in afferent arteriolar resistance resulting in a large compensatory increase in glomerular blood flow and filtration rate in the remaining nephrons. This is associated with a considerable rise in capillary hydrostatic pressure and an increase in the permeability of the capillary wall. These changes cause more of the plasma's *non diffusable* contents to be pushed into and through the capillary walls. Some of this material is disposed of by the mesangial cells, and some appears as proteinuria. It has been suggested that glomerulosclerosis occurs when the mesangial cells become overloaded and can no longer 'clean up' the capillary walls. These changes are more marked the higher the protein intake perhaps because there is a direct relation between protein intake and renal blood flow.

*Direct effect of hypertension on glomerular structure and function.* Reduction in renal mass leads to vasodilatation and hypertrophy, it also tends to cause salt and water retention and a rise plasma angiotensin II which lead to hypertension (p. 261). The rise in arterial pressure superimposed on the dilated afferent arterioles aggravates the glomerulosclerotic process described above. This process will occur in those areas of the renal vasculature that remain fully dilated. In other areas however, in which the arterioles and smaller renal arteries are partially occluded by hypertensive intraluminal proliferation the glomeruli become sclerosed from ischaemic shrinkage.

*Phosphate retention.* The progress of renal failure in an experimental animal with a remnant kidney is less rapid if the animal's phosphate intake is reduced. Some of this beneficial effect may be due to the low phosphate diet preventing secondary hyperparathyroidism (p. 192) with which is associated a laying down of calcium and phosphorus in the kidney.

A loss of nephrons brings out many other adaptive mechanisms. It is remarkable, for instance, that though a patient's glomerular filtration rate may fall to 10 ml/min plasma sodium, potassium, phosphate, bicarbonate, phosphate and uric acid may be in the normal range. In order to achieve this constancy the tubular handling of each of these substances has to be adjusted by specific mechanisms, most of which have not yet been identified. It is possible, however, that the presence of some of these adaptive mechanisms, persistently acting at an abnormal rate may have secondary harmful effects, e.g. the raised concentration of parathyroid hormone which helps control plasma phosphate.

## CAUSES OF CHRONIC RENAL FAILURE

1. Destructive disease due to some immunological disturbance
   Glomerular nephritis
   Polyarteritis nodosa
   Disseminated lupus erythematosus
   Subacute bacterial endocarditis
   Anaphylactoid purpura

2. Infection
   Reflux nephropathy
   Tuberculosis

3. Obstruction to the urinary tract
   Prostatic obstruction
   Bilateral calculi
   Urethral valves, etc.

4. Congenital lesions
     Polycystic disease
     Tubular abnormalities (final stages)

5. Hypertension
     Malignant
     Non-malignant

6. Others
     Phenacetin nephropathy.
     Amyloid
     Gout
     Diabetic nephropathy
     Hypercalcaemia
     Chronic intermittent haemoglobinuria: (a) sickle cell; (b) nocturnal
     Renal vein thrombosis
     Myelomatosis

Any other renal diseases which eventually destroy the nephrons, e.g. tubular changes associated with metallic cation loss.

There are certain selective disturbances of tubular function in which initially there is little or no evidence of a decline in the number of nephrons. These syndromes are usually named after the particular disturbance of tubular function involved, i.e. familial nephrogenic diabetes insipidus, they are discussed elsewhere (p. 350).

## SIGNS AND SYMPTOMS

Chronic renal failure is characterised by a wide variety of biochemical disturbances and numerous clinical signs and symptoms. It is one of the outstanding peculiarities of chronic renal failure that some of the biochemical abnormalities do not appear to cause any symptoms, while most of the clinical abnormalities have no known biochemical cause.

The following account of chronic renal failure is divided into two parts. The first describes the biochemical abnormalities that have been identified and the clinical manifestations that they cause; the second describes the many clinical features of unknown cause.

### Biochemical features and their clinical manifestations

*Water metabolism*

Thirst and nocturia occur frequently, polyuria is less common. The symptoms are due to a diminished capacity to concentrate the urine and to a loss of the normal diurnal rhythm of urinary excretion. Often the ability to make the urine hypotonic remains for some time after the ability to concentrate has almost disappeared; later the urine concentration remains fixed at the same osmolality as plasma, a phenomenon known as isosthenuria.

Though inability to make the urine hypertonic may be due in part to a diminished functional capacity of the nephrons which remain, it is mainly due to an increased rate of solute excretion per nephron. This is an explanation which has been advanced earlier (p. 70) but which can be elaborated here. It is evident that in chronic renal failure the total solute output remains almost unchanged, for the patient is usually in normal electrolyte and water balance, and yet nearly always there is a considerable reduction in the number of functioning nephrons. It follows, therefore, that each surviving nephron must be handling much larger quantities of solutes and water than normally. This is a situation similar to that obtaining in each nephron of a dehydrated normal person who has been given a large quantity of a solute, such as sucrose, mannitol or urea which is then promptly excreted in the urine: the rate of solute excreted per nephron increases, and there is a concomitant rise in urine flow and *fall in urine concentration*, i.e. there is an osmotic diuresis (p. 70). The impaired ability to concentrate the urine in chronic renal failure is mainly due to an osmotic diuresis. It follows that this apparent impairment in the kidney's ability to concentrate the urine is not necessarily an indication that the nephrons are diseased but that they are less numerous.

In chronic renal failure there is frequently an increased turnover of water and the ability to dilute the urine remains normal or better than normal for a considerable time. But there is diminished ability to excrete a water load rapidly. This occurs before, as well as after, the ability to make the urine hypotonic has disappeared. When it is present before, it is presumably due to the diminished number of nephrons, for even if each nephron forms a hypotonic urine at a normal rate there is an insufficient number to increase the total urine flow adequately. This is the reason why polyuria is never gross in chronic renal failure and seldom exceeds 3–4 1/24 hours, in contrast to the 8–10 litres found in diabetes insipidus, or compulsive polydipsia. When the kidneys can no longer form a hypotonic urine the inability to excrete a water load is easier to understand.

These disturbances make patients suffering from chronic renal failure vulnerable to acute changes in water balance. Diarrhoea and vomiting may quickly cause severe dehydration, for the output of water and salt does not drop as sharply as in the normal; conversely, an impetuous intravenous administration of water (5% glucose) may cause overhydration. Sometimes slight nausea with a distaste for eating and drinking is sufficient to cause dehydration, when a vicious circle of increasing renal failure, more pronounced nausea, and further dehydration then occurs.

*Sodium metabolism*

It has already been pointed out that as the number of nephrons diminishes each remaining nephron reabsorbs a smaller proportion of the filtered sodium so that urinary sodium excretion remains unchanged and the patient's sodium balance is undisturbed. The fall in sodium reabsorption is associated with and may be due to a rise in a natriuretic hormone/circulating sodium transport inhibitor. The diminution in sodium reabsorption is certainly not due simply to a convenient deterioration of function of the nephrons that remain, for urinary sodium excretion can be altered by changing the dietary salt intake, or by heart failure and haemorrhage.

As renal failure advances, however, disturbances of sodium balance may occur. The ability to adjust to sudden changes in salt and water loss becomes progressively less efficient. An attack of diarrhoea or a spell of anorexia and vomiting do not cause a compensatory reduction in urinary sodium output. There is instead a continued urinary loss of sodium and water, a contraction of the extracellular fluid volume, an intense renal vasoconstriction and thus a severe deterioration of renal function. This sudden sequence of relatively gross changes is easily recognised. It may cause death.

An insidious change in sodium balance, however, is more common and is usually far more difficult to discern. There may be a very slow but progressive overall loss of sodium. This causes a reduction of extracellular fluid volume and a very gradual reduction of renal function. A mild negative sodium balance in chronic renal failure is associated with an increased secretion of aldosterone, a tendency to a low plasma potassium, and a normal blood pressure. It is, in fact, a useful generalisation that if a patient with advanced renal failure has a normal blood pressure he probably has a urinary sodium leak. In other words, in contrast to the majority of patients with renal failure in whom the loss of nephrons causes an increasing difficulty in excreting sodium these patients have renal lesions which in spite of the nephron loss causes them to have a difficulty retaining sodium.

Severe urinary sodium leaks which give rise to severe sodium deficiency cause hypotension, rapidly advancing renal failure, thirst and anorexia. The syndrome is then called 'salt losing nephritis'. Patients with urinary sodium leaks often have polyruria. The diseases which tend to cause this syndrome include phenacetin nephropathy, polycystic kidneys, chronic urinary obstruction, and occasionally, when the urine is infected, reflux nephropathy. Disturbances of sodium metabolism are best detected clinically along the lines outlined in Section 17. Some patients with chronic renal failure may slide from a state of sodium retention to one of urinary sodium leak or vice versa (Figs 13.1 and 13.2). It is important to be aware of this possibility for the treatment of the two conditions is diametrically opposed. It must also be stressed that disturbances of sodium metabolism are poorly reflected by changes in the concentration of plasma sodium which more often reflect changes in hydration. The concentration of plasma sodium is therefore not a guide to the size of the extracellular fluid volume, or the exchangeable sodium.

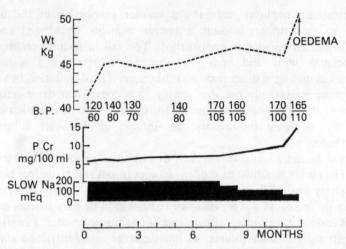

**Fig. 13.1** Changes in weight and blood pressure in a patient with chronic renal failure and a sodium leak. Terminally the blood pressure and the weight rose though the sodium supplements were diminished. Conversion: traditional units to SI creatinine 1 mg/100ml = 88 μmmol/l.

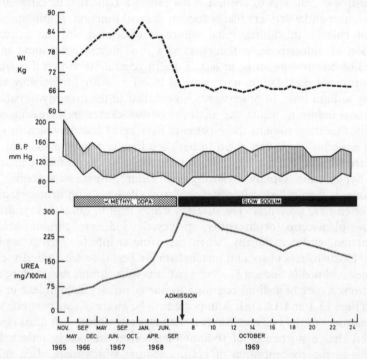

**Fig. 13.2** Weight and blood pressure in a patient with chronic renal failure. At first the patient needed methyl dopa to control hypertension. The patient then developed a sodium leak and needed supplemental sodium to control hypotension. Conversion: tradition to SI units—urea 10 mg/100 ml = 1.7 mmol/l.

It is interesting that even in those patients who have a tendency to retain sodium, and in whom there is a rise in the concentration of the natriuretic hormone/circulating sodium transport inhibitor, plasma aldosterone levels tend to be raised due presumably to the raised levels of ansiotensin II. The rise in aldosterone may also be due, in part, to the known direct stimulatory effect of sodium transport inhibition on the adrenal gland.

*Potassium metabolism*

Overall potassium homeostasis is maintained remarkably well up to the terminal stages of renal failure. The kidney is the main organ responsible for this phenomenon, urinary potassium excretion being maintained by an increasing amount of potassium being excreted by each remaining nephron. Though this compensatory phenomenon is sometimes aided by increased levels of aldosterone, particularly when there is a tendency to hyper-kalaemia, it can occur in the absence of such a rise. The underlying mechanism is therefore unkown.

Potassium balance varies markedly from patient to patient. There may be true potassium *deficiency*, often with hypokalaemia due to decreased dietary intake, the use of potassium losing diuretics, diarrhoea and vomiting. Such a loss can be corrected by appropriate treatment, multiple plasma potassium estimations being made if potassium supplements are given. There is, in addition, a tendency for intracellular potassium to fall due, perhaps, to the overall inhibition of $Na^+$-$K^+$-ATPase caused by the circulating sodium transport inhibitor. This disturbance in potassium metabolism is sometimes known as potassium *depletion*, but as it is not primarily due to loss of potassium it cannot be corrected by the administration of potassium. It does respond to haemodialysis.

Plasma potassium is usually maintained within the normal range but the concentration of potassium in the plasma is a poor indicator of the potassium stores. Acute hyperkalaemia in chronic renal failure occurs when there is a sudden deterioration in renal function, a fall in plasma pH, a rise in plasma osmolality (hyperglycaemia), and of course following an increased exogenous (or 'endogenous') load of potassium. Persistent hyperkalaemia can be due to an absence of aldosterone, a resistance of the tubules to mineralo-corticoids, the administration of spironolactone or potassium sparing diuretics, or to a persistently high dietary intake of potassium (e.g. dried fruits and chocolate). A persistently low plasma aldosterone is mainly seen in diabetic patients over the age of 50 years. It is due to a lowered plasma renin of unknown cause. The condition responds well to the administration of fludrocortisone.

*Hydrogen ion metabolism*

On a normal diet the kidney has to excrete about 40 to 60 mmol a day of hydrogen ions to prevent the internal environment from becoming acid (p. 83). In chronic renal failure there is an impaired ability to eliminate hydrogen ions which results in a systemic acidosis with a fall in plasma pH and bicarbonate. This is due to (1) a reduced ability to excrete ammonia caused by the diminished number of nephrons (Fig. 13.3), and (2) a reduced titratable acid excretion because of a diminished excretion of buffer phosphate mainly due to a diminished intake of phosphate. The urine pH is usually below 5.0 and there is therefore no impairment in the ability to maintain a hydrogen ion gradient. Nevertheless, if the plasma bicarbonate and pH are raised to normal by an intravenous infusion of sodium bicarbonate or lactate, and the patient is observed thereafter as he returns to his original acidotic state, it is evident that the urine pH does not fall in a normal manner. In some patients with chronic renal failure the urine pH does not fall below 5.0 until the plasma bicarbonate is less than 20 mmol/l whereas in a normal individual the urine pH falls below 5.0 when the plasma bicarbonate is less than 24 mmol/l. It is apparent that in chronic renal failure, therefore, the ability to acidify the urine in response to a standard rise in plasma hydrogen ion concentration is in fact below normal. This is due to the nephrons' depressed ability to reabsorb bicarbonate, which in turn is due in part to their reduced ability to secrete hydrogen ions, and this stems directly from their reduced number. There is also some evidence to suggest that the slightly expanded extra cellular fluid volume (p. 86) and the raised level of plasma PTH also impair bicarbonate reabsorption in the proximal tubule. This inhibition of bicarbonate reabsorption is sometimes known as bicarbonate wastage or leak. It is to be noted that it can only be detected if the ability to acidify (when the plasma bicarbonate is low) is normal.

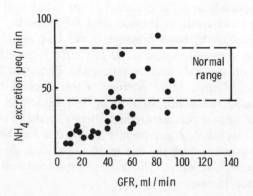

**Fig. 13.3** The relationship between ammonium excretion and glomerular filtration rate after the administration of an acid load to patients with renal disease. Each point represents a separate individual (adapted from Wrong & Davies 1959 Quart J Med 28: 259).

The most remarkable phenomenon about hydrogen ion metabolism in chronic renal failure is that though the plasma bicarbonate and pH may be depressed it remains at the same level for many weeks or months. Or in other words, though the patient can only get rid of fraction of the hydrogen ions he is producing each day, and he is thus in positive hydrogen ion balance every day, the plasma *does not become increasingly* acidotic. The probable explanation is that the hydrogen ions are being neutralised by calcium carbonate and other calcium buffers in bone.

Kussmaul respiration is the only clinical feature undoubtedly due to the acidosis; its severity is determined as much by the rate of fall in pH as by the extent of its reduction. It is also possible that the osteopenia of chronic renal failure (p. 200) is due to the retention of hydrogen ions. Finally, there is a long list of signs and symptoms, particularly of the alimentary, and central nervous systems, which some consider may possibly be caused by the acidosis. But it is possible that these clinical features are due instead to the pharmacological actions of the retained unidentified 'renal failure anions'.

## Calcium Metabolism

There are multiple abnormalities of calcium metabolism. Urinary calcium excretion falls to very low values, 10 mg/day (0.25 mmol) or less, and there is little or no calcium absorbed from the gut. Overall therefore the patient may be in calcium equilibrium, though often there is a mild negative calcium balance. Plasma calcium is either normal or low.

The diminution of calcium absorption from the gut is due, primarily, to a diminution in plasma 1,25-dihydroxycholecalciferol (1,25(OH)$_2$vit D, a metabolite of 25OHvit D manufactured only in the kidney) and to the tendency of patients with chronic renal failure to eat very little calcium (Fig. 13.4). The hypocalcaemia is due in part to a resistance of the bone to the action of parathyroid hormone for it is associated with high concentrations of circulating parathyroid hormone. This resistance of the bone to the action of parathyroid hormone stems mainly from the low plasma concentrations of 1,25(OH)$_2$vit D, for the calcium mobilising action of both of these hormones is dependent on the presence of the other. It is also probable that the resitance of the bone to parathyroid hormone may also be due to the plasma's increased capacity to inhibit sodium transport. It must be stressed that in advanced renal failure though the plasma parathyroid hormone levels may be very high, serum calcium is often *below* normal, and that concentrations above 12 mg per 100 ml (3 mmol/l) do not occur unless there is an adenoma of the parathyroid. When a high serum calcium coexists with renal failure the high calcium is not the result of the failure, it is usually its cause, particularly if the failure is not very severe.

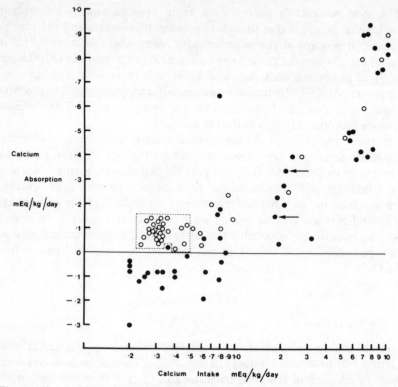

**Fig. 13.4** Calcium absorption plotted against calcium intake in patients with chronic renal failure (●) and normal subjects (○). The normal intake of calcium varies from approximately 0.5 to 1.0 mEq kg day (0.25 to 0.5 mmol). 1 mEq of calcium = 0.5 mmol. (Reproduced from Clarkson, Eastwood, Koutsaimanis et al 1973 Kidney Int 3: 258, with kind permission).

## Renal bone disease

Renal bone disease sometimes known as 'renal osteodystrophy', occurs in patients who have suffered from chronic renal failure for some time. The histological lesions can be discerned after a few months of renal failure, the radiological changes appear after a few years, and the clinical features develop even later. Renal bone disease is a variable mixture of hyperparathyroidism, osteosclerosis, osteopenia and osteomalacia, the latter due either to vit D deficiency or to aluminium intoxication.

Histologically, hyperparathyroidism, osteosclerosis, osteomalacia and osteopenia are usually present at the same time, though it is usual for one of these to predominate. The overall effect is one of osteopenia. It is not known whether this apparent decalcification is due to negative calcium balance or to redistribution of calcium within the bone; it is probably a combination of both. Figure 13.5 illustrates some of the possible mechanisms responsible for these abnormalities.

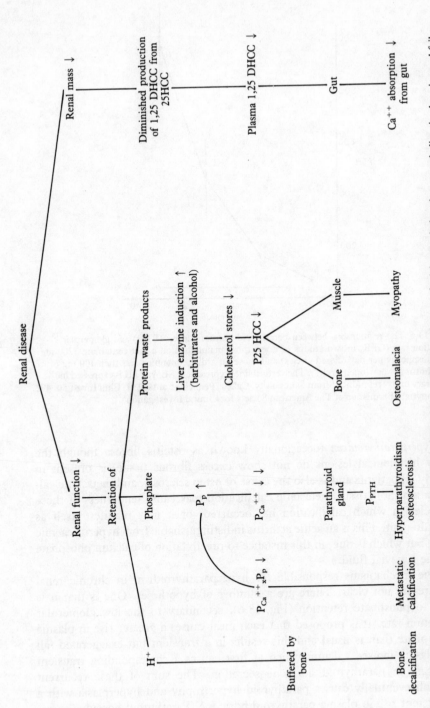

**Fig. 13.5** Schema of mechanisms involved in the aetiology of the various disturbances of calcium and phosphate metabolism in chronic renal failure. 1,25 DHCC = 1,25 dihydroxycholecalciferol; 25 HCC = 25 hydroxycholecalciferol; P = plasma.

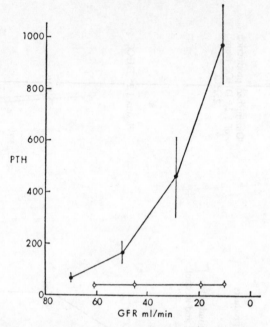

**Fig. 13.6** The relationship between parathyroid hormone levels (PTH) and glomerular filtration rate (GFR) in two groups of dogs: those maintained on a diet containing 1200 mg of phosphorus per day (closed circles) and those on a diet containing less then 100 mg of phoshorus per day (open circles). The vertical lines represent ± SEM; PTH is expressed in arbitrary units (reproduced from Saltopolsky, Calgar, Pennell et al 1971; J, Clini Invest 50: 492, by copyright permission of The American Society for Clinical Investigation).

*Hyperparathyroidism* (occasionally known as osteitis fibrosa though the early histological lesions do not show excess fibrous tissue) is present in nearly all patients and is also the cause of osteo sclerosis, and metastatic calcification. Soft tissue metastatic calcification may cause tenderness of those muscles in which calcification has occurred; or it may manifest itself as pseudo-gout. This is an acute arthritis indistinguishable from hyperuricaemic gout but which is due, in this instance to precipitation of calcium phosphate in the synovial fluid.

The mechanisms responsible for hyperparathyroidism in chronic renal failure are not clear. There are a number of hypotheses. One is that it is due to phosphate retention (Fig. 13.6), secondary to the low glomerular filtration rate. It is proposed that each meal causes a greater rise in plasma phosphate than is usual and this results in a transient but exaggerated fall in plasma ionised calcium which at first causes a corresponding transient increase in parathyroid hormone secretion. The sum of these recurrent stimuli eventually causes parathyroid hypertrophy and hyperplasia with a persistent rise in plasma parathyroid hormone. Parathyroid hormone secretion is also stimulated by the absence of 1,25(OH)$_2$vit D (see below).

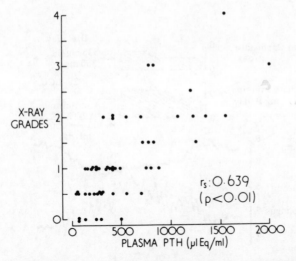

**Fig. 13.7** Correlation between radiographic grades of severity of hyperparathyroidism in the hand X-rays of patients suffering from chronic renal failure on maintenance haemodialysis and plasma concentrations of parathyroid hormone (reproduced from Memmos, Eastwood, Talner et al 1981 Brit Med J i: 1919, with kind permission).

All four parathyroid glands enlarge, occasionally one becomes ademomatous, at which time the other three become smaller. The raised concentration of parathyroid hormone causes the bony lesions of hyperparathyroidism (Fig. 13.7) including osteoclastic resorption, osteitis fibrosa and osteosclerosis, and it increases phosphate excretion which tends to return plasma phosphate towards normal.

Unfortunately for patients with chronic renal failure parathyroid hormone not only increases urinary phosphate excretion but it also, mobilises phosphate, as well as calcium, from the bone. If renal failure is very advanced, therefore, so that the increase in plasma parathyroid hormone can increase urinary phosphate excretion no further, the mobilisation of phosphate from the bone by the raised parathyroid hormone causes a *rise* in plasma phosphate, as opposed to the fall which usually occurs when renal function is normal. Thus, in chronic renal failure, hyperparathyroidism more often causes a rise in the product of plasma calcium × plasma phosphate ($PCa \times P_p$) by raising the plasma phosphate rather than by raising the plasma calcium. And it is the rise in $PCa \times P_p$ which is responsible for metastatic calcification.

*Vit D deficiency osteomalacia* is mainly diagnosed histologically. There is an accumulation of osteoid due to an impaired mineralization of the osteoid seam which lies next to the trabecular bone. This seam in which mineralization takes place is known as the calcification front. As it is possible to measure the rate and extent of the mineralizing activity taking place at the

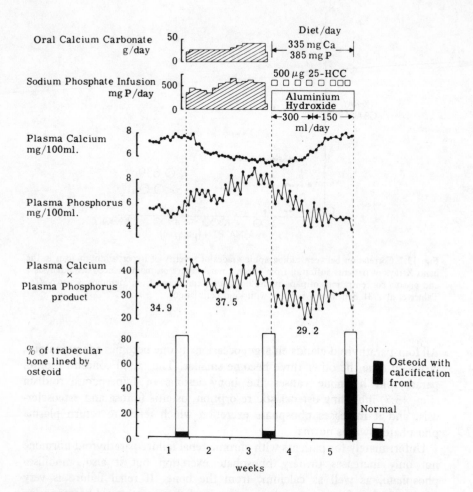

**Fig. 13.8** Demonstration that 25OH vit $D_3$ acts directly on the bone. Changes in plasma calcium, plasma phosphorus, plasma calcium × plasma phosphorus product and in the amount of trabecular bone covered with osteoid together with the amount of calcification front in a patient with chronic renal failure and osteomalacia before and during the administration of calcium and phosphate and after the administration of vit D. The extent of the calcification front did not rise during the administration of calcium carbonate and sodium phosphate though there was a rise in plasma calcium × plasma phosphorus product. But it did rise during the administration of vitamin D though there was a fall in plasma calcium × plasma phosphorus product. Aluminium hydroxide was given to stop the plasma phosphorus rising. The numbers immediately below the plotted values of plasma calcium × plasma phosphorus product are the mean values for each period. Individual injections of 25-hydroxycholecalciferol (25-HCC) are denoted by each of the boxes (top right). Conversion: SI to traditional units — calcium 1.5 mmol/l = 6.0 mg/100 ml: phosphorus 2.0 mmol/l = 6.2 mg/100 ml (reproduced from Eastwood, Bordier, Clarkson et al 1974 Clin Sci Mol Med 47: 23, with kind permission).

calcification front it is now possible to detect the presence of osteomalacia with some precision. The calcification front is under the control of 25OHvit $D_3$. The enzymes concerned with the mineralizing process at the calcification front can be inhibited by phosphate depletion, prolonged severe acidosis, and intoxication with aluminium and fluoride. 25OHvit D acts directly on the bone and not through any accompanying change in the concentration of plasma calcium and phosphate (Fig. 13.8). The two main causes of osteomalacia in chronic renal failure are a lack of 25OHvit D before maintenance haemodialysis is begun, and aluminium intoxication (see below) after it has started.

Using the sensitive and precise histological criteria mentioned above a third to half of the patients with terminal renal failure, but before they are placed onto dialysis, have some degree of osteomalacia. There is always an associated hyperparathyroidism, and in those patients with the most severe osteomalacia plasma parathyroid hormone and alkaline phosphatase are raised. As renal failure becomes terminal the increased incidence of osteomalacia is associated with a progressive fall in plasma 25OHvit D (Fig. 13.9). The patients with the most overt osteomalacia have the lowest plasma 25OHvit D (Fig. 13.9). The fall in plasma 25OHvit D is probably due to a diminshed dietary intake of vit D, and in the most severe symptomatic cases there is often, in addition, a high alcohol intake or a regular consumption of barbiturates. Both increase liver enzyme induction which increases the hydroxylation of cholecalciferol to 25OHvit D and eventually depletes the stores of cholcalciferol. Upon being placed onto maintenance haemodialysis, plasma 25OHvit D rises again to normal (Fig. 13.9) and in dialysis centres free from aluminium problems, the incidence of histological osteomalacia diminishes and clinical osteomalacia is a rarity.

The osteomalacia of chronic renal failure is not related to the plasma concentration of $1,25(OH)_2$vit D which begins to fall relatively early in the progress of renal failure and continues to fall thereafter both before and after the onset of maintenance dialysis. Furthermore anephric patients who have the lowest concentration of $1,25(OH)_2$vit D do not have a greater tendency to develop osteomalacia than other patients on maintenance dialysis. These findings are consistent with the observation that in nutritional osteomalacia due to vit D deficiency the plasma concentration of 25OHvit D is low and the plasma concentration of $1,25(OH)_2$vit D is normal.

At one time it was considered that the osteomalacia of chronic renal failure was due to a resistance of the uraemic osteoid to vit D. This concept mainly stemmed from the observation that the *radiological* appearances of the bones of most children with renal bone disease are indistinguishable from those of nutritional rickets. Not unnaturally therefore the bone disease was assumed to be due to vit D deficiency. It is now recognised, however, that in children with renal bone disease though the radiological appearances are the same as those of children with nutritional vit D deficiency, the

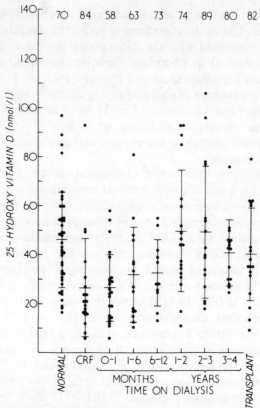

**Fig. 13.9** Plasma 25 hydroxy vitamin D in normal subjects (Normal), in patients with terminal renal failure (CRF), in patients who have been on maintenance haemodialysis for up to 11 years and in renal transplant patients. The 213 results illustrated are single estimations obtained from 213 different individuals (reproduced from Eastwood, Daly, Carter et al 1979 Clin Sci 57: 473, with kind permission).

*histological* appearances are those of hyperparathyroidism and not of osteo-malacia. It was not surprising therefore that 'renal rickets' (a radiological diagnosis) did not respond to normal amounts of vit D. The confusion was further compounded when it was found that the radiological appearances of 'renal rickets' did improve when very large doses of vit D were given. But the improvement was due to these enormous amounts of vit D causing large increases in the intestinal absorption of calcium, which in turn caused a rise in plasma calcium and thus a fall in plasma parathyroid hormone. The vit D, however was not correcting a defect of mineralization at the calcification front. Instead it caused a diffuse, scattered and haphazard calcification of the osteoid.

Very rarely osteomalacia, in a patient on maintenance haemodialysis is due to phosphate depletion. This is due to an abnormal faecal loss of phosphate which together with the usual dialysis loss of phosphate causes a fall

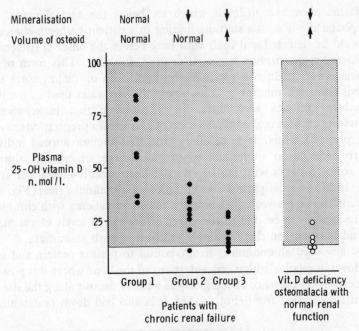

**Fig. 13.10** Plasma 25 OH vit D in 22 patients with renal failure, divided into 3 groups, and in 6 patients with vitamin D deficiency osteomalacia without renal failure (reproduced from Eastwood, Harris, Stamp et al 1976 Lancet 2: 1209, with kind permission).

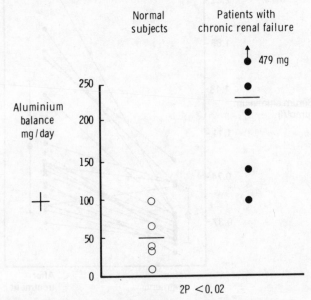

**Fig. 13.11** Aluminium balance in normal subjects (○) and patients with chronic renal failure (●) ingesting 100 ml of aluminium hydroxide gel per day. Conversion: SI to traditional units — aluminium 1 mmol = 27 mg (reproduced from Cam, Luck, Eastwood et al 1976 Clin Sci Mol Med 51: 407, with kind permission).

in plasma phosphate to levels which are below the normal range. Hypophosphataemia is such a startling finding in a patient on haemodialysis that it should be detected and dealt with long before the onset of osteomalacia.

*Aluminium intoxication osteomalacia (and dementia).* This form of osteomalacia occurs mainly in patients who have been on maintenance haemodialysis for a few months in areas where the tap water used in the dialysis procedure contains aluminium. It is probable that intoxication also follows the chronic oral administration of aluminium preparations to control hyperphosphataemia. It is certainly true that though normal individuals absorb little or no aluminium when given large amounts of aluminium hydroxide, patients with chronic renal failure absorb substantial amounts (Fig. 13.11) and the plasma concentration of aluminium rises (Fig. 13.12). This difference between normal individuals and patients with chronic renal failure appears to be due to the effect of the raised levels of plasma parathyroid hormone on the intestine's ability to absorb aluminium.

The absorbed aluminium is firmly bound to plasma protein and is then laid down in relatively high concentrations in the bone where it is possible to demonstrate its presence histologicaly as a linear deposit along the site of the absent calcification front (Fig. 12.13). It is also laid down preferentially in

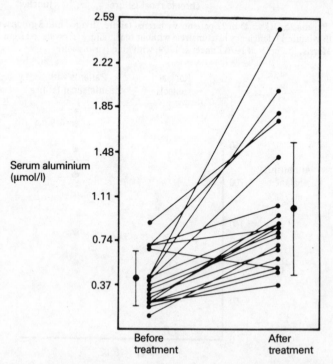

**Fig. 13.12** Serum aluminium concentrations in 20 patients with chronic renal failure before and after treatment with oral aluminium hydroxide 3.8 g daily (alucaps) in three divided doses with meals for four weeks (reproduced from Biswas, Arze, Ramos et al 1982 Brit Med J 284: 776, with kind permission).

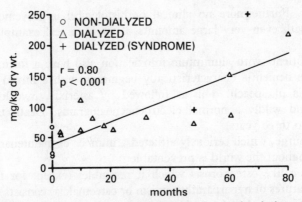

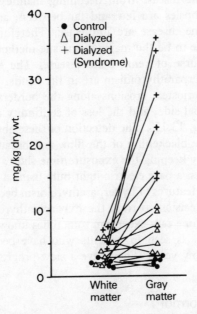

**Fig. 13.13** Correlation between duration of dialysis (months) and trabecular bone aluminium levels (reproduced from Alfrey, Legendre & Kaehny 1976 New Eng J Med 294: 184, with kind permission).

**Fig. 13.14** Aluminium levels in grey and white matter of control subjects and uremic patients with and without the encephalopathy syndrome (reproduced from Alfrey, Legendre & Kaehny 1976 New Eng J Med 284: 184, with kind permission).

the grey matter of the cerebral cortex (Fig. 13.14). The osteomalacia which results progresses rapidly and gives rise to severe bone softening with much bone pain and alarming deformities. This form of osteomalacia has many features which distinguish it from the osteomalacia of vit D deficiency. Plasma parathyroid hormone and alkaline phosphatase are normal or low due to the direct inhibiting effect of aluminium on the parathyroid gland and the osteoblasts. Furthermore no clinical or histological improvement can be obtained with even very large amounts of vit D (a real example of vit D resistance).

Many patients with aluminium intoxication also have a form of rapidly progressive dementia characteristically beginning with a mixed dysarthria and apraxia of speech. This is followed by asterixis, myoclonus, focal seizures and wildly abnormal electroencephalograms. Death takes place after one to three years.

This scourge, which seriously afflicted a number of maintenance dialysis units throughout the world is preventable.

*Osteopenia* like osteoporosis which it resembles (except for the accompanying features of hyperparathyroidism or osteomalcia) consists of loss and thinning of bone trabeculae and tends to occur in all patients.

*Radiological and clinical features.* It should be the aim to avoid the clinical features of renal bone disease from becoming manifest, but facilities for quantitative bone biopsies are few and far between, and the biochemical features of renal bone disease are imprecise. Therefore radiology of the skeleton will continue to be the major diagnostic method for detecting and following up the course of renal bone disease. The earliest radiological abnormalities of hyperparathyroidism are in the hands. The most useful to follow are the sub-periosteal erosions along the borders of the phalanges, particularly their radial side, and the loss of continuity of the cortex of the terminal phalanx (Fig. 13.15). The detection of these abnormalities is made easier by an adequate blackening of the film, and because patients tend to have a fine tremor, by keeping the exposure time short. It is also helpful to look at the film against a bare electric light bulb using a hand lens. Most of the other radiological features of hyperparathyroidism become manifest later, by which time the decision to treat the hyperparathyroidism should have been taken. There is one rare exception sometimes known as the 'shrinking man syndrome'. This is seen in patients who have been on maintenance haemodialysis for many years. They have a slow progressive loss of height

Normal             Abnormal

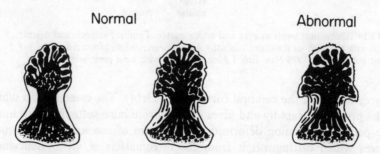

**Fig. 13.5** Comparison of microradioscopic and morphometric findings in the hand bones with densitometric findings in the proximal radius in thyrotoxicosis and renal osteodystrophy (reproduced from Meema & Meema 1972 Invest Radiol 7, 88 with kind permission).

due to kyphosis of the upper thoracic spine. The vertebral bodies have an increased translucence, but compression fractures are unusual. Because of the mild non progressive evidence of hyperparathyroidism in the hands and the lack of rise in plasma akaline phosphatase it is assumed that the syndrome is due to osteopenia. Bone biopsy however, reveals very severe hyperparathyroidism with erosive tunnelling of the trabecuale and osteitis fibrosa.

The only characteristic radiological lesions of osteomalacia are pseudo-fractures known as Looser's zones, which occur late in the progress of the disease. They consist of narrow bands of translucency, perpendicular or oblique to the bone surface. On either side of the band the presence of an increase number of cells may give rise to shadows which are denser than the surrounding bone. The lesions are often bilateral and symetrical.

Osteopenia, like osteoporosis is difficult to diagnose radiologically and is probably best quantified with the use of an index such as the metacarpal index which relates the width of the bone to that of the marrow at a particular place along one particular metacarpal. It is interesting that the osteopenia of chronic renal failure rarely gives rise to compression fractures of the vertebral bodies.

## Magnesium metabolism

Plasma magnesium and magnesium balance are normal in chronic renal failure whatever the creatinine clearance. There is reduced alimentary absorption and urinary excretion of magnesium due in part at least to the reduced intake of magnesium consequent upon increasing anorexia and medical advice. The ability to excrete a sudden load of magnesium, however, is severely impaired so that the use of magnesium sulphate as a purgative may be lethal. The persistent use of magnesium trisilicate for chronic dyspepsia can also raise plasma magnesium and at least on death from hypermagnesaemia from this cause has been documented.

## Phosphate metabolism

In contrast to calcium, phosphate absorption from the gut, and urinary excretion, are unimpaired in chronic renal failure. As glomerular filtration rate falls urinary phosphate excretion remains normal because the rising plasma parathyroid hormone leads to a diminution in the proportion of the filtered phosphate that is reabsorbed. Plasma phosphate therefore does not rise until the creatinine clearance is approximately 10–20 ml/min, and even then the rise is usually a modest one. This stability is also due in part to a fall in phosphate intake which accompanies a reduction of protein intake. Occasionally, however, particularly in patients who drink much milk, plasma phosphate may rise to more than 6.5 mmol/l (20 mg/100 ml). This may cause tissue calcification including acute arthritis from precipitation of calcium in the synovial fluid (pseudo-gout, see above).

## Fat metabolism

Chronic renal failure is accompanied by hypertriglyceridemia with a normal plasma cholesterol. This is due to the raised plasma insulin concentration and an impairment of lipoprotein lipase activity. These changes have been claimed to be associated with premature atherosclerosis and an increased incidence of death from cardiovascular accidents. Others have denied this assertion with some vigour. Recently however, there is one report that the mortality from myocardial infarction in men on maintenance haemodialysis is 9 to 20 times greater than in normal men of comparable age.

## Carbohydrate metabolism

An abnormal glucose tolerance test, a mild degree of hyperglycaemia and hyperinsulinaemia often occur in chronic renal failure. These disturbances are mainly due to resistance of the hepatic cells to insulin.

It is interesting however, that insulin dependent diabetics have a decrease in their requirements of insulin when they develop renal failure. This may be due to depressed renal metabolism of insulin and a diminished renal glyconeogenesis.

## Protein metabolism

The stools of both normal man and uraemic patients do not contain urea. This is because the urea in intestinal juice is continually being hydrolysed to ammonia by bacterial ureases. The ammonia nitrogen which is reabsorbed from the gut is then reutilised. It can be found incorporated into serum albumin. In patients with chronic renal failure with a high blood urea, the urea of the intestinal juices is high and therefore the magnitude of this recycling of nitrogen is very great. It has been calculated that with a blood urea of (200 mg/100 ml) about 1.0 mol (15 g) of endogenous ammonia nitrogen is available for protein synthesis.

As chronic renal failure advances there is often a progressive negative nitrogen balance due mainly to a diminished intake of protein. This may be due either to anorexia or to the therapeutic use of a low protein diet. In addition it may be aggravated by urinary protein loss or losses into the peritoneal fluid during peritoneal dialysis. As the nitrogen balance becomes negative several adaptive compensatory mechanisms come into play, for instance, the incorporation of ammonia nitrogen into albumin. But these compensatory mechanisms are not so efficient in chronic renal failure as they are in normal man. For instance, whereas normal man can stay in nitrogen balance with a dietary protein intake as low as 0.25 g/kg/day (i.e. about 18 g for a 70 kg man) patients with chronic renal failure need about 0.5 g/kg/day (i.e. 35 g/kg/day) (Fig. 13.16).

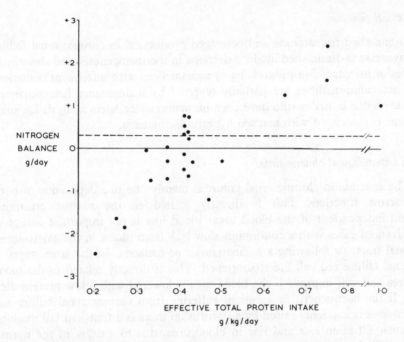

**Fig. 13.16** Nitrogen balance in 24 patients with chronic renal failure on varying intakes of protein. The interrupted horizontal line denotes average nitrogen loss per day in sweat in a moderate climate Conversion: traditional units to SI units — nitrogen 1.0 g = 70 mmol (reproduced from Ford, Phillips, Toye et al 1969 Brit Med J i: 735, with kind permission).

## Thyroid metabolism

Many patients with chronic renal failure have some of the appearances of myxoedema. They have pale, pigmented puffy faces and, in very advanced renal failure, they tend to be cold and slow. Others have exophthalmos, tachycardia, moist hands and may arouse suspicion that they are suffering from thyrotoxicosis. These features are accompanied by many abnormalities of thyroid function. There may be a diminished rise in plasma TSH in response to an injection of thyroid releasing factor, there is an increased frequency of goitre and the plasma concentrations of $T_4$ and $T_3$ tend to be low. Maintenance dialysis improves the patient's 'myxoedematous' appearance but does not affect the biochemical abnormalities, whereas these are reversed by transplantation. The relevance of the biochemical abnormalities is unclear, for except in those few patients who were known to be myxoedematous before the development of renal failure the onset of unequivocal myxoedema in patients on maintenance haemodialysis is unusual. Furthermore the administration of thyroid to patients with renal failure who look myxoedematous produces no obvious clinical improvement.

## Sexual function

Diminished testosterone and oestrogen production in chronic renal failure gives rise to diminished libido, a decrease in spermatogenesis, and abnormalities of menstruation progressing to amenorrhoea with infrequent ovulation. These abnormalities are partially reversed by maintenance haemodialysis. Impotence in males who have been on maintenance haemodialysis for some time is associated with marked hyperprolactinaemia.

## Haematological abnormalities

The anaemia in chronic renal failure is mainly due to a depression of bone marrow function. This is directly related to the plasma creatinine and independent of the blood urea. Blood loss is not important except in advanced cases with a continuous slow leak from ulcers in the gastro-intestinal tract, or following a haematemesis or melaena. In the later stages of renal failure red cell life is shortened. This is directly related to the blood urea and will improve if the blood urea is lowered with a low protein diet.

If the haematocrit in a patient suffering from chronic renal failure and anaemia is suddenly raised by a transfusion there is a transient fall in glomerular filtration rate and rise in blood urea, due to a delay in the normal vasodilating response to a rise in haematocrit (p. 118). This sharp fall in glomerular filtration rate, which often takes place upon transfusing cases of renal failure, may sometimes be fatal if the presence of kidney disease is unsuspected. If transfusions are continued until the haemoglobin is normal the blood urea rises rapidly and the patient may die of acute renal failure. Nevertheless, as acute haemorrhage causes intense renal vasoconstriction, transfusions are occasionally inevitable. When chronic anaemia is sufficiently severe to cause or contribute to the onset of cardiac failure, the associated renal vasoconstriction will cause an additional depression of renal function which may respond to small transfusions of packed cells.

Chronic renal failure is also accompanied by a leucocytosis and a raised sedimentation rate, both of unknown cause.

## Urea retention

The rise in blood urea is due to the diminished glomerular filtration rate. There is much evidence that urea itself is not responsible for any of the symptoms of renal failure. It has been shown that uraemic patients can be greatly improved by the use of an artificial kidney without necessarily changing the level of blood urea; and it is well known that in acute renal failure, where the blood urea rises to a plateau and then falls, the patient's general condition may be critical as the blood urea is rising, but that at an identical value a week later there may be a vast improvement.

*Retention of other substances*

It is well established that the longer the blood urea has been raised the greater the discrepancy between the plasma concentration of non-protein nitrogen and urea. This is due to a rise in the concentrations of uric acid, creatinine, phenol derivatives, amines and other nitrogenous metabolites of protein metabolism. Plasma urate rises relatively steeply to about 500 $\mu$mol/l (8 mg/100 ml) until the plasma creatinine is about 250 $\mu$mol/l (3 mg/100 ml), it then tends to remain between 500 to 600 $\mu$mol/l (8 to 10 mg/l) however severe the renal failure. Very occasionally if the concentration rises above 600 to 900 $\mu$mol/l (10–15 mg/100 ml) it may precipitate an acute attack of gout. The rise in plasma creatinine is not thought to produce any symptoms. The importance of the rise in plasma creatinine is that in advanced renal failure it is a far better guide to the extent of accumulation of protein metabolites than is the level of blood urea. A blood urea of 17 mmol/l (100 mg/100) ml may be associated with plasma creatinine levels of 3 to 20 mg/100 ml depending mainly on the diet the patient is having, the duration of his illness and the glomerular filtration rate. A plasma creatinine of 260 $\mu$mol/l (3 mg/100 ml) is of no immediate prognostic importance, whereas with a plasma creatinine of 1800 $\mu$mol/l (20 mg/100 ml) the patient is likely to die within a few days from a gastro-intestinal haemorrhage, a haemorrhagic pericarditis or some other calamitous complication.

It has been claimed that the increased quantity of circulating phenols is responsible for some of the features of renal failure, such as lassitude, nausea and anaemia but there is not significant correlation between the blood concentrations of phenol and any particular symptom. The rise in amines is probably of more consequence.

There is also a retention of sulphate, some unidentified anions and urochromogen. The retention of sulphate and unidentified anions together with phosphate is responsible for the fact that as the serum bicarbonate falls with the increasing retention of hydrogen ions, there is no compensatory rise in plasma chloride, there may even be a fall. This is in contrast to what takes place in the tubular disorder known as 'renal tubular acidosis' (p. 362) where there is hydrogen ion retention with little disturbance in glomerular filtration rate and therefore no retention of phosphates, etc. The fall in plasma bicarbonate which accompanies the accumulation of hydrogen ions is then associated with a compensatory rise in plasma chloride, i.e. hyperchloraemic acidosis.

The diminished excretion of urochromogen is one reason why the urine is pale, even in subjects without polyuria. Urochromogens are lipid soluble pigments which are therefore known as lipochromes. They darken in the sunlight. In chronic renal failure their deposition in the subcutaneous fat causes the characteristic dirty yellow pigmentation of uraemia. And this explains why some patients with chronic renal failure take on such a good tan in the summer and also why it remains relatively unchanged during the subsequent winter. It is more difficult to understand why some patients never become pigmented.

## Clinical features of unknown cause

### Gastro-intestinal

The tongue in renal failure is classically described as being brown and dry. Though it is true that such an appearance is frequently seen, it is a change which is by no means confined to those suffering from renal failure. It may occur in any patient who breathes through his mouth, particularly if he has pyorrhoea and bleeding gums, and it is almost inevitable if he is also dehydrated and hyperpnoeic. A foul taste in the mouth is a frequent complaint in chronic renal failure and the patient may notice a taste of ammonia, particularly on waking due to the decomposition of urea by anaerobes under the gums.

The breath may smell of urine. This is characteristic of advanced renal failure and is sometimes the first sign to be noticed. It is not present in every case, and often when it has been noticed, it turns out that the smell has orignated from urine in the trousers of a patient with prostatic difficulties, whose blood urea is normal. A person with a normal blood urea but suffering from severe pyorrhoea may also have a uraemic breath.

Hiccough is almost invariably present in advanced chronic renal failure and may cause much fatigue and distress; it appears in episodic attacks of varying length and is usually brought on by eating and drinking.

Eventually anorexia, nausea and vomiting are almost always present. They are often the most prominent and, occasionally, the only symptoms; they are responsible in part, for the extensive loss of weight of chronic renal failure. Nausea and retching may be particularly pronounced in the early morning. All severities or vomiting occur, from two to three times a day to an almost continuous series of painful retches; and both small and large quantities of fluid are brought up. Dehydration follows more or less rapidly and is due to a combination of circumstances which reinforce each other; there is a distaste for fluids by mouth, combined with a loss of fluid from the stomach and an inability to concentrate the urine, so that urine flow tends to remain high. Dehydration in turn causes a further reduction in renal blood flow and glomerular filtration rate, and these aggravate the renal failure so that anorexia, nausea and vomiting become worse.

Sometimes the first complaint is one of fullness after meals with or without vomiting. Such patients are often suspected of having some local stomach condition such as a peptic ulcer. These do occur, mainly just before the patient is placed onto haemodialysis when the plasma gastrin is raised because of diminished renal metabolism of gastrin. After the onset of maintenance haemodialysis the plasma gastrin falls towards normal values. The presence of a gastric ulcer is likely if the patient first appears with a severe gastro-intestinal haemorrhage. Haematemesis and melaena are most frequent towards the terminal phase of renal failure and should not therefore cause any confusion, for by this time the presence of renal failure is usually known. Nevertheless, it is remarkable how often renal failure may progress to an advanced state before the patient decides, or is forced by circumstances, to see a doctor. Gastro-intestinal haemorrhages are due to a combination of increased capillary fragility and local ulceration; the latter is particularly pronounced in the large bowel. The effect of haemorrhage in chronic renal failure is extremely serious, for the accompanying renal vasoconstriction and fall in blood pressure lower the glomerular filtration rate even further and cause a preciptious rise in blood urea (p. 116). When the haemorrhage is from the gastro-intestinal tract, some of the blood is digested and absorbed so that there is in addition a large ingestion of protein at a time of diminishing renal function.

Constipation is common, but occasionally severe diarrhoea may occur and may quickly cause death from dehydration.

### Neurological

*Cerebral.* The commonest complication is an intellectual deterioration. In some patients this is associated with a reluctance to enter into conversation, whereas in others there is a circumlocution which rarely reaches a conclusion. Mental concentration and the making of decisions are difficult. Frequently there are recurrent bouts of depression and apathy, but the tenacity with which most patients will try and overcome their disabilities is remarkable. Headaches, lassitude, languor, muscular fatigue and weakness are all present in the final stages of renal failure. They may occur much earlier. Terminally the patient may become torpid during the day and yet not be able to sleep during the night, when instead he is restless and confused. Finally, there is loss of consciousness, but often even at this late stage there may be short lucid intervals; not infrequently the patient retains a complete understanding of what is happening to him right up to few hours before death.

Epileptic convulsions in chronic renal failure may be due either to sudden increases in blood pressure in patients with established hypertension, or they may occur without any change in blood pressure. Both types are very rare; the first is called hypertensive encephalopathy; the other has no particular designation. The latter variety is seen mainly in young adults in whom the fits may be the only complaint and yet the blood urea is extraordinarily high, e.g. 70 mmol/l (approx 400 mg/100 ml).

In advanced renal failure muscle twitches are often seen; they are caused by anterior horn cell discharges of unknown cause, and are unrelated to any apparent change in calcium metabolism, though they can often be relieved by the intravenous administration of calcium. A few patients have involuntary twitchings and choreiform movements of both legs, a phenomenon appropriately called the 'restless leg syndrome'. It may herald a fit. A 'flapping tremor' which is more frequently described in hepatic failure, often occurs in the terminal stages of chronic renal failure.

The rapidly progressive form of dementia due to aluminium intoxication that occurs in patients on maintenance haemodialysis has been described above.

*Peripheral nerves.* Uraemic polyneuropathy is a rare syndrome which occurs mainly in men who have been inadequately dialysed. It is due to a destruction of the myelin sheath and axons of medullated fibres in the peripheral nerves. The first signs of uraemic nephropathy are impaired vibratory sense in the lower limbs and loss of deep tendon jerks first of the ankles and then of the knees. The onset of symptoms may be painful burning feet followed by a progressive numbness and weakness. The feet and legs and affected more than the arms, and the distal segments more than the proximal. Eventually ataxia is prominent with a wide based steppage gait. Sometimes there may be no subjective sensory disturbances. The cause is unknown. It is not due to a deficiency of vitamin $B_1$. It is cured by increasing the duration of dialysis, so that it is presumably due to the retention of some injurious substance.

*Myopathy.* An unusual condition in which there is a weakness of the proximal muscles, particularly the shoulder girdle, hip flexion and spinal muscles. There is a waddling gait, difficulty climbing stairs and standing upright from the squatting position. Some patients have to go upstairs on their hands and knees. The condition is most often seen in association with osteomalacia and very occasionally with severe hyperparathyroidism. The deep tendon reflexes are normal and brisk.

*Muscle cramps* of the legs is a common condition in chronic renal failure and may be a cause of much misery and fatigue in some patients on maintenance haemodialysis, particularly during dialyses.

### Cardiovascular

*Hypertensive vascular disease.* Hypertension and chronic renal failure are closely related (p. 260) and, though hypertension may occasionally cause renal failure, the reverse is much more common. The probable cause for the rise in blood pressure in chronic renal failure is discussed later. The blood pressure frequently rises in chronic renal failure, but its rise may produce few symptoms. When they occur they are due to widespread vascular changes or cardiac failure.

The vascular lesions may be acute or chronic. Some can nearly always be observed on inspection of the ocular fundus where they produce certain characteristic disturbances of the retinal arteries and of the retina. The acute changes (i.e. those found in malignant hypertension) produce an appearance called *hypertensive retinopathy*, while the chronic changes are called *arterio-sclerotic retinopathy*.

Hypertensive retinopathy is distinguished primarily by the presence of papilloedema which at first may be unilateral. There are also flame-shaped or blotchy haemorrhages fanning out from the optic disc, and multiple areas of white discoloration known as exudates. These have indefinite margins and are of uneven size and colour; a lack of precision and uniformity which has caused them to be called 'soft' exudates. They consist of collections of oedema fluid. Sometimes the oedematous retina lies in folds radiating from the macula towards the optic disc, an appearance referred to as a macular star. Soft exudates and haemorrhages may precede the development of papilloedema.

In arteriosclerotic retinopathy the retinal arteries become tortuous and narrow, either irregularly or evenly along their whole length. They characteristically cross the veins at right angles, as opposed to the more usual oblique direction, and at these crossings the veins appear to be compressed by the artery, an appearance known as arterio-venous nipping. It is due to an accumulation of connective tissue between the artery and the vein, so that in fact the vein, as it approaches the artery, is not compressed but obscured. Exudates are also seen, but they are 'hard' as opposed to those seen with the acute vascular changes. They are small and compact, they have definite, sharp margins, and are of a dense yellowish-white colour. Eventually they are found in clusters particularly spreading out radially from the macula; another form of macular star. As chronic vascular changes frequently precede by several years the onset of the acute changes it is not unusual to find arteriosclerotic and hypertensive retinopathy combined.

Hypertensive retinopathy may cause varying degrees of visual impairment, depending on the degree of papilloedema and the site and extent of the haemorrhages and exudates (particularly if the macula has been involved). The striking clinical finding, however, is that often both fundi may be severely affected without the patient being aware of any change in vision; with arteriosclerotic retinopathy visual symptoms are even less frequent.

The changes which hypertensive vascular disease may produce upon renal structure and function are described on p. 260. When they are super-imposed upon chronic renal disease, they will intensify the severity of the renal failure. If cardiac failure occurs there is an additional sharp deterioration in renal function. With malignant hypertension cardiac failure is often one of the presenting clinical features. There are acute attacks of paroxysmal nocturnal and postural dyspnoea, and eventually oedema with a permanently raised venous pressure. Deterioration in renal function is due to (1) the reversible renal vasoconstriction associated with cardiac failure, and (2) the local vascular lesions.

The onset of *acute* vascular changes in the kidney is revealed not only by the sudden change in renal function but also by the onset of haematuria and increased proteinuria. The deterioration in renal function due to the vascular changes associated with malignant hypertension is partially reversible if it has not progressed too far before treatment is started. How far the functional changes produced by chronic vascular changes are reversible is uncertain.

*Pericarditis.* An aseptic, fibrinous pericarditis often develops in the terminal phase of chronic renal failure. Its cause is unknown. It may be painless or excruciatingly painful. Occasionally it is associated with a large bloody effusion, which may cause tamponade.

*Increased capillary permeability.* This manifests itself in many ways. Retinitis in the absence of hypertension; transient attacks of reversible blindness due to cerebral oedema; pulmonary oedema (the uraemic lung) in the absence of a raised pulmonary capillary pressure; skin purpura; and the presence in most patients of a slight excess of peritoneal fluid containing a concentration of protein close to that found in the plasma. One minor contributing cause for the increased permeability may be an increased concentration of circulating renin which is known to cause increased capillary permeability in experimental animals.

## Respiratory

The deep sighing respirations of acidosis have already been mentioned. The other respiratory complications of renal failure are (1) 'uraemic lung' and (2) infection.

'Uraemic lung' is a radiological diagnosis. It consists of dense bilateral opacities radiating from the hilum into the lung substance, while the upper and lower zones and the outer rim of the middle zones are clear. These appearances are usually due to left heart failure but there is a group of patients in whom they are associated with a normal pulmonary artery pressure, when they are presumably due to increased transudation from abnormal capillaries.

Pneumonia is frequently the immediate cause of death, but it usually develops only when the patient is already moribund. It is not improbable that this late onset is because the deep respirations of acidosis and the rapid respiration of left heart failure prevent the bronchioles from becoming blocked, and the lungs from collapsing, the usual preliminaries to pneumonia in semiconscious patients.

## Cutaneous

The characteristic pigmentation of renal failure, together with the anaemia, give patients suffering from chronic renal failure a characteristic colour. The eyelids tend to be slightly swollen and an expression of tiredness and depression is common. It is not known why the eyelids should be swollen, this usually occurs in the absence of generalised oedema. Relatively often, patients will develop a moon face like that seen in Cushing's disease but it is not associated with an excess secretion of cortisone.

In advanced renal failure there may be purpura, usually preceded and accompanied by bleeding gums; this is associated with gross abnormalities in platelet function, though the number of platelets is normal. (This deterioration in platelet function is related to the retention of guanadino succinic acid.)

Pruritus is common and there may also be a variety of unspecific rashes, erythema, vesicles and urticaria. The skin is often very dry because of dehydration; recurrent boils, carbuncles, and slowly healing scratches and abrasions are not infrequent.

*Joints*

More than 50% of patients on maintenance haemodialysis either are suffering, or have suffered relatively recently, from pain and stiffness of one or more joints. The hands and feet are the ones most involved and the hips the least. Most of the symptoms are non specific but there are some definite features including metastatic calcification, persistent haemarthrosis resulting in chronic capsulitis, carpal tunnel syndrome, ruptured peripheral tendons and avascular necrosis (usually of the hips). There is a close association between these complaints and hyperparathyroidism but there are sufficient anomalies to suggest that this is not the only cause of the problem.

*Increased incidence of cancer*

It has been recognised for some time that the incidence of cancer in patients after transplantation is raised, and that this is probably due to the prolonged use of immunosuppressive drugs given to prevent rejection. Uraemic patients also have a defective humoral and particularly cell mediated immunity. It is not surprising therefore that the incidence of cancer in patients with chronic renal failure is also raised. For example in one group of 148 men who had been on maintenance haemodialysis for some years, 9 developed a cancer whereas the expected incidence was 3.6, a very significant difference. In another study of 1651 patients on dialysis, there was a raised incidence of non-Hodgkin's lymphoma, though not of other tumours.

*Proteinuria and urinary cell content*

Proteinuria is nearly always present in chronic renal failure, but the concentration of protein in the urine is no guide to the severity of the failure; there are even reports of advanced chronic renal failure without proteinuria. At first protein may appear intermittently and then only after standing in the upright posture. If a nephrotic syndrome has preceded the onset of renal failure the daily protein excretion will sometimes diminish as the glomerular filtration rate falls.

Granular casts and an excess number of red and white cells are also found. The characteristic though uncommon finding of advanced renal failure is the appearance of broad casts; evidence of dilated nephrons.

## TREATMENT OF CHRONIC RENAL FAILURE

Treatment of chronic renal failure consists of dealing promptly with any potentially reversible cause, and delaying the progressive deterioration of renal function with conservative measures. When these measures are no longer able to keep the patient at work and leading a normal life the patient has entered the stage of terminal renal failure (or end stage renal disease (ESRD) as it is known in the United States). Now, the only effective forms of treatment are dialysis and transplantation.

Clearly it is of the utmost importance to try and identify the primary cause of the persistent renal failure, for in some instances (see list below) it may be possible to treat the immediate cause of failure and so prevent any further deterioration of function. Often it may even be possible to obtain a large measure of improvement.

*Some potentially reversible causes of chronic renal failure*

Urinary tract obstruction
Infections of the renal parenchyma
Analgesic nephropathy
Hypertension
Hypercalcaemia
Hypokalaemia
Hyperuricaemia

Subacute bacterial endocarditis
Nephrotoxic drugs
Systemic lupus erythematosus
Polyarteritis nodosa

Unfortunately, in most instances the cause of chronic renal failure is not treatable, for it is either unknown, or structurally irreversible, as with chronic glomerular nephritis, and congenital polycystic kidneys.

### Conservative treatment

This may be very rewarding, for often much of the disturbance in renal function is reversible, having been caused by a vicious circle in which the disturbed renal function causes a change in the internal environment, which in turn leads to a further depression in renal function, e.g. renal failure → polyuria and nausea → dehydration → renal vasoconstriction → diminished glomerular filtration rate.

Conservative treatment consists mainly in preventing or correcting disturbances of water and electrolyte balance, controlling the rise in arterial pressure, and delaying the rate of rise of the end products of protein metabolism.

## Treatment of biochemical abnormalities

### Waste products of protein metabolism

The concentration of urea in the blood is controlled by the rate of protein intake and the glomerular filtration rate. In chronic renal failure glomerular filtration rate falls, the blood urea rises and there is a concomitant deterioration in the patient's general condition. As it is clear that urea is not directly responsible for this change, presumably it is due to the accumulation of other end-products of protein metabolism. For this reason alone the patient will feel better, and may survive longer, if protein intake is limited.

Another, more debatable reason has been advanced for reducing protein intake. It has been pointed out that in chronic renal failure each remaining nephron increases its renal blood flow and glomerular filtration rate and that the extent of this increase is in part determined by the protein intake. It has been demonstrated in the rat that extensive glomerular vasodilatation leads to an increase in glomerular permeability, an increased leak of protein and eventually to glomerular sclerosis possibly due to mesangial overload. It is certainly true, and has been known for many years that the renal lesions of senescence can be accelerated by a high protein diet; and that following unilateral nephrectomy and the removal of large portions of the other kidney, structural changes in the remaining renal tissue can be hastened by the administration of large quantities of protein. If these results are applicable to man then once renal failure has been diagnosed, protein intake should be reduced, whatever the initial concentration of blood urea. But the therapeutic implications of these observations have tended to be ignored because (1) the demoralising effect of a greatly reduced protein intake (2) the very obvious dangers of protein deficiency (see below) and (3) the lack of evidence at present, that in man the progress of renal failure can be retarded by a low protein diet. On the whole therefore protein intake tends to be lowered only to control established symptoms late in the course of events. If, however, as seems likely, it will be demonstrated that the rate of functional deterioration early in the disease can be influenced by a moderate reduction in protein intake, it is inevitable that such a reduction will be advised. The difficulty then will be to persuade an otherwise fit person with a prognosis of 10–20 years to reduce his intake of the most appetising component of his diet for the rest of his life.

*Low protein diet to control symptoms in the late stages of the disease.* The consequences of a persistent negative nitrogen balance are a fall in the albumin pool, hypoalbuminaemia, weight loss, muscle wasting and fatigue. Though a very low protein diet prolongs the patient's life, for a variety of reasons, it also gives time for the insidious development of many complications including those due directly to protein deficiency. For instance when patients are placed on maintenance haemodialysis they recover their health more quickly if they have not been on a very low protein diet (less than 0.5 g/kg/day) for a long time before dialysis is begun. Full recovery, in protein deficient patients, may take up to a year.

The aim therefore of a reduced intake of protein to control symptoms is to bring about a reduction in the concentration of nitrogenous waste products without producing a prolonged negative nitrogen balance. On a palatable diet this is achieved by giving about 0.5 g/kg/day of protein (i.e. 35 g per day to a 70 kg man) with as high a calorie intake as is comfortable. It is difficult to be precise when a low protein diet to control symptoms should be started. Perhaps anorexia and lassitude are the two best guides. In young patients these may not develop until the blood urea is 50 to 70 mmol/l (300 to 400 mg/100 ml) whereas in older patients they appear earlier.

If when a patient is first seen, he is anorexic and vomiting it is usually necessary first to give some saline intravenously. As a result, appetite often returns. It may then be worth while to give a very low protein (i.e. 0.2 g/kg/day) for two to three weeks to lower the blood urea. It is important to remember to give at least 100 to 150 mmol of sodium per day at the same time, particularly if the patient is not hypertensive. The blood urea will often fall to below 17 mmol/l (100 mg/100 ml) even with creatinine clearances of 5 ml/min. Mental faculties become clear and lassitude diminishes. When the blood urea has stabilised the dietary intake of protein should be increased to 0.5 g/kg/day. This will produce some rise in the blood urea, e.g. from 13 to 20 mmol/l (80 to 120 mg/100 ml) but usually the improvement in the patient's appetite and wellbeing will remain. Thereafter treatment depends on whether the patient is eventually going to be treated with maintenance haemodialysis. If he is, the protein intake should not be lowered below 0.5 g/kg/day. If he is not to be treated with maintenance haemodialysis then the protein intake is progressively lowered to control the anorexia and vomiting. Commercial preparations of essential amino acids for oral use are available and are sometimes most useful. The patients who do best are those with normal blood pressures, and they are the ones who tend to have large urine volumes. Patients with severe hypertension do badly. Progress is assessed by measuring plasma creatinine. Whatever the level of blood urea and however satisfactory the patient's clinical condition the outlook is poor if the plasma creatinine continues to rise. Often the plasma creatinine rises while the blood urea remains unchanged. When the plasma creatinine reaches 1300 mmol/l (15 mg/100 ml) the patient is liable to die at any moment from a haemorrhage. At this level of plasma creatinine, and as it rises further, the patient's physical wellbeing begins to be marred by an increasing sense of anxiety, restlessness and insomnia. Nevertheless, protein intake as low as 0.2 g/kg/day have certainly done much to shorten the period of severe ill-health which used to accompany the last stages of renal failure.

A transitory fall in blood urea can sometimes be induced by the administration of anabolic steroids. This effect, however, is least noticeable in patients on a low intake of protein, or if there has been much loss of weight.

Protein catabolism is less the higher the calorie intake. Therefore it is reasonable to suppose that the minimal protein intake needed to maintain nitrogen balance could be lower if the diet includes a high intake of calories. Within the range of calorie intake which are practical, however, these considerations do not seem important. It is also known that the higher the intake of proteins of high biological value (i.e. those which contain a large proportion of essential amino acids) the lower the total protein intake needed to maintain nitrogen balance. Again, however, within the limits imposed in trying to keep the diet palatable this is not an important factor. On the other hand, if it is decided to renounce normal food, the intake of protein can be so arranged that it only contains essential amino acids and then the total protein intake can be drastically reduced.

### Water

In normal man the amount of urea excreted in the urine is proportional to the urine flow up to urine flows of 2 ml/min (i.e. approximately 3 1/24 hr) (p. 42). In chronic renal failure this relationship is still present and even appears to hold at greater urine flows. There is also evidence that a high turnover of water increases glomerular filtration rate. Unfortunately in many patients thirst is not a sufficient stimulus to prevent their becoming dehydrated. Some patients, particularly women, habitually drink very little. They must be advised to drink rather more than they are accustomed to, i.e. an extra three to four glasses of water a day. In the average case it is sufficient to point out that the fluid intake should be generous. The dangers of overhydration are minimal when water is being taken by mouth.

### Electrolyte and acid base balance

When hypovolaemia has occurred through nausea, vomiting or diarrhoea it must be corrected immediately by the intravenous administration of saline, and bicarbonate when indicated. Gross sodium chloride deficiency arising from excess urinary loss is rare in chronic renal failure; its treatment is dealt with on p. 323. Minor sodium chloride deficiency due to a urinary sodium leak, excess sweating, mild diarrhoea, or glycosuria can be avoided by ensuring that the salt intake is liberal or by giving a slow release sodium chloride tablet (Slow Sodium, Ciba). The latter are extremely useful for they ensure a constant intake of sodium even during periods of anorexia. It is always dangerous to restrict the salt intake of patients suffering from chronic renal failure, particularly if the blood pressure is normal, e.g. the use of a salt-free diet in the treatment of Menière's syndrome. The ability to conserve salt is limited and a contraction of the extracellular fluid space may develop insidiously with all its complications, particularly renal vasoconstriction, *hypotension* and deterioration of renal function. Major surgery, in patients with chronic renal failure, is usually considered to be contraindicated, unless it is to save life. This is particularly applicable to patients who tend to have a 'sodium leak' as in obstructive uropathy and phenacetin nephropathy. Nevertheless if such patients are given saline IV before, during and after the operation (approx. 3 to 8 litres in 2 to 4 days) major surgical procedures can be undertaken without any deterioration of renal function (Fig. 13.17).

Retention of sodium chloride is associated either with cardiac failure or the nephrotic syndrome. Treatment of the nephrotic syndrome when combined with renal failure is awkward and difficult. A high protein diet must not be given, for it will raise the blood urea as will the administration of prednisone. The only procedures which are likely to be useful are the administration of diuretics and a low salt diet.

The acidosis of chronic renal failure rarely causes any generalised symptoms. The main reason for trying to correct it is to prevent the bone changes which a persistent and accumulating retention of hydrogen ions may cause osteopemia. In addition, the administration of the sodium ion (if sodium bicarbonate is given) will greatly improve the wellbeing of those patients who may be in negative sodium balance.

Acidosis can be controlled by the oral administration of sodium bicarbonate 3–9 g/day. Calcium carbonate 6–10 g/day can also be given though it is less effective than sodium bicarbonate in raising plasma bicarbonate, but it is useful when the intake of sodium must be restricted as in heart failure or severe hypertension. Calcium carbonate also gives rise to a positive calcium balance which may also be of value. When there is a sudden fall in plasma bicarbonate due to a sudden deterioration of renal function and it is thought necessary to treat the acidosis promptly, it may be corrected by the intravenous administration of sodium bicarbonate. The speed of infusion, however, should be carefully controlled for otherwise there may be a sharp fall in the pH of the cerebro-spinal fluid with giddiness, nausea, vomiting and disturbances of consciousness. This is due to the same mechanism as that which causes a similar syndrome during a rapid dialysis for acute renal failure (p. 158).

It should be remembered that sometimes ammonium chloride is given to test renal function, (p. 97) it is best avoided in chronic renal failure for it may precipitate or aggravate a state of acidosis.

Potassium retention with hyperkalaemia is uncommon in chronic renal failure (in contrast to acute renal failure). It tends to occur only as a terminal event, or when there are acute incidents such as diarrhoea and vomiting which cause sudden deterioration in renal function. Persistent hyperkalaemia is treated with advice about the dietary content of potassium and the administration of oral cation exchange resins, either 15–60 g of a sodium containing resin or if the sodium ion is contraindicated, the same quantity of a resin that contains calcium. The treatment of acute hyperkalaemia is described on page (329). Postassium deficiency and hypokalaemia is most

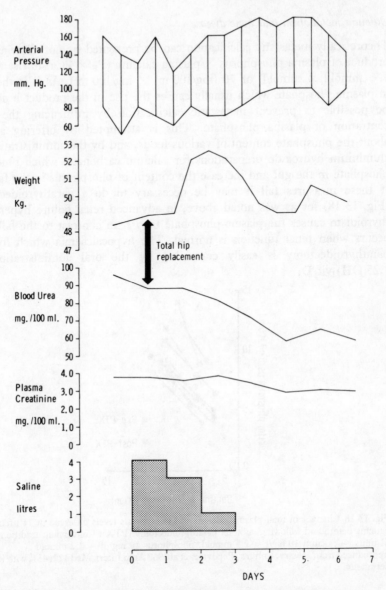

**Fig. 13.17** Arterial pressure, weight, and renal function in a patient suffering from phenacetin nephropathy undergoing total hip replacement with saline given prophylactically. Renal function improved during and after operation. Conversion: traditional to SI units — urea 10 mg/100 ml = 1.7 mmol/l: creatinine 1 mg/100 ml = 88 $\mu$/l (reproduced from Tasker, MacGregor & de Wardener 1974 Lancet 2: 911, with kind permission).

unusual in chronic renal failure unless it is the cause of the renal failure (e.g. the surreptitious self administration of diuretics or laxatives) (page 327).

*Calcium metabolism and bone disease*

Theoretically metastatic calcification can be prevented by not allowing the product of plasma phosphorus × plasma calcium ($P_P$ × PCa) to rise above 5.7 (mmol/l × mmol/l) or 70 (mg/100 ml × mg/100 ml). As it is the rise in plasma phosphate which usually causes the rise in the product it should be possible to prevent metastatic calcification by influencing the concentration of plasma phosphate. This is attempted by offering advice about the phosphate content of various foods, and by the administration of aluminium hydroxide preparations (or calcium carbonate) which bind the phosphate in the gut and increase the content of phosphorus in the faeces. If these measures fail it may be necessary to do a parathyroidectomy (Fig. 13.18) for as was noted above, in advanced renal failure hyperparathyroidism causes the plasma phosphate to *rise*, in contrast to the fall that occurs when renal function is normal. The hypocalcaemia which follows parathyroidectomy is easily controlled by the oral administration of 1,25(OH)$_2$vit D$_3$.

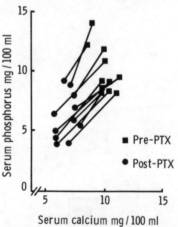

**Fig. 13.18** Changes in total plasma calcium and phosphorus levels observed in 11 uremic patients before and following subtotal parathyroidectomy (PTX). Conversion: traditional to SI units — calcium 10 mg/l = 2.5 mmol/l: phosphorus 10 mg/dl = 3.2 mmol/l (reproduced from Massry, Coburn, Popovtzer et al 1969 Arch Intern Med 124: 431, with kind permission).

The progress of hyperparathyroidism in some patients on maintenance haemodialysis can be retarded and perhaps prevented by the administration of 1,25(OH)$_2$vit D$_3$. This is illustrated in Figure 13.19. In patients who had little or no evidence of hyperparathyroidism radiologically, and in whom the rise in plasma parathyroid hormone was least pronounced, the oral administration of 1,25(OH)$_2$vit D$_3$ prevented its appearance. The initial dose should be 0.25 µg/day. Plasma phosphorus and calcium must be monitored with great vigilance because patients with mild hyperparathy-

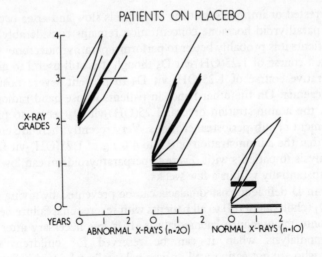

PATIENTS ON PLACEBO

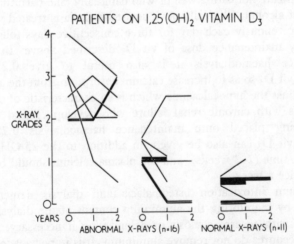

PATIENTS ON 1,25(OH)₂ VITAMIN D₃

**Fig. 13.19** Radiographic grades of severity of hyperparathyroidism in hand X-rays initially and one and two years after treatment with either placebo (above) or 1,25(OH)₂vit D₃ (below). The hyperparathyroidism became more marked with the placebo. It tended to improve, or more particularly, not to develop with 1,25(OH)₂vit D₃ (reproduced from Memmos, Eastwood, Talner et al 1981 Brit Med J: 1919, with kind permission).

roidism are particularly liable to develop hyperphosphataemia or hypercalcaemia. This liability makes it hazardous to use 1,25(OH)₂vit D₃ in patients with chronic renal failure before they are placed onto maintenance haemodialysis, for then the rise in plasma phosphorus and calcium may cause a fall in glomerular filtration rate.

In patients on maintenance haemodialysis who have unequivocal radiological changes of hyperparathyroidism and in whom the plasma parathyroid hormone is much higher the administration of 1,25(OH)₂vit D₃ by mouth is unsatisfactory (Fig. 13.19). There is a tendency for the radiological changes to be arrested or improved but the response is slow and after two years the plasma parathyroid hormone concentration remains considerably raised. In such patients it is probably better to perform a parathyroidectomy than give a prolonged course of $1,25(OH)_2$vit $D_3$ though it is still useful to give a short pre-operative course of $1,25(OH)_2$vit $D_3$ to prevent severe post-operative hypocalcaemia. On the other hand, in patients whose hand radiographs are normal, the administration or oral $1,25(OH)_2$vit $D_3$ seems to prevent the development of sub-periosteal erosions. Very recently there are encouraging reports that the administration of 0.5 to 4.0 $\mu$g of $1,25(OH)_2$vit $D_3$ IV after each dialysis to patients with severe hyperparathyroidism can lower plasma. PTH substantially within a few weeks.

Vitamin D deficiency osteomalacia can be prevented by giving 50 $\mu$g/day of Vit $D_3$ (cholecalciferol) to all patients with severe renal failure before being placed onto maintenance haemodialysis. It is less necessary after the onset of haemodialysis when it can be reserved for children and those patients who are not eating well or who habitually take barbiturates or large amounts of alcohol. Clinically obvious osteomalacia is treated with 1 mg of vit $D_3$ intravenously each day for three consecutive days followed by the small daily maintenance dose of vit $D_3$ described above. In patients on maintenance haemodialysis it is also useful to give 0.25 $\mu$g/day of $1,25(OH)_2$vit $D_3$ so as to increase calcium absorption from the gut and more quickly adjust the hypocalcaemia which is so characteristic of osteomalacia. In patients with chronic renal failure who develop clinical osteomalacia before being placed onto maintenance haemodialysis 0.25 $\mu$g/day of $1,25(OH)_2$vit $D_3$ can also be given, in addition to the 25 OH vit $D_3$, but for a short time (2–3 weeks), and the plasma calcium should be monitored at least twice a week.

Aluminium intoxication osteomalacia and dialysis dementia can be prevented by monitoring the aluminium content of the dialysis water and treating it with reverse osmosis or deionization if necessary. Water 'softening' procedures do not remove aluminium. It is important to be continuously thinking about the amount of aluminium hydroxide the patient is ingesting and not to give large amounts routinely and continuously. Plasma aluminium levels can also be measured. Once aluminium intoxication has occurred it is most efficiently and quickly reversed by renal transplantation. Otherwise recovery can be induced by removing aluminium from the patient at each dialysis by means of intravenous desferrioxamine.

Phosphate depletion osteomalacia in patients on maintenance haemodialysis is cured by making the diagnosis. The routine administration of aluminium hydroxide is stopped, oral sodium phosphate is given and the patient is encouraged to drink milk.

*Treatment of pruritus*

Parathyroidectomy cures some patients. Others may obtain some relief with cholestyramine 5 mg b.d.

## Treatment of hypertensive vascular disease

*Malignant hypertension.* If the patient has malignant hypertension the blood pressure must be lowered immediately; otherwise the prognosis is less than two years. The success of treatment depends not only on the ability of the hypotensive drug to lower the blood pressure but also on the ability of the kidneys to function at the lower pressure (p. 120); the latter probably depends on the extent of irreversible arteriolar narrowing present before treatment is begun. If the blood pressure is lowered too quickly it may precipitate a sudden deterioration of renal function which may need treatment with haemodialysis, or more importantly the hypotension causes a severe cerebral complication which may be irreversible (Fig. 13.20). In order to avoid these complications it is best to lower the pressure gently over a matter of days in order to allow the renal and cerebral circulation time to adjust. Propranolol, hydralazine, captopril and nifedipine are well tolerated anti hypertensive drugs. Occasionally several drugs have to be given in full dosage to lower the blood pressure. In an emergency (e.g. acute pulmonary oedema) the blood pressure can be lowered with an intravenous injection of hydralazine or nifedipine. The response to treatment, and survival is slightly better in those patients whose malignant hypertension

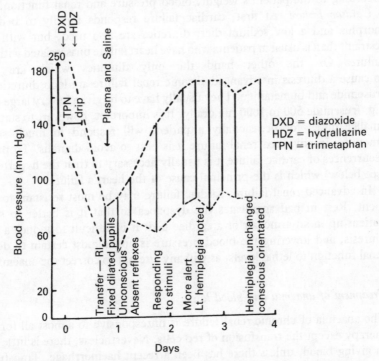

**Fig. 13.20** Man aged 33 with severe hypertension. A precipitous fall in arterial pressure, induced therapeutically, caused a persistent hemiplegia (reproduced from Ledingham & Rajagopolan 1979 Quart J Med 48: 25, with kind permission).

and impaired renal function is superimposed upon chronic renal disease. A few patients in whom the treatment of the hypertension has suddenly pitched them onto maintenance haemodialysis have subsequently recovered sufficient renal function to be able to stop dialysis.

*Non-malignant hypertension.* Both in man and animals there is a close association between hypertension and sclerotic vascular lesions. In man the progress of renal damage from 'non-malignant' hypertension is so slow that it rarely causes death from renal failure. It is generally agreed, however, that renal function in chronic renal disease deteriorates more rapidly once there is a pronounced rise in blood pressure. Accordingly it is considered reasonbale and justifiable to try and lower even a symptomless hypertension if there is any cause to believe that there is underlying renal disease.

The blood pressure can often be brought under control most effectively by combining the administration of hypotensive drugs with a low intake of sodium. In chronic renal failure this causes a substantial sodium depletion more quickly than in a normal peron and may lower the blood pressure but it may also induce a rapid deterioration of renal function. Nevertheless, if one is alert and is closely monitoring the patient's progress it is worth attempting. As soon as the blood pressure is under control the intake of sodium must be increased towards normal, the intake then being adjusted according to the patient's weight, blood pressure and renal function.

*Cardiac failure.* At first, cardiac failure responds rapidly to bed rest, morphia and a low sodium diet; diuretics are also used, but with more restraint than is usual in patients who have heart failure unassociated with renal failure. On the other hand the only diuretics which are likely to cause a diuresis in advanced chronic renal failure are loop diuretics like frusemide and bumetanide. They usually have to be given in very large doses, e.g. frusemide 500 to 1000 mg orally. It is important, however, to start with smaller doses for occasionally a patient will respond to much smaller amounts. In advanced renal failure it is best to avoid digitalis. To prevent recurrences of cardiac failure it is usually necessary to treat the hypertension (see below) which is the principal cause of the heart's failure.

In advanced renal failure, cardiac failure may be most resistant to treatment. Rest in bed aggravates the dyspnoea so that it is better to sit the patient up in an armchair or a cardiac bed; it is difficult to induce a saline diuresis; and lowering the blood pressure is now almost certain to depress renal function to lethal levels, as will any attempt to correct the anaemia.

## Treatment of anaemia and blood loss

The anaemia of chronic renal failure is unresponsive to almost all forms of therapy except the transfusion of red cells. Nevertheless, there is little point in giving blood, unless there has been a recent haemorrhage. Transfusions inhibit the bone marrow's production of red cells so that the packed cell volume usually quickly falls to its previous level. It is customary to give

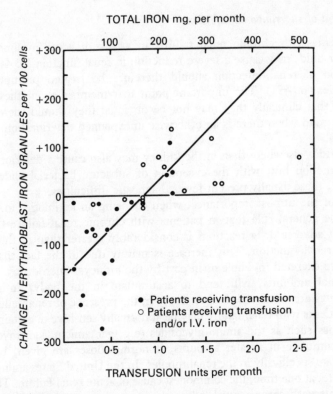

**Fig. 13.21** Relation between number of transfusions per month, or the total amount of iron administered per month, for 8–25 months and the change in the iron content of bone marrow erythroblasts which occurred during that time (reproduced from Edwards, Pegrum & Curtis, 1970 Lancet 2: 491; with kind permission).

iron preparations by mouth. These are effective in the few patients who are iron deficient, and it is particularly useful in patients on maintenance haemodialysis in whom it prevents iron deficiency developing (Fig. 13.21).

It has been reported that non-androgenic steroids such as oxymethalone are of value in men on maintenance haemodialysis. Few centres now use this form of treatment the advantages of which are marginal, difficult to reproduce, short lasting and liable to cause complications such as jaundice. Cobaltous chloride is very effective in treating the anaemia of maintenance haemodialysis but it tends to be retained and cause sudden death from acute cardiomyopathy.

Haemorrhage must be treated as rapidly as possible with transfusions of whole blood. The dangers to renal function of under- and overtransfusion have already been mentioned. It is essential that patients with chronic renal failure should not become carriers of Hepatitis B. Blood for transfusion must therefore be screened for the presence of Hepatitis B surface antigen.

## Treatment of superimposed infection

In patients with chronic renal failure an attack of acute pyelonephritis, however mild, may cause a severe reduction in renal function (p. 446). Any suspicion of renal infection should therefore be treated promptly with antibiotics (p. 451). The important point to remember about these infections is that clinically they may not be obvious; they should therefore be kept in mind when there is an otherwise unexplained deterioration of renal function.

Infections elsewhere than in the kidney may also cause a deterioration of renal function but, with the exception of subacute bacterial endocarditis (p. 424), these usually present fewer diagnostic difficulties.

It is of the utmost importance, when choosing an antibiotic, to keep in mind the general rule that in patients with chronic renal failure the incidence of adverse drug reactions is considerably greater than in those with normal renal function. This increase is mainly due to the fact that many drugs are excreted in whole or in part by the kidneys. Such drugs, if given in normal amounts, will tend to accumulate in the body. In addition some drugs are metabolised more slowly in the presence of renal failure, and some patients with renal failure may be abnormally sensitive to certain drugs. Antibiotics such as the amino glycosides (e.g. gentamicin, kanamycin) not only accumulate in greater amounts, if normal doses are given, but they accumulate specifically in the renal tubules. In the United States amino glycosides were, at one time, the commonest cause of acute renal failure. Their use in patients with chronic renal failure therefore is extremely hazardous. The dose must be adjusted according to the severity of the renal failure and blood levels should be monitored. Obviously nephrotoxicity is less important when the patient is on maintenance haemodialysis.

## Treatment of hiccough

There are many methods of treating hiccough, including the inhalation of carbon dioxide, and the administration of chlorpromazine or mepyramine. The latter can be given in doses of 100 mg four-hourly by mouth or by injection; it is sometimes useful when all else has failed. Occasionally a drop of oil of peppermint on a piece of sugar is sufficient to stop an attack.

## Treatment of nausea, vomiting and dyspnoea

Some of the gastrointestinal symptoms such as dyspepsia and flatulence may respond to metaclopramide. Endoscopically evident lesions should be treated with a reduced dose of cimetidine (200 mg 12 hourly). When nausea and vomiting become persistent the simplest treatment is to reduce the intake of protein. Sometimes, if the patient is first seen in an advanced uraemic state, it may be useful to perform one or two peritoneal diaslyses in order to obtain an initial return of appetite. If this is unsuccessful the patient should be placed onto some form of persistent dialysis or transplanted.

In those patients who cannot eat a very low protein diet and for whom maintenance dialysis or transplantation are not available nausea and vomiting can be best controlled by the administration of thiethylperazine or chlorpromazine. In the terminal stages chlorpromazine not only abolishes nausea and vomiting, but it calms the patient's anxiety. It also reduces the quantity of drugs needed to control the other two distressing features of terminal renal failure, dyspnoea, and physical and mental restlessness. Morphia is useful for dyspnoea, and in combination with chlorpromazine is less likely to cause nausea and vomiting. Restlessness and distress can often be controlled with diazepam, if not, chlorpromazine and morphine may be necessary. Barbiturates also useful in this respect, but they sometimes cause a persistent unhappy, confused drowsiness which aggravates the restlessness. The repeated administration of short and medium acting barbiturates should be avoided because of contamination with barbital which accumulates in patients with renal failure.

## Maintenance dialysis and Transplantation

It is important to decide whether a patient is to be treated with maintenance dialysis or transplantation before he is moribund. The optimum time to place most patients on maintenance dialysis is when conservative treatment has either failed to enable the patient to stay at work or failed to prevent the plasma creatinine rising to around 1300 mmol/l /15 mg/100 ml). Patients suffering from diabetes are placed onto dialysis much earlier.

### Maintenance dialysis

This can be carried out with either haemodialysis or peritoneal dialysis.

*Maintenance haemodialysis.* Either a subcutaneous arterior-venous fistula is made by anastamosing the radial artery to a nearby superficial vein, or an arterio-venous shunt is established into one of the patient's limbs with teflon and silicone rubber tubes. These measures allow repeated, quick, atraumatic access to the patient's arterial and venous circulation at all times. Dialyses are performed by pumping the patient's blood through a dialyser. This consists of an apparatus in which the blood passes on one side of a semi premeable membrane, such as cellophane or cuprophane, whilst a dialysis fluid containing electrolytes and glucose passes on the other. Diffusion, ultrafiltration and osmosis occur across the membrane. Low molecular weight substances (<1000 Daltons) pass through the pores of the membrane by diffusion. The amount of ultrafiltration that occurs is controlled by adjusting the pressure gradient across the membrane and occasionally by using especially permeable membranes.

Dailyses are performed two to three times a week, the overall survival and rehabilitation being the same whichever frequency is chosen but the control of blood pressure is easier with three dialyses a week. It is the total number of hours of dialyses per week which appears to be important. The optimum number is uncertain and of course will depend on the residual renal function and the properties of the dialyser. Dialysers have now become so efficient that the diffusional aspects of dialysis can be performed very rapidly (2–4 hours). And it is true that in that time it is usually possible by ultrafiltration to remove the excess fluid that the patient has retained since the last dialysis. But it is often a great strain on the patient to have such rapid changes in the composition and volume of the extracellular fluid. The obsession to shorten the duration of dialysis may be partly responsible for the twenty fold increase in the incidence of myocardial infarction which has been recorded in Federal Germany in patients aged 35–54 who have less than 12 hours of dialysis per week. Dietary restrictions are necessary. Their extent depend to a large extent on the daily urine volume, residual renal function, and the blood pressure.

The aim of treatment is to keep the weight gain between dialyses below 1.5 kg, and to keep the blood pressure normal. Water and sodium intake are therefore regulated accordingly. Sodium intake has to be regulated more strictly at the beginning of treatment than after a year or two; it is usually limited to 20–50 mmol/day. Potassium intake is limited to around 50 mmol/day, and protein intake to between 40 and 70 g/day depending on the patient's weight. The calory intake is raised to the maximum possible, e.g. 3,000 calories or more. The bone marrow depression of chronic renal failure is relieved to a certain extent by maintenance haemodialysis and many patients will keep packed cell volumes of 20 to 25 per cent without transfusion. Hypertension is brought under control by reducing the patient's weight by 1 or 2 kg at each dialysis by ultrafiltration. Initially as much as 20 kg may have to be gradually removed before the blood pressure is controlled.

*Contraindication.* As the alternative is death there are not many contraindications to dialysis though occasionally peritoneal dialysis may be more suitable (see below) than haemodialysis. The patient should be sane and not suffering from a terminal malignancy. A preceding cerebrovascular accident or myocardial infarction make it likely that the patient will either be difficult to teach or suffer from severe hypotension during dialysis. Nevertheless many such patients can be treated. Except in the United Kingdom, most 'Western' countries do not consider that age is a contra-indication to dialysis. It has to be admitted, however, that the elderly do find it difficult to remember what they have recently been taught, and may therefore be difficult to train for home dialysis.

*Complications.* The fistula or shunt may clot or become infected, and peripheral neuropathy, metastatic calcification, calcium 'gout', hyperpara-thyroidism, hypertension and anaemia may cause symptoms. Insufficient dialysis causes the 'under dialysis syndrome' which consists of lassitude, anor-exia, weight loss, depression and a high incidence of 'complications' (see below). Acute pulmonary oedema and cerebrovascular accident are the commonest cause of death. The former is due either to carelessness about fluid removal or more often to the patient's incontinent intake of fluid despite multiple warn-ings of the possible consequences. Patients on dialysis are particularly liable to infection with hepatitis B and hepatitis non A-non B viruses. Prophylactic measures in the United Kingdom however had reduced the incidence of these infections to a total of 7 and 2 respectively in 1981. Many of the patients infected with hepatitis B and non A-non B viruses in the preceding years have developed chronic hepatitis subsequently.

*Bicarbonate haemodialysis.* It is not possible to manufacture dialysate concentrates containing bicarbonate. It is the custom therefore to substitute acetate for bicarbonate, and the acetate is then rapidly metabolised to bicar-bonate. Nevertheless acetate is a potent vasodilator, depresses myocardial contractility and causes hypoxaemia. It is also possible that some of the acetate is metabolised to fats and thus contributes to the incidence of hyperlipidaemia. It is highly probable that acetate is sometimes responsible for many of the unpleasant side effects of dialysis. A few patients appear to be very sensitive to the usual plasma concentrations of acetate which occur, while others may have some difficulty in metabolising the sudden influx of acetate so that the plasma acetate rises to much higher levels than normal. This is seen particularly in patients with diabetes. It has been claimed that in certain patients the use of bicarbonate dialysis had signifi-cantly lowered the incidence of such symptoms as nausea, hypotension and post dialysis fatigue. There are now commercially available methods of preparing a bicarbonate dialysate.

*Chronic haemofiltration.* The principle of this technique is to remove the toxic substances by a convective process similar to that occurring through the glomerular capillaries. A highly permeable membrane is used so that ultrafiltrate is formed at rates of up to 25 litres in 3 to 4 hours. An infusate, the composition of which is changed during the course of the procedure, is injected intra-venously at the same rate as the ultrafiltrate is formed. This technique is much more complicated and expensive than that of the stan-dard form of haemodialysis and it is unsuitable for home dialysis. It is claimed however, that with chronic haemofiltration it is much easier to control hypertension and that the incidence of nausea, vomiting, cramps, headaches and hypotension is greatly reduced. And that in addition there is higher clearance of larger molecular weight substances.

This treatment is seldom used routinely but modifications of it are often employed for patients who are habitually overloaded with fluids.

*Quality of survival.* If maintenance dialysis is properly carried out most of the patients are well, active and at work. If maintenance haemodialysis is only an adjunct to prepare patients for transplantation it is apt to be incompetently performed and the patients tend to be unwell, inactive and unhappy.

*Maintenance peritoneal dialysis.* This may be performed in one of three ways:

1. *Intermittent peritoneal dialysis (IPD).* A fresh disposable peritoneal catheter is inserted into the peritoneal cavity two to three times a week or more usually a silastic peritoneal catheter is kept in situ. Peritoneal dialysis is then performed two to three times per week for 18 hours each time. Automated cycling devices allow the patient to be at home.

2. *Continuous ambulatory peritoneal dialysis (CAPD).* A permanently placed peritoneal catheter is connected at all times to a 2 litre bag of dialysate fluid. The fluid is run into the peritoneal cavity and allowed to stay *in situ* for about five to six hours during which time the patient carries the empty bag rolled up next to his person. The dialysate fluid which has now come into equilibrium with the patient's extracellular fluid volume is then allowed to run back into the bag. This bag is then exchanged for a fresh bag and the procedure repeated. The average CAPD regimen consists of four exchanges per day, three during the day and one during the night. Because of its low efficiency CAPD is best used after a patient's renal failure has been brought under control by some other form of dialysis. One advantage is that dietary intake of sodium, potassium and water tends to be unrestricted and the patient is encouraged to eat a large amount of protein.

3. *Continuous cycling peritoneal dialysis (CCPD).* This modification was introduced to avoid the high risk of peritonitis inherent in the multiplicity of bag exchanges in CAPD, or the long constraining dialysis sessions of IPD. The indwelling peritoneal catheter is joined to an automated cycling device each evening when the patient goes to bed for four exchanges of 2 litre each. In the morning a fresh 2 litre of dialysate is placed into the peritoneal cavity and the patient is disconnected from the machine. In this way the catheter is only handled twice in 24 hours and the patient has nothing to do during the day.

Peritoneal dialysis is useful in some patients with acute renal failure. In the treatment of terminal renal failure it is invaluable as a holding manoeuvre when the renal centre is overcrowded. CAPD is the only form of peritoneal dialysis which has been attempted in a large number of patients as a long term substitute for maintenance haemodialysis. But because of the risk of peritonitis it has mainly been offered to debilitated patients who have either been unable to stand up to the cardiovascular rigours of haemodialysis or were unlikely to be able to learn how to haemodialyse themselves at home. This may explain the poor results obtained with CAPD. In Europe only 28% of 4525 patients placed on CAPD by the end of 1981 were still on this form of treatment at the end of two years. The other 72% had either died (35%) or dropped out because of peritonitis, abdominal pain, back pain, inadequate dialysis or a distaste for the procedure. For these reasons the initial enthusiasm for CAPD, which was always difficult to understand, for the risk of peritonitis was well known and the recurrent costs no less than those of haemodialysis, is now more muted.

## Renal transplantation

A kidney is removed from either a living donor or a corpse and transplanted into the patient suffering from terminal renal failure. The functional efficiency of the transplanted kidney mainly depends on the compatibility of the tissue antigens of the corpse and the patient. The greater the incompatibility the quicker the patient's immunological mechanisms cause the kidney to be rejected. If they are completely compatible, as in identical twins, there will be no rejection.

To minimise rejection ABO compatibility is always observed, and many (though not all) units also attempt to match the HLA-A, HLA-B and HL-DR antigens of the donor and recipient as closely as possible (Fig. 13.22). Direct cross matching of donor cells and recipient serum is performed to detect whether the recipient's serum contains circulating antibodies to the donor's cells. It is interesting however that the presence of such antibodies against the donor's B lymphocytes does not appear to affect the survival of the graft.

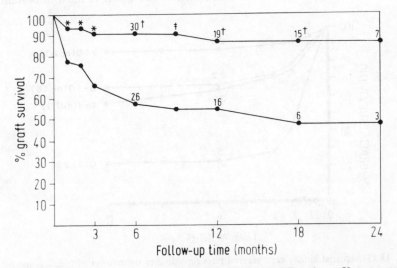

**Fig. 13.22** Kidney-graft survival and matching for A, B, and DR antigens. Upper curve represents grafts with ≤ 1 mismatch at A and/or B loci and ≤ 1 mismatch at DR; lower curve represents other grafts. Figures above curves are the number of surviving grafts. *Difference between points on upper and lower curves is significant P < 0.05; †P < 0.01; ‡P < 0.01 (reproduced from Persijn, Gabb, van Leeuwen et al 1978 Lancet 1: 1278, with kind permission).

In addition it has now been established that the survival of the graft is favourably related to the number of transfusions the recipient receives before transplantation (Fig. 13.23). Patients awaiting a transplantation therefore tend to be transfused. The nature of the immunological benefit this bestows is difficult to understand. It is possible that blood transfusions stimulate patients to form antibodies against certain HLA specific antigens. Transfusions may thus select those patients who will respond to these HLA antigens so that a direct cross match of such a patient's serum against a potential donor's cells, before a transplantation, then screens those patients who have responded in this way. In other words the benefit of blood transfusions may be that it is better to be sensitized by being transfused before the graft is put into place, than it is to be sensitized by the graft itself and suffer its loss from rejection.

The surgical technique involved in cadaveric renal transplantation is relatively simple. The prospective patient has usually been kept fit and well by maintenance haemodialysis beforehand. The principal difficulty is to bring the kidney and the patient together rapidly after the donor dies. A variety of techniques have been evolved to prevent the kidney from deteriorating in the interval. Immunological rejection of the transplanted kidney may be particularly violent a few days after the transplant operation. Rejection is suppressed by the administration of immunosuppressive drugs such as azathioprine and prednisone, or cyclosporin A. Antilymphocytic serum and most recently monoclonal anti T cell antibody preparations are also used, and sometimes local irradiation of the graft. A most important

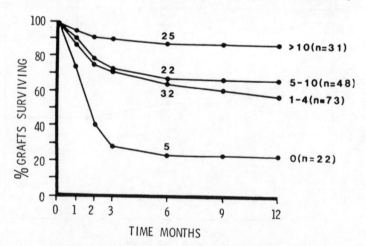

**Fig. 13.23** Actuarial kidney graft survival rates according to the number of transfusions received before transplantation. Numbers of transfusions are indicated at end of each curve and numbers of patients are given in parentheses. Numbers of graft survivals for each group at 6 mo are as indicated. Number of patients at risk at 6 mo are as indicated. p (by weighted regression analysis) was < 0.0001 at 3, 6, and 12 months indicating that the improvement in graft outcome was dependent on an increased number of pre-transplant transfusions (reproduced from Opelz, Graver & Terasaki 1981 Lancet 1: 1223, with kind permission).

advance has been the recognition that it is unnecessary to use large amounts of prednisone. The following regimen has been used with success. The day after the transplant operation azathioprine 1.5 mg/kg/day and prednisone 20 mg/day are given until the creatinine clearance exceeds 20 ml/min when the azathioprine is increased to 3.0 mg/kg/day. After six months the prednisone dose is gradually reduced to about 10 mg/day during the next year. Acute rejection episodes are treated with 200 mg of prednisone/day for 2–3 days after which the dose is reduced to 20 mg/day in the next 2–5 days. With this reduced dosage of prednisone the incidence of opportunistic infection is much lower and the results achieved have been among the best in the world (e.g. 80% cadaver graft survival at 5 year).

Cyclosporin A also has to be given with great caution for it is both hepatotoxic and nephrotoxic. The nephrotoxicity may be difficult to distinguish from graft rejection. It is interesting and useful that graft rejection which may be resistant to treatment with prednisone and azathioprine may respond to cyclosporin A and vice versa. But these two forms of treatment should not be given together for there is then an increased incidence of lymphoma and other malignancies.

If rejection is difficult to overcome immunosuppressive treatment should be tailed off, the kidney removed and the patient returned to dialysis.

*Contraindications.* The contraindications to transplantation are: (1) history of a recently treated neoplasm, (2) aseptic bone necrosis, (3) angina, myocardial infarction and heart failure, (4) the presence of circulating glomerular basement membrane antibody, (5) recent exacerbation of tuberculosis, (6) bronchiectasis, (7) hepatitis B antigenaemia (8) the patient is being dialysed at home, is well and at work and is reluctant to be transplanted, or (9) he is over 55 years.

*Complications.* The complications of renal transplantation are those which affect the transplanted kidney or its ureter, and those which are due to the drugs used to suppress rejection. Apart from infection and infarction the kidney may suffer any of five pathological processes. Acute tubular necrosis may occur. It appears immediately after the operation and is due to deterioration of the kidney before it is transplanted. Acute rejection may develop a few days later and is characterised by a heavy infiltration of mononuclear cells, plasma cells and eosinophils together with acute destruction of the renal parenchyma. If these acute hazards are avoided other more gradual changes may occur, including a slowly progressive interstitial nephritis and an occlusive arteritis. The rate at which the arteries become occluded is the main determinant of the graft's survival. If the recipient initially suffered from glomerular nephritis there is about a 1 in 5 chance that the same lesion will recurr in the graft. The following lesions have recurred, dense deposit disease, membrano proliferative, extra membranous, IgA, crescentic, proliferative, and focal sclerosing glomerular nephritis. A recurrence of minimal change glomerular nephritis with nephrotic syndrome has also been observed. These lesions may recur a few months to several years after the transplantation. Necrosis of the ureter at its insertion into the bladder also appears to be due to a rejection phenomenon.

The complications which stem from the use of cytotoxic drugs are those of immunological and bone marrow suppression including fulminating infections with agranulocytosis, multiple haemorrhages from thrombocyto-poenia and the appearance of malignant tumours. The patient may die of infections with various fungi or viruses which are rarely pathogenic in other circumstances. The administration of large amounts of prednisone in the past often caused the classical florid facies of Cushing's disease. Prednisone may also reactivate pulmonary tuberculosis and cause hypertension, cata-racts, or a devastating gastro-intestinal haemorrhage from an acute peptic ulcer. It may also cause ischaemic bone necrosis particularly at either end of the femur. Patients with hepatitis B antigenaemia tend to develop chronic active hepatitis, cirrhosis, and hepatomas, and die of liver failure.

Persistent hypercalcaemia and hypophosphataemia due to continuing hyperparathyroidism following transplantation may take several years to settle down.

*Quality of survival.* If the graft is successful and there are no serious symp-tomatic complications the patients' physical and occupational rehabilitation is better than that of patients on maintenance haemodialysis. Subjective assessment, however, of the quality of life (frequency of boredom, range of interests, facility for excitement and pleasure in accomplishment) is about the same in the two groups. But the physical condition, rehabilitation and subjective assessment of those patients who have had a failed transplant (the majority of those who have had a cadaveric transplant) are significantly below that of patients with a successful transplant or of patients on dialysis. In addition one has to add the often prolonged periods of illness which precede and follow the rejection of the graft. It is interesting, in this connection, that two physicians who have been on maintenance haemodi-alysis for over 15 years, mainly at home, have preferred, so far, not to have a cadaveric transplant.

*Duration of survival.* The best way to organise the treatment of terminal renal failure is to have closely knit teams who can offer either dialysis or transplantation depending on which is the most suitable for the patient at any one time.

Overall, combining the results of all forms of haemodialysis and trans-plantation, survival is gradually improving with the years. It is directly related to age; 85% survival at 3 years between the ages of 20–25 years falling to 60% survival between the age of 60–65 yr (Fig. 13.24). On the other hand the majority of patients suffering from terminal renal failure are over 50 years of age, whereas transplantation is mainly carried out in patients below the age of 40 years. The survival of patients who have received a live related donor kidney is much better than if the kidney comes from a corpse. Survival of patients (of all ages) on home dialysis is the same

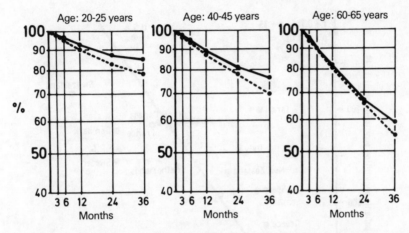

**Fig. 13.24** Overall survival on renal replacement therapy, 1974–1976 (●----●) and 1979–1981. (●———●) Numbers of patients for 1974–1976 and 1979–1981 were: age 20–25 years 1792 and 2217 respectively, age 40–45 years 3323 and 4316, age 60–65 years 2050 and 3799 (reproduced from European Dialysis and transplant association registration committee. Chairman: A. J. Wing. Combined report on regular dialysis and transplantation in Europe XII, 1981. Proceedings of the European Dialysis and Transplant Association, 1982, XIX, Pitman, London, with kind permission).

as that of patients (mainly below 40 years) who have received a kidney from a living related donor (approximately 75% at 5 years). Whereas patients (mainly below 40 years) receiving a kidney from a corpse have a lower survival (about 58% at 5 years). As the survival of the grafts is 20 to 30% less than that of the patients, it is clear that the excellence of a transplant centre, as regards its concern for its patients, can be gauged by the ratio of patient survival to graft survival. The further away from unity the better, for this then indicates that the centre is more concerned with the survival of the patients than of the graft. There is a temptation, when rejection threatens, to continue to increase the dose of immunosuppressive drugs indefinitely. If this is not resisted the graft may survive but the patient dies from one of the many complications of immunosuppression.

## THE NEED FOR AND DISTRIBUTION OF FACILITIES FOR THE TREATMENT OF TERMINAL RENAL FAILURE

The incidence of terminal renal failure in Western countries is about 90 per million per year. At least 50 per million below the age of 65 are suitable for treatment. If patients above the age of 65 are included the total number who could benefit from treatment rises rapidly. The provision of services, however, and consequently the number of patients on treatment, does not correlate with need but with gross national product (GNP) (Fig. 13.25). The intercept of the regression line, at 2700 US dollars per capita in Figure 13.25

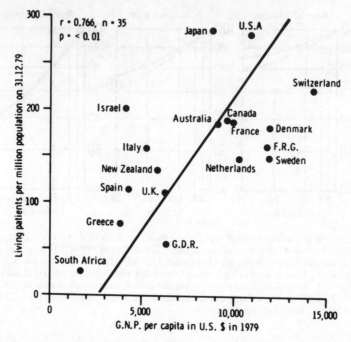

**Fig. 13.25** Correlation between number of patients treated for terminal renal failure and gross national product in 1979 (reproduced from Wing & Selwood 1982 In: Recent Jones NF, Peters DK (eds) Advances in renal medicine. Churchill Livingstone, Edinburgh, p. 103, with kind permission).

suggests that countries with a per capital GNP of less than this will find it either very difficult or more possibly, inappropriate, to try and put many patients on this form of treatment. In 1979 three quarters of the world's population lived in countries which had a per capita gross national product below this amount.

It is interesting to note that in those countries that can afford to treat terminal renal failure some are clearly more concerned with their sick than others. For instance in 1979 Spain and Italy, the GNP of which was less than that of the UK, were treating a larger number of patients. By 1981 the position in Great Britain had deteriorated further and other much less affluent nations such as Greece, Cyprus and Austria had more patients on treatment per million population than Great Britain.

Hospital maintenance dialysis centres are the mainstay of the treatment available, for they train, and support the large number of patients who dialyse at home, they also make the patients fit for transplantation and again provide treatment when the graft fails. The staff patient ratio of nephrology centres in the UK is far below that of any other western country so that the 'productivity' of nephrologists in the UK is correspondingly greater. This has been achieved by stretching the available facilities to the utmost by concentrating on home dialysis and transplantation. More recently the use of clinical computers had made it easier for the same number of staff to treat an increasing number of patients. By the end of 1981 the total number of transplantations performed in the UK was almost double that of any other European country. Even more patients could be transplanted if the supply of kidneys became more plentiful. This in turn depends on all doctors becoming aware of the large numbers of deaths that take place from which suitable kidneys could be obtained. Nevertheless the more patients are transplanted the greater the facilities needed to rescue the failures. An increase in the number of transplants performed therefore does not necessarily lower the requirements for dialysis facilities.

BIBLIOGRAPHY

**General**
Anderson R J, Gambertoglio J G, Schrier R W 1976 Clinical uses of drugs in renal failure. Thomas, Springfield
Bricker N S, Fine L G 1981 The renal response to progressive nephron loss. In: Brenner B M, Rector F C (eds) The kidney, vol 1. Saunders, Philadelphia, 1056
Curtis J R, Williams G B 1975 Clinical management of chronic renal failure. Blackwell Scientific, Oxford
Gottschalk C W 1971 Function of chronically diseased kidney. Circ Res 28 & 29: 1
Ibels L S, Alfrey A C, Haut L et al 1978 Preservation of function in experimental renal disease by dietary restriction of phosphate. New Engl J Med 298: 122
Montgomerie J Z, Kalmanson G M, Guze L B 1968 Renal failure and infection. Medicine 47: 1
Newberry W M, Sanford J P 1971 Defective cellular immunity in renal failure: Depression of reactivity of lymphocytes to phytohemagglutin in by renal failure serum. J Clin Invest 50: 1262
Taylor C M, Mawer E B, Wallace J E et al 1967 The contribution of residual nephrons within the chronically diseased kidney to urate homeostasis in man. Amer J Med 43: 876
Touraine J L, Touraine F, Revillard J P et al 1975 T-lymphocytes and serum inhibitors of cell-mediated immunity in renal insufficiency. Nephron 14: 195
Tsaltas T T 1969 Studies of lipochromes (Urochromes) in uraemic patients and normal controls 1. The elimination of plasma lipochromes by haemodialysis. Trans Amer Soc Artif Inter Organ XV: 321
**Cancer**
Kinlen L J, Eastwood J B, Kerr D N S et al 1980 Cancer in patients receiving dialysis. Brit Med J 280: 1401
**Sodium**
Clarkson E M, Curtis J R, Jewkes R J et al 1971 Slow sodium. An oral slowly released sodium chloride preparation. Brit Med J 3: 604
Espinel C H 1975 The influence of salt intake on the metabolic acidosis of chronic renal failure. J Clin Invest 56: 286
*Goodwin T J, James H T, Peart W S 1974 The control of aldosterone secretion in nephrectomised man. Clin Sci Mol Med 47: 235
Hayslett J P, Kashgarian M, Epstein F H 1969 Mechanism of change in the excretion of sodium per nephron when renal mass is reduced. J Clin Invest 48: 1002
Schambelan M, Sebastian A, Biglieri E G 1980 Prevalence, pathogenesis and functional significance of aldosterone deficiency in hyperkalaemic patients with chronic renal insufficiency. Kidney Int 17: 89
Stanbury S W, Mahler R F 1959 Salt-wasting renal disease. Quart J Med 28: 425
Tasker P R W, MacGregor G A, de Wardener H E 1974 Prophylactic use of intravenous saline in patients with chronic renal failure undergoing major surgery. Lancet 2: 911

**Potassium**

Schon D A, Silva P, Hayslett J P 1974 Mechanism of potassium excretion in renal insufficiency. Amer J Physiol 227: 1323

**Bone disease**

Bloom W L, Flinchum D 1960 Osteomalacia with pseudofractures caused by the ingestion of aluminium hydroxide. J Amer Med Assoc 174: 1327

Bordier Ph J, Tun Chot S, Eastwood J B et al Wardener H E 1973 Lack of histological evidence of Vit D abnormality in the bones of anephric patients. Clin Sci 44: 33

Canterbury J M, Gavellas G, Bourgoignie J J et al 1980 Metabolic consequences of oral administration of 24,25-dihydroxy-cholecalciferol to uremic dogs. J Clin Invest 65: 571

de Vernejoul P, Crosnier J 1980 Effect of parathyroidectomy on left-ventricular function in haemodialysis patients. Lancet i: 112

Eastwood J B 1977 Renal osteodystrophy — a radiological review. C.R.C. Critical Reviews in Diagnostic Imaging 9: 77

Eastwood J B, Bordier P J, Clarkson E M et al 1974 The contrasting effects on bone histology of Vit D and of calcium carbonate in the osteomalacia of chronic renal failure. Clin Sci 47: 23

Eastwood J B, Bordier P, de Wardener H E 1971 Comparison of the effect of vitamin D and calcium carbonate in renal osteomalacia. Quart J Med 40: 569

Eastwood J B, Harris E, Stamp T C B et al 1976 Vitamin D deficiency in the osteomalacia of chronic renal failure. Lancet 2: 1209

Eastwood J B, de Wardener H E, Gray R W et al 1979 Normal plasma 1,25(OH)$_2$ Vitamin D concentrations in nutritional osteomalacia. Lancet i: 1377

Ellis H A, Peart K M 1973 Azotaemic renal osteodystrophy: a quantitative study on iliac bone. J Clin Path 26: 83

Kaye M, Frueh A J, Silverman M et al 1970 A study of vertebral bone powder from patients with chronic renal failure. J Clin Invest 49: 442

Krieger N S, Tashjian A H 1981 Inhibition by ouabain of parathyroid hormone — stimulated bone resorption. J Pharmacol Exp Ther 217: 586

Mehls O, Ritz E, Kreusser W et al 1980 Renal osteodystrophy in uraemic children. Clin Endocrinol Metab 9: 151

Memmos D E, Eastwood J B, Harris E et al 1982 Response of uremic osteoid to Vitamin D. Kidney Int Suppl 11, 21: S50

Memmos D E, Eastwood J B, Talner L B et al 1981 Double blind trial of oral 1,25 (OH)$_2$ Vit D$_3$ versus placebo in asymptomatic hyperparathyroidism in patients receiving maintenance haemodialysis. Brit Med J 1: 1919

Pellegrino E D, Biltz R M 1965 The composition of human bone in uraemia. Medicine 44: 397

Pierides A M, Ellis H A, Ward M et al 1976 Barbiturate and anticonvulsant treatment in relation to osteomalacia with haemodialysis and renal transplantation. Brit Med J i: 190

Rickers H, Nielsen A H, Smith Pedersen R et al 1978 Bone mineral loss during maintenance haemodialysis. Acta Med Scand 204: 263

Ritz E, Rambausek M, Kreusser W et al 1982 Bone metabolism in renal disease. In: Jones N F, Peters D K (eds) Recent advances in renal medicine 2. Churchill Livingstone, London, p 151

Rasmussen H, Baron R, Broadus A et al 1980 1,25(OH)$_2$D$_3$ is not the only D metabolite involved in the pathogenesis of osteomalacia. Amer J Med 69: 360

Slatopolsky E, Caglar S, Pennell J P et al 1971 On the pathogenesis of hyperparathyroidism in chronic experimental renal insufficiency in the dog. J Clin Invest 50: 492

Slatopolsky E, Gradowska L, Kashemsant C et al 1966 The control of phosphate excretion in uremia. J Clin Invest 45: 672

Slatopolsky E, Martin K, Hruska K 1980 Parathyroid hormone metabolism and its potential as a uremic toxin. Amer J Physiol 239: F1

Somerville P J, Kaye M 1978 Resistance to parathyroid hormone in renal failure: Role of Vit. D metabolites. Kidney Int 14: 245

Stanbury S W 1972 Bone complications of renal diseases. In: Black D A K (ed) Renal disease. Blackwell Scientific Pub, Oxford

Stanbury S W 1978 Vitamin D and the syndromes of Azotaemic osteodystrophy. Contrib Nephrol 13: 132

Taylor C M, Mawer E B, Wallace J E et al 1978 The absence of 24,25-dihydroxycholecalciferol in anephric patients. Clin Sci Mol Med 55: 541

Ward M K, Ellis H A, Feest T G et al 1978 Osteomalacic dialysis osteodystrophy; evidence for a water — borne aetiological agent, probably aluminium. Lancet i: 841

**Aluminium**

Alfrey A C, Legendre G R, Kaehny W D 1976 The dialysis encephalopathy syndrome. New Engl J Med 294: 184

Biswas C K, Arze R S, Ramos J M et al 1982 Effect of aluminium hydroxide on serum ionised calcium, Immunoreactive parathyroid hormone, and aluminium in chronic renal failure. Brit Med J 284: 776

Boukari M, Rottembourg J, Jaudon M-C et al 1978 Influence de la prise prolongée de gels d'alumine sur les taux sériques d7 d'aluminium chez les patients atteints d'insuffance rénal chronique. Nouv Press Med 7: 85

**Calcium and magnesium**

Clarkson E M, McDonald S J, de Wardener H E 1965 Magnesium metabolism in chronic renal failure. Clin Sci 28: 107

Clarkson E M, McDonald S J, de Wardener H E 1966 The effect of a high intake of calcium carbonate in normal subjects and patients with chronic renal failure. Clin Sci 30: 425

Wallach S, Rizek J E, Dimich A et al 1966 Magnesium transport in normal and uremic patients. J Clin Endocrinol 26: 1069

**Hydrogen ions**

Goodman A D, Lemann J, Lennon E J et al 1965 Production, excretion, and net balance of fixed acid in patients with renal acidosis. J Clin Investig 44: 495

Schwartz W B, Hall P W, Hays R M et al 1959 On the mechanism of acidosis in chronic renal disease. J Clin Invest 38: 39

Elkington J R 1963 Hydrogen ion turnover in health and in renal disease. Ann Intern Med 57: 660

**Central nervous system**

Blagg C R, Kemble F, Travener D 1968 Nerve conduction velocity in relationship to the severity of renal disease. Nephron 5: 290

Raskin N H, Fishman R A 1976 Neurologic disorders in renal failure. New Engl J Med 294: 143, 204

Richet G, Novalez de E L, Verroust P 1970 Drug intoxication and neurological episodes in chronic renal failure. Brit Med J 2: 394

**Gastro intestinal**

Mason E E 1952 Gastrointestinal lesions occurring in uraemia. Ann Int Med 37: 96

Shepherd A M M, Stewart W K, Wormsley K G 1973 Peptic ulceration in chronic renal failure. Lancet i: 1357

**Joints**

Brown E A, Gower P E 1982 Joint problems in patients on maintenance haemodialysis. Clin Nephrol 18: 247

**Protein**

Coles G A, Peters D K, Jones J H 1970 Albumin metabolism in chronic renal failure. Clin Sci 39: 423

Ford J, Phillips M E, Toye F E et al 1969 Nitrogen balance in patients with chronic renal failure on diets containing varying quantities of protein. Brit Med J i: 735

Jones N F, Peters D K 1982 Recent advances in renal medicine. Churchill Livingstone, Edinburgh p 103

Nitrogen and amino acid metabolism in uremia 1 and 2 1975 Clin Nephrol 3, No 5 and 6, 166, 228

Nutrition in renal disease 1968 In: Berlyne G M (ed) Williams and Wilkins, Baltimore

Richards P, Houghton B J, Path M C et al 1969 Ammonia metabolism in renal failure. Brit J Urol 41, suppl No 103

Waterlow J C 1968 Observations on the mechanisms of adaptation to low protein intakes. Lancet 2: 1091

Wolthuis F H 1961 Balance studies on protein metabolism in normal and uraemic man. Acta Med Scand Suppl 373

**Fat and carbohydrates**

Cramp D G, Moorhead J F, Wills M R 1975 Disorders of blood-lipids in renal disease. Lancet i: 672

de Fronzo R A, Andres R, Edgar P et al 1973 Carbohydrate metabolism in uremia: a review. Medicine 52, Baltimore 469

Drücke T, Fauchet M, Fleury J et al 1973 Hypertriglyceridemia in chronic non nephrotic renal failure. Amer J Clin Nutrit 26: 165

Lundin A P, Friedman E A 1978 Vascular consequences of maintenance haemodialysis — an unproven case. Nephron 21: 177

**Blood**

Edwards M S, Pegrum G D, Curtis J R 1970 Iron therapy in patients on maintenance haemodialysis. Lancet 2: 491

Eschbach J W, Cook J D, Scribner B H et al 1977 Iron balance in haemodialysis patients. Ann Intern Med 87: 710

**Cardiovascular**

Cordingley F T, Jones N F, Wing A J, Hilton P J 1980 Reversible renal failure in malignant hypertension. Clin Nephrol 14: 98

Cuthbert M F, Peart W S 1970 Studies on the identity of a vascular permeability factor of renal origin. Clin Sci 38: 309

Ledingham J G G, Rajagopalan B 1979 Cerebral complications in the treatment of accelerated hypertension. Quart J Med 48: 25

Lewis B S, Milne F J, Goldberg B 1976 Left ventricular function in chronic renal failure. Brit Heart J 38: 1229

Man in't Veld A J, Schicht I M, Derkx F H M et al 1980 Effects of an angiotensin-converting enzyme inhibitor (Captopril) on blood pressure in anephric subjects. Brit Med J i: 288

**Hormones**

Holdsworth S, Atkins R C, Kretser de D M 1977 The pituitary-testicular axis in men with chronic renal failure. New Engl J Med 296: 1245

Korman M G, Laver M C, Hansky J 1972 Hypergastrinaemia in chronic renal failure. Brit Med J i: 209

Lim V S, Fang V S, Katz A I et al 1977 Thyroid dysfunction in chronic renal failure: A study of pituitary-thyroid axis and peripheral turnover kinetics of thyroxine and tri iodothyronine. J Clin Invest 60: 522

**Dialysis and transplantation**

Advances in dialysis 1980 Edited by del Greco F, Ivanovich P, Krumlovsky F A Kidney Int, suppl 10

Burke J F, Francos G C, Moore L L et al N 1978 Accelerated atherosclerosis in chronic-dialysis patients — another look. Nephron 21: 181

Cohen J, Pinching A J 1982 Infection and immunosuppression. In: Jones N F, Peters D K (eds) Recent advances in renal medicine, Churchill Livingstone, London, 87

Conceicao S C, Wilkinson R, Feest T G et al 1981 Hypercalcaemia following renal transplantation: causes and consequences. Clin Nephrol 16: 235

Continuous ambulatory peritoneal dialysis in Australia, Europe and the United States 1983 Edited by Gahl G M, Boen F S T, Nolph K D Kidney Int 23: 1

Cyclosporin A as sole immunosuppressive agent in recipients of kidney allografts from cadaver donors 1982 Preliminary results of a European multicenter trial. Lancet II: 57

European dialysis and transplant association registration committee 1982 Chairman: Wing A J. Combined report on regular dialysis and transplantation in Europe XII, 1981. Proceedings of the European Dialysis and Transplant Association XIX. Pitman Books, London

Galbraith R M, Dienstag J L, Purcell R H, Gower P H et al 1979 Non-A, Non-B Hepatitis associated with chronic liver disease in a haemodialysis unit. Lancet i: 951

Gingell J C, Burns G P, Chisholm G D 1968 Gastric acid secretion in chronic uraemia after renal transplantation. Brit Med Jour 4: 424

Manis T, Friedman E A 1979 Dialytic therapy for irreversible uremia. New Engl J Med 301: 1260, 1321

McGeown M G, Kennedy J A, Loughridge W G G et al 1977 One hundred kidney transplants in the Belfast City Hospital. Lancet 2: 648

Morzycka M, Croker B P, Siegler H F et al. 1982 Evaluation of recurrent glomerulonephritis in kidney allografts. Amer J Med 72: 588

Opelz G, Graver B, Terasaki P I 1981 Induction of high kidney graft survival rate by multiple transfusion. Lancet i: 1223

Oreopoulos D G, Khanna R, Williams P et al 1982 Continuous ambulatory peritoneal dialysis — 1981. Nephron 30: 293

Persijn G G, Gabb B W, Van Leeuwen A et al 1978 Matching for HLA antigen of A.B. and D.R. loci in renal transplantation by Eurotransplant. Lancet i: 1278

Wing A J, Brunner F P, Brynger H et al 1980 Dialysis dementia in Europe. Lancet ii: 190

Wing A J, Selwood N H 1981 Achievements and problems in the treatment of end stage renal failure. In: Jones N F, Peters D K (eds) Recent Advances in renal medicine. Churchill Livingstone, Edinburgh, p 103

Zuckerman A S 1980 Acute viral hepatitis. J Roy Coll Phys 15: 88

Zuckerman A J 1982 Priorities for immunisation against hepatitis B. Brit Med J i: 686

Additional reading on maintenance haemodialysis and renal transplantation: Transactions of the American Society for Artificial Internal Organs. Proceedings of the European Dialysis and Transplant Association.

# 14

# Acute nephritic syndrome

The acute nephritic syndrome consists of a sudden onset of oliguria, oedema, hypertension, raised jugular venous pressure and proteinuria, due to an abrupt generalised disturbance which involves the kidneys. In some patients one or more of these features may be absent, e.g. there may be no proteinuria.

The acute nephritic syndrome may develop in a previously normal person, it may occur as a transient complication in chronic renal failure, or be superimposed upon a nephrotic syndrome. It may also precede chronic renal failure, the nephrotic syndrome or acute renal failure. It is seen in a variety of diseases which affect the kidney, including all stages of glomerular nephritis, polyarteritis nodosa, anaphylactoid purpura, disseminated lupus erythematosus, and following irradiation of the kidneys (Fig. 14.1). It occurs most commonly in acute glomerular nephritis.

## Structural changes in the kidneys

The glomeruli usually show diffuse proliferation of mesangial and endothelial cells with narrowing of the capillary lumen, and widening of the capillary walls, with varying degrees of inflammatory cell reaction. In the more severe cases the tubules show focal areas of degeneration associated with clumps of inflammatory cells. On occasion an acute nephritic syndrome may occur with only minimal changes in Bowman's capsule.

## Functional changes

Proteinuria is rarely greater than 2–5 g per day, and there is an increased urinary excretion of red and white cells, granular casts and blood casts. The number of white cells sometimes is as great as the number of red cells. As the urine is usually acid the haemoglobin in the red cells changes to acid haematin and, if there is sufficient blood, the urine becomes dark brown. Lesser quantities of blood cause a smokey turbulence when the urine is gently shaken; the presence of blood is confirmed microscopically. These urinary changes are directly related to the histological changes in the glom-

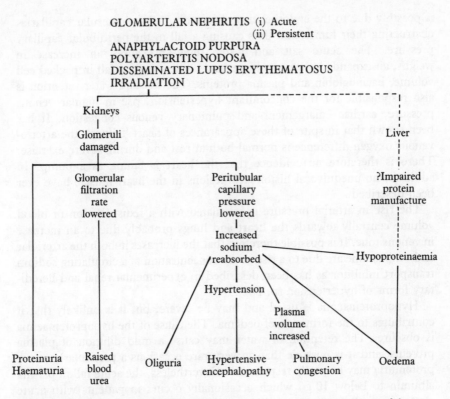

GLOMERULAR NEPHRITIS (i) Acute
(ii) Persistent
ANAPHYLACTOID PURPURA
POLYARTERITIS NODOSA
DISSEMINATED LUPUS ERYTHEMATOSUS
IRRADIATION

Kidneys

Glomeruli damaged

Glomerular filtration rate lowered

Peritubular capillary pressure lowered

Increased sodium reabsorbed

Hypertension

Plasma volume increased

Liver

?Impaired protein manufacture

Hypoproteinaemia

Proteinuria Haematuria

Raised blood urea

Oliguria

Hypertensive encephalopathy

Pulmonary congestion

Oedema

**Fig. 14.1** Diseases in which the acute nephritic syndrome may develop and some of the physiological disturbances which take place.

erular tufts, for when there is no proteinuria the glomerular capillaries are normal.

Glomerular filtration rate is often reduced, but it is remarkable how frequently the blood urea concentration remains within normal limits, if the patient previously had normal kidneys. In those with pre-existing renal disease and long-standing impairment of filtration rate, the further depression in filtration rate associated with the acute nephritic syndrome causes a substantial rise in blood urea. The renal blood flow is usually unaffected except in the most severe cases and in those with pre-existing renal disease; when the blood flow is reduced the decrease is always proportionately less than that of the glomerular filtration rate, i.e. there is a fall in filtration fraction.

The ability to concentrate the urine varies with the degree of tubular damage; if the syndrome complicates established chronic renal failure there is nearly always a complete inability to concentrate.

Salt and water retention is due to an excessive tubular reabsorption of salt and manifests itself as oedema. The increase in tubular sodium reabsorption is possibly due to the endothelial proliferation of the glomerular capillaries obstructing their lumen and thus causing a fall in the peritubular capillary pressure. The acute salt and water retention causes an increase in weight, an expanded plasma volume, and consequently a fall in packed cell volume, haemoglobin and plasma proteins. The salt and water retention is also responsible for the concomitant hypertension, rise in jugular venous pressure, cardiac enlargement and pulmonary venous congestion. It has been shown that in spite of these appearances of heart 'failure', the arterio-venous oxygen difference is normal both at rest and during severe exercise. There is therefore no evidence that the heart is failing as a pump. In addition, no unequivocal histological lesions in the heart muscle have ever been described.

The rise in arterial pressure is associated with a redistribution of blood volume centrally towards the heart and lungs probably due to an increase in venous tone. It is possible therefore that the increases in both the arteriolar and venous tone are due to a rise in the concentration of a circulating sodium transport inhibitor as has been described in experimental renal and heredi-tary forms of hypertension (p. 261).

Hypoproteinaemia is usual and may be severe, but it is unlikely that it contributes to the formation of oedema. The cause of the hypoproteinaemia is obscure. The retention of water may cause a mild dilution of plasma proteins, and it is possible that on very rare occasions a particularly heavy proteinuria may be partly responsible. Nevertheless, the acute fall in plasma albumin to below 10 g/l which occasionally occurs in patients with acute *anuria* from glomerular nephritis makes it extremely likely that, at least in these cases, there has been a considerable diminution in production. It is possible, therefore, that a diminished protein production is a contributory factor in the mild hypoproteinaemia which is usually found in the acute nephritic syndrome. When there is severe hypoproteinaemia there is also a marked rise in serum cholesterol.

The rise in jugular venous pressure, cardiac enlargement and pulmonary venous congestion occurs in nearly all patients. Paroxysmal attacks of postural and nocturnal dyspnoea are rare, but milder degrees of dyspnoea are relatively common. The heart rate is often either unchanged or slower than normal. In fact this combination of raised jugular venous pressure and bradycardia can be one of the most diagnostic features of the acute nephritic syndrome.

The sudden onset of hypertension probably causes the bradycardia. The extent of the rise in blood pressure varies a great deal and often it is so small that it is only noticed retrospectively, particularly in children. The cause of the rise in blood pressure appears to be related to the salt and water retention, for it does not occur without oedema and a gain in weight; it also seems to be related to the histological changes in the glomeruli, though occasionally the blood pressure may be normal in the presence of extensive glomerular proliferation and exudative inflammation.

## Clinical features

At the onset the patient notices that the face, hands or feet are swelling or that the urine has changed colour to dark brown, or red. Very occasionally dyspnoea may be the presenting symptom; this is more likely in children or when there is pre-existing renal disease. There are few other complaints, though upon direct questioning it may be possible to obtain a history of a recent gain in weight, oliguria, and lassitude. Severe pain in the back often occurs with polyarteritis nodosa, and an ache in the loins seems to be a genuine feature of acute glomerular nephritis. Feverish symptoms and the extent of the rise in temperature vary with the cause of the syndrome. Children often present with loss of appetite, and pallor.

Progress depends a great deal on the disease with which the syndrome is associated, but in the majority of cases the signs and symptoms subside within 7–14 days. There is a brisk diuresis and hypertension and oedema quickly disappear. When the syndrome is superimposed upon pre-existing renal disease, recovery may be much slower and some additional impairment of renal function may be permanent. In patients with previously normal kidneys, recovery is often complete, particularly with acute glomerular nephritis. Death during the acute phase of the syndrome is unusual, but may be caused by pulmonary oedema, acute renal failure or hypertensive encephalopathy.

## Treatment

Occasionally it may be possible to influence directly the disease which has precipitated the acute nephritic syndrome; for instance, the use of adrenal steroids in polyarteritis nodosa. Otherwise treatment is symptomatic and is aimed at preventing or minimising the effects of pulmonary oedema, acute renal failure, and hypertensive encephalopathy until there is a spontaneous recovery.

It is convenient to keep a day-to-day chart of the fluid intake, urinary output, blood pressure, weight and 24-hour urinary protein excretion; plasma urea and creatinine should be estimated twice a week.

### Pulmonary oedema and congestion

In most patients there is no necessity to treat this by any other means than the salt and water restriction mentioned above. The dyspnoea of the onset usually settles after a few hours bed rest, but if it increases it may be necessary to use morphia, and to sit the patient up in an armchair or cardiac bed throughout the 24 hours. Hypotensive drugs are useful when there is a considerable rise in blood pressure. During a paroxysm of acute pulmonary oedema with deepening cyanosis, 25 mg of either hydralazine intravenously or nifedipine intramuscularly may be life-saving. On general principles the use of diuretics is not advised and, in any case, they rarely succeed in producing a diuresis in an acute nephritic syndrome.

*Renal failure.*

As renal failure is usually minimal and of short duration its treatment is not difficult. During the oliguric phase the patient is placed on a salt-and protein-free diet, and the daily fluid intake is limited to a volume equal to the urine passed in the previous 24 hours, plus 500 ml to replace insensible loss. As soon as a diuresis starts, and the glomerular filtration rate returns to normal, these restrictions are relaxed.

In the rare cases when there is acute renal failure with either complete anuria or a daily urine output below 400 ml with a specific gravity around 1.010, treatment is as described for acute renal failure from any other cause, except that measures taken to avoid acute pulmonary congestion have to be more carefully observed than usual.

*Hypertensive encephalopathy*

This exceedingly rare complication responds to the intravenous administration of barbiturates (sodium amylobarbitone or thiopentone). After the initial injection it is usually sufficient to continue sedation with large intermittent doses of barbiturates by mouth. These measures are combined with the administration of hypotensive drugs.

BIBLIOGRAPHY

Black D A K, Platt R, Rowlands E N et al 1948 Renal haemodynamics in acute nephritis. Clin Sci 6: 295
Cameron J S 1975 Acute nephritic syndrome. Am Acad Med Singapore 4 (2): 1
Earle D P, Farber S J, Alexander J D 1950 Renal function and edema in acute glomerulo-nephritis. J Clin Invest 29: 810
Earle D P, Taggart J V, Shannon J A 1974 Glomerulonephritis: a survey of functional organisation of the kidney in various stages of diffuse glomerulonephritis. J Clin Invest 23: 119
Farber S J 1957 Physiologic aspects of glomerulo nephritis. J Chronic Dis 5: 87
Glassock R J, Cohen A H, Bennett C M 1981 The major clinical syndromes. In: Brenner BM, Rector FC (eds) The kidney, 2nd edn. Sauders, Philadelphia
Guz A, Noble M I M, Trenchard D, Garnett E S et al 1966. The significance of a raised central venous pressure during sodium and water retention. Clin Sci 30: 295
Hilden T 1943 Diodrast clearance in acute nephritis. Acta med Scand 116: 1
Peters J P 1953 Edema of acute nephritis. Amer J Med 14: 448
Schwartz W B, Kassirer J P 1971 Clinical aspects of acute poststreptococcal glomerulonephritis. In: Strauss M B, Welt L G (eds) Diseases of the kidney, 2nd edn. Little Brown, Boston

# 15

# Hormones and the kidney

The kidney, (1) releases some hormones which are carried in the blood to other sites where they have their effect, (2) releases other hormones which only have an intrarenal effect, (3) is itself profoundly influenced by certain hormones which are released elsewhere, (4) and is involved in the catabolic destruction of many hormones. One way or another therefore chronic renal failure influences the function of most hormones.

## CIRCULATING HORMONES HAVING THEIR MAIN SITE OF ORIGIN IN THE KIDNEY AND THEIR EFFECTS AT OTHER SITES

### Renin

In the kidney, renin is synthesised in the cells of the afferent arteriole of the glomerulus where it forms a part of the juxta glomerular apparatus. Renin acts on the circulating 15 amino acid substrate angiotensinogen to form the inactive decapeptide angiotensin I. This is further cleaved by a converting enzyme to the active decapeptide angiotensin II which is destroyed by angiotensinase. The control of renin secretion is outlined in Figure 15.1. It is probable that the most important stimulants to renin release are sympathetic stimulation of the renin secreting cells, vasodilatation of the afferent arteriole and a fall in the ionic concentration of calcium in the renin secreting cells. As however, all forms of vasodilatation are usually associated with a diminution in the intracellular concentration of ionic calcium it is possible that a final common path for renin release is the intracellular concentration of calcium.

The main functions of angiotensin II are to control arteriolar tone and thus arterial pressure, aldosterone secretion, tubular sodium reabsorption and thirst. Clinically most changes in plasma renin activity are either due to some intrinsic, usually ischaemic, renal lesion, or they are due to changes in extracellular fluid or blood volume. The ischaemic lesions consist either of multiple partial distal occlusions of the renal arterial tree secondary to any disease which destroys the renal cortex (e.g. glomerular nephritis) or

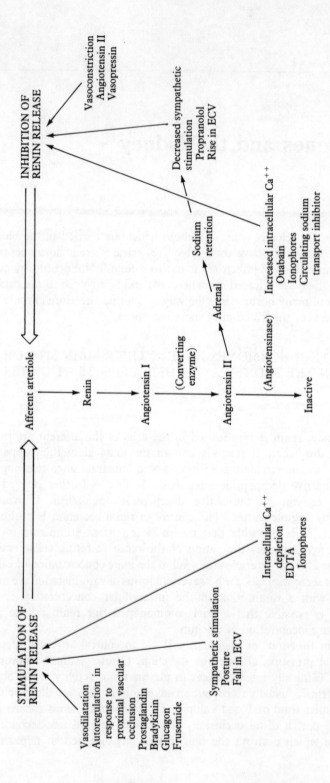

**Fig. 15.1** Control of renin secretion from juxta glomerular apparatus.

to one or more discreet partial occlusive lesions of the renal artery itself or of the main branches (e.g. renal artery stenosis). Such partial occlusions increase plasma renin activity because, via the mechanism responsible for circulatory autoregulation, they cause vasodilatation of that portion of the vascular tree, including the afferent arteriole, which is situated distal to the lesion.

Plasma renin activity also responds to changes in extracellular fluid volume or blood volume even when they are so small that they are difficult, or impossible to detect by other means e.g. the fall in volume which may occur in poorly controlled Addison disease, the sureptitious self administration of diuretics or purgatives, or the rise in volume which occurs so often in a patient on maintenance haemodialysis. The height to which the plasma renin rises is dependent in part by the duration of the stimulus for renin release, as well as it's intensity for if the stimulus is prolonged it may cause considerable hypertrophy of the renin secreting cells.

### 1,25(OH)$_2$Vit D$_3$

Vit D$_3$, the natural form of vit D, is either formed in the skin from the UV irradiation of 7 dehydrocholesterol, or it is absorbed from the intestinal tract. Vit D$_3$ then travels to the liver where it is hydroxylated in the 25 position to form 25OHvit D$_3$ which is then further hydroxylated in the kidney at either the 1 or the 24 position to produce 1,25(OH)$_2$vit D$_3$ or 24,25(OH)$_2$vit D$_3$. 25OHvit D$_3$ and 1,25(OH)$_2$vit D$_3$ are the active metabolites. 25OHvit D$_3$ appears to be responsible for the calcification of osteoid and for muscle contraction whereas 1,25(OH)$_2$vit D$_3$ the plasma concentration of which is about 1000 times less than that of 25OHvit D$_3$ controls calcium absorption from the gut, parathyroid hormone secretion, and the effectiveness of parathyroid hormone in mobilising calcium from the bone (Fig. 15.2). In addition the presence of 1,25(OH)$_2$vit D$_3$ within the proximal tubule cell controls many of its metabolic functions including the reabsorption of amino acids, phosphate and glucose.

The hydroxylation of 25OHvit D$_3$ to 1,25(OH)$_2$vit D$_3$ in the adult kidney occurs in the convoluted portion of the proximal tubule. The hydroxylase responsible for the hydroxylation at the 1 position is only found in the kidney. In chronic renal failure the plasma concentration of 1,25(OH)$_2$vit D$_3$ begins to fall when glomerular filtration rate is below approximately 40 ml/min; it is nil when the filtration rate is less than 1ml/min and in the anephric patient. The hydoxylase responsible for hydroxylation at the 24 position however is not only present in the kidney but it can also be found in the gut. It will hydroxylate any metabolite of Vit D which contains a 25 hydroxyl group and can thus form not only 24,25(OH)$_2$vit D$_3$ but also 1,24,25(OH)$_3$vit D$_3$. Clinically this may be important for in chronic renal failure the fall in plasma 1,25(OH)$_2$vit D$_3$, which accompanies it's impaired production by the kidney may be aggra-

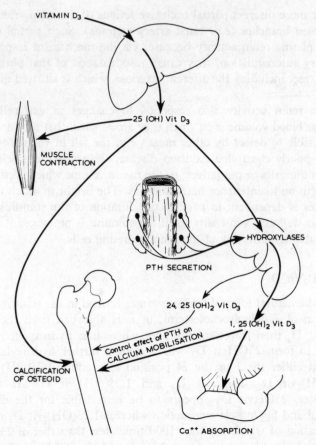

**Fig. 15.2** Metabolism of Vitamin D. The recent finding that 1,25(OH)₂vit D₃ also influences PTH secretion is not shown.

vated by the continual conversion of the little active 1,25(OH)₂vit D₃ that there is to the inactive 1,24,25(OH)₃vit D₃.

The hydroxylation of vit D₃ to 25OHvit D₃ in the liver is controlled by the plasma level of 25OHvit D₃. The hydroxylation of the 25OHvit D₃ to 1,25(OH)₂vit D₃ in the kidney is regulated by the need for calcium and phosphorus. This is illustrated in Figure 15.3, which demonstrates the effect of changes in serum calcium on the relative production of 1,25(OH)₂vit D₃ and 24,25(OH)₂vit D₃. At calcium concentrations above 2.25 mmol/l little or no 1,25(OH)₂vit D₃ is formed whereas 24,25(OH)₂vit D₃ is being produced in large amounts. When the serum calcium falls below 2.2 mmol/l there is an abrupt reversal with a brisk rise in the production of 1,25(OH)₂vit D₃ and a reciprocal fall in that of 24,25(OH)₂vit D₃. The stimulation of 1,25(OH)₂vit D₃ synthesis is due to the direct action of parathyroid hormone on the proximal tubule cell. Small changes in plasma calcium having produced a significant change in the concentration of plasma

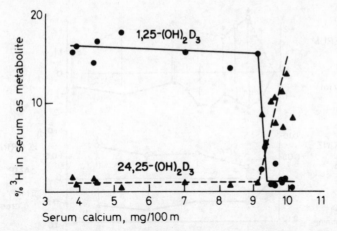

**Fig. 15.3** The relationship between serum calcium concentration and plasma 1,25-(OH)$_2$D$_3$ or 24,25-(OH)$_2$D$_3$ in the rat. Hypocalcemia increases plasma 1,25-(OH)$_2$D$_3$ and reduces plasma 24, 25-(OH)$_2$D$_3$. Hypercalcemia lowers 1,25-(OH)$_2$D$_3$ and raises plasma 24,25-(OH)$_2$D$_3$ Conversion: Traditional to SI units-calcium 10 mg/100 ml = 2.5 mmol/l; (reproduced from de Luca HF, 1981 Contr Nephrol 13: 81, with kind permission).

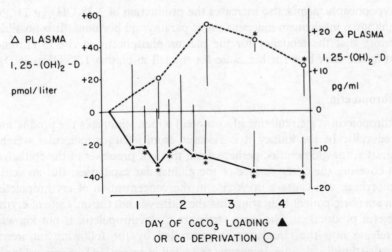

**Fig. 15.4** The mean changes from control in plasma 1,25(OH)$_2$vit D concentration during CaCO$_3$ loading or dietary Ca deprivation in man (reproduced from Adams, Gray & Lenann 1979 J Clin Endocrinol & Metab 48: 1008, with kind permission).

parathyroid hormone. This is illustrated in Figure 15.4 which depicts the changes in plasma 1,25(OH)$_2$vit D$_3$ which occur in man during a short period of calcium deprivation and the oral administration of large amounts of calcium carbonate. The associated changes in plasma parathyroid hormone and urine cAMP are shown in Figure 15.5.

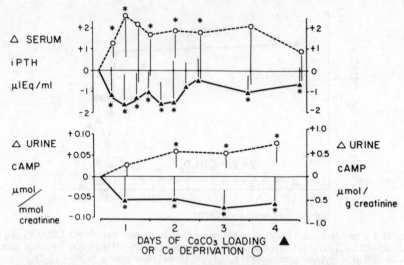

**Fig. 15.5** The mean changes from control in serum PTH concentrations and urinary cAMP/creatinine during CaCO₃ loading and dietary Ca deprivation in man (reproduced from Adams, Gray & Lenann 1979 J Clin Endocrinol & Metab 48:1008, with kind permission).

Hypophosphataemia also increases the production of $1,25(OH)_2vit\ D_3$ by an unknown mechanism independent of parathyroid hormone. It is possible therefore that the tendency for the plasma phosphorus to rise in chronic renal failure may be a further cause for the fall in plasma $1,25(OH)_2vit\ D_3$.

## Erythropoietin

Erythropoietin is a circulating glycoprotein which stimulates the production of red cells. In the kidney it is released from a larger molecular weight material at the glomerulus, perhaps from the foot processes of the epithelial cells covering the outer surface of the glomerular capillaries. But an acute haemorrhage will cause a brisk rise in the concentration of erythropoietin in an anephric patient indicating that the kidney is not the only site of erythropoietin production. The exact structure of erythropoietin is not known. Its release into the circulation is controlled by the following intrarenal hypoxic stimuli, anaemia, ischaemia and a fall in arterial $pO_2$. Some evidence suggests that the hypoxic increase in the production of intrarenal prostaglandins may be an important step in the release of erythropoietin.

When renal function is normal plasma erythropoietin is directly related to the haemoglobin concentration. In the anaemia of chronic renal failure however, the plasma erythropoietin concentration, may be low, normal or raised. Presumably in those patients in whom it is low the absolute fall in erythropoietin below normal, in spite of the anaemia, is an important factor in the multiple aetiology of the anaemia of chronic renal failure. For instance anephric patients who have the most severe anaemia have the lowest

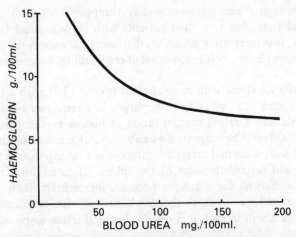

**Fig. 15.6** Schema of the mean relationship between the haemoglobin concentration and the blood urea; individual plots show a considerable scatter. Conversion: traditional to SI units — blood urea 100 mg/100 ml = 17 mmol/l.

concentration of plasma erythropoietin. The normal or raised concentrations of plasma erythropoietin in chronic renal failure (Fig. 15.6, 15.7) are probably due to a greatly raised production of erythropoietin per surviving glomerulus. Some destructive processes of the renal parenchyma are more apt to demonstrate this phenomenon than others, e.g. patients with polycystic

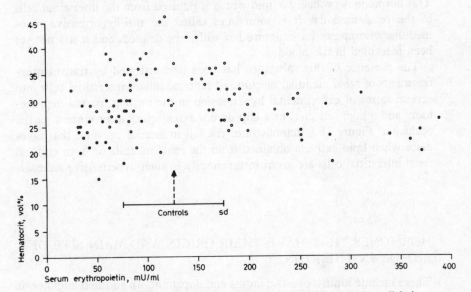

**Fig. 15.7** Serum erythropoietin concentration and hematocrit in 100 regular hemodialysis patients. Mean ± SD of 30 healthy controls is indicated by the dotted line. o = males (n = 73); ● = females (n = 27) (reproduced from Koch & Radtke 1978 Contr Nephrol 13: 60, with kind permission).

kidneys have higher haemoglobins and erythropoietin levels at comparable reductions of renal function than patients with chronic renal failure from other causes. It is interesting however, that many patients in the early stages of glomerular nephritis, before the onset of renal failure, have an *increased* red cell mass.

Occasionally a patient with normal renal function but with a local lesion of the kidney such as a cyst, a hydronephrosis or a renal carcinoma will have polycythaemia and a raised concentration of plasma erythropoietin. Renal polycythaemia should be suspected when a polycythaemia of unknown cause is associated with a normal arterial saturation but no increase in white cells or platelets and no enlargement of the spleen. If in addition there is an episode of haematuria the diagnosis becomes increasingly likely. Occasionally there is a tendency to think that the haematuria has been caused by the polycythaemia when, in fact, it is due to the renal lesion responsible for the polycythaemia. About 1% of all patients with an initial diagnosis of polycythaemia vera are subsequently found to have renal polycythaemia. A few of these have a palpable spleen, which is misleading. Polycythaemia also occurs in some patients following transplantation when it is probably due to the administration of steroids and the vascular damage in the transplanted kidney caused by immunological rejection.

### Blood pressure lowering hormone

This hormone is probably a lipid which is released from the interstitial cells of the renal medulla. It is sometimes called the anti-hypertensive reno-medullary hormone. Its structure has still to be defined, and it has not yet been identified in the blood.

The presence of this substance has been demonstrated by transplanting fragments of renal medulla, or cultured reno medullary interstitial cells into several forms of experimental hypertension in the rat, e.g. partial nephrectomy and a high salt diet, or a clip on one renal artery to produce a partial occlusion. Figure 15.8 demonstrates the fall in arterial pressure that takes place when lipid extracts obtained from the renal medulla or from cultural renal interstitial cells are given intravenously to such hypertensive animals.

## HORMONES THAT HAVE THEIR ORIGIN AND MAIN SITE OF ACTION IN THE KIDNEY

These include kinins, prostaglandins and dopamine. In addition angiotensin II, the systemic action of which was discussed above, probably has an important local vasoconstrictive action, and a direct effect on tubular sodium reabsorption.

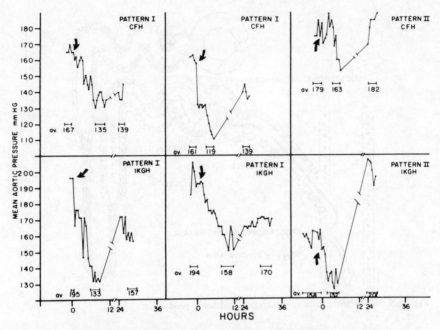

**Fig. 15.8** Transplants of cultured renomedullary interstitial cells (RIC) in partial nephrectomy+salt (CFH) and one kidney Goldblatt (IKGH) hypertension. These are individual results. The transplant (~ 30 M viable cells) was introduced at the arrow. The arterial pressure was lowered to a minimum by 16–12 h. The figures under the bars are averages for the interval of the bar (reproduced from Muirhead, Rightsel, Leech et al 1977 Lab Invest 36: 162 with kind permission).

## The kallikrein-kinin system

There are several forms of kallikreins and kinins depending on their site of origin. Kallikreins are peptidases which act on the plasma globulin substrate kininogen to release peptide kinins. These are rapidly destroyed by plasma and tissue peptidases (kininases), which are the same enzymes as those responsible for the conversion of angiotensin I to II. Kininogens are present in tubule fluid whereas renal kallikrein is secreted into the fluid by the cells of the distal tubule (Fig. 15.9). Kinin is therefore formed in the distal tubule and is probably at its highest concentration in the fluid entering the collecting duct. Both aldosterone and prostaglandins increase the production of kinin.

Kinins are powerful local vasodilators and like all vasodilators have natriuretic properties. But the role of kinins in the normal control of urinary sodium excretion is unclear. The vasodilating properties of kinins may be due to their ability to stimulate prostaglandin synthethis. The presence of kinins in the tubule fluid also stimulates the intracellular production of prostaglandin in the cells of the distal tubule and collecting duct and this renders these cells less permeable to water. In other words the renal kallikrein-kinin

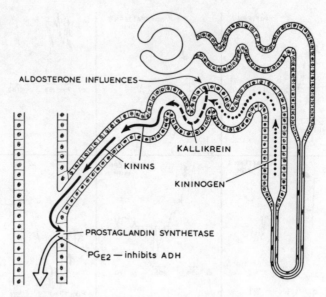

**Fig. 15.9** Site of renal kallikrein secretion and kinin production.

system through its effect on prostaglandin production inhibits the action of ADH.

Patients with established essential hypertension and their normotensive children excrete subnormal amounts of kallikreins in the urine. If this abnormality reflects a reduced concentration of intrarenal kinins it may be connected to the inherited defect in the control of urinary sodium excretion which it is thought may be the primary disturbance in the aetiology of essential hypertension.

## Prostaglandins

Prostaglandins are unsaturated lipid acids formed from the action of prostaglandin synthetase on arachidonic acid. They are rapidly destroyed locally. Prostaglandin production is highest in the medulla and papilla but an appreciable amount also takes place in the cortex. Prostaglandins are potent vasodilators and natriuretics, though their contribution to the normal control of urinary sodium excretion is tenuous.

As mentioned above, prostaglandins inhibit the action of ADH (Fig. 15.10). It is therefore interesting that ADH itself stimulates prostaglandin synthetase. Prostaglandin synthetase is also stimulated by angiotensin and noradrenaline so that their vasoconstricting action is opposed by the vasodilating effect of the prostaglandins, the concentration of which they have themselves increased. Prostaglandins therefore are modulators of ADH and renal vasoconstrictors. Prostaglandins also stimulate the release of eryth-

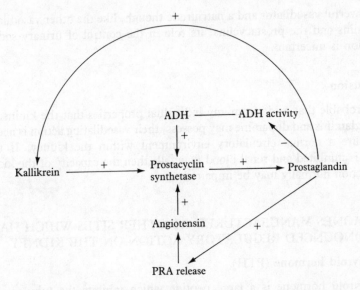

**Fig. 15.10** The relation of prostacyclin synthetase activity and prostaglandins to some other hormones.

ropoietin (see above) and possibly kallikrein which themselves increase prostaglandin synthetase.

Clinically there are three situations in which prostaglandins seem to play an obvious role. The first is Bartter's syndrome (p. 355) in which there is a renal leak of salt of unknown cause, a reduced extracellular fluid volume, a high plasma renin activity and plasma aldosterone and a greatly increased excretion of prostaglandins in the urine. All these changes also occur with the excess use of diuretics. The administration of indomethacin, a prostaglandin synthetase inhibitor causes much improvement, though sometimes this is only temporary. The third clinical setting in which prostaglandins are involved is in advanced chronic renal failure when the administration of indomethacin may accidentally precipitate a rapid shut down of renal function. Presumably the removal of the prostaglandin's normal vasodilatory action, at such a time is sufficient to jeopardise the precarious blood flow that remains. Occasionally this phenomenon has been used deliberately to abolish all secretory renal function in a patient on maintenance dialysis whose urinary output of salt and water is so excessive that it leads to recurrent hypotension.

## Dopamine

The amount of dopamine in the renal vein exceeds the amount delivered into the kidney via the renal artery. In addition there is dopamine in the urine. The kidney therefore manufactures large quantities of dopamine. It is a powerful vasodilator and a natriuretic though, like the other vasodilators the kinins and the prostacyclins, its role in the control of urinary sodium excretion is uncertain.

## Conclusion

It is probable that aside from any individual properties that the kinins, the prostaglandins and dopamine may possess, their vasodilating action is needed to ensure a normal circulatory environment within the kidney. If their action is inhibited and renal blood flow falls then the capacity of the kidney to function normally may be impaired.

## HORMONES MANUFACTURED AT OTHER SITES WHICH HAVE A PRONOUNCED REGULATORY ACTION ON THE KIDNEY

### Parathyroid hormone (PTH)

Parathyroid hormone is a large peptide which inhibits the tubular reabsorption of phosphate and bicarbonate thus increasing their excretion into the urine, but it stimulates the reabsorption of calcium and thus tends to reduce urinary calcium excretion. These actions are accompanied by an increased urinary excretion of cyclic AMP.

When renal function is normal, an excess of PTH leads to hypophosphataemia and a mild metabolic acidosis. In chronic renal failure the plasma concentration of PTH rises to very high levels, often much higher than in primary hyperparathyroidism. This counteracts the tendency of retain phosphate but the associated increase in bicarbonate excretion may in part contribute to the metabolic acidosis which accompanies chronic renal failure. The raised plasma concentration of PTH is also responsible for the increased osteoclastic activity in the bone which is the commonest bone lesion in renal bone disease. It may also be responsible for a wide variety of other complications of chronic renal failure.

### Antidiuretic hormone (ADH)

Andidiuretic hormone is a small peptide which is produced in the hypothalamus and released from the posterior pituitary. It increases the permeability of the distal tubule and collecting duct to water and urea thus increasing their reabsorption and diminishing their excretion in the urine. It is also a vasoconstrictor which in certain circumstances may contribute to the control of the arterial pressure (hence the original name 'vasopressin'). The importance of this vasoconstricting action in normal circumstances is uncertain but it is probable that it is in part responsible for the fall in the flow of blood through the countercurrent system in the medulla which occurs when the urine is hypertonic. Such a reduction in flow would increase the osmolality of the medulla which would increase the osmolality of the urine.

## Aldosterone

Aldosterone is a steroid synthetised in the zona glomerulosa of the adrenal gland. It increases the permeability of the distal tubule and collecting duct to sodium and therefore increases sodium reabsorption. This phenomenon is associated with an increased tubular secretion of potassium. Normally therefore the effect of aldosterone on the kidney is to prevent sodium depletion on the one hand and potassiun retention on the other.

When there is a rise in the plasma concentration of aldosterone due to a tumour of the adrenal (primary aldosteronism) the increased tendency to reabsorb sodium causes a rise in the ratio of the body's sodium to potassium content but there is no oedema. This is because the tendency for the extra-cellular fluid volume to increase causes a rise in the plasma concentration of the natriuretic/sodium transport inhibitor. This phenomenon, sometimes called mineralocorticoid 'escape' prevents a serious accumulation of sodium. It is interesting that the changes in blood volume that occur are similar to those found in essential hypertension; another condition in which it is prob-able that there is a persistent tendency to retain sodium (Fig. 15.11). A

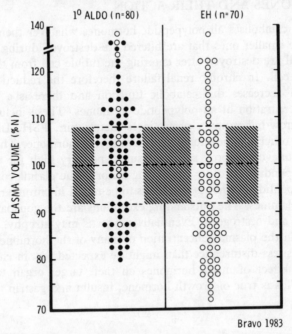

**Fig. 15.11** Plasma volumes during normal dietary sodium intake in 80 patients with primary aldosteronism and 70 with essential hypertension. The crossed hatched area represents normal range (reproduced from Bravo, Tarazi, Dustan et al 1983 Amer J Med 74: 641, with kind permission).

minority of patients in both conditions have a raised blood volume while in the majority the blood volume is either normal or low. Compensatory mechanisms to control the associated urinary loss of potassium however are less effective than those against sodium retention. When plasma aldosterone rises either primarily, or secondarily the increase in potassium excretion may cause a serious depletion of body potassium and symptomatic hypokalaemia.

Alternatively when there is a fall in the concentration of plasma aldosterone due either to a diminished secretion of renin or a disease of the adrenal the urinary loss of sodium causes a loss of weight and hypotension and the diminished urinary excretion of potassium leads to hyperkalaemia.

## Natriuretic hormone/sodium transport inhibitor

The natriuretic hormone/sodium transport inhibitor was discussed on page 80. Its effects, other than to increase urinary sodium excretion are uncertain but as its plasma concentration appears to be raised in both essential hypertension and secondary hypertension associated with salt retention it is possible that it has vasoactive properties.

## THE RELATION OF RENAL FUNCTION TO THE TURNOVER OF HORMONES AND THEIR ACTION

The kidney catabolises all polypeptide hormones whatever their molecular weight. The smaller ones that are filtered are destroyed during their reabsorption. All are destroyed after entering the tubule cell from the capillary side of the cell. In chronic renal failure therefore the reduction in renal parenchyma decreases this catabolic function and there is a rise in the plasma concentration of all polypeptide hormones. These include insulin, glucagon, growth hormone, prolactin, somatotropin, FSH, LH, βMSH, gastrin and other gut hormones and parathyroid hormone. The extent of this rise is uneven, approx x 2 for insulin and very high for parathyroid hormone depending on other controlling factors. The plasma concentration of non-polypeptide hormones also tends to be raised in chronic renal failure e.g. catecholamines. The outstanding exceptions are the gonadal hormones testosterone and oestrogens. Eventually the testis may atrophy.

The rise in the plasma concentration of many of the hormones discussed above causes less disturbance than might be expected for, in chronic renal failure, the effect of many hormones on their target organ tends to be impaired. This is true of growth hormone, insulin and gastrin.

BIBLIOGRAPHY

Ardaillou R, Paillard F 1979 Métabolisme rénal des hormones polypeptidique. Actualités nephrologiques de l'hôpital Necker. Flamarion, p 187

Bonomini Y, Orsoni G, Stefoni S et al 1979 Hormonal changes in uremia. Clinical Nephrology 11: 275

Brunette M G, Chan M, Ferriere C et al 1978 Site of 1,25(OH)$_2$vit D$_3$ synthethis in the kidney. Nature 276: 287

Distiller L A, Morley J E, Sagel J et al 1975 Pituitary-gonadal function in chronic renal failure. The effect of luteinizing hormone — releasing hormone and the influence of dialysis. Metabolism 24: 711

Doherty C C, Buchanan K D, Ardill J et al 1980 Gut hormones and renal failure. Dialysis & Transplantation 9: 245

Drueke T 1981 Endocrine disorders in chronic haemodialysis patients (with the exclusion of hyperparathyroidism). In: Hamburger J, Crosnier J, Grunfeld J et al (eds) Advances in nephrology, 10. Year Book Medical Publishers, Chicago, p 351

Eastwood J B, Bordier P J, Clarkson E M et al 1974 The contrasting effects on bone histology and of Vitamin D and of calcium carbonate in the osteomalacia of chronic renal failure. Clin Sci Mol Med 47: 23

Eastwood J B, Harris E, Stamp T C B et al 1976 Vitamin-D deficiency in osteomalacia of chronic renal failure. Lancet ii: 1209

Einsenback G M, Brod J 1978 Vasoactive renal hormones. In: Contributions to Nephrology 12: Karger S, Basel

Eisenback G M, Brod J 1978 Non-vasoactive renal hormones. In: Contributions to Nephrology 13: Karger S, Basel

Fisher J W 1980 Prostaglandins and kidney erythropoietin production. Nephron 25: 53

Fisher J W, Ohno Y, Barona J et al 1978 Role of erythropoietin and inhibitors of erythropoiesis in the anaemia of renal insufficiency. Dialysis and transplantation 7: 472

Gilkes J J H, Eady R A, Rees L H et al 1975 Plasma immunoreactive melanotrophic hormones in patients on maintenance haemodialysis. Brit Med J 1: 656

Haussler M R, McCain T A 1977 Basic and clinical concepts related to Vitamin D metabolism and action (in two parts). New Eng J Med 297: 974, 1041

Jones N F, Payne R W, Hyde R D et al 1960 Renal polycythaemia. Lancet 1: 299

Klahr S, Delinez J, Harter H 1982 Endocrine and metabolic consequences of chronic renal failure. Cardiovascular Reviews & Reports. 3: 613

Margolius H S 1982 Kallikrein as a participant in renal and circulatory function. Cardiovascular Reviews and Reports 3: 559

Norman A W 1974 1,25 Dihydroxyvitamin D$_3$: A kidney-produced steroid hormone essential to calcium homeostasis. Amer J Med 57: 21

Slatopolsky E, Martin K, Hruska K 1980 Parathyroid hormone metabolism and its potential as a uremic toxin. Amer J Physiol 239: F1

# 16

# The kidney and blood pressure

## The effect of hypertension on renal structure

Hypertension, however caused, eventually leads to changes in renal structure and function: the structural changes are sometimes known as nephrosclerosis. Initially the structural changes occur mainly in the vessels, but, as the lesions progress, there are secondary ischaemic changes in the nephrons. The vascular changes may be either acute or chronic. The acute changes are found in association with malignant hypertension; they consist of gross thickening of the intima of the smaller arteries, and focal necrosis of arterioles. The chronic lesions are found in association with non-malignant hypertension, they consist of a less marked thickening of the whole wall of the smaller arteries.

### Acute changes

The most important change is a thickening of the intima of the comparatively large intralobular arteries so that their lumens become extremely small. In younger patients this is due to a cellular hyperplasia with no increase in collagen or elastic fibres. In older patients it is due to an increased quantity of fibro-elastic tissue similar to that found in much smaller quantities in non-malignant hypertension. There is little doubt that this subintimal proliferation is due directly to the rise in blood pressure. Teleologically it is reasonable that the normal mechanism whereby the rise in blood pressure induces a renal functional vasoconstriction (circulatory autoregulation, p. 120) should be reinforced by a structural narrowing, but the intensity of this phenomen may cause the patient's death.

The other acute vascular change consists of localised areas of necrosis of the whole thickness and circumference of an arteriole. These necrotic lesions contain large amounts of fibrin so that the change is often called fibrinoid necrosis.

Subintimal proliferation occludes the smaller arteries and afferent arteroles to the glomerulus. At first this produces a secondary thickening of the glomerular capillary walls but subsequently the glomeruli atrophy and are replaced by collagen. Arteriolar necrosis may be associated with focal areas of acute necrosis in the glomeruli which can be recognised as collections of structureless eosin-staining material containing disintegrating nuclei and narrow capillary lumens.

There is a strong suggestion that the principal factor which determines whether the lesions accompanying the rise in blood pressure are acute or chronic is a difference in the state of the vessels and not just the height of the pressure. The nature of this difference is unknown. Acute changes are more likely if the rate of rise in blood pressure is rapid or if the hypertension is initially caused by a renal disease such as glomerular nephritis or pyelonephritis.

*Chronic changes*

The chronic vascular changes which are found characteristically in prolonged hypertension may also be found in patients with normal blood pressure. There is a generalised narrowing of the arterioles and intralobular arteries with fibroelastic tissue and the deposition of an eosinophilic structureless material. Gradually complete occlusion of the lumen may occur and a patchy ischaemia of increasing severity develops throughout the renal parenchyma. This process may develop in previously normal kidneys, and may very occasionally be severe enough to cause renal failure. Because of the association of renal disease with hypertension it also complicates most longstanding cases of renal disease, when it then contributes to, and accelerates, the kidney's eventual destruction. In the larger arteries these chronic vascular lesions eventually cause focal wedge-shaped areas of degeneration situated between relatively normal renal tissue. Such areas have a characteristic appearance for while the tubules tend to disappear the glomeruli seem to survive preferentially and are crowded together. At first, the tubules between the glomeruli lose their lumens, but the cells show little change so that the glomeruli appear to be packed in solid wedges of relatively normal cells. Later the tubule cells atrophy and there is fibrous tissue replacement. The glomerular tufts show a diffuse thickening with collagen accompanied by a similar thickening of the glomerular capsule; eventually the collagenised tuft and capsule become fused, the capillary lumens are obliterated and the glomerulus is replaced by fibrous tissues. When these vascular changes are far advanced there may be no normal tissue left and it may then be impossible, histologically, to distinguish them from the end stages of such renal diseases as glomerular nephritis or chronic interstitial nephritis, in which vascular changes are only a complication.

## The role of the kidney in the aetiology of hypertension

The kidney is intimately linked to the control of blood pressure through its ability to secrete renin and to control urinary sodium excretion. The secre-

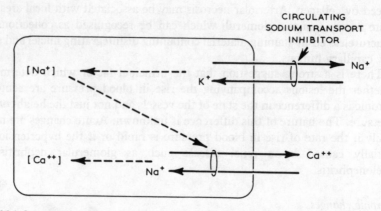

**Fig. 16.1** Suggested hypothesis to explain how a circulating sodium transport inhibitor might raise the intracellular concentration of ionised calcium (see script). (Derived from Blaustein 1977 Amer J Physiol 232(3): C165.)

tion of renin is directly related to the plasma concentration of the rapidly acting vasoconstrictor angiotension II. How a change in urinary sodium excretion affects the blood pressure is less obvious. Changes in sodium balance produce changes in the concentration of angiotension II and in the volume of extracellular fluid and blood. These changes in volume produce parallel changes in (1) the plasma's natriuretic properties, (2) the plasma's capacity to inhibit sodium transport and (3) the plasma's capacity to increase vascular tone and reactivity. Theoretically the rise in the concentration of a circulating sodium transport inhibitor could be responsible for the increase in vascular reactivity and the tone of vascular smooth muscle. The exact mechanism is debatable

The schema illustrated in Figure 16.1 delineates one possibility. The intracellular concentration of ionic calcium determines the tension of smooth muscle, and the intracellular concentration of ionic calcium is controlled in part by the intracellular concentration of ionic sodium. Furthermore one of the factors which controls the intracellular concentration of ionic sodium is the activity of the $Na^+-K^+$-ATPase pump. Any interference with net sodium transport therefore, including a diminution of $Na^+-K^+$-ATPase activity, which leads to a rise in the intracellular concentration of ionic sodium will increase the intracellular calcium concentration and arteriolar tone. As the circulating sodium transport inhibitor inhibits $Na^+-K^+$-ATPase it is possible that a diminution in urinary sodium excretion which leads to a slight expansion of the extracellular fluid volume and blood volume, and thus to a compensatory increase in the plasma's natriuretic and sodium transport inhibiting capacity may cause an increase in vascular reactivity and tone and eventually a rise in arterial pressure.

Angiotension II, like other vasoconstrictors such as noradrenaline and vasopressin also increases the tone of vascular smooth muscle by inducing a rise in the concentration of ionic calcium. Therefore the kidney's control of vascular tone may be mediated by two hormones which control the intracellular ionic calcium concentration of vascular smooth muscle, angiotensin II and the circulating sodium transport inhibitor. In *normal circumstances*, there is a reciprocal relationship between the plasma concentration of angiotensin II and the circulating sodium transport inhibitor. When sodium balance tends to become negative there is a rise in plasma angiotensin and a fall in the circulating sodium transport inhibitor, and vice versa (p. 80, 247). There is a strong possibility, however, that one of the functions of the circulating sodium transport inhibitor is to control the vascular reactivity of vascular smooth muscle to vasoconstrictors such as angiotensin and noradrenaline. It is certainly true that when sodium balance becomes negative and there is a fall in the plasma concentration of the sodium transport inhibitor, the reactivity of vascular smooth muscle to the rising level of angiotensin is greatly reduced. And conversely when sodium balance becomes positive, and there is a rise in the circulating concentration of the sodium transport inhibitor, the reactivity of the smooth muscle to the lowered concentration of angiotensin is increased. At such a time plasma concentrations of angiotensin which would have no effect during sodium depletion induce a powerful vasoconstriction. In other words the circulating sodium transport inhibitor, by its effect on the intracellular calcium concentration, may set the scene for the superimposed effect of angiotensin.

These interlocking mechanisms which would appear to counterbalance each other so nicely in normal circumstances are potentially dangerous when the kidney is under abnormal influences or is diseased. (Fig. 16.2). Either the kidney has a normal architecture but it has a difficulty in excreting sodium (e.g. in essential hypertension and primary aldosteronism) when the tendency to retain sodium may lead to a fall in angiotensin II, but the persistent compensatory rise in the sodium transport inhibitor may be responsible for the rise in blood pressure. Or the kidney's architecture is so disturbed by disease (e.g. glomerular nephritis) that the lowered number of nephrons causes a difficulty in excreting sodium, and the associated haphazard distortion of the vascular tree reduces the perfusion pressure to a sufficient number of juxta glomerular cells to increase the output of renin. There is then a most abnormal situation. A rise in plasma angiotensin II together with *increase* in vascular reactivity due to a simultaneous rise in the concentration of the circulating sodium transport inhibitor. Eventually the natriuretic effect of the rise in arterial pressure overcomes the kidney's difficulty in excreting sodium. A natriuresis then takes place which lowers the blood volume. But this further increases the plasma renin concentration to even higher levels so that the blood pressure either remains raised or rises further, even if there is a profound fall in blood volume and possibly of the concentration of the circulating sodium transport inhibitor.

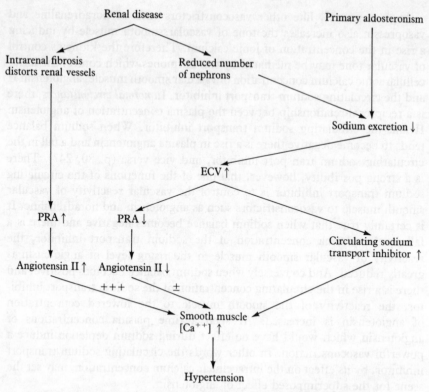

**Fig. 16.2** Possible relation between angiotensin II and the circulating sodium transport inhibitor in the aetiology of hypertension in renal disease and primary aldosteronism.

## Essential hypertension

### Aetiology

The cause of essential hypertension is unknown. The following hypothesis, based on some of the considerations outlined above proposes that the rise in pressure in essential hypertension is due to an increase in peripheral resistance due largely to the observed increase in the concentration of the circulating sodium transport inhibitor. As Figure 16.3 illustrates it is proposed that the underlying abnormality is an inherited renal difficulty in excreting sodium of unknown cause which is more apparent the higher the sodium intake.

The difficulty in excreting sodium may initially cause a transient increase in total blood volume with a rise in intrathoracic blood volume. It is suggested that this increases the plasma's ability to increase sodium excretion and to inhibit sodium transport, possibly via an afferent reflex incorporating the vagus and the hypothalamus. These changes adjust sodium excretion so that sodium balance is normal, but at the cost of having a persistently high

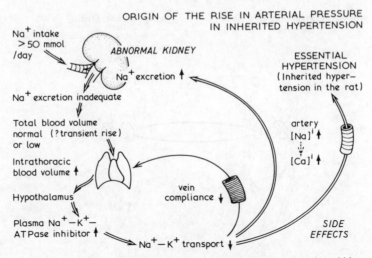

ORIGIN OF THE RISE IN ARTERIAL PRESSURE
IN INHERITED HYPERTENSION

**Fig. 16.3** Possible mechanism linking a congenital functional abnormality of the kidney, salt intake and a circulating sodium transport inhibitor to essential hypertension. (Derived from de Wardener & MacGregor 1980 Kidney Int 18: 1.)

level of the circulating sodium transport inhibitor. This raises the tone and vascular reactivity of the smooth muscle of both arteries and veins thus causing the observed rise in arterial pressure and diminution in venous compliance. The increase in venous tone causes the observed shift of blood from the periphery to the centre, which it is proposed raises the intrathoracic pressure and perpetuates the stimulus for greater secretion of the sodium transport inhibitor, even if the adjustments to sodium excretion have caused the total blood volume to fall to, or below, normal.

There are several lines of evidence which support the suggestion that in essential hypertension there is an impairment in the kidney's ability to excrete sodium. The most direct evidence, unfortunately, can only be obtained from rats with hereditary hypertension; an animal form of hypertension which most closely resembles essential hypertension. In such rats cross transplantation experiments have demonstrated that 'the hypertension follows the kidney' i.e. if a kidney from a young normotensive strain rat is placed into a young hypertensive strain rat, before the development of the hypertension, hypertension now does not develop in the latter (Fig. 16.4). The reverse also obtains. This experiment demonstrates that the kidney in hereditary hypertensive rats carries the genetic abnormality that leads to hypertension. Other experiments in these animals demonstrate that the abnormality is a difficulty in excreting sodium.

In man it is not possible to obtain direct experimental evidence that the kidney carries the hereditary abnormality. Nevertheless it is interesting that observations made among patients with renal grafts does suggest that the incidence of hypertension in the recipient is greatest if the kidney comes

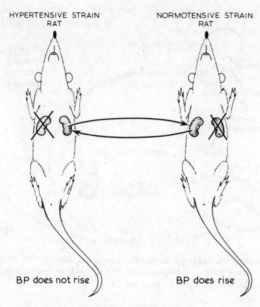

HYPERTENSIVE STRAIN
RAT

NORMOTENSIVE STRAIN
RAT

BP does not rise

BP does rise

**Fig. 16.4** Cross transplantation experiment between an inherited hypertensive strain rat and a control normotensive strain rat demonstrating that the kidney carries the genetic abnormality which causes the blood pressure to rise. Both kidneys are removed from each rat and one kidney is then cross transplanted into the other rat. The experiments are performed before the arterial pressure has risen in the hypertensive strain rat.

from a donor with a familial predisposition to hypertension. There is some evidence that, as in the rats, patients with essential hypertension have a difficulty in excreting sodium, but of course, this need not necessarily be due to a renal abnormality. Having established that in normal subjects the renal excretion of a standard *small* intravenous sodium load is genetically determined it has been demonstrated that the normotensive children of hypertensive parents excrete less sodium following such a load than do the normotensive children of normotensive parents. Population studies have also shown that in man there is a highly significant relation between arterial pressure and salt intake (Fig. 16.5). In populations with sodium intakes of approximately 400 mmol/day the incidence of hypertension, as age advances, is approximately 40% whereas populations which consume less than 60 mmol/day have no rise in arterial pressure with age. Finally in the inherited forms of hypertension in the rat and in essential hypertension the natriuresis which follows a *large* intravenous infusion of saline comes on much more quickly than in normal subjects. This accelerated natriuresis is often referred to as an 'exaggerated' natriuresis. Such an accelerated natriuresis strongly suggests a state in which there is a continuing need to oppose a persistent tendency to retain sodium. It occurs in primary aldosteronism and in normal subjects given aldosterone or prednisone even when, as in essential

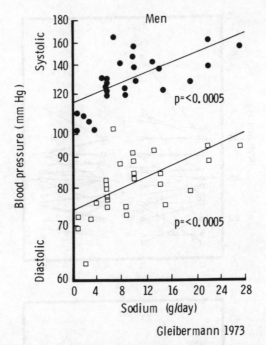

Gleibermann 1973

**Fig. 16.5** Relation between salt intake and mean arterial pressure in 27 populations. (Reproduced from Gleiberman 1973 Ecol Food Nutr 2: 143, with kind permission.)

hypertension the compensatory matriuretic mechanisms may have ensured that there is no measurable increase in extracellular fluid volume.

Patients with essential hypertension also have a remarkable tendency to excrete abnormally large quantities of sodium and water in response to many other stimuli including the insertion of a catheter into the bladder and certain emotional situations (Fig. 16.6). It has certainly been established that the faster natriuretic response of hypertensive patients to a large intravenous infusion of saline is not, due to a difference in peritubular oncotic or hydrostatic pressure (Fig. 16.7). Normotensive relatives of hypertensive patients also have an accelerated natriuresis when given a large intravenous load of saline.

The increased concentration of the circulating sodium transport inhibitor in the plasma of patients with essential hypertension has been demonstrated in several ways (Figs 16.7, 16.8). In association with the increase in the plasma concentration of the sodium transport inhibitor there are widespread abnormalities of sodium transport in red cells, white cells, and blood vessels. And it has been shown that some of the abnormalities in these circulating cells are reversed by the administration of diuretics.

Once the hypertension is established the hypertensive occlusive changes described above will tend to aggravate the hypertension. But by themselves widespread hypertensive vascular occlusive changes do not perpetuate the

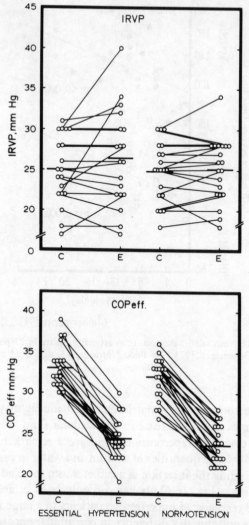

**Fig. 16.6** Individual values for intrarenal venous pressure (IRVP) and estimated efferent arteriolar colloid osmotic pressure (COP eff) in normal controls and patients with essential hypertension given a large intravenous infusion of saline. (Reproduced from Willassen & Ofstad 1981 Hypertension 2: 771, with kind permission.)

hypertension (with the exception of the vascular changes present in the kidneys). This is evident in patients who have had severe essential hypertension for many years and who have eventually developed terminal renal failure from advanced nephrosclerosis. If the kidneys of such patients are removed and they are given a renal transplant the blood pressure will return to normal in spite of the generalised advanced arterial occlusive changes. Similarly the removal of a pheochromocytoma from a patient who has had hypertension for many years may cause a permanent fall in arterial pressure.

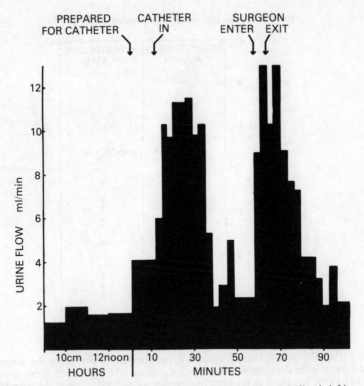

**Fig. 16.7** The effect on urine flow of (1) catheterising the bladder and (2) a brief interview with a surgeon; in a patient suffering from hypertension. The sudden increase in urine flow was associated with a sudden increase in sodium excretion. (Reproduced from Miles & de Wardener 1953 Lancet 2: 539, with kind permission.)

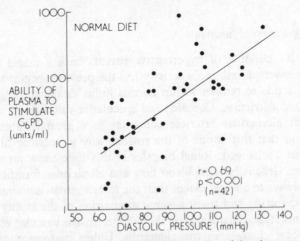

**Fig. 16.8** Diastolic arterial pressure plotted against the ability of the plasma to stimulate G6PD (an index of the plasma's ability to inhibit Na⁺-K⁺-TPase) in normotensive subjects and hypertensive patients demonstrating that the plasma of hypertensive patients have a greater ability to inhibit sodium transport. (Reproduced from MacGregor, Fenton, Alaghband-Zadeh et al 1981 Brit Med J 283: 1355, with kind permission.)

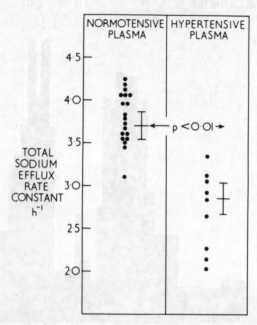

White cells from normotensives incubated in :-

Fig. 16.9 The effect of incubating leucocytes from normotensive subjects in the plasma of normal subjects or in the plasma of hypertensive patients. The sodium efflux rate constant of the white cells incubated in the hypertensive plasma decreased to about the same level as that of leucocytes obtained from hypertensive patients. Therefore the plasma contains a sodium transport inhibitor which inhibits sodium transport of white cells. (Derived from Poston, Sewell, Wilkinson et al 1981 Brit Med J 282: 847, with kind permission.)

## Other changes in renal function

Normotensive children of hypertensive parents have a raised renal blood flow and a lower plasma renin activity. As the pressure begins to rise renal blood flow tends to remain within normal limits demonstrating that there is renal vasoconstriction. Complex and speculative calculations suggest that the efferent glomerular arteriole constricts to a greater extent than the afferent, and that this is one of the reasons why glomerular filtration rate also remains unchanged. Renal biopsies at this time show no abnormality of structure. Gradually renal blood flow and glomerular filtration decrease, the latter always to a lesser extent than the former; small amounts of protein appear in the urine and there is some diminution of the ability to concentrate. At this stage renal biopsies show hypertensive vascular changes with scattered local changes in the glomeruli. Unless malignant hypertension supervenes it is unusual for these changes to become sufficiently extensive to cause symptomatic renal failure. With malignant hypertension proteinuria increases and the urine contains many red cells and granular casts;

tubular capacity to concentrate is lost; renal blood flow and glomerular filtration rate fall precipitously, and renal failure rapidly develops. The extent of the proteinuria is greatest in those who rapidly develop renal failure, and daily excretion rates above 5 g/day may occur together with a nephrotic syndrome. Whatever the rate of proteinuria (and occasionally malignant hypertension may present without proteinuria) the high levels of plasma renin activity and angiotensin II levels give rise to such hyperaldosteronism that the increased potassium excretion results in hypokalaemia.

## Renal hypertension

The term renal hypertension is given to those forms of hypertension in which it is considered that the initial rise in arterial pressure is due to an histologically identifiable pathological process within the kidney or the renal artery. It is probable, however, that as in essential hypertension the rise in arterial pressure is usually associated with a rise in the plasma concentration of a circulating sodium transport inhibitor.

Most of the work which has demonstrated the increase in the concentration of the circulating sodium transport in renal hypertension has been obtained from animal experiments (Fig. 16.10). The rise is presumably due to the diseased kidney's tendency to retain sodium. This is due either to occlusive arterial lesions causing a fall in the hydrostatic pressure in the peritubular venous capillary bed, which is a powerful sodium retaining stimulus, or to loss of nephrons. It is probable that sodium retention is also due, in part to a raised plasma aldosterone, due to the high plasma angiotensin II. The latter is due to multiple partial occlusions of the renal arterial tree caused by the pathological process destroying the kidney. It can also be due to a single

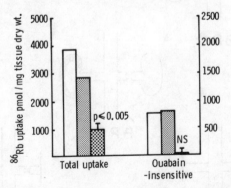

**Fig. 16.10** Sodium transport inhibitor in renal hypertension. Total $^{86}$Rb uptake (left panel, n = 10) and ouabain-insensitive $^{86}$Rb uptake (right panel, n = 5) by tail arteries taken from normal rats when incubated in supernates of boiled plasma from control normotensive rats drinking water ☐ , or drinking saline ▨ ; and hypertensive rats with reduced renal mass ▧ . (Reproduced from Huot, Pamnani, Clough et al 1983 Amer J Nephrol 3: 92, with kind permission.)

occlusive process in the main renal artery. The fall in perfusion pressure distal to the occlusions causes a reflex vasodilatation of the distal side of the partially occluded artery which is a potent stimulus for renin release. The consequent increase in blood volume which, by its effect on the intrathoracic blood volume, is probably the stimulus for the plasma's increased concentration of sodium transport inhibitor, is accentuated by another phenomenon. It is that there is a fall in the extracellular fluid volume to plasma volume ratio, i.e. the plasma volume increases at the expense of the extracellular volume. This change is probably due to the secretion from the kidney of a substance which effects the ability of the extracellular fluid space to contain fluid.

Once the hypertension is established the occlusive changes which it superimposes on the arteries in general, and the renal arterial tree in particular perpetuate the hypertension. Experimentally this is demonstrated in a rat by partially occluding one renal artery for a few months. After the blood pressure has been elevated for a period of time the occlusion is removed. Whether or not the arterial pressure then returns to normal depends on the extent of the hypertensive vascular damage present in the untouched kidney (Fig. 16.11). If the lesions are sufficiently severe the blood pressure remains elevated. It is presumed that the multiple nephrosclerotic arterial lesions throughout the renal arterial tree are now producing the same effect as the single experimentally produced initial occlusion of the main renal artery. It is probable that such a self perpetuating hypertensive mechanism occurs in man.

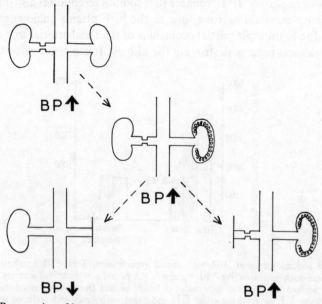

**Fig. 16.11** Perpetuation of hypertension by secondary nephrosclerotic changes induced by hypertension.

Renal hypertension can be due to unilateral, or bilateral, destructive lesions, or to an intrarenal renin secreting tumour.

## Bilateral renal disease associated with hypertension

80% of patients with chronic renal failure have hypertension. In general all renal diseases that primarily affect the renal cortex (e.g. glomerular nephritis) eventually cause hypertension whereas in those that primarily affect the medulla (reflux nephropathy and obstructive uropathy) the arterial pressure often remains normal or occasionally becomes lower than normal. There is however, much blurring between these two categories for the disease processes which primarily involve the medulla eventually affect the cortex. The onset of hypertension in a patient with a chronic destructive process of the renal parenchyma heralds an acceleration in the rate of functional deterioration.

Most patients on maintenance haemodialysis continue to fight a relentless battle against hypertension. The mechanisms causing the rise are the same as those operating before but they are now greatly magnified. On the one hand the gross reduction in daily urine volume inevitably causes a rapid increase in extracellular fluid volume to occur between each dialysis (easily

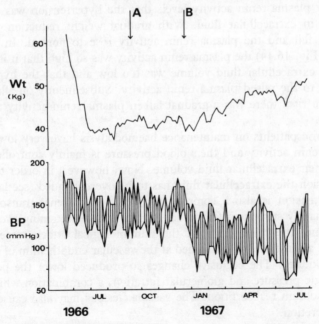

**Fig. 16.12** The effect of bilateral nephrectomy (B) on uncontrollable hypertension in a patient on maintenance haemodialysis with a very high plasma renin. There is an immediate fall in blood pressure which is maintained though there is a rise in weight. At point (A) the patient had an attack of acute infectious hepatitis. (Reproduced from Curtis, Lever, Robertson et al 1969 Nephron 6: 329, with kind permission.)

monitored as a gain in weight), and on the other hand the severely diseased kidneys tend to secrete large amounts of renin. Furthermore the need to lower the patients weight at each dialysis by rapidly removing a considerable amount of fluid may cause a brisk rise in plasma renin activity. If this recurring see saw reciprocal movement of extracellular fluid volume and renin release is sufficiently violent it eventually seems to resonate. Then the more one attempts to control the blood pressure by fluid removal the greater the rise in renin and ansiotensin II so that the blood pressure instead of falling, rises and becomes uncontrollable. This is well illustrated in Figure 16.12 which depicts the changes that occurred in a patient placed onto haemodialysis in the days before the whip-lash effect of weight reduction on plasma renin activity was properly appreciated. In an attempt to control the hypertension the patient's weight was lowered from 60 kg to 40 kg in about two months. This so reduced the extracellular fluid and blood volume that the patient fainted when he stood up, but his renin secretion was now so great that when he lay down he had severe hypertension with intolerable headaches and a tendency to develop acute pulmonary oedema. The problem was resolved by bilateral nephrectomy, an operation which is now rarely performed to control hypertension. Figures 16.13, 16.14 illustrate more contemporary problems in two further patients with hypertension on maintenance haemodialysis. In Figure 16.13 it is clear from the very low plasma renin activity levels that the hypertension was due to an increase in extracellular fluid. With gradual weight reduction the blood pressure fell and the plasma renin activity rose to normal. In the other patient (Fig. 16.14) the plasma renin activity was so high that it is probable that the extracellular fluid volume was too low and that the hypertension was due to the raised plasma renin activity. Subsequently on allowing the weight to rise, there was a gradual fall in plasma renin activity and blood pressure.

Anephric patients on maintenance haemodialysis have very low levels of plasma renin activity and their blood pressure is mainly controlled by the size of their extracellular fluid volume. Now, however, in order to prevent hypotension the extracellular fluid has to be overexpanded (see later).

Hypertension is also a common complication of renal transplantation. This is hardly surprising for, in addition to the salt retaining properties of prednisone, the main brunt of the immunological attack waged by the recipient against the graft is aimed at the vascular endothelium of the transplanted kidney. The occlusive changes so produced lower the peritubular hydrostatic pressure and glomerular filtration, a combination which causes intense sodium reabsorption. The vascular lesions may also cause a rise in renin secretion.

*Unilateral renal disease associated with hypertension*

The importance of this group of patients is that in a few the hypertension

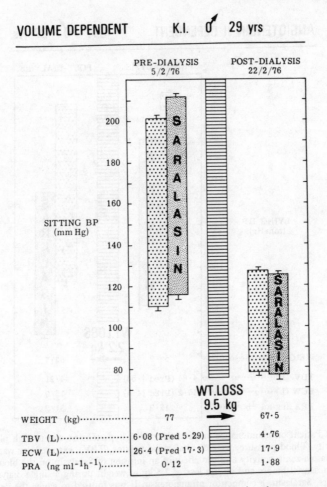

**Fig. 16.13** Patient on maintenance haemodialysis with hypertension due to excess volume. Blood pressure, weight, total blood volume (TBV), extracellular water (ECW), plasma renin activity (PRA) and the effect of an infusion of Saralasin on the blood pressure, measured before and after the loss of 9.5 kg of weight in 17 days. Saralasin, a competitor of angiotensin II, was infused to gauge the dependency of the blood pressure on angiotensin II. On the first occasion, when the blood pressure was 200/100 mmHg, the blood volume was obviously high and there was a gross expansion of extracellular water, plasma renin activity was abnormally low and the lack of effect of the infusion of Saralasin on the blood pressure indicated that the blood pressure was not dependent on the plasma level of angiotensin II. On the second occasion, after the loss of weight, when the blood pressure was 128/78 mmHg, blood volume, extracellular water and plasma renin activity were now normal and the Saralasin infusion again demonstrated that the blood pressure was not dependent on angiotensin II. (Unpublished data by kind permission of Dr G A MacGregor.)

may be due to the renal lesion, and that nephrectomy, or correction of an obstruction or by-pass of a renal arterial occlusion may cure the hypertension. On the other hand, only approximately 0.25 per cent of all patients with a raised diastolic pressure are found to have a unilateral renal lesion

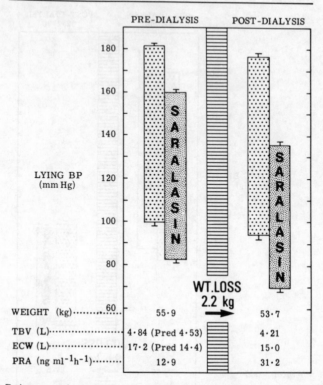

**Fig. 16.14** Patient on maintenance haemodialysis with hypertension due to high plasma renin activity. Blood pressure, weight, total blood volume (TBV), extracellular water (ECW), plasma renin activity and the effect of an infusion of Saralasin on the blood pressure measured before and after a loss of 2.5 kg of weight during a single dialysis of seven hours. Saralasin, a competitor of angiotensin II was infused to gauge the dependency of the blood pressure on angiotensin II. Before dialysis, when the blood pressure was 180/100 mmHg, the blood volume was normal, though the extracellular water was 2.5 kg greater than predicted (a not unusual gain in weight between dialyses), plasma renin activity was greatly raised and the fall in blood pressure induced by the infusion of Saralasin indicated that the blood pressure was under the influence of angiotensin II. After dialysis, having lost a 'normal' amount of weight, the blood pressure was 170/95 mm Hg, the blood volume and extracellular water were normal but the plasma renin activity was now extremely high, and the greater fall in blood pressure induced by Saralasin infusion indicated that the blood pressure was even more dependent on angiotensin II. (Unpublished data by kind permission of Dr G. A. MacGregor.)

which surgery can benefit. It is also important to note that demonstrable partial occlusion of the renal artery may not be associated with hypertension; or that if partial occlusion of the renal artery is associated with hypertension, occlusion may not be its cause. Occlusion of the renal arterial tree may be either in the main renal artery or its main segmental branches before they enter the parenchyma of the kidney, or in the smaller arteries within the renal parenchyma. The lesions in the main artery and its branches include atheromatous plaques, 'fibromuscular hyperplasia', aneurysm embolism, and external compression from a tumour. Unilateral parenchymatous renal lesions include reflux nephropathy, irradiation, and tuberculosis of a kidney and the rare renin producing tumour.

*Mechanisms.* The hypertension is due to a combination of salt and water retention and a rise in renin secretion. This is most easily distinguished in renal artery stenosis. The intense sodium and water reabsorption of the stenosed kidney is blunted by a compensatory increase in urinary sodium excretion from the other 'normal' kidney, perhaps due in part to a rise in the plasma concentration of the natriuretic hormone sodium transport inhibitor. The partial occlusion of the renal artery also increases renin secretion by the mechanism described above. Occasionally plasma renin activity is so high that the associated increase in plasma aldosterone causes potassium deficiency and hypokalaemia i.e. secondary aldosteromism.

*Renal function.* Experimental partial occlusion of a renal artery perfusing functioning renal parenchyma causes a variable fall in renal plasma flow and glomerular filtration rate. The most characteristic change, however, is a great increase in tubular reabsorption of sodium in the proximal tubule. This is due to the lowering of the peritubular venous capillary pressure (p. 74). The increase in sodium reabsorption causes a marked increase in water reabsorption from the proximal tubule. This has two consequences, it reduces the urine flow and raises the concentration of those substances in the tubule lumen which are not reabsorbed, i.e. creatinine, inulin, PAH or Hypaque. A kidney being perfused by a partially occluded renal artery therefore will produce urine at a slow rate which nevertheless contains a lower concentration of sodium than that from the opposite kidney but a higher concentration of creatinine, inulin or PAH. Clearly, the pattern is only discernible if the process is unilateral or at least more pronounced on one side than the other. If this phenomenon can be demonstrated it is highly probable that a considerable proportion of functioning proximal tubules are being perfused at a low pressure. It is then justifiable to imply that a similar proportion of functioning juxta-glomerular apparati are also being perfused at a low pressure and to conclude therefore that at least part of the hypertension is probably due to partial occlusion of the renal arteries. The opposite also holds. The unequivocal demonstration of a unilateral renal abnormality or renal artery stenosis in the absence of this characteristic functional pattern implies that either the occlusion to the renal arteries is not sufficient to lower the perfusion pressure, or that the low perfusion pressure is not affecting functioning proximal tubules and therefore functioning juxta-glomerular apparati.

*Renal structure.* The characteristic appearance in the parenchyma is best seen in occlusion of the main renal artery or its branches. The tubules become small with narrow lumens and shrunken cuboidal cells. The glomeruli remain relatively unchanged but are crowded together because of the tubular atrophy. On the other hand, the arterioles are normal, in striking contrast to the arterioles from the opposite kidney which is being perfused with a raised arterial pressure.

*Clinical features.* On the whole there is little to distinguish these patients from the other 99.75% of patients suffering from hypertension. There may be a recent history of abdominal trauma, emboli or thrombi in other sites, or of pain in the flank or loin. The diastolic pressure may have been noted to rise rapidly and when there is potassium deficiency there may be a complaint of thirst and polyuria. Very occasionally the extent of the proteinuria is such that the patient presents with a nephrotic syndrome. Stenosis of the renal artery is sometimes associated with a sytolic murmur which is heard best posteriorly over the affected artery.

*Diagnosis.* The intensity with which the following maneouvres are pursued depends on how suggestive are the clinical features, the age of the patient, and what is considered it might be appropriate to do if occlusive renal arterial disease were found.

*IVU.* It is imperative that an intravenous pyelogram be performed on any patient in whom one or more of the clinical features described above is present. An IVU in such a patient must be performed with a rapid infusion of contrast medium and the taking of films at 15 sec, 1, 2 and 3 min after the injection, in addition to the other films taken at 5, 10 and 20 min. Ureteric compression must not be used during the first few minutes. If there is unilateral occlusion of the renal arterial tree the contrast medium appears first in the pelvis and ureter of the unaffected kidney, and in the first few minutes the contrast medium on the affected side is *less dense* than in the 'normal' side. This is due to the slow urine flow and reduced glomerular filtration rate of the affected kidney. Ten to 20 min later, however, the picture is reversed. Because of the increased sodium and water reabsorption which accompanies the vascular occlusion, the contrast medium on the affected side is now *denser* than on the normal side. At this time it is possible to compare the lengths of the two kidneys; a difference greater than 1.5 cm is abnormal and nearly always accompanies partial occlusion of the renal artery.

These characteristic findings can sometimes be made more distinct by performing the pyelogram during a water or a urea-saline diuresis. If the I.V.U. is normal and the clinical features not particularly suggestive of occlusive arterial disease no further test need be carried out.

*Aortogram and renal arteriogram.* Occlusive lesions situated at the origins of the renal arteries, usually atheromatous plaques, are best delineated by aortography, while lesions in the renal artery and its branches are best seen if the radio-opaque dye is injected directly into the renal artery.

*Renin concentration in the renal vein and vena cava.* Blood is obtained from both renal veins and from the vena cava above and below the renal veins. Unilateral occlusive renal arterial disease can be considered to be causing the rise in blood pressure if the following conditions are satisfied: (1) that the renin concentration on the affected side is at least 1.5 times greater than on the unaffected side and (2) that the renin concentration in the vena cava above the renal veins is greater than the concentration of renin in the venous blood of the unaffected kidney. If these criteria are satisfied surgical interference is likely to lower the blood pressure. Occasionally the amount of salt and water retention associated with the renal artery stenosis is sufficiently great to partially suppress the rise in plasma renin activity. It may then be difficult to interpret the measurement of plasma renin activity. This uncertainty can sometimes be resolved if the measurements are repeated after the patient's weight has been reduced one to two kilograms by means of a low sodium diet and diuretics.

*Isotope renogram as a tool to diagnose occlusive vascular disease.* The popularity of this technique for this purpose was more due to its non invasiveness and convenience than to it's reliability.

*The use of the isotope renogram and gamma camera to study individual renal blood flow or glomerular filtration rate.* It is essential that the contribution of each kidney to total renal function is assessed before performing a nephrectomy for the relief of hypertension. The tradition of relying on the intravenous urogram for this information is hazardous. Individual function studies can be measured either with excretion renography with a radioactive substance (p. 16).

*The use of bilateral ureteric catheterisation.* In this hazardous technique ureteric catheters are introduced via a cystoscope into each ureter and urine collected from each kidney during the intravenous administration of urea, saline and vasopressin. The characteristic finding with renal artery stenosis is that the affected kidney has a urine flow 50% less than on the other side, with at least a 20% increase in creatinine concentration and 20% reduction in sodium concentration. This highly invasive technique is difficult to perform, is liable to unpleasant complications, and unless it is carried out by a team of individuals to whom it is familiar it usually goes wrong because of some technical incompetence e.g. one of the ureteric catheters slips down into the bladder. Even when it is successfully performed the results are often difficult to interpret, particularly if there is any degree of renal failure.

*Treatment.* Overall the influence of operation on blood pressure and survival is disappointing. If the patient is young and the disease is unilateral it is justifiable to attempt either to correct or by-pass the occlusion or to perform a nephrectomy. Nephrectomy is the more satisfying procedure in terms of both immediate and long term mortality. In the majority of instances, however, the patients are middle-aged or elderly and the cause of the occlusion is atheroma. If the hypertension can be controlled satisfactorily with hypotensive drugs the patient should not be subjected to an operation. Treatment with spironolactone alone may be sufficient.

It is also possible, sometimes, to dilate the stenosis by blowing up a balloon placed in the lumen of the artery under radiological control. This procedure, which has acquired the name of 'angioplasty' may give a temporary respite and can be repeated. It is most useful in cases of fibro-mucular hyperplasia. Its success is very dependent on the skill and experience of the radiologist. Restenosis with a recurrence of the hypertension often occurs, when the procedure can be repeated. Alternatively, a favourable response can be used as an indication that surgical treatment will be successful.

## Hypertension due to excess mineralocorticoids or glucocorticoids

Primary aldosteronism, in which the adrenal gland is secreting an excess of aldosterone, or Cushing's disease in which there is an increase in glucocorticoids, and the administration of prednisone are all associated with hypertension. The rise in pressure is due in part to the salt and water retention, and occurs in spite of a compensatory fall in plasma renin. It is possible that, in addition, the excess aldosterone or glucocorticoids contributes to the hypertension in some other way (see below). The diagnosis is based on the association of hypertension, raised plasma aldosterone, hypokalaemia with a raised urinary potassium excretion, a low plasma renin activity and a raised total exchangeable potassium to sodium ratio. Contrary to expectations only a minority of patients have a raised plasma volume. In the majority it is either normal or *reduced* (p. 257).

## Renal hypotension

Renal hypotension is a rare complication of some forms of renal disease, and usually follows bilateral nephrectomy.

The renal diseases which are most prone to this unusual complication are those which predominantly affect the renal medulla e.g, reflux nephropathy, obstructive uropathy and phenacetin nephropathy. Though the condition is sometimes referred to as 'salt losing nephritis' is is rarely due to glomerular nephritis. The fall in arterial pressure is due to a urinary leak of sodium and only occurs with bilateral renal disease, after the onset of renal failure. It is associated with a gross generalised hypertrophy of the juxta glomerular apparati and of the adrenals. Plasma renin activity and aldosterone are raised. Often there is hypokalaemia due in part to the aldosteronism and in part to the renal disease. The condition tends to fluctuate wildly. Exacerbations are often caused by an upper urinary infection when the combination of infection, hypotension, fall in extracellular fluid volume and hypokalaemia may cause severe but usually entirely and easily reversible reductions in renal function. In spite of these alarming episodes these patients survive much longer than other patients with renal failure whose progress is calmer but who develop hypertension. Survival of the patients with renal hypotension depends on the skill and speed of reaction of those who look after them. The continuous administration of oral supplements of sodium chloride such as Slow Sodium (Ciba), the repeated monitoring of the urine for infection and the prompt treatment of a relapse may prevent any progressive deterioration in renal function.

Renal hypotension is such a serious and frequent complication of the anephric state that together with the accompanying extremely severe anaemia, with haemoglobin concentrations often below 5 g/100 ml, bilateral nephrectomy is no longer used for the treatment of intractable hypertension in patients on maintenance haemodialysis. After bilateral nephrectomy the relation between the arterial pressure and the blood volume is such that the volume has to be much greater than normal to maintain a normal blood pressure (Fig. 16.15). Many anephric patients therefore live precarious lives of fluctuating hypotension in spite of an overexpanded extracellular fluid volume, sometimes to the point of demonstrable clinical oedema and breathlessness. The low arterial pressure is presumably due primarily to the almost total absence of renin and angiotensin II, but there is suggestive evidence that it may also be due in part to the associated reduction in plasma aldosterone.

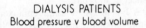

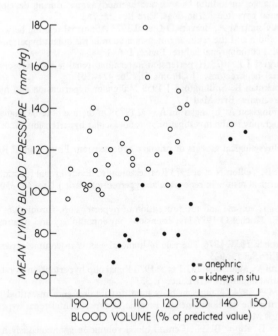

**Fig. 16.15** Blood volume versus mean lying blood pressure in patients on maintenance haemodialysis. At normal blood volumes the blood pressure of anephric patients (○) was lower than in patients whose kidneys were still *in situ* (●). (Unpublished data by kind permission of Dr G. A. MacGregor.)

These two forms of hypotension beautifully illustrate the interdependence of angiotensin and the extracellular fluid volume, and possibly therefore of the circulating sodium transport inhibitor, in the control of blood pressure. On the one hand in 'salt losing nephritis' the urinary leak of sodium and decrease in extracellular fluid volume are so great that the arterial pressure falls in spite of enormous rises in plasma renin activity. On the other hand, in the absence of angiotensin, gross overexpansion of the extracellular fluid volume barely prevents the arterial pressure from being intolerably low.

BIBLIOGRAPHY

Barraclough M A 1966 Sodium and water depletion with acute malignant hypertension. Amer J Med 40: 265
Berlyne G M, Tavill A S, de C Baker S B 1964 Renal artery stenosis and the nephrotic syndrome. Quart J Med 33: 325
Bianchi G, Brown J J, Lever A F et al 1968 Changes plasma renin concentration during pressor infusions of renin in the conscious dog: the influence of dietary sodium intake. Clin Sci 34: 303
Blaustein M P 1977 Sodium ions, calcium ions, blood pressure regulation and hypertension: a reassessment and a hypothesis. Amer J Physiol 232(3): C165
Borst J G G, Borst-de Geus A 1963 Hypertension explained by Starling's theory of circulatory homeostasis. Lancet 1: 677–682
Brown J J, Curtis, J R, Lever A F et al 1969 Plasma renin concentration and the control of blood pressure in patients on maintenance haemodialysis. Nephron 6: 329
Conway J 1968 Changes in sodium balance and haemodynamics during development of experimental renal hypertension in dogs. Circ Res 22: 763
Davies D L, Schalekamp M A, Beevers D G et al 1973 Abnormal relation between exchangeable sodium and the renin-angiotensin system in malignant hypertension and in hypertension with chronic renal failure. Lancet I: 683
Del Greco F, Burgess J L 1973 Hypertension in terminal renal failure. Observations pre and post bilateral nephrectomy. J Chronic Dis 26: 471–501
Dollery C T, Shackman R, Shillingford J 1959 Malignant hypertension and hypokalaemia cured by nephrectomy. Brit Med J 2: 1367
Erikson U, Hemmingsson A, Ljungstrom A et al 1975 On the use of renal angiography and intravenous urography in the investigation of renovascular hypertension. Acta Med Scand 198: 39
Folkow B 1982 Physiological aspects of primary hypertension. Physiological Reviews 62: 348
Fournier A, Safar B, Veillon N et al 1973 Reassessment of divided renal function study in prediction of surgical results in renovascular hypertension. Brit J Urol 45: 350 Urol 45: 350
Freis E D 1976 Salt, volume and the prevention of hypertension. Circulation 53: 589
Genest J, Koiio E, Kuchel O 1977 Hypertension: physiopathology and treatment. McGraw-Hill, New York
Haddy F J, Overbeck H W 1976 The role of humoral agents in volume expanded hypertension. Life Sci 19: 935
Louis W J, Renzini V, MacDonald G J et al 1970 Renal clip hypertension in rabbits immunised against angiotensin II Lancet i: 333
Lucas J, Floyer M A 1974 Changes in body fluid distribution and interstitial tissue compliance during the development and reversal of experimental renal hypertension in the rat. Clin Sci Mol Med 47: 1
Lundin S, Folkow B, Rippe B 1981 Central blood volume in spontaneously hypertensive rats and Wistar-Kyoto normotensive rats. Acta Physiol Scand 112: 257
McNeil B J, Varedy P D, Burrows B A et al 1975 Measure of clinical efficiency; lost effectiveness calculations in the diagnosis and treatment of hypertensive reno-vascular disease. New Eng J Med 293: 582

MacGregor G A 1977 Diseases of the urinary system. High blood pressure and renal disease. Brit Med J 2: 624

Maxwell M H, Bleifer K H, Franklin S S et al 1972 The co-operative study of renovascular hypertension. Demographic analysis of the study. J Amer Med Assoc 220: 1195

Owen K 1973 Results of surgical treatment in comparison with medical treatment of renovascular hypertension. Clin Sci Mol Med 45: 95S

Poston L, Jones R B, Richardson P J et al 1981 The effect anti-hypertensive therapy on abnormal leucocyte sodium transport in essential hypertension. Clin Exp Hyper 3: 693

Stockigt J R, Collins R D, Noakes C A et al 1972 Renal-vein renin in various forms of renal hypertension. Lancet i: 1194

Strong C G, Hunt J C, Sheps S G et al 1971 Renal venous renin activity enhancement of sensitivity of lateralization by sodium depletion. Amer J Cardiol 27: 602

Swales J D 1976 The hunt for renal hypertension. Lancet i: 57

Vaughan E D, Buhler, F R, Laragh J H et al Renovascular hypertension: renin measurements to indicate hypersecretion and contralateral suppression, estimate renal plasma flow, and score surgical curability. Amer J Med 55: 402

Wilson C, Byrom F B 1941 The viscious circle in chronic Bright's disease. Experimental evidence from hypertensive rat. Quart J Med N S 10: 65

Wardener de H E, MacGregor G A 1982 The natriuretic hormone and essential hypertension. Lancet i: 1450

# 17

# The kidney's control of urinary sodium excretion in disease

## NORMAL CONTROL OF THE VOLUME AND CONCENTRATION OF BODY FLUIDS

Water is added to body fluids principally by oral intake, but there is also a small contribution of 200–300 ml a day which is an end product of metabolism. Water is lost via the skin, lungs and kidneys; loss from the gut is negligible unless there is vomiting, diarrhoea or a fistula. The intake of water is controlled by thirst, while its output is adjusted by the kidneys; the amount of water lost from the skin and respiratory tract in mainly dependent on atmospheric conditions and is thus beyond the body's internal authority.

### Thirst

The sensation of thirst appears to originate in the hypothalamus; it is influenced by a wide variety of factors, the two most important being the osmolality of the extracellular fluid, and the blood volume. The first can easily be demonstrated by administering hypertonic saline, and the second by performing a substantial venesection. It is probable that the thirst centre is directly stimulated by changes in osmolality, but it is not known how it is aware of changes in blood volume.

### Renal control of extracellular fluid tonicity

The control of water output by the kidney is intimately connected with the control of sodium chloride excretion, both varying with the need to keep the tonicity of body fluids and the blood volume within normal limits. It is probable that the osmolality of the intra- and extracellular fluids is the same, so that it is possible for the kidney to maintain tonicity of body fluids simply by adjusting the osmolality of the extracellular fluid. Theoretically this could be achieved by altering the urinary excretion of either water or salt, but in practice it is done mainly by altering the excretion of water. The neurohypophysis responds to changes in plasma osmolality by rapid alterations in the rate at which the antidiuretic hormone (ADH) is secreted into the circulation, and ADH in turn controls the concentration of the urine and therefore, the volume of urine that is excreted. For instance, a drink of water lowers plasma osmolality; this inhibits ADH production by the neurohypophysis and within 20–30 min the urine becomes hypotonic, whereas with fluid deprivation and a rise in plasma osmolality the mechanism is reversed.

## Renal control of extracellular fluid and blood volume

Changes in blood volume induce alterations in both sodium and water excretion. It is clear that if the tonicity of body fluids is to remain constant the ratio of salt to water released or retained must be in isotonic proportions. This synchronisation of the different mechanisms which control salt and water excretion can be demonstrated by bleeding a normal subject, when there is a prompt and simultaneous *decrease* in both salt and water excretion; or, conversely, by administering blood or a 'plasma expander' such as albumin when there is a simultaneous *increase* in salt and water excretion.

The efferent mechanism responsible for changes in water excretion consists mainly in altering the rate of secretion of antidiuretic hormone (ADH). Changes in sodium excretion which originate from a change in blood volume are due almost entirely to changes in tubular reabsorption of sodium. The mechanisms responsible for changing the reabsorption of sodium have been outlined earlier (p. 72). They include changes in sympathetic activity, renal blood flow, peritubular hydrostatic pressure and oncotic pressure, renin secretion and plasma angiotensin II, and aldosterone. It is clear however, that, while an acute injection of aldosterone indubitably increases tubular sodium reabsorption, a persistent excess of aldosterone does not cause oedema. This is evident in primary aldosteronism, during the prolonged administration of aldosterone or other mineralocorticoids and following a prolonged infusion of angiotensin II (secondary hyperaldosteronism). When aldosterone is administered there is an initial increase in sodium reabsorption associated with a small gain in weight, but within a few days the 'escape' phenomenon takes place, i.e. urinary sodium excretion rises to match the intake and the weight levels out (Fig. 17.1). Often at this time, there is an overshoot with a temporary increase in urinary sodium excretion to a rate greater than the intake so that the weight that is eventually attained is very close to that obtained before the aldosterone was administered. It is clear therefore that an excess of aldosterone can only contribute to the development of generalised oedema if the 'escape' phenomenon does not occur. As, however, the escape appears to be, due at least in part, to an increase in the plasma's natriuretic activity, it is possible that aldosterone can only cause oedema if either this compensatory increase does not occur or the kidney has become resistant to its action.

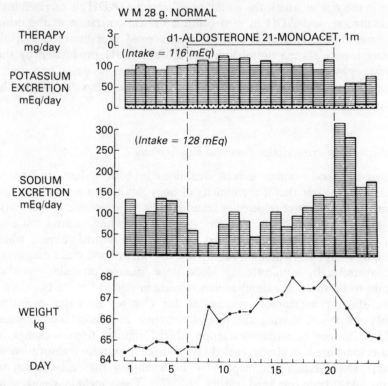

**Fig. 17.1** Effect of 1 mg of aldosterone given intramuscularly at 8 hourly intervals on urinary sodium and potassium excretion in a normal man receiving a constant diet. Stippled areas indicate potassium excretion in the stool. (Reproduced from August, Nelson & Thorn 1958 The J Clin Invest 37: 1958, by copyright permission of The American Society for Clinical Investigation.)

## DISCUSSION OF THE POSSIBLE MECHANISMS RESPONSIBLE FOR SODIUM RETENTION IN VARIOUS DISEASES ASSOCIATED WITH GENERALISED OEDEMA

Whatever the condition that initiates generalised oedema, the increase in extracellular fluid volume and consequential gain in weight has to be due to a retention of salt and water by the kidney. This occurs in an acute nephritic syndrome, a nephrotic syndrome, cardiac failure, chronic liver failure, diuretic abuse (sometimes known as idiopathic oedema) and malnutrition.

### Acute nephritic syndrome

The cause of the sodium retention and oedema in this condition is not known. It is not due to heart failure for there is no evidence that the heart is failing as a pump. There is usually some degree of hyproproteinaemia and a fall in glomerular filtration rate which is greater than the fall in renal blood flow. There is therefore a fall in filtration fraction and plasma protein osmotic pressure in the peritubular capillaries, which would tend to *decrease* sodium reabsorption and thus increase urinary excretion of sodium. Renal biopsy however shows that the glomerular tufts tend to be obliterated by cellular proliferation. It is possible therefore that the cause of the increased reabsorption of sodium is a diminished hydrostatic pressure in the peritubular capillaries, which is a powerful stimulus to sodium reabsorption. Occasionally there is considerable interstitial oedema which may possibly contribute to an increase in sodium reabsorption.

## Nephrotic syndrome

In the nephrotic syndrome there is heavy proteinuria, hypoproteinaemia and generalised oedema. The increase in sodium reabsorption appears to be due to some intrarenal disturbance. Until recently it was thought that a fall in blood volume initiated sodium retention and that this reduction in volume was due, not only to the negative nitrogen balance diminishing the total num-

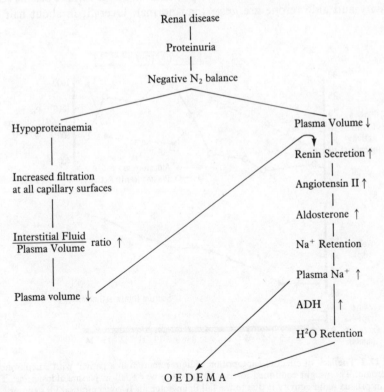

**Fig. 17.2** One hypothesis to explain the mechanisms responsible for oedema in the nephrotic syndrome.

ber of albumin molecules available to keep the plasma volume normally expanded but that in addition it was due to the fall in the plasma protein concentration. It was suggested that the latter increased the filtration of solute and water from the plasma into the interstitial space at all capillary surfaces and thus lowered the plasma volume (Fig. 17.2). It is unlikely however, that in a relatively young person this second explanation is of any importance for an increase in filtration is normally matched by an increase in lymphatic flow and a return of the fluid back into the circulation via the thoracic duct at the same rate as it is being filtered. It was also believed that the fall in blood volume caused a rise in plasma renin activity, angiotensin II and aldosterone which in turn caused an increase in sodium reabsorption (Fig. 17.2).

This sequence, though probably correct in some aspects has probably little to do with the increased sodium reabsorption in the nephrotic syndrome. It has now been established that in a substantial number of patients with a nephrotic syndrome, who are actively retaining sodium and gaining 0.5 to 1 kg of weight per day, the blood volume is either normal or *raised*, and that though, in a few patients with low blood volumes plasma renin activity and aldosterone may be raised, their concentration is often normal, while in those patients who have a raised blood volume plasma renin activity and aldosterone are *lower* than normal. Overall, in about half the

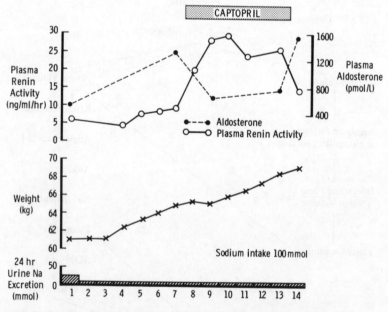

**Fig. 17.3** The lack of effect of captopril on sodium retention in a patient with a nephrotic syndrome. The weight continued to rise though there was a fall in plasma aldosterone. The rise in plasma renin activity is due to the fall in angiotensin II concentration for captopril inhibits the conversion of angiotensin I to angiotensin II. (Reproduced from Brown, Markandu, Sagnella et al 1982 Lancet 2: 1237, with kind permission.)

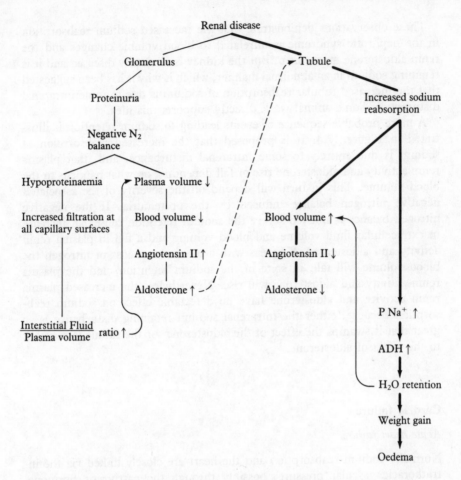

Renal disease

Glomerulus                                    Tubule

Proteinuria                                   Increased sodium
                                              reabsorption

Negative N₂
balance

Hypoproteinaemia      Plasma volume ↓         Blood volume ↑

Increased filtration at
all capillary surfaces    Blood volume ↓      Angiotensin II ↓

                      Angiotensin II ↑        Aldosterone ↓

                      Aldosterone ↑

                                              P Na⁺ ↑

Interstitial Fluid
─────────────  ratio ↑                        ADH ↑
Plasma volume

                                              H₂O retention

                                              Weight gain

                                              Oedema

**Fig. 17.4** A more contemporary hypothesis to explain the mechanisms responsible for the oedema in the nephrotic syndrome.

patients the increased sodium reabsorption is demonstrably not due to a raised plasma renin activity and aldosterone. And it can also be shown that even in those in whom plasma renin activity and aldosterone are raised the increase in sodium reabsorption is due to some other mechanism. For instance the administration of captopril (a converting enzyme inhibitor which prevents the conversion of angiotensin I to II and thus reduces aldosterone secretion) to such patients lowers plasma aldosterone and angiotensin II but sodium retention and the daily increase in weight continues unabated (Fig. 17.3). Plasma renin activity and aldosterone can also be lowered by the daily intravenous administration of salt free albumin for three days. This also tends to correct the low blood volume and the hypoproteinaemia, yet sodium retention and the increase in weight continue.

These observations demonstrate that the increased sodium reabsorption in the nephrotic syndrome is unrelated to blood volume changes and the renin aldosterone mechanism. But the kidney is obviously diseased and it is retaining sodium in an abnormal manner, which is why it has been suggested that the increased tubular reabsorption of sodium is due to some intrarenal disturbance. Some animal work directly supports this idea.

A more probable sequence of events leading to sodium retention is illustrated in Figure 17.4. It is proposed that the increased reabsorption of sodium is due entirely to some intrarenal disturbance, and, that plasma renin activity and aldosterone rise or fall depending on what happens to the blood volume. This in turn will depend on the severity of the associated negative nitrogen balance induced by the proteinuria. If the negative nitrogen balance is not too severe the sodium retention causes an increase in extracellular fluid volume and blood volume and a fall in plasma renin activity and aldosterone. Whereas with a more severe loss of nitrogen the blood volume will fall, in spite of the sodium retention, and the plasma renin activity and aldosterone will rise. Nevertheless the increased plasma renin activity and aldosterone have no detectable effect on sodium reabsorption because, either the intrarenal sodium retaining disturbance is so great that it swamps the effect of the aldosterone, or the tubule is resistant to the effect of aldosterone.

## Cardiac failure

### Acute heart failure

Normally sodium reabsorption and the heart are closely linked via the intrathoracic vascular pressure, possibly through the natriuretic hormone. On physiological grounds an acute rise in intrathoracic blood volume due to a failing left ventricle should be associated with an *increase* in sodium excretion. And so, rather surprisingly, it is. For 24 to 48 hours immediately after a myocardial infarction there is an increase in renal blood flow, glomerular filtration and urinary sodium excretion. During this time peripheral vasoconstriction due to a reflex from the injured heart produces a shift of blood volume from the periphery to the center so that the intrathoracic and left auricular pressure rise and there may be pulmonary oedema in spite of sodium depletion. The administration of diuretics for the breathlessness then causes a further loss of sodium. This further depletion of the extracellular fluid volume may then perpetuate the peripheral vasoconstriction, or as the heart improves and the vasoconstriction diminishes, the reduced blood volume may cause the blood pressure to fall. Both the hypovolaemia and the hypotension now tend to cause sodium retention. Or if the heart failure persists the mechanisms for sodium retention detailed below come into operation.

## Chronic heart failure

Chronic cardiac failure is associated with an increase in sodium reabsorption and an accumulation of oedema which, in the absence of diuretics, will first cripple and then destroy the patient. The exact mechanisms responsible for this fatuous response to a failing heart are not clear. There are probably several contributory causes. There is renal vasoconstriction and fall in glomerular filtration so that most patients have some degree of renal failure. The vasoconstriction is due in part to an increase in sympathetic activity, and a rise in the plasma concentration of angiotensin II. Sometimes this is associated with an increase in plasma aldosterone but most of the sodium and water retention does not appear to be related to the increased plasma aldosterone. Sodium retention is more likely to be due to a fall in hydrostatic pressure in the peritubular capillaries caused by the renal vasoconstriction and possibly by the direct effects of catecholamines and angiotensin II on tubular sodium reabsorption. In addition, as the fall in glomerular filtration rate is greater than the fall in renal blood flow there is a rise in the filtration fraction and therefore a rise in the plasma oncotic pressure in the peritubular

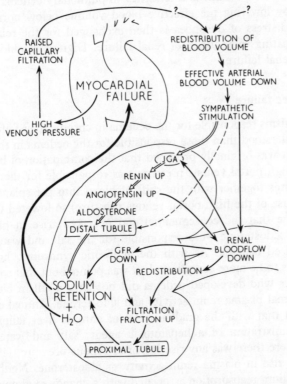

**Fig. 17.5** Possible mechanisms involved in the sodium retention in cardiac failure. The diminution in peritubular hydrostatic pressure associated with renal vasoconstriction has been omitted for simplification. N.B. Salt and water retention makes the heart failure worse.

capillaries, which may also increase sodium reabsorption to a small extent. The importance of angiotensin II in the aetiology of the oedema is evident from the natriuresis obtained with the converting enzyme inhibitor captopril. It is not clear however if this is due to the fall in angiotensin II diminishing the increased sodium reabsorption directly or whether the beneficial effect of captopril is entirely due to the improvement in cardiac function produced by the diminution of peripheral vasoconstriction. There is no reason to believe that the rise in renal venous pressure associated with heart failure is an important factor in the increased sodium reabsorption for it has been shown in animals that urinary sodium excretion is not influenced by renal venous pressure until it exceeds a threshold of about 20 cm of water.

Oral diuretics control the oedema and breathlessness of heart failure but to do this it may be necessary to reduce the blood volume to such an extent that the patient may slip from a state in which the renal failure of heart failure is exchanged for the renal failure of volume depletion. It is therefore necessary to monitor renal function from time to time. Occasionally the heart's pumping action is so severely compromised that the increase in intrathoracic blood volume and tendency to pulmonary oedema can only be controlled by lowering the effective blood volume below normal deliberately. The distress of dyspnoea is then exchanged for the relatively preferable nauseating somnolence of renal failure. Digitalis should be avoided if there is renal failure.

## Chronic liver failure

The mechanisms responsible for the oedema in chronic liver failure are even less well understood than those responsible for the oedema in the nephrotic syndrome. It was originally proposed that the combination of hypoproteinaemia and high portal venous pressure was responsible for the ascites, and that the ascites together with the shift of blood into the splanchnic circulation (because of the high portal venous pressure) so lowered the effective blood volume that the consequential and observed, rise in plasma renin activity and aldosterone were responsible for the salt and water retention and generalised oedema. As with the nephrotic syndrome, however, the truth appears to be more complicated. It was pointed out that some patients with cirrhosis who developed oedema did not have a fall in blood volume and had normal plasma renin activity and aldosterone. Animal experiments then showed that with the gradual onset of chronic liver failure, induced by the administration of a hepatotoxic agent, salt and water retention occurred before there was any rise in portal venous pressure, fall in plasma protein or a rise in plasma renin activity or aldosterone. Neither was the increased sodium reabsorption associated with a change in glomerular filtration rate or renal blood flow. These observations have led to the proposal that the oedema of chronic liver failure is due primarily to a renal retention

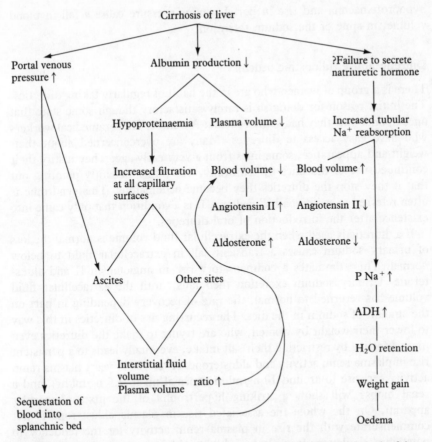

**Fig. 17.6** Possible mechanism responsible for sodium and water retention in cirrhosis of the liver. There is an important contribution from an increased tubular reabsorption of unknown cause.

of sodium, the so called 'overflow'hypothesis; which is due to a sodium retaining stimulus originating directly from the diseased liver.

The nature of this stimulus remains a mystery. There is some evidence obtained in man that cirrhotic patients have a defective capacity to raise their plasma concentration of natriuretic sodium transport inhibitor. For instance they tend to have an inability to escape from the salt retaining effects of prolonged mineralocorticoid administration, and at such a time their urine does not show the normal rise in the concentration of natriuretic substances. Figure 17.6 illustrates a sequence of events in chronic liver failure which tries to include the various mechanisms outlined above which may be involved in the associated sodium retention. As in the nephrotic syndrome, sodium and water retention appear to be independent of changes in protein metabolism, portal venous pressure or aldosterone. And the concentration of plasma aldosterone will depend on whether the primary sodium retention is causing a rise in blood volume, or the severity of the hypoproteinaemia and rise in portal venous pressure cause a fall in blood volume, in spite of the sodium retention.

### Diuretic abuse (idiopathic oedema)

There is a group of women who are in the habit of regularly taking diuretics. The initial reason for doing so is rarely satisfactory though some state that once upon a time they had some oedema. A number are paramedical workers who have easy access to diuretics. Many are overconcerned about their weight and appearance, sometimes from a very early age. They justify their continued use of diuretics by truthfully, but rather defiantly pointing out that if they stop the diuretics they become oedematous. This syndrome is often referred to as 'idiopathic' oedema. It is a condition that only came into existence after the introduction of oral diuretics.

If a diuretic is used when the extracellular fluid volume is normal the loss of urinary sodium causes a transient fall in extracellular fluid to below normal. This stimulates a compensatory rise in angiotensin II and aldosterone. Urinary sodium excretion then falls, until the extracellular fluid volume has returned to normal, the rate of recovery depending in part on the amount of sodium in the diet. The recurring use of diuretics in this way to lower their weight by women, who are trying to make the diuretics even more effective by restricting their salt intake, eventually leads to a persistent rise in plasma renin activity and aldosterone. After 10–15 years plasma renin activity can rise to around 10 ng/ml/hr (normal up to 2.5 ng/ml/hr), and a renal biopsy will show a striking hypertrophy of the juxta glomerular apparati. On the whole the associated rise in plasma aldosterone is not commensurate with the rise in plasma renin activity for the tendency to potassium depletion fortunately inhibits aldosterone production. These patients tend to be thirsty and some have an extraordinary craving for salt. From time to time they suffer from postural hypotension, tiredness, anorexia and very occasionally from symptomatic hypokalaemia or gout.

If in such patients the diuretics are stopped suddenly there is an initial rapid gain in weight of up to 5 kg in 3–4 days associated with a characteristic feeling of bloatedness and a tightness across the abdomen and ankles. At 5–6 days the fall in plasma renin activity and aldosterone is usually accompanied by a sodium diuresis and a brisk loss of weight towards control values (Fig. 17.7). In a few women the recent gain in weight and overt oedema is not lost though plasma renin activity and aldosterone fall to below normal. The persistence of oedema and weight gain despite a fall in plasma renin activity and aldosterone to below normal demonstrate that in such patients sodium continues to be retained by some other mechanism than the renin aldosterone system. There is some fragmentary evidence which suggests that such patients have become insensitive to the natriuretic hormone, the plasma concentration of which has presumably been well below normal for many years. These patients can be controlled by placing them on a low

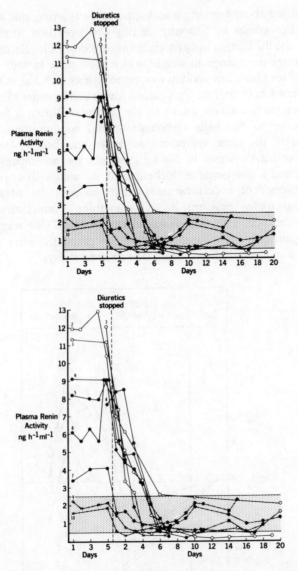

**Fig. 17.7** Plasma renin activity and urinary aldosterone excretion before and after stopping diuretics in 10 patients with diuretic induced oedema ('idiopathic oedema'). (Reproduced from MacGregor, Roulston, Markandu et al 1979 Lancet 1: 397, with kind permission.)

sodium diet (approximately 30 mmol/day) when the oedema gradually subsides. The sodium intake is then increased gradually, over a year, back to normal (approximately 150 mmol/day) without the reappearance of oedema.

It is not known why these patients initially become 'hooked' onto diuretics. Some women may suffer relatively large changes in weight during the menstrual cycle. Possibly if such a change occurs in a woman who is already worried about her weight and appearance at a time that she is trying to reduce her weight by 'starving' during the week and 'stuffing' at the weekends, the fluctuation in her weight may become quite alarming. Figure 17.8 illustrates the change in weight which took place in four nurses who were first placed on a low sodium low carbohydrate diet and then suddenly switched onto a high sodium high carbohydrate diet in order to mimmic the sudden changes in sodium intake of the patients. Within a few hours of changing over to the high carbohydrate and sodium diet, the nurses complained of the same symptoms as those described by patients with 'idiopathic oedema'. A gain of 2–4 kg in weight was accompanied by gross discomfort and a questionable thickening of the ankles. It is possible that such a sequence of events causes patients to seek the advice of their doctor, who under pressure 'to do something', reluctantly agrees to prescribe a diuretic. This now magnifies the problem. One way to solve it, relatively painlessly, is to stop the diuretics gradually, after placing the patient on a moderately low sodium diet (50 mmol/day).

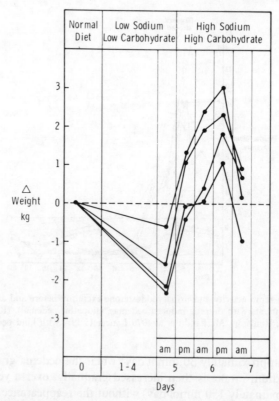

**Fig. 17.8** Changes in weight in 4 normal young women upon changing from their normal diet to a low sodium, low carbohydrate diet, and then to a high sodium, high carbohydrate diet. (Reproduced from MacGregor, Roulston, Markandu et al 1979 Lancet 1: 397, with kind permission.)

## Malnutrition

The cause of the oedema of malnutrition is not known. In a population suffering from malnutrition the hypoproteinaemia, reduction in blood volume, renal blood flow and plasma aldosterone levels are no different in the oedematous than in non oedematous individuals. One of the earliest abnormalities of sodium metabolism evident before there are any changes in plasma proteins, is an inverted diurnal rhythm of urine excretion which greatly 'disturbs the night's repose'. This is also seen in many other conditions in which there is a continuous need to overcome a tendency to retain sodium, e.g. in primary aldosteronism, the prolonged administration of prednisone, the nephrotic syndrome and to a lesser extent in most forms of hypertension.

## COMPENSATORY CHANGES IN SOME DISEASES IN WHICH THERE IS A TENDENCY TO RETAIN SODIUM BUT NO OEDEMA

In essential hypertension, renal vascular hypertension, renal artery stenosis, primary and secondary aldosteronism the urinary excretion of sodium takes place against a persistent tendency to retain sodium. These conditions were discussed in Chapter 16 in relation to the rise in blood pressure with which they are usually accompanied. There is also an increased tendency to retain sodium in many forms of chronic renal failure.

## Chronic renal failure

As chronic renal failure develops sodium intake remains relatively unchanged but there is little overt evidence of oedema. Therefore the urinary excretion of sodium must remain the same as the intake. The only way this can be done is for each remaining nephron to excrete a much greater fraction of the sodium that is filtered into it than was excreted when there were a normal number of nephrons. In chronic renal failure therefore sodium balance is maintained by a gross reduction in fractional sodium reabsorption. It has been conclusively demonstrated that this reduction in tubular reabsorption of sodium is independent of the accumulation of toxic waste products such as hippurates which take place in chronic renal failure, some of which are known to inhibit sodium transport.

Figure 17.9 illustrates one of the experiments on which this conclusion is based. Dogs were made progressively uraemic in a step-wise fashion by the gradual surgical removal of renal parenchyma. When this was done in animals in which the intake of sodium remained unchanged there was a substantial fall in fractional sodium reabsorption whereas if the sodium intake was reduced in proportion to the fall in glomerular filtration, fractional sodium reabsorption did not fall. The rise in blood urea and other waste products was the same in both groups of animals.

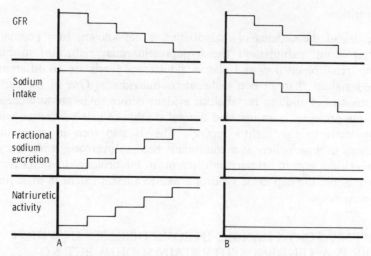

**Fig. 17.9** Schematic presentation of the effect of a progressive fall in renal function on fractional sodium reabsorption and natriuretic activity of the plasma when the sodium intake remains constant (A) and when it is proportionally reduced (B). (Reproduced from Bricker, Schmidt, Weber et al 1972 Modern diuretic therapy in the treatment of cardiovascular and renal disease. Excerpta Medica, Amsterdam, p 40, with kind permission.)

There is much evidence which suggests that the compensatory diminution in tubular sodium reabsorption is probably due to a progressive rise in the concentration of a circulating natriuretic sodium transport inhibitor. In the experiment just described the plasma was shown to contain a higher concentration of the natriuretic sodium transport inhibitor when the dogs were on a constant sodium intake than when the sodium intake was lowered as the glomerular filtration rate fell.

As renal failure progresses, however, it is not uncommon for patients to lose control and develop either a tendency to leak sodium in excess or to retain a large quantity of sodium. Sometimes a patient may slide from one tendency to the other for no clear reason (p. 186). It is of the utmost importance to be aware of this possibility for obviously the two conditions are dramatically opposed. A tendency to retain sodium is associated with hypertension, while a tendency to lose sodium with either a normal or a low arterial pressure gives rise to a further deterioration in renal failure. The first is treated with diuretics and the second with sodium supplements. Selective tubular disturbances of sodium reabsorption of unknown cause are discussed on p. 354.

Patients with chronic renal failure can adapt to changes in sodium balance but they do so more slowly than normal subjects. The delay may be dangerous particularly when the patient develops acute diarrhoea and vomiting during a holiday in some hot climate. The normal rapid reduction in urinary sodium excretion does not occur. The patient develops a reduction in extracellular fluid volume and such a rapid deterioration in renal

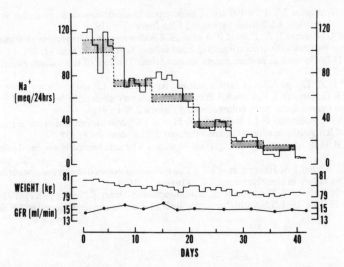

**Fig. 17.10** Changes in urinary sodium excretion, body weight and glomerular filtration rate in a patient with chronic renal failure during a gradual reduction in sodium intake (interrupted lines). The shaded areas represent the range of dietary sodium intake. (Reproduced from Danovitch, Bourgoignie & Bricker 1977 New Eng J Med 296: 14 with kind permission.)

function that his life is endangered. Nevertheless it *is* possible to lower sodium intake in a patient with chronic renal failure to very low levels without causing a fall in glomerular filtration rate if the intake is reduced gradually over 3 to 4 months (Fig. 17.10). This is the only safe way to reduce sodium intake when trying to control hypertension.

BIBLIOGRAPHY

Bernard D B, Alexander E A, Couser W G et al 1978 Renal sodium retention during volume expansion in experimental nephrotic syndrome. Kidney Int 14: 478

Bricker N S, Schmidt R W, Weber H et al 1973 The modulation of sodium excretion in chronic renal disease; the possible role of a natriuretic hormone. In: Modern diuretic therapy in the treatment of cardiovascular and renal disease. Excerpta Medica, Amsterdam, p 40

Brown E A, Markandu U D, Roulston J E et al 1982 Is the renin-angiotensin-aldosterone system involved in the sodium retention in the nephrotic syndrome. Nephron 32: 102

Chonko A M, Bay W H, Stein J H et al 1977 The role of renin and aldosterone in the salt retention of oedema. Amer J Med 63: 881

Epstein M 1979 Deranged sodium homeostasis in cirrhosis. Gastroenterology 76: 622

Guz A, Noble M I M, Trenchard D et al 1966 The significance of a raised central venous pressure during sodium and water retention. Clin Sci 30: 295

Kruck F, Kramer H J 1978 Third factor and edema formation. Cont Nephrol 13: 12

Kuroda S, Aynedjian H S, Bank N 1979 A micropuncture study of renal sodium retention in nephrotic syndrome in rats: Evidence for increased resistance to tubular fluid flow. Kidney Int 16: 561

Levy M 1977 Sodium retention and ascites formation in dogs with experimental portal cirrhosis. Amer J Physiol 233(6): F 572

Nelson D H, August J T 1958 Failure of aldosterone to maintain sodium retention in normal subjects and addisonian patients. J Clin Invest 37: 919

Nicholls M G, Espiner E A, Donald R A et al 1974 Aldosterone and its regulation during diuresis in patients with gross congestive heart failure. Clin Sci Mol Med 47: 301

Patrick J 1979 Oedema in protein energy malnutrition: The role of the sodium pump. Proc Nutr Soc 38: 61

Peters J P 1952 The problem of cardiac edema. Amer J Med 12: 66

Schneider E G, Dresser T P, Lynch R E et al 1971 Sodium reabsorption by proximal tubule of dogs with experimental heart failure. Amer J Physiol 220(4): 952

Torrente A de, Robertson G L, McDonald K M et al 1975 Mechanism of diuretic response to increased left atrial pressure in the anaesthetized dog. Kidney Int 8: 355

Verney E B 1946 Absorption and excretion of water. The antidiuretic hormone. Lancet 2: 739

Watkins L, Burton J A, Haber E et al 1976 The renin-angiotensin-aldosterone system in congestive failure in conscious dogs. J Clin Invest 57: 1606

Wardener H E de 1978 The control of sodium excretion. Amer J Physiol 235(3): F163

Wardener H E de 1981 'Idiopathic' oedema: Role of diuretic abuse. Kidney Int 19: 881

# 18

# Clinical disorders accompanying disturbances of water metabolism

The control of water balance depends on (1) the intake of water which itself is dependent on the integrity of the thirst center in the hypothalamus, and the availability of water; (2) the plasma concentration of antidiuretic hormone (ADH) secreted from the supra-optico and para-ventricular areas of the hypothalamus; and (3) the kidney's ability to concentrate the urine.

Thirst can either be blunted by various cerebral conditions such as coma or trauma to the hypothalamic area, cerebral haemorrhage or tumours or it may be stimulated by angiotensin II (particularly with volume depletion) and by certain metabolic abnormalities such as hypercalcaemia and hypokalaemia. It is probable that the thirst center is also under the influence of baroreceptor reflexes.

ADH is secreted from two independent but closely adjacent sites in the hypothalamus. One responds to changes in plasma osmolality and the other to afferent stimulation from the baroreceptors (Fig. 18.1). Plasma osmo-

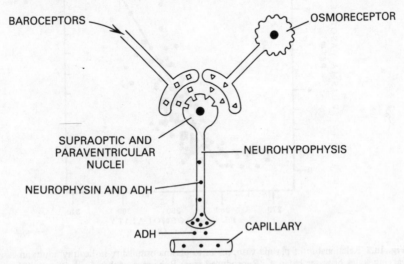

**Fig. 18.1** Possible arrangement of the neurohypophysis and the osmo-and baro-receptors. (Robertson, Athor & Shelton 1977 In: Andreoli T E, Grantham J J, Rector F C (eds) Disturbances in body fluid osmolality. Amer Phys Soc: 125, with kind permission.)

lality mainly depends on the concentration of sodium. Baroreceptors are particularly influenced by changes of blood volume.

The effect of changes in plasma osmolality on plasma vasopressin in normal man is illustrated in Figure 18.2 in which it can be seen that the threshold plasma osmolality at which the plasma vasopressin begins to rise is about 280 mosmol/kg (normal plasma osmolality 275 to 290 mosmol/kg). The influence of the baroreceptors on plasma vasopressin in illustrated in Figure 18.3 which shows the effect of plasma osmolality on plasma vasopressin in normal rats compared to rats made either hypotensive or hypovolaemic. At any one plasma osmolality, hypotensive, or hypovolaemic rats had a substantially higher plasma concentration of vasopressin (e.g. at a plasma osmolality of 290 mosmol/kg the plasma vasopressin in the control rats was below 1 pg/ml whereas in the hypovolaemic or hypotensive rats it was 20 pg/ml.

With dehydration the rise in plasma sodium concentration and the reduction in blood volume both cause a rise in ADH secretion. With haemorrhage the secretion of ADH is stimulated by the fall in blood volume alone. The effect of blood volume changes on water excretion are paralleled by its effect on sodium excretion, the adjustment to the plasma osmolality being controlled by the osmoreceptors. Nevertheless if hypovolaemia is persistent,

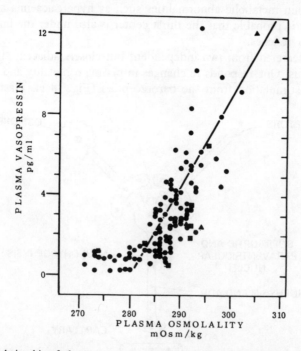

**Fig. 18.2** Relationship of plasma vasopressin to plasma osmolality in healthy adults in varying states of water balance. (Reproduced from Robertson, Athar & Shelton 1977 In: Andreoli T E, Grantham J J, Rector F C (eds) Disturbances in body fluid osmolality. Amer Phys Soc: 125, with kind permission.)

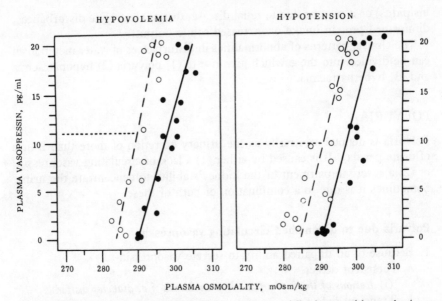

**Fig. 18.3** Relationship of plasma vasopressin to plasma osmolality in normal hypovolemic, or hypotensive rats. Blood volume was reduced by intraperitoneal injection of polyethylene glycol and the blood pressure was reduced with a subcutaneous injection of isoproterenol; • = control rats, ○ = hypovolaemic or hypotensive rats. (Reproduced from Robertson, Athar & Shelton 1977 In: Andreoli T E, Grantham J J, Rector F C (eds) Disturbances in body fluid osmolality. Amer Phys Soc: 125, with kind permission.)

baroreceptor stimulation of ADH secretion will raise the concentration of plasma ADH even though this results in a fall in plasma osmolality which is presumably informing the osmoreceptors to diminish ADH secretion. In other words persistent blood volume contraction may be associated with hyponatraemia. This was first demonstrated in a clear cut manner by McCance in 1936 who placed himself on a very low sodium intake for 11 days. He ensured that be became increasingly deprived of sodium, even though his urine soon became virtually free of sodium, by taking vigorous exercise every day, thereby losing much sodium in the sweat. In the first four days he lost about 2 kg in weight and his plasma remained isotonic but thereafter he started to retain water in spite of the gradual fall in plasma sodium that this occasioned. This prevented further loss of weight but his plasma sodium fell from 148 to 131 mmol/l. In this way he underwent the more gradual and less prominent symptoms of hyponatraemia instead of the catastrophic vascular collapse he would otherwise have suffered if he had tried to maintain the isotonicity of his plasma.

In normal man the kidney's ability to concentrate the urine is mainly dependent on the concentration of vasopressin in the plasma. In disease there may either be an abnormality of vasopressin secretion or more commonly the distal and collecting ducts are unable to respond normally to vasopressin. This may be a congenital abnormality (nephrogenic diabetes insipidus) or it may be due to renal disease, drugs, electrolyte disturbances, diminished protein intake or increased solute output.

The clinical patterns of abnormalities in disturbances of water metabolism can be divided into those which give rise to (1) polyuria (2) hyponatraemia and (3) hypernatraemia.

## POLYURIA

Polyuria is defined arbitrarily as the urinary excretion of more than 2 litre of urine per day. It is caused by either (1) a lack of circulating vasopressin, or (2) a severe impairment of the kidney's ability to concentrate the urine. Sometimes it is due to a combination of both of these.

### Polyuria due to diminished circulating vasopressin

1. Because of an impaired ability to secrete vasopressin
   a. Persistent defect
       (i) *Lesions of the supraoptico-hypothalamus, i.e. diabetes insipidus*
   b. Transient defect
       (i) Compulsive water drinking
       (ii) ? Potassium deficiency.
2. Because of a diminished need to secret vasopressin due to an increased intake of water due to increased thirst
   a. *Compulsive water drinking*
   b. *Potassium deficiency*
   c. *Lesion of thirst centre*
   d. Hypercalcaemia.
3. Because of a circulating antibody to vasopressin.

### Polyuria due to a severe impairment in the kidney's ability to concentrate the urine

1. Congenital
   a. Single tubular lesion; nephrogenic diabetes insipidus
   b. One of several tubular lesions; renal tubular acidosis
   c. 'Fanconi syndrome'.
2. Excess water intake
   a. Compulsive water drinking
   b. Diabetes insipidus.
3. Chronic renal disease
   a. Medullary cystic disease
   b. Obstructive uropathy.
4. Electrolyte abnormalities
   a. Potassium deficiency
   b. Hypercalcaemia and hypercaliuria.

5. Osmotic diuresis; increased solute output per nephron
   a. Chronic renal failure (rarely)
   b. Glycosuria.
   c. Salt diuresis following relief of urinary obstruction

Polyuria due to glycosuria is easily diagnosed by a routine test of the urine. Polyuria due to an antibody to vasopressin appears in pregnancy. Spontaneous recovery occurs after delivery.

The other causes of polyuria can be subdivided into those that are associated with a moderate rise in blood urea and in which the urine volume is usually only increased to about 3–4 litres per 24 hours, and those that have a normal or low blood urea, and in which the urine volume is usually above 5 litres per 24 hours (often up to 10–12 litres).

Those conditions in which there is a rise in blood urea and only a moderate rise in urine volume include chronic renal failure, potassium deficiency, some cases of hypercalcaemia, and renal tubular acidosis; while those with a normal blood urea and the excretion of large volumes of urine include diabetes insipidus compulsive water drinking, some cases of hypercalcaemia, and familial nephrogenic diabetes insipidus:

| A<br>*Polyuria with urine volume usually less than*<br>*3–4 l/24 hr and blood urea raised* | B<br>*Polyuria with urine volume often greater*<br>*than 5 l/24 hr and blood urea normal* |
| --- | --- |
| 1. Chronic renal failure (p. 183) | 1. Diabetes insipidus |
| 2. Potassium deficiency (p. 324) | 2. Compulsive water drinking |
| 3. Hypercalcaemia (p. 331) | 3. Hypercalcaemia (p. 331) |
| 4. Fanconi's syndrome (p. 360) | 4. Familial nephrogenic diabetes insipidus |

The disturbances included in Group A are discussed elsewhere. Those in Group B are discussed below, except for hypercalcuria which is discussed on page 331.

## Causes of polyuria in which the urine volume is usually greater than 5 1/24 hr and the blood urea is normal

### Familial nephrogenic diabetes insipidus

This is a rare sex-linked condition which occurs in males and with such a marked familial incidence that sometimes there are several patients under the same roof with the same symptoms. The onset of symptoms is during infancy or childhood. Occasionally chronic dehydration with plasma hypertonicity in infancy may lead to severe and permanent mental retardation. Investigation of entire families has shown that they may contain symptomless heterozygous female carries, in whom there is a mild impairment of maximum concentrating capacity.

The evidence that the primary defect is an inability of the tubules to utilise vasopressin is obtained by giving vasopressin intravenously. In nephrogenic diabetes insipidus the amount of vasopressin that then appears unchanged in the urine is much greater than in normal subjects. It must also be pointed out that microdissection of nephrons has revealed that in nephrogenic diabetes insipidus the proximal tubules are shorter than normal. The relevance of this finding to the inability of the tubule to utilise vasopressin is not clear. If, however, the shortening results in an increased amount of glomerular filtrate reaching the loop of Henle and the distal tubule it may be an additional cause for the hypotonicity of the urine.

The disease is characterised by an almost complete inability to raise the urine concentration above the concentration of plasma with either vasopressin, or moderately severe fluid deprivation sufficient to cause a loss of up to 5% of body weight; in both instances the urine usually remains around S.G. 1.004 (an osmolality of around 150 mosmol/kg). If the vasopressin dosage is raised to toxic levels (i.e. 2 units/min of the aqueous solution intravenously), or the dehydration is so severe that it gives rise to distress and fever, the urine concentration may then rise to much higher levels; this is sometimes seen terminally in nephrogenic diabetes insipidus of infancy.

Treatment consists mainly in early recognition and the adequate administration of water. Infants also greatly benefit from a low electrolyte diet, for this produces a quicker return to normal plasma osmolality. Diuretics which cause much sodium loss such as frusemide or chlorothiazide can reduce the extent of the polyuria. They are useful for special occasions, but their prolonged administration may cause potassium deficiency. It is not known how they reduce the urine volume. It has been pointed out that this only occurs when the patient is in a negative sodium balance, and it has been suggested that this causes such an increased reabsorption of sodium from the proximal tubule that the quantity of tubular fluid which travels into the loop of Henle and emerges into the distal tubule as hypotonic fluid is greatly reduced.

### Diabetes insipidus

It has been mentioned above that diabetes insipidus is due to a diminished ability of the supraopticohypophyseal system to secrete vasopressin. This is usually an acquired defect associated with fracture of the base of the skull, tumours, infections and lipoid storage diseases. Not infrequently the cause is unknown. It is more common in men than in women. A few familial congenital cases have been described.

The onset of symptoms is usually gradual and, once polyuria and polydipsia have developed, the daily water exchange remains relatively constant. Sometimes 12–15 litres of fluid are ingested and excreted each day for many years; yet in spite of the great disturbance to sleep, there may be no other symptoms or signs. Loss of weight, exhaustion and constipation occur if the urine volumes become astronomical, i.e. 20–30 litres a day.

*Differential diagnosis*

The main difficulty in the differential diagnosis is to distinguish between diabetes insipidus and compulsive water drinking. Sometimes diabetes insipidus can be distinguished with relative certainty by finding other evidence of structural disease in the area of the neurohypophysis; or a diagnosis of compulsive water drinking can be inferred from the patient's disturbed mental state and previous history of psychiatric peculiarities.

*Treatment*

The analogue of vasopressin DDAVP (1 deamino-8-arginine vasopressin) has a higher antidiuretic potency, less pressor activity and a longer duration of action than lysine vasopressin. It may be administered intranasally or by injection. 2 $\mu$g intravenously has an effect for 10 hours. 10–15$\mu$g intranasally twice a day induces a normal urine flow throughout the 24 hours.

In acute diabetes insipidus (following hypophysectomy) it may be preferable to use acqueous pitressin (20 units/ml). Its short duration of action permits more careful monitoring and diminishes the risk of water intoxication.

Chlorpropamide 250 mg b.d. is also useful in some cases. It acts by enhancing the effect of vasopressin in some manner which is not clear. It probably increases the sensitivity of the distal and collecting ducts to trace amount of vasopressin. The dangers of chlorpropamide are hypoglycaemia and toxic reactions such as rashes and nausea.

**Compulsive water drinking**

This is a much more common condition than diabetes insipidus. It is seen principally in middle-aged women. The onset of polydipsia and polyuria is often sudden and not infrequently it coincides with medical advice to drink more fluid (e.g. for constipation). The quantity of water which is consumed is apt to vary erratically from one day to the next, and frequently there is also a slow periodicity, with relapses and remissions varying from several weeks to months. Hysterical manifestations and depression are a part of the syndrome, and there is nearly always a long previous history of psychological disturbances; occasionally these patients are discovered to be magnifying the extent of their polyuria by pouring jugs of water into the bedpan.

A diagnosis of compulsive water drinking is usually suspected from the history and appearance of the patient, and often it is soon apparent that polydipsia and polyuria are the least of the patient's troubles. The differential diagnosis between diabetes insipidus and compulsive water drinking is discussed below.

*Treatment*

The only treatment which is likely to succeed is one that controls the

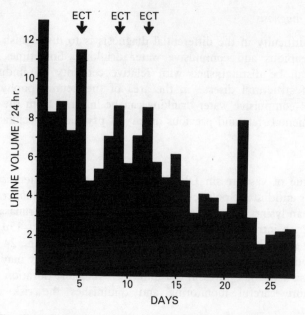

**Fig. 18.4** The effect of electro-convulsive therapy (ECT) on a patient with compulsive water drinking and severe depression. (Reproduced from Barlow & de Wardener Quart J Med 28: 235, with kind permission.)

particular psychological disturbance involved. Sometimes reassurance and encouragement are sufficient. Occasionally a rest in hospital will produce marked improvement and, if such a remission coincides with the administration of vasopressin, an erroneous diagnosis of diabetes insipidus may be made. Usually stronger measures have to be employed, such as electroconvulsive therapy for the depression (Fig. 18.4) and continuous narcosis for hysteria. Substantial remissions may be induced but the tendency to relapse is very great.

*Diagnostic tests used to distinguish between diabetes insipidus and compulsive water drinking*

As diabetes insipidus is due to a persistent defect in the ability to secrete ADH because of an abnormality of the neurohypophysis, and compulsive water drinking is simply an increased intake of fluid because of a mental abnormality, it should be possible to distinguish the two conditions by estimating the concentration of antidiuretic hormone in the blood during a period of fluid deprivation. From the results illustrated in Figure 18.5 it is clear that a distinction can be made, but only if the period of dehydration is sufficient to raise the plasma osmolality to at least 295 mosmol/kg.

The difficulty arises because (1) the majority of patients with diabetes insipidus have an incomplete lesion and are able to secrete some vasopressin under the stress of severe dehydration and (2) though patients with

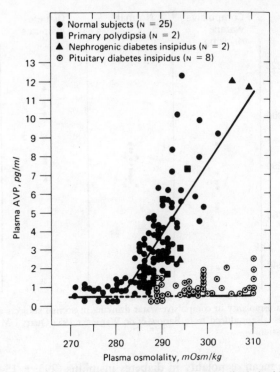

**Fig. 18.5** The relationship of plasma vasopressin to plasma osmolality in healthy adults and patients with different types of polyuria. Primary polydipsia = compulsive water drinking. (Reproduced from Robertson, Shelton & Athar 1976 Kidney Int 10: 25, with kind permission.)

compulsive water drinking should secrete vasopressin normally some patients on some occasions do less well than a normal subject. As a result it turns out that to distinguish between diabetes insipidus and compulsive water drinking by stimulating vasopressin secretion and measuring plasma ADH is somewhat less than totally satisfactory. Furthermore the measurement of plasma vasopressin is difficult, the expertise necessary appears to be confined to very few centres, and the manner a blood sample is handled on the way to the laboratory is critical. For these reasons other methods to distinguish between diabetes insipidus and compulsive water drinking continue to be used. These are (1) estimating the osmolality of the plasma (2) comparing the kidney's ability to concentrate the urine following dehydration and after the administration of vasopressin and (3) observing the generalised effects of prolonged vasopressin administration.

*Plasma osmolality*

The plasma osmolality of patients suffering from diabetes insipidus and compulsive water drinking is compared in Fig. 18.6 with that of normal

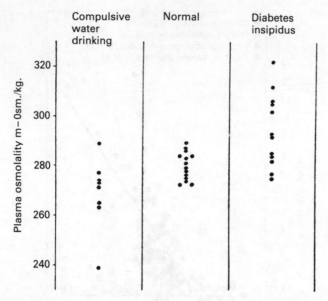

**Fig. 18.6** Plasma osmolality in compulsive water drinking in normal subjects and in diabetes insipidus. (Reproduced from Barlow & de Wardener 1959 Quart J Med 28: 235, with kind permission.)

subjects. The mean osmolality in diabetes insipidus (295 ± 15 mosmol/kg) is significantly higher than in the normal subjects (280 ± 6 mosmol/kg), whereas in compulsive water drinking (269 ± 14 mosmol/kg) it is significantly lower. These findings are in keeping with the aetiology of the two conditions. In patients with diabetes insipidus the initial disturbance is polyuria and the excessive drinking is a normal response to the contraction and concentration of body fluids, whereas in compulsive water drinking the initial disturbance is excessive drinking and the polyuria is the normal response to expansion and dilution of body fluids. There is a considerably overlap between the groups, but it appears that if the plasma osmolality of a patient with polyuria is greater than 290 mosmol/kg the diagnosis is likely to be diabetes insipidus, and if it is less than 275 mosmol/kg it is more likely to be compulsive water drinking.

*Comparison of the kidney's ability to concentrate the urine after a period of fluid deprivation and after the administration of vasopressin*

The period of fluid deprivation immediately precedes the administration of vasopressin which takes place while the patient is still dehydrated.

A period of fluid deprivation stimulates ADH production because of the negative balance of water that results. The duration of such a period therefore is of secondary importance. For instance, a period of 12 hours' fluid deprivation is a stronger stimulus to ADH production in a polyuric patient unable to concentrate the urine, and who therefore excretes 3 to 5 litres of urine, than is a 24-hour period of fluid deprivation in a normal person who only loses one litre. The most satisfactory method is to be guided by the weight that is lost during fluid deprivation (or the rise in plasma osmolality), and to estimate the urine concentration after the loss of 3 to 5% of the initial weight. If greater losses are allowed the urine may become concentrated by mechanisms other than the neurohypophyseal secretion, and the test becomes pointless.

When the plasma osmolality has risen to above 290 mosmol/kg or preferably when the patient has lost the required weight the bladder is emptied and the osmolality of the urine recorded. Now aqueous vasopressin is given either intravenously 100 m units in 20 seconds followed by 5 m units per min thereafter for one hour or until the next sample of urine collected. Alternatively the vasopressin can be given intramuscularly (DDAVP 10 μg).

The interpretation of this test depends on an appreciation of two independent phenomena. The first is that the ability of the normal kidney to concentrate urine is impaired by the polyuria which accompanies a high water intake (Fig. 18.7) whatever its cause. This is because the concerntration of the urine, under the influence of a large amount of vasopressin in dependent on the osmolality of the renal medulla, which is 'washed out' by a water diuresis. As a result patients with diabetes insipidus and

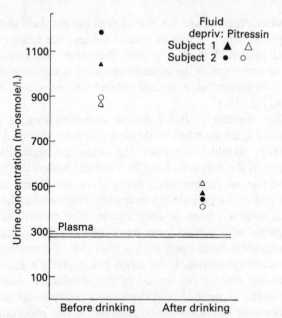

**Fig. 18.7** Urine concentrations following the intravenous administration of vasopressin, and after a 26-hour period of fluid deprivation, before and at the end of drinking about 10 litres of water a day for 11 days. The plasma osmolarity varied between the limits indicated by the two parallel horizontal lines. (Reproduced from de Wardener & Herxheimer 1957 J Physiol 139: 42, with kind permission.)

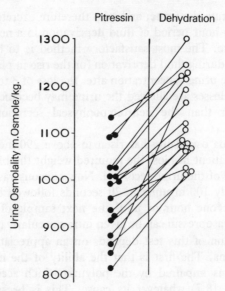

**Fig. 18.8** Urine osmolality after dehydration and after the administration of vasopressin tannate in oil in normal subjects. (Reproduced from Jones & de Wardener 1956 Brit Med J i: 271, with kind permission.)

compulsive water drinking are not able to concentrate their urine normally. The second phenomenon is that in normal kidneys the urine concentration after a period of dehydration is greater than after the administration of vasopressin. In other words the administration of vasopressin at the end of a period of dehydration in a normal subject has no effect on the urine concentration (Fig. 18.8).

Theoretically, therefore, after a period of dehydration, a patient with compulsive water drinking who should have raised his plasma ADH concentration normally, should concentrate the urine less well than a normal person, because of the polyuria, but like a normal person the urine concentration should rise no further upon being given a maximal dose of vasopressin at the end of the period of dehydration. On the other hand the urine concentration, after a period of dehydration, of a patient suffering from diabetes insipidus who should have some difficulty in raising his plasma ADH's concentration should also be less than that of a normal subject but the urine concentration should rise upon being given a large amount of vasopressin at the end of the period of dehydration, a totally abnormal response. Though, in general, the distinction between diabetes insipidus and compulsive water drinking can be achieved by this procedure, occasionally, as with the estimation of plasma vasopressin the interpretation of the test can be difficult.

*Results of fluid deprivation and vasopressin in diabetes insipidus.* Some patients with diabetes insipidus are indeed unable to concentrate their urine normally following fluid deprivation or vasopressin. But after vasopressin the specific gravity or osmolality of the urine in *all* patients rises to a concentration which is *much greater than with* dehydration alone.

*Results of vasopressin and fluid deprivation tests in compulsive water drinking.* These patients may respond in a variety of ways. The following responses are seen:

1. The kidney's ability to concentrate the urine following fluid deprivation is normal, i.e. urine concentration rises to levels found in normal individuals and, what is more important, the concentration does not rise after the administration of vasopressin. This indicates that both tubular function and the ability to secrete antidiuretic hormone are normal. Such a response is only found in patients whose daily urine volume is less than five litres.
2. The kidney's ability to concentrate the urine following fluid deprivation and vasopressin is impaired but the concentration does not rise after the administration of vasopressin.

This indicates that tubular function is impaired but the ability to produce ADH is normal. In these patients the urine concentration with fluid deprivation may be S. G. 1.014 or below.

3. The kidney's ability to concentrate the urine following fluid deprivation is impaired but it rises to normal following administration of vasopressin (i.e. the response is the same as patients with diabetes insipidus).

This indicates that tubular function is normal, but that there is some inhibition to ADH production which is not overcome by fluid deprivation. It may be difficult to differentiate such a patient from one suffering from diabetes insipidus, particularly if aqueous vasopressin preparation has been used. If a more long acting preparation has been given the distinction is usually easier (see below).

4. The response is the same as in 3, but the urine concentration does not rise to normal levels after the administration of the vasopressin.

This indicates that there is a combination of tubular impairment and diminished ability to secrete ADH. This is the same response as some patients with diabetes insipidus.

The cause of the impaired ADH secretion (3 & 4) in a patient with compulsive water drinking is not obvious, perhaps it is the emotional stress of the fluid deprivation. This conclusion is strengthened if after treating the patient with some suitable psychotherapeutic maneouvre a normal response to fluid deprivation is now obtained.

## Discussion

The patient's ability to secrete ADH is sometimes tested by other means than fluid deprivation. For instance, the supraopticohypophyseal system can be stimulated by intravenous nicotine, or by suddenly raising the plasma osmolality with an infusion of hypertonic saline. Nicotine acid tartrate (3 to 6 mg) is given intravenously; it is only effective if it induces severe nausea and vomitting, but even if these unpleasant symptoms are produced some normal subjects may fail to respond. The hypertonic saline test is performed by infusing 2.5 g NaCl per 100 ml $H_2O$ at a rate of 0.25 ml/kg of body weight per minute, an hour after the oral ingestion of 20 ml/kg of water. The urine flow should fall, but occasionally the water diuresis is replaced by a saline diuresis and the urine flow does not change materially (particularly in hypertensive women). Another disadvantage is that in elderly patients the large infusion of saline may precipitate heart failure. Neither of these two manoeuvres gives as much information as a properly controlled period of fluid deprivation, which is in any case a more physiological stimulus to ADH secretion.

It is interesting to note that patients with long-standing polyuria and polydipsia excreting hypotonic urine may also have a reversible impairment in their ability to acidify the urine. To the unwary this combination of polyuria and polydipsia with an impaired ability to concentrate and acidify may suggest a diagnosis of renal tubular acidosis secondary to renal disease. This is a diagnostic trap into which only the sophisticated who measure these various tubular functions may fall. On the other hand, they are the ones best qualified to interpret these findings correctly.

*General effects following the administration of a long-acting vasopressin preparation*

If a patient suffering from compulsive water drinking is given a long-acting vasopressin preparation, there is a considerable decrease in urine flow even if the tubule's capacity to concentrate is seriously impaired* (see above). But usually thirst continues unabated, the intake of water exceeds the output, and overhydration develops (Fig. 18.9). There is abdominal distension, headache, drowsiness, and sometimes nausea and vomitting. In striking contrast, therefore, to patients suffering from diabetes insipidus, cases of compulsive water drinking complain of long acting vasopressin agents often with much vehemence and bitterness. Occasionally, both the patient and his attendants are unaware that the onset of nausea, headache and drowsiness is related to the administration of vasopressin. Instead, these symptoms are considered to be additional evidence in favour of an intracranial lesion in the vicinity of the neurohypophysis, and therefore of a diagnosis of diabetes insipidus.

## HYPONATRAEMIA

Hyponatraemia is due to the kidneys not being able to dilute the urine

---

* Vasopressin can lower the urine flow from 10 to 3 ml/min without the concentration of the urine rising above S.G. 1.012; higher concentrations only occur at lower urine flows.

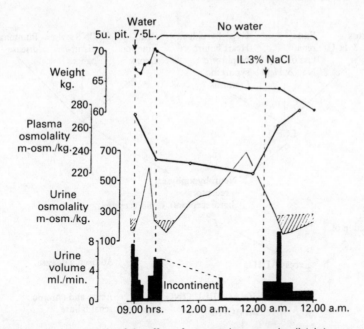

**Fig. 18.9** An extreme example of the effect of vasopressin tannate in oil (pit.) on a compulsive water drinker. Urine flow decreased, but the patient continued to drink large volumes of water, and in seven hours she gained 3.5 kg (●—●) in weight and the plasma osmolality (○—○) fell from 272 to 232 mosmol/kg. Initially the urine was hypotonic (hatched area), and it then became hypertonic. At the peak of the gain of weight after seven hours the urine became hypotonic, and its volume increased; the patient vomited, became incontinent, developed a hysterical fugue, and stopped drinking. A few hours later urine became hypertonic once more, and remained so for the next two days, so that the plasma osmolality continued to fall though the weight returned towards normal. On the third day one litre of three per cent saline given intravenously raised the plasma osmolality from 218 to 275 mosmol/kg., and induced a brisk diuresis of hypotonic urine. Hatched areas below dotted horizontal line indicate hypotonic urine. (Reproduced from Barlow & de Wardener 1959 Quart J Med 28: 235, with kind permission.)

normally (Fig. 18.10). Either the plasma concentration of ADH is raised or the kidney is so diseased that its ability to excrete a sufficient quantity of dilute urine is overcome by an increased intake (or administration) of water, or a normal kidney's diluting capacity has been impaired by a drug. Plasma ADH is raised by (1) a persistently low blood volume (2)certain cerebral conditions, drugs and lung disease and (3)ectopic production of ADH in a malignant tumour.

There are many pathological instances in which baroreceptor stimulation of ADH secretion in response to a fall in blood volume, causes retention of water and hyponatraemia (the McCance phenomenon p. 303).

1. Renal loss of salt and water from the use of diuretics; 'salt losing nephritis', renal tubular acidosis, mineralocorticoid deficiency and glycosuria.
2. Extrarenal loss of salt and water from vomiting or diarrhoea.

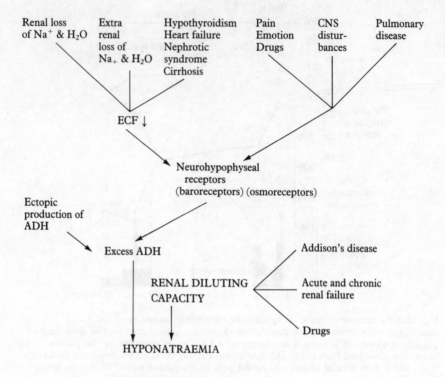

**Fig. 18.10** Causes and mechanisms of hyponatraemia.

3. A shift of extracellular fluid and plasma into a 'third space' as in burns or pancreatitis.
4. A decrease in 'effective' blood volume in heart failure due to splanchnic pooling.
5. Loss of plasma albumin into the extracellular fluid due to increased capillary permeability in hypothyroidism.
6. Diminished albumin production in cirrhosis.

The central nervous disorders which may cause an increase in ADH secretion and hyponatraemia include meningitis, encephalitis, acute psychosis, cerebral vascular accidents, tumours, abscess, trauma to the head and emotional stress. Certain pulmonary diseases also raise plasma ADH e.g. pneumonia, tuberculosis and pulmonary abscess. Pain and morphine are also powerful stimuli to ADH secretion, while some drugs may impair the ability of the kidney to excrete hypotonic water e.g. indomethocin, cyclophosphamide and vincristine. Addison's disease is also associated with an impaired ability to excrete a dilute urine. On the whole renal disease does not impair the kidney's ability to dilute urine. Malignant tumours particularly of the lung, may manufacture vasopressin like material.

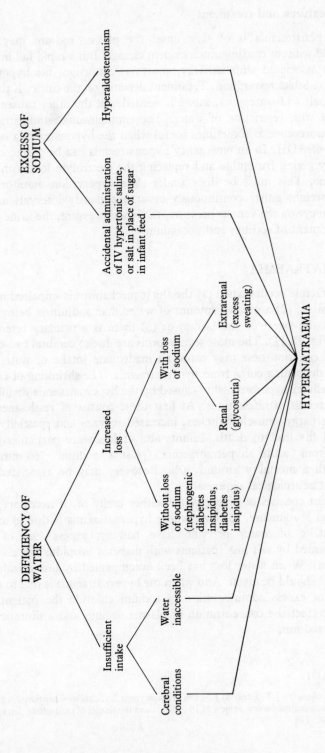

**Fig. 18.11** Causes and mechanisms of hypernatraemia.

### Clinical features and treatment

If the hyponatraemia is of slow onset the plasma sodium may fall to 110 mmol/l without causing much evident change. But a rapid fall in plasma sodium is associated with lethargy, anorexia, confusion, fits hypothermia and Cheyne-Stoke respiration. Treatment depends on the cause. If the cause is due to salt and water loss, saline is needed. All the other causes should be treated with restriction of water. The simultaneous administration of demeclochlorcycline is sometimes useful when the hyponatraemia is due to an excess of ADH. In an emergency hyponatraemia can be corrected more quickly by giving frusemide and replacing the electrolyte loss with hypertonic saline. This must be done under close supervision monitoring the patient's weight either continuously or at one hourly intervals and also keeping an eye on the venous pressure, the blood pressure, the urine volume and it's content of sodium and potassium.

## HYPERNATRAEMIA

Hypernatraemia occurs when (1) the thirst mechanism is impaired or water is inaccessible; (2) a greater amount of water than sodium is being lost in the urine, the sweat or the faeces; or (3) there is a primary retention of sodium (Fig. 18.11). The most severe forms are due to cerebral causes when a blunted consciousness may cause an inadequate intake of water which leads to a deepening coma from hypernatraemia. The shrinking of cells and the intracellular hyperosmolality caused by the hypernatraemia mainly gives rise to cerebral manifestations. At first these consist of restlessness, irritability, lethargy, muscle twitches, increased reflexes and spasticity. Later coma and fits lead to death. Infants· and children are particularly liable to die from acute hypernatraemia (plasma sodium 160 mmol/l or more) with a mortality around 50%. Recovery may be associated with permanent neurological sequelae.

Treatment consists of giving water, either orally or, if necessary, intravenously as 5% glucose, to those whose hypernatraemia is due to an inadequate intake of water or who have had an excess loss of water unaccompanied by salt loss (patients with diabetes insipidus are also given vasopressin). When water loss has been accompanied by loss of salt hypotonic saline should be given. And when the hypernatraemia is due to sodium retention or excess administration of sodium chloride the patient needs water to correct the concentration of plasma sodium and a diuretic to get rid of the sodium.

BIBLIOGRAPHY

Avioli L V, Lasersohn J T, Lopresti J M 1963 Histiocytosis X (Schüller-Christian disease): a clinico-pathological survey, review of 10 patients and the results of prednisone therapy. Medicine 42: 119

Barlow E D, de Wardener H E 1959 Compulsive water drinking. Quart J Med N S 28: 235

Berl T, Anderson R J, McDonald K M et al 1976 Clinical disorders of water metabolism. Kidney Int 10: 117

Berl T, Cadnapaphornchai P, Harbottle J A et al 1974 Mechanism of suppression of vasopressin during alpha-adrenergic stimulation with norepinephrine. J Clin Invest 53: 219

Better O S, Schrier R W 1983 Disturbed volume homeostasis in patients with cirrhosis of the liver. Kidney Int 23: 303

Bisset G W, Black A, Hilton P J et al 1976 Polyuria associated with an antibody to vasopressin Clin Sci Mol Med 50: 277

Carone F A, Epstein F H 1960 Nephrogenic diabetes insipidus caused by amyloid disease. Amer J Med 29: 539

Carter C, Simpkiss M 1956 The "carrier" state in nephrogenic diabetes insipidus. Lancet 2: 1069

Daniel P M, Treip C S 1961 The pathology of the pituitary gland in head injury. In: Gardiner Hill H (ed) Modern trends in endocrinology, 2nd series, Butterworths, London, p 58

Dicker S E, Eggleton M G 1963 Nephrogenic diabetes insipidus. Clin Sci 24: 81

Editorial 1977 Diabetes insipidus-turning off the tap. Brit Med J 1: 1050

Epstein F H, Rivera M J, Carone F A 1958 The effect of hypercalcaemia induced by calciferol upon renal concentrating ability. J Clin Invest 37: 1702

Hickey R C, Hare K 1944 The renal excretion of chloride and water in diabetes insipidus. J Clin Invest 23: 768

Jones N F, de Wardener H E 1956 Urine concentration after fluid deprivation or pitressin and annate in oil. Brit Med J 1: 271

McCance R A 1936 Experimental sodium chloride deficiency in man. Proc Roy Soc, London, S B: 119, 245

Manitius A, Levitin H, Beck D et al 1960 On the mechanism of impairment of renal concentrating ability in potassium deficiency. J Clin Invest 39: 684

Martin F I R 1959 Familial diabetes insipidus. Quart J Med N S 28: 573

Miller M, Dalakos T, Moses A M et al 1970 Recognition of partial defects in antidiuretic hormone secretion. Ann Intern Med 73: 721

Panitz F, Shinaberger J H 1965 Nephrogenic diabetes insipidus due to sarcoidosis without hypercalcaemia. Ann Internal Med 62: 113

Robertson G L, Athar S 1976 The interaction of blood osmolality and blood volume in regulating plasma vasopressin in man. J Clin Endocrinol 42: 613

Robertson G L, Athar S, Shelton R L 1977 Osmotic control of vasopressin function. In: Andreoli T E, Grantham J J, Rector F C (eds) Disturbances in body fluid osmolality. Amer Physiol Soc: p 125

Robinson A G 1976 D.D.A.V.P. in the treatment of central diabetes insipidus. New Eng J Med 294: 507

Roussak N J, Oleesky S 1954 Water-losing nephritis. A syndrome simulating diabetes insipidus. Quart J Med N S 23: 147

Schrier R W, Berl T 1980 Disorders of water metabolism. In: Schrier R W (ed) Renal and electrolyte disorders. Little Brown, Boston, p 1

Schrier R W, Berl T, Anderson R J 1979 Osmotic and nonosmotic control of vasopressin release. Amer J Physiol 236(4): 321

Shannon J A 1942 The control of the renal excretion of water (1) The effect of variations in the state of hydration on water excretion in dogs with diabetes insipidus. J Exp Med 76: 371

Statius Van Eps L W, Pinedo-Veels C, de Vries G H et al 1970 Nature of concentrating defect in sickle cell nephropathy. Lancet 1: 450

Stephens W P, Coe J Y, Baylis P H 1978 Plasma arginine vasopressin concentrations and antidiuretic action of carbamazepine. Brit Med J 1: 1445

Troyer de A D, Demanet J C 1975 Correction of antidiuresis by demeclocycline. New Eng Med J 293: 915

Ufferman R C, Schrier R W 1972 Importance of sodium intake and mineralocorticoid hormone in the impaired water excretion in adrenal insufficiency. J Clin Invest 51: 1639

Verney E B 1946 Absorption and excretion of water: the antidiuretic hormone. Lancet 2: 739, 781

Wardener de H E 1960 Polyuria. J Chron Dis 11: 199

Wardener de H E, Herxheimer A W 1957 The effect of a high water intake on the kidney's ability to concentrate the urine in man. J Physiol 139: 42

Webster B, Bain J 1970 Antidiuretic effect and complications of chlorpropamide therapy in diabetes insipidus. J Clin Endocr Metab 30: 215

Zerbe R L, Robertson G L 1981 A comparison of plasma vasopressin measurements with a standard indirect test in the differential diagnosis of polyuria. New Eng J Med 305: 1539

# 19

# Renal function and some electrolyte disturbances

Impairment of renal function may be responsible for various electrolyte abnormalities including negative balances of sodium, potassium, calcium and magnesium. Alternatively negative balances or changes in the plasma concentration of various constituents of the extracellular fluid may lead to changes in renal function. These may vary from deterioration in renal function to vigorous renal compensatory adjustments e.g. to maintain arterial pH.

## SODIUM

### Sodium deficiency due to renal disease

The following renal diseases may sometimes be responsible for an excess urinary loss of sodium:
1. Renal disease of moderate severity combined with dietary salt restriction
2. Advanced chronic renal failure
3. During recovery from acute tubular necrosis
4. Renal tubular acidosis
5. Reflux nephropathy during a urinary infection
6. Phenacetin nephropathy.

### Sodium deficiency as a cause of renal failure

The following conditions may occasionally cause such a loss of sodium that its deficiency contributes materially to the onset of renal failure:
1. Severe diarrhoea and vomiting (e.g. pyloric stenosis)
2. Post-operative gastric suction without replacement
3. Intestinal and biliary fistulae
4. Diabetes
5. Acute pathological processes involving the brain
6. Hypo-adrenalism (Addison's disease)
7. Diuretics, particularly frusemide.

## Clinical features of sodium, chloride and water deficiency

Sodium loss is usually accompanied by chloride and water loss, the deficiency of the chloride is usually proportional to that of sodium, but the negative balance of water is usually smaller, for the patient often continues to drink and the reduced extra cellular fluid volume increases ADH secretion. The extracellular fluid, therefore, tends to become hypotonic, and there is a transfer of water into the cells. The eventual signs and symptoms of sodium deficiency are thus a combination of those due to intracellular overhydration, and decreased extracellular fluid volume. The former gives rise to cerebral and the latter to cardiovascular abnormalities.

The patient is drowsy, restless, apathetic, and sometimes uncooperative. There is thirst (despite the hypotonic plasma), headache, anorexia, nausea and postural giddiness; vomiting may occur and there is a liability to faint on standing; eventually muscle and abdominal cramps develop and the patient may pass into a muttering delirium. There is loss of weight, the face is haggard and the eyes sunken, the skin is clammy and cold and, on pinching it, tends to remain raised; the superficial veins are thin and constricted; the tongue is dry and the eyeballs soft; the pulse is rapid and both the mean arterial and the pulse pressures are decreased. The circulating haemoglobin concentration is raised, but plasma sodium and chloride are lowered. If salt deficiency is not corrected the patient may die rapidly from peripheral circulatory failure.

It must be emphasised, however, that *there may be a considerable loss of salt before there is much clinical evidence of deficiency*. But even a subclinical deficiency is sufficient to cause renal vasoconstriction with a fall in renal blood flow and glomerular filtration rate, and an increase in blood urea. When salt deficiency is secondary to renal failure the urinary specific gravity is around 1.010 and the urine contains some sodium; whereas if the kidneys were previously healthy, tubular function remains normal, the specific gravity will at first be greater than 1.020 and the urine will contain no sodium. Proteinuria is nearly always present.

### Aetiology and diagnosis

*Sodium, chloride and water deficiency due to renal disease*

Reflux nephropathy and phenacetin nephropathy, during an acute flare-up of infection, are the most common renal diseases to cause florid salt and water deficiency. It has also been reported with chronic glomerular nephritis and polycystic disease. The syndrome is sometimes known as 'salt losing nephritis' (p. 280). Very rarely sodium deficiency may also occur during the recovery stage of acute tubular necrosis (p. 150). The chronic renal diseases which cause sodium deficiency may give rise to serious diagnostic difficulties but the salt and water loss following acute tubular necrosis should be anticipated.

*Sodium, chloride and water deficiency as a cause of renal failure*

Salt and water deficiency following post-operative gastric suction, intestinal and biliary fistulae should also be anticipated; the onset of renal failure in these conditions is often an indication of mismanagement.

The risk of precipitating renal failure by giving low salt diets to patients suffering from renal disease has been mentioned earlier.

Renal failure from loss of water and salt caused by diarrhoea and vomiting or diabetic ketosis does not usually present any diagnostic difficulties. But when loss of water and salt complicates a cerebral condition it may easily be overlooked.

The greatest diagnostic difficulty is in differentiating the sodium chloride deficiency and renal failure of Addison's disease from sodium chloride deficiency due to chronic renal disease. In both there is a urinary leak of salt and in both there may be nausea, weakness, loss of weight, pigmentation, hypotension, and a raised plasma potassium. In an emergency the two conditions can be distinguished by the fact that the administration of hydrocortisone and $9\alpha$ fluorohydrocortisone to patients with renal disease has little effect on the high rate of urinary salt excretion, while recovery occurs rapidly upon giving large amounts of salt and water. When there is more leisure to make the diagnosis it will be found that in sodium chloride deficiency due to renal disease, the concentration of plasma cortisol is normal or raised while that of aldosterone is raised. Plasma renin activity will be raised in both Addison's disease and renal disease.

If the patient is severely ill treatment consists simply in the rapid intravenous administration of large amounts of isotonic (1/6 molar) saline preferably with isotonic (1/6 molar) sodium bicarbonate in a proportion of 2 to 1. Isotonic saline contains 150 mmol/l of sodium and 150 mmol/l of chloride, whereas the extracellular fluid contains 140 mmol/l of sodium but only 100 mmol/l of chloride; the administration of one litre of isotonic sodium bicarbonate (150 mmol of sodium) for every two of saline ensures that sodium and chloride are given in physiological proportions. If acute renal failure has already occured, the rate of infusion must be more moderate, for great care is needed to prevent the onset of pulmonary oedema; it is also essential that sodium bicarbonate be given, for the kidneys are unable to excrete the excess chloride in the sodium chloride solutions. Tablets of slow release sodium chloride (Slow-Sodium, Ciba), 10 mmol per tablet can be given orally with water when the need for sodium replacement is less urgent, or as a prophylatic measure.

*Sodium and chloride deficiency with excess water intake*

Occasionally patients who are suffering from salt deficiency and oliguria are inadvertently given water (5% glucose) intravenously, but because of the persistent rise in plasma ADH due to the hypovolaemia they cannot excrete the water (p. 303). They then develop acute overhydration with nausea, vomiting and mental confusion. Treatment consists in giving a slow intravenous administration of about 300 ml of hypertonic (3%) saline.

## POTASSIUM

### Hypokalaemia

*Potassium deficiency due to renal disease*

The following renal diseases may sometimes cause an excess urinary loss of potassium:
1. Chronic glomerular nephritis
2. Reflux nephropathy, during a relapse of infection
3. During recovery from acute tubular necrosis
4. Renal tubular acidosis (p. 362)
5. Renal artery stenosis (p. 274)
6. Polyarteritis nodosa.

*Potassium deficiency as a cause of renal failure*

The following conditions may cause such a loss of potassium that its deficiency contributes materially to the onset of renal failure:
1. Prolonged vomiting, e.g. pyloric obstruction
2. Prolonged diarrhoea, e.g. small bowel insufficiency, excessive use of purgatives or enemas, pancreatic adenomata, and villous tumours of the large bowel
3. Post-operative gastric suction
4. Intestinal and biliary fistulae
5. Uncontrolled diabetes
6. Injudicious use of ion exchange resins
7. Aldosteronism
8. Diuretics.

### Clinical features of potassium deficiency

Until potassium deficiency is advanced its signs and symptoms are vague and indefinite. The outstanding and characteristic feature of advanced potassium deficiency is the development of muscular weakness which progresses to paralysis and death from respiratory failure. Otherwise there may be thirst, irritability, nausea, confusion and paralytic ileus. The physical signs are apathy, loss of reflexes, loss of motor power, tetany, gasping respirations and occasionally irregularity of the heart rate. The severity and localisation of the effects of potassium deficiency are influenced to a certain extent by the patient's age. The elderly appear to be more susceptible and tend to have predominantly renal and cardiac complications, whereas the young are less susceptible and tend to have the muscular changes. If the potassium loss is due to renal disease the presence of which is unsuspected, many of these features may at first be thought to be due to hysteria.

A certain diagnosis of low serum potassium can only be made by direct estimation, though some information can be obtained from an electrocardiograph which shows flattened T waves, often with prominent U waves and ST depression. Though the serum concentration of potassium is sometimes of value when the loss of body potassium is severe, it is sometimes misleading, particularly when rapid shifts of potassium are taking place from one fluid compartment to another. The cells may then be severely deficient in potassium though the plasma concentrations are normal or even high. In relatively steady conditions a serum potassium of 3 mmol/l implies a potassium deficit of about 200–300 mmol. Below 3 mmol/l every 1 mmol/l fall represents another 200 to 400 mmol deficit in total body potassium. Therefore a plasma potassium of 1.5 mmol and a normal arterial pH may have a potassium deficit of 500 to 800 mmol. With changes in acid-base states an alteration in plasma potassium can occur without a net change in total body potassium. As an approximation 0.1 unit change in pH is associated with an inverse change in plasma potassium of about 0.6 mmol/l.

When potassium deficiency is primary and renal failure its consequence, the plasma bicarbonate is usually raised; but when potassium deficiency is due to renal disease the plasma bicarbonate may be reduced because of the impaired ability to secrete hydrogen ions and ammonia which accompanies chronic renal failure. Alkalosis is initially caused by the diminished amount of potassium in the tubule cells. Sodium reabsorption is then associated with a rather greater secretion of hydrogen than potassium ions from the tubule cells into the tubule lumen. This in turn generates larger quantities of bicarbonate than normal and the plasma bicarbonate rises. A larger load of bicarbonate thus has to be filtered at the glomerulus and a larger reabsorption of bicarbonate results. This active process of bicarbonate reabsorption automatically reduces the passive reabsorption of chloride. Chloride excretion therefore rises. In the final stage there is therefore, a combination of potassium and chloride deficiency and bicarbonate retention. Alkalosis is also due in part to a shift of hydrogen ions into the intracellular fluid, in exchange for intracellular potassium which is released into the extracellular fluid which prevents its concentration from falling to a lethal level. Sodium ions also cross into the intracellular fluid in exchange for potassium so that in pure potassium deficiency there is an overall intracellular sodium retention. Chronic potassium deficiency is often associated with oedema without evidence of heart failure or rise in jugular venous pressure.

Presumably the renal failure which follows potassium deficiency is due to lack of potassium within the tubule cells, for both functional and histological changes are mainly found in the tubules. The ability to concentrate the urine is lost at an early stage though the ability to dilute remains for a considerable time; occasionally the urine may remain at a fixed concentration which is hypotonic to plasma. The loss of the ability to concentrate is probably due to the potassium deficiency impairing the sodium pump in the ascending loop of Henle. Polyuria and particularly nocturia are distinctive features of renal failure associated with potassium deficiency. In some patients there is a complete inversion of the normal diurnal rhythm. The polyuria is due to the potassium deficiency stimulating the thirst centre. Following the administration of ammonium chloride, the ability to form a highly acid urine, and to excrete hydrogen ions at a normal rate is impaired though the ability to excrete ammonium remains normal or raised for a considerable time. Changes in glomerular filtration rate follow and are less severe than the tubular changes. The rise in blood urea is also due in part to an increased permeability of the proximal tubule to urea. Nearly always there is a trace of protein in the urine.

The most characteristic histological change found in potassium deficiency in man is extensive vacuolation of the cells of the proximal tubule; this change is rapidly reversible after potassium administration. The more advanced appearances are those of interstitial nephritis and are not reversible. In animals there are also extensive changes in the collecting ducts.

## Aetiology and diagnosis

### Potassium deficiency due to renal disease

This rare phenomenon is characterised by the continued excretion of substantial amounts of potassium in the urine despite depleted body potassium and low plasma potassium. The renal disease responsible for such a deficiency is easy to diagnose when it occurs during recovery from acute tubular necrosis, but it is more difficult to distinguish when it is due to chronic glomerular nephritis, infected reflux nephropathy, polyarteritis nodosa or a selective defect of tubular function.

The early stages of potassium deficiency due to a renal tubular acidosis may sometimes be differentiated from chronic destructive renal disease such as glomerular nephritis by the fact that with the former the impairment in glomerular filtration rate is moderate, and the ability to produce a highly acid urine and to excrete ammonia in response to ammonium chloride is grossly abnormal (p. 97). With chronic destructive lesions, though there is also an impaired ability to excrete ammonia, glomerular filtration rate is severely reduced and the ability to excrete a highly acid urine appears normal until potassium deficiency itself impairs the ability to excrete an acid urine (see above).

### Potassium deficiency as a cause of renal failure

This syndrome is more frequent than its converse and its cause is usually more easily diagnosed. When potassium deficiency causes renal failure the loss of potassium is nearly always from the alimentary tract. Vomiting, gastric suction, diarrhoea, intestinal fistulae and the misuse of ion exchange resins are easily identifiable causes of excessive loss of potassium. Long-continued use of purgatives and small bowel insufficiency may be more obscure, but there is usually some looseness of the bowels. In all these conditions the urine contains only minimal amounts of potassium (p. 98) and except with ion exchange resins, the plasma bicarbonate is raised (p. 86). This combination of renal failure, low plasma potassium and low urinary excretion of potassium, proves that the renal failure is indeed due to *extrarenal* loss of potassium.

Very, very occasionally when severe potassium deficiency has been present for some time, the severity of the renal damage which results may impair the reabsorption of potassium. Urinary potassium excretion then rises in spite of the hypokalaemia and it may now be difficult to distinguish whether the renal failure is due to the potassium deficiency or vice versa. Compulsive, depressed, post-menopausal women, who obtain satisfaction and relief by secretly taking large quantities of purgatives, are those most likely to damage themselves in this way. They are characteristically evasive or downright misleading about their use of purgatives, so that the true cause of the potassium deficiency and renal failure may not be detected for a considerable time, even with the patient in hospital. Others with abnormal personalities who pose the same problems may have anorexia nervosa or there may be surreptitious vomiters or secret users of diuretics (Fig. 19.1).

There are two other situations in which renal failure is caused by excessive *renal* loss of potassium, diabetic ketosis and primary aldosteronism. In diabetic ketosis (p. 344) the potassium deficiency is only an incidental cause of renal failure and no diagnostic confusion is likely.

Clinically, renal failure due to primary hyperaldosteronism may be extremely difficult to distinguish from renal disease causing secondary hyperaldosteronism, when the associated renal ischaemia causes a release of renin and stimulation of the adrenal glands by angiotensin. In both there may be polyuria and thirst, low plasma potassium, hypertension and a raised blood urea. The blood urea is usually much higher, i.e. about 30 mmol/l (200 mg/100 ml) if renal disease is causing secondary hyperaldosteronism. In primary aldosteronism, the hypertension is not usually malignant, whereas it is more often malignant with renal ischaemia. In addition the plasma sodium is higher (137–160 mmol/l) in primary aldosteronism than in secondary aldosteronism (125–141 mmol/l) though there is some overlap. On the other hand, the plasma potassium is lower (1.4 to 3.2 mmol/l) in primary aldosteronism than in secondary aldosteronism (3.1 to 4.2 mmol/l). These two conditions can be distinguished by measuring the plasma renin before and after three days on a low sodium diet; the second blood being taken on the third day, after standing for four hours. In primary aldosteronism the control plasma renin is low and it remains low. In secondary

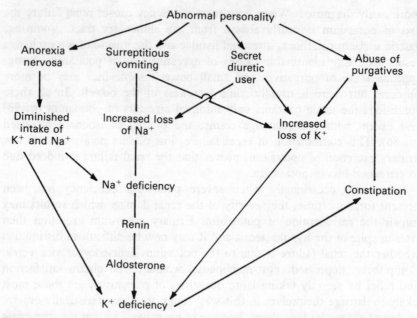

**Fig. 19.1** Some causes of potassium deficiency and consequential renal failure in patients with abnormal personalities. (Reproduced from Wolff, Vecsei, Kruck et al 1968 Lancet 1: 257, with kind permission.)

aldosteronism the control renin should be higher but the most characteristic finding is that it rises further after a low sodium diet and standing. A renal biopsy can sometimes help. If the structural changes are characteristic only of potassium deficiency, i.e. there is vacuolation of the tubule cells, particularly of the distal tubules, the hypokalaemia and renal failure may be due to primary aldosteronism. If the lesions are more extensive and include those of interstitial nephritis renal biopsy is of relatively little help, for such changes can follow potassium deficiency or they may be due to a long-standing chronic renal disease which may be the cause of the potassium deficiency.

## Treatment

When renal disease is the cause of the potassium deficiency the only effective treatment is potassium replacement followed by the daily oral administration of sufficient potassium to balance the excess urinary loss.

Potassium chloride is clearly what is needed in nearly all instances, particularly at the beginning of treatment when there is a potassium and chloride deficit to be corrected. Solutions of oral potassium chloride however, have an unpleasant taste, and enteric coated tablets produce sharply delineated zones of cicatricial narrowing of the small bowel which may cause complete or partial obstruction. Slow release tablets of 'wax' impregnated with potassium chloride (Slow K, Ciba) are the most suitable preparations to use. Once the initial potassium and chloride deficiency has been corrected, the administration of supplemental potassium chloride may have to be continued to prevent a deficiency of potassium recurring. Other salts of potassium which are also used include a mixture of potassium acetate, citrate and bicarbonate, 1 g of each in 8 ml of water, four times a day which supplies 116 mmol of potassium in a relatively palatable form. Mist. Pot. Cit. (B.P.) contains 3 g of potassium citrate, i.e. 28 mmol of potassium per 15 ml which is about half an ounce; this is also well tolerated.

To prevent the onset of potassium deficiency during the early diuretic phase of acute tubular necrosis, it is usually only necessary to give plenty of orange and tomato juice, figs, apricots, dates and meat extract, all of which contain high quantities of potassium (p. 570).

When potassium deficiency is due to excess alimentary loss all that is required is to replace the potassium and stop any further loss; if the latter is not possible (e.g. intestinal fistulae, gastric suction) potassium should be given intravenously at the same rate as it is being lost.

Potassium is best given intravenously when there is a good urine flow, in order that an excess plasma potassium may more easily spill over in the urine. It is also wise to avoid intravenous administration for 24 hours after any particular stress such as an operation, for at these times the plasma potassium is apt to be raised whatever the concentration in the cells. It should also be borne in mind that in normal circumstances, though the total body potassium is about 2500 mmol, the amount in the extracellular fluid is only 75 mmol and that death occurs if it rises to 150 mmol. Cardiac arrest from hyperkalaemia occurs at plasma levels of 9–10 mmol/l; it is generally wise not to give potassium intravenously at a greater rate than 25 mmol per hour. It is also best to limit the concentration of the fluid to 40 mmol/l, for higher concentrations are liable to cause painful spasm of the vein.

If a patient suffering from a pure potassium deficiency is given saline instead of potassium there is likely to be increased sodium retention with oedema and an increased urinary excretion of potassium. The administration of sodium bicarbonate should also be avoided for this induces a severe alkalosis.

## HYPERKALAEMIA

Hyperkalaemia due to a decreased renal excretion of potassium can occur in acute and chronic renal failure, Addison's disease, hyporeninaemic hypoaldosteronism, systemic lupus erythematosus, and occasionally in a transplanted kidney. It is interesting that, on the whole, hyperkalaemia does not occur in chronic renal failure until the patient is near death, unless there is a sudden rise in the transfer of intracellular potassium to the extra-cellular fluid (e.g. acidosis), or an excess intake of potassium, particularly if it is sudden. Therefore, if hyperkalaemia does develop in a patient before the plasma creatinine is 1000 $\mu$mol/l, it is usual to find that there has either been a worsening of the metabolic acidosis, an increase in catabolism (e.g. an infection) or a gastro-intestinal bleed. Potassium-sparing diuretics such as Triamterene or Spironolactone may induce a fatal hyperkalaemia, particularly in diabetic patients presumably because they already tend to have hyperkalaemia from hyporeninaemic hypoaldosteronism, the inability to raise plasma aldosterone making it difficult for them to control the rise in plasma potassium. Hyperkalaemia may also be due to a selective isolated defect in urinary potassium excretion; a condition sometimes seen in a transplanted kidney and in systemic lupus erythematosus.

Hyperkalaemia (like hypokalaemia) can cause marked weakness, paralysis, and cardiac arrest. But is has a stimulating effect on the pancreas and the adrenal increasing the secretion of glucagon, insulin, adrenaline and aldosterone (Fig. 19.2).

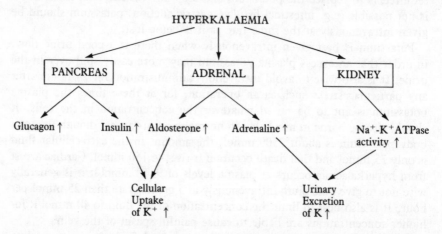

**Fig. 19.2** Adaptive response to hyperkalaemia. The increased release of glucagon, insulin, and adrenaline move the potassium from the plasma and extracellular fluid into the cells while the rise in plasma aldosterone and the direct effect of the hyperkalaemia on the kidney move the potassium from the plasma into the urine. (Adapted from Gabow & Peterson 1980 In: R W Schrier (ed) Renal and electrolyte disorders p 211, with kind permission.)

## Treatment

*Remember to stop the administration of potassium supplements.* The most rapid countermeasure is a bolus intravenous injection of calcium gluconate 20 ml of a 10% solution. It antagonises the neuromuscular effects of the hyperkalaemia within minutes but it is only effective for 20–30 min. An IV infusion of sodium bicarbonate 250 ml of a 2.4% solution in four hours (look out for hypocalcaemia) or 250 ml of a 10% glucose solution together with 10 units of insulin in 30 min will redistribute the potassium from the plasma and extracellular fluid into the cells within 30 min and the effect will last several hours. Another relatively quick method, the effect of which is more lasting is the rapid removal of potassium by the gut, with the oral administration of Sorbitol 100 ml of 70% solution orally hourly until the diarrhoea starts. The method is less unpleasant than it sounds and is extremely effective. There is a rapid loss of water, sodium, potassium and bicarbonate and it is particularly indicated when the patient is salt and water loaded and threatened with pulmonary oedema. The administration of resins is the slowest method and is most useful as a long term method, or if the plasma potassium is less than 6.5 mmol/l. If the patient is not overloaded a sodium resin can be given, 15–30 g two to three times a day orally or rectally. If the patient is overloaded a calcium resin is used in rather larger quantities, e.g. 20–40 g two to three times a day orally, and/or rectally. Occasionally, long term use of resins can cause severe constipation and this may be responsible for the rupture of a diverticulum into the peritoneal cavity.

Sometimes it is necessary to use dialysis. Haemodialysis is preferable, for peritoneal dialysis is even less effective for the removal of potassium than resins.

## CALCIUM

A raised urinary excretion of calcium may cause renal failure irrespective of the overall calcium balance. The reason for this is not known, but it is probably related to an intracellular accumulation of calcium ions in the tubules. This is in contrast to the renal failure of potassium deficiency (see above), which is due to an intracellular deficiency of potassium ions, or the renal failure of sodium deficiency which is due to contraction of the extracellular fluid volume and renal vasoconstriction.

The following conditions are associated with a high urinary calcium excretion and renal failure.

### Increased urinary excretion of calcium due to renal disease

The only renal disease known to cause an increase in urinary calcium excretion is renal tubular acidosis (p. 362) which may induce a mild impairment of renal function.

### Increased urinary excretion of calcium as a cause of renal failure

1. Following increased calcium absorption:
    a. Compulsive milk drinking
    b. excess vitamin D intake
    c. sarcoidosis
    d. idiopathic hypercalcaemia of infants.

2. Following an increased rate of bone decalcification:
   a. Hyperparathyroidism
   b. Malignancy including myelomatosis
   c. Immobilisation
   d. Paget's disease.

## Effect of hypercalcaemia on renal structure and function

In the early stages renal biopsy may show no abnormality, but later, precipitated calcium can be seen as clumps between and across the nephrons, and as a fine dusting of the tubule cells and their basement membranes. The early lesions are in the collecting ducts, distal tubules and ascending loops of Henle. Later the whole nephron is involved. Some tubules eventually atrophy, and varying numbers of glomeruli become structureless round eosin-staining masses. In long-standing cases the deposition of calcium in the kidney can be seen radiologically (nephrocalcinosis).

Hypercalcaemia increases urinary hydrogen ion excretion. Ammonia excretion therefore rises and urine pH falls, while plasma bicarbonate and pH rise and there is an alkalosis. (This acceleration of hydrogen ion secretion by the tubule is paralleled by an increase in hydrogen ion secretion by the gastric mucosa so that hypercalcaemia is often associated with epigastric pain, dyspepsia and peptic ulcers.) The acceleration of hydrogen ion secretion, may be due to stimulation of carbonic anhydrase activity. In early hypercalcaemia therefore (with the exception of hyperparathyroidism), there may be the paradoxical finding of a raised plasma bicarbonate with a low urine pH. On the other hand, parathormone inhibits hydrogen ion excretion and increases bicarbonate excretion so that when hypercalcaemia is due to hyperparathyroidism there is a rise in urine pH and a tendency for the plasma bicarbonate to fall and the plasma chloride to rise.

Hypercalcaemia and hypercalcuria from any cause profoundly impair the kidney's ability to concentrate the urine; frequently the urine concentration remains fixed at a concentration well below that of plasma. The impaired ability to concentrate is related to the hypercalcuria as well as the hypercalcaemia and may therefore occur without hypercalcaemia. It is probably due to the excess intracellular calcium impairing the sodium pump in the ascending loop of Henle. If hypercalcaemia persists there is a fall in glomerular filtration rate, a rise in blood urea and proteinuria. At first the blood urea is only moderately raised to 8–10 mmol/l (50–60 mg/100 ml), and there is then a marked discrepancy between the severe impairment in concentrating ability and the modest rise in blood urea. Gradually so many nephrons are destroyed that eventually the findings are the same as those in chronic renal failure from any cause. At this point the increasing impairment of hydrogen ion secretion and ammonia production of renal failure is superimposed upon the effect of hypercalcaemia and if the plasma bicarbonate was raised it now falls to normal or below.

## Clinical features associated with hypercalcuria and hypercalcaemia

As the renal failure is only related to the high urinary excretion of calcium and not to negative calcium balance (unlike potassium and sodium), the general signs and symptoms vary widely from one cause to another. For instance, if the hypercalcuria is secondary to bone disease there will be a negative calcium balance and signs and symptoms of bone softening or fractures, whereas if hypercalcuria is due to excessive intestinal absorption of calcium there will be calcium equilibrium and no signs or symptoms of bone disease.

There is always thirst, polydipsia and polyuria. These are often of such severity that the patient may at first be thought to be suffering from diabetes insipidus (p. 304). As in potassium deficiency this is mainly due to the hypercalcaemia stimulating the thirst centre.

Hypercalcuria is usually present when the serum calcium is raised; it may also be present without such a rise. Alternatively, if glomerular filtration rate is sufficiently depressed there may be hypercalcaemia with hypocalcuria. Occasionally, when the urinary excretion of calcium is extremely high, i.e. around 25 mmol (1000 mg) a day (on a normal diet the usual range is 2 to 10 mmol 80–400 mg), the urine upon standing will develop a thin white chalky precipitate which is characteristic.

## Aetiology and diagnosis

*Increased urinary excretion of calcium as a cause of renal failure*

   *a. Following increased calcium absorption.* In compulsive milk drinking, vitamin D intoxication, sarcoidosis and idiopathic hypercalcaemia of infants there is an increased alimentary absorption of calcium with the following consequences: hypercalcaemia → hypercalcuria → renal failure.

Compulsive milk drinking is a rare condition which, initially, can easily be overlooked, for the patient may fail to disclose his idiosyncrasy, or he minimises its extent. Frequently the milk drinking begins because of recurrent dyspepsia, but as the amount taken increases and hypercalcaemia develops, the dyspepsia becomes worse. The fact that these patients are also apt to take large quantities of alkalis, which often contain calcium carbonate, may increase the liability of calcium to be deposited in the kidney. Compulsive milk drinkers are frequently admitted with advanced renal failure and alkalosis. Diagnosis may be difficult for by this time glomerular filtration rate is so depressed that there is no hypercalcuria, and in addition the patient is now so ill and nauseated that his compulsion for milk is less pressing. Hypercalcaemia is usually present and often there are widespread deposits of calcium in the skin, joints, corneae and lungs.

Excess vitamin D intake is not uncommon. In adults it occurs as a form of food fad, or more usually from taking vitamin D supplements to avoid colds. In infants and children excess vitamin D intake derives from oversolicitous motherly attention. At one time infants and children normally ingested larger quantities of vitamin D than necessary. Not only was it given as concentrated cod and halibut liver oil, but much of the food they ate, such as milk preparations and cereals, often had vitamin D added in substantial quantities. This excess may have been the precipitating cause of the increased calcium absorption of idiopathic hypercalcaemia of infants. In recent years however, the vitamin D content of commercial milk preparations and cereals has been reduced. Recently there have been attempts to use the oral administration of 1,25(OH)₂vit D₃ to prevent the development of renal bone disease in patients with advanced renal failure before they are placed onto maintenance haemodialysis. This practice can also cause a sudden deterioration of renal function.

The increased intestinal absorption of calcium in sarcoidosis is due to a raised plasma concentration of 1,25(OH)₂vit D₃. The site of the increased manufacture of 1,25(OH)₂vit D₃ is not known. Hypercalcaemia and a raised plasma 1,25(OH)₂vit D₃ can occur in an anephric patient suffering from sarcoidosis; it is thus possible that the sarcoid lesions themselves can produce 1,25(OH)₂vit D₃. Hypercalcaemia tends to be precipitated by sun bathing, or a mild excess of vitamin D in the diet (Fig. 19.3).

  *b. Following increased rate of bone decalcification.* There are three principal

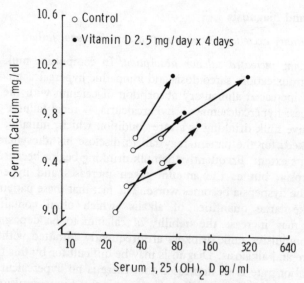

**Fig. 19.3** Effect of vitamin D₂ on serum 1,25(OH)₂vit D and serum calcium in six patients with sarcoidosis. There was a brisk rise in serum 1,25(OH)₂vit D and calcium. Normal subjects given the same amount of vit D, would have had no change in serum 1,25(OH)₂vit D or serum calcium. Conversion: traditional to SI units — calcium 10 mg/dl = 2.5 mmol/l: 1,25(OH)₂vit D 100 pg/ml = 230 pmol/l. (Reproduced from Stern, Olazabal & Bell, 1980 J Clin Invest 66: 852 by copyright permission of The American Society for Clinical Investigation.)

conditions to be considered: hyperparathyroidism, diffuse carcinomatosis of bone and myelomatosis.

In addition to finding a raised plasma parathyroid hormone the diagnosis of hyperparathyroidism depends on the finding of a raised plasma total calcium but more importantly a raised plasma ionised calcium, a low plasma phosphate, and hypercalcuria; the characteristic periosteal erosions in the bones of the hands, bone cysts, and a raised alkaline phosphatase. Recurrent renal calculi may also occur. Hyperparathyroidism gives rise to the highest serum calcium concentrations; sometimes over 5 mmol/l (20 mg/100 ml). Acute hyperparathyroidism with severe prostration, muscular weakness, pains and tenderness, vomiting, cardiac failure, dyspepsia, polyuria and polydipsia may not be recognised, unless the diagnosis is suspected on every occasion that there is unexplained thirst and polyuria. Radiological bone lesions may be absent both in acute and chronic hyperparathyroidism, which makes the differentiation from sarcoidosis difficult. The confusion is greatest if renal failure is moderately advanced, for this occasionally causes the plasma phosphate to rise and thus obscures one of the most characteristic alerting signs of hyperparathyroidism.

Diffuse carcinomatosis of bone is identified by X-rays and scans of the skeleton and by bone marrow biopsy; and there may also be a leucoerythroblastic anaemia. The hypercalcaemia associated with malignancy is sometimes due to circulating substances which may either resemble parathyroid hormone, or though they are not parathyroid hormone they stimulate osteoclastic resorption. In some instances the increased resorption appears to be prostaglandin mediated. Renal failure associated with myelomatosis is sometimes due to increased urinary calcium excretion. Hypercalcaemia may precipitate a rapid deterioration of renal function.

**Treatment**

The treatment of renal tubular acidosis is discussed in Section 18.

The increased absorption and hypercalcaemia of sarcoidosis can be controlled by adrenal steroids. 150 mg of cortisone per day for 10 days causes a fall in plasma calcium and in urinary calcium excretion. As the tendency to develop hypercalcaemia is often phasic, treatment should be interrupted now and again to see if it is still necessary.

Idiopathic hypercalcaemia of infants will usually respond in a few weeks when treated with either a low calcium diet or cortisone; the latter allows a much greater flexibility in the diet, and calcium ingestion need only be controlled to a limited extent.

Hyperparathyroidism is treated by removal of adenomata or hyperplastic glands. Acute renal failure following operation may occur and is particularly dangerous, for the falling serum calcium and rising potassium summate in their ill effects. Patients suffering from compulsive milk drinking or vitamin D intoxication are usually only in need of advice.

Severe symptomatic hypercalcaemia (usually associated with malignancy) is treated by the IV administration of large amounts of saline at the rate of one to two litres in four hours to correct the dehydration, and to increase the urinary excretion of calcium. The latter can be speeded up by placing frusemide into the saline so that approximately 20 mg is given per four hour period. The plasma potassium must be monitored, at frequent intervals and the weight must also be monitored preferably continuously on a weigh bed, otherwise, at hourly intervals. Indomethacin 25–50 mg t.d.s. and prednisone 80 mg per day are also useful in some patients with malignancy and hypercalcaemia. Dialysis with calcium-free solutions has occasionally been used. Calcitonin is slow to work and rarely effective.

## MAGNESIUM

### Increased urinary excretion of magnesium due to renal disease

Very occasionally a severe upper urinary infection in a patient with chronic renal failure due to reflux nephropathy may cause a reversible urinary leak of magnesium. This is nearly always associated with a simultaneous equally reversible leak of sodium, potassium and calcium with a profound hypocalcaemia. The diagnosis is most easily made by measuring the plasma magnesium which will be low. Symptoms of magnesium deficiency develop at plasma levels of magnesium well below 0.5 mmol/l. These consist of gross tremors, confusion with panic attacks, vomiting, fasciculation, hyporeflexia and usually, but not always, positive Trousseau's and Chvostek's signs.

Chronic renal failure from other causes such as persistent glomerular nephritis has on rare occasions been associated with a persistent urinary leak of magnesium.

### Hypomagnesaemia due to urinary loss of magnesium

By far the most important cause of this condition is the use of diuretics either too vigorously or in a patient who is not eating well, particularly if he is an alcoholic, for a high alcohol intake also increases urinary magnesium excretion. In such patients the diagnosis may first be suspected because of a refractory hypokalaemia with an atrial fibrillation which does not respond to digoxin. A high excretion of magnesium also occurs in ketoacidosis, and in hyperaldosteronism, which may be sufficient to cause hypomagnesaemia.

A cause of severe persistent hypomagnesaemia from urinary loss which may be difficult to treat, is the occasional harmful effect of cytotoxic drugs on the tubule. Figure 19.4 illustrates the findings in this unusual but well known complication in a patient treated for a choriocarcinoma. It illustrates the major electrolyte abnormalities which have been described in experimental dietary magnesium deficiency in man. They are: (1) hypomagnesaemia which in this patient, in contrast to the dietary deficient cases, was associated with

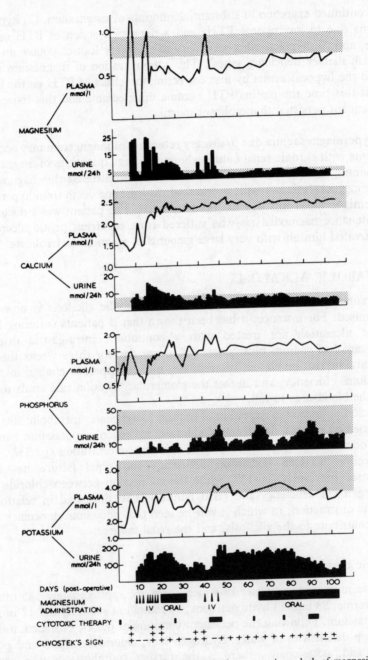

**Fig. 19.4** Details of a patient with hypomagnesaemia due to a urinary leak of magnesium following treatment of a choriocarcinoma with cytotoxic drugs (see text). Conversion: SI to traditional units — magnesium 1 mmol/l = 2.4 mg/100 ml; 5 mmol/24 hr = 120 mg/24 h: Calcium 2.5 mmol/l = 10 mg/100 ml; 5 mmol/24 hr = 200 mg/24 hr: phosphorus 1 mmol/l = 3.1 mg/100 ml; 10 mmol/24 hr = 310 mg/24 hr. (Reproduced from Moloney, Eastwood & de Wardener 1982 Nephron 30: 51, with kind permission.)

the continued excretion of substantial amounts of magnesium, (2) hypocal-caemia due to low plasma PTH, and a depressed action of PTH on the bone, and (3) hypokalaemia secondary to a urinary leak of potassium (also seen in dietary deficiency cases). The administration of magnesium alone cured the hypocalcaemia by first correcting the effect of PTH on the bone, for at this time the plasma PTH became undetectable and this caused the subsequent persistent hyperphosphataemia.

**Hypermagnesaemia due to urinary retention of magnesium** may occur in patients with chronic renal failure who ingest large quantities of magnesium containing antacids. As these are often self administered the diagnosis of hypermagnesaemia is usually overlooked. At least one death from hypermag-nesaemia induced this way has been recorded. The patient was a doctor on maintenance haemodialysis who suffered from recurrent peptic ulceration and treated himself with very large amounts of magnesium trisilicate.

## METABOLIC ALKALOSIS

The normal kidney's ability to prevent a metabolic alkalosis is now well recognised. For instance, it has been shown that if patients suffering from peptic ulceration are treated with a continuous intra-gastric drip of 1000 mmol of sodium bicarbonate (84 g) per day for three weeks there is a persistent rise in plasma bicarbonate, but no apparent change in renal functional efficiency, and in fact the glomerular filtration rate tends to rise and the blood urea to fall.

Excluding increased ingestion of sodium bicarbonate, metabolic alkalosis is caused by either a deficiency of chloride, hydrogen or potassium ions, or very occasionally by a rise in plasma calcium concentration (p. 332). The connection between potassium deficiency and renal failure has been discussed previously (p. 187) while the connection between chloride and hydrogen ion deficiency and renal failure is best discussed in relation to pyloric obstruction, in which it will be seen that potassium deficiency may also contribute to the alkalosis, and the renal failure.

### Pyloric obstruction

Gastric juice contains water in which there are approximately 145 mmol/l of chloride, 83 mmol/l hydrogen ions, 50 mmol/l of sodium, and 12 mmol/l of potassium. Following the persistent vomiting of pyloric obstruction there develop deficiencies of water, hydrogen ions, chloride, sodium and potas-sium and, occasionally, there is the further complication of a gastro-intestinal haemorrhage. Each of these gives rise to its own sequence of disturbance in body fluids, and renal function. It is important to realise that the direction of some of the renal functional disturbances depend on the pattern of the deficiencies, i.e. there may be oliguria or polyuria, an alkaline urine or an acid urine. The relative proportions of these deficiencies determine which functional changes will predominate.

Figure 19.5 illustrates the changes which may occur.

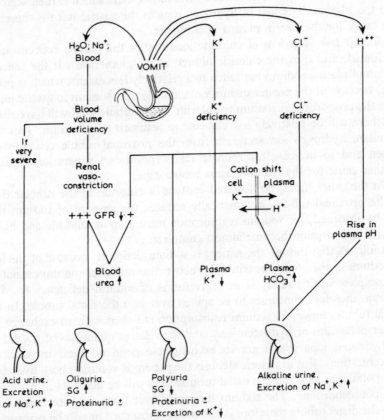

**Fig. 19.5** Changes in plasma concentrations and renal function which may occur as a consequence of the persistent vomiting of pyloric obstruction.

## Factors involved in the renal failure of pyloric obstruction

*Water and blood loss.* The continuous loss of water (with sodium and chloride) reduces the extra cellular fluid volume and the blood volume, and this is followed by consequences which have been described previously, i.e. renal vasoconstriction → reduced glomerular filtration rate → rise in blood urea. These changes will be more pronounced if there is also gastrointestinal bleeding. In rare instances acute renal failure develops. Usually the renal ischaemia stops short of tubular necrosis and there is only *oliguria* with a urine concentration which tends to be raised.

*Hydrogen ion loss.* The loss of hydrogen ions raises the plasma pH, slows respiration and raises $pCO_2$. The rise in $pCO_2$ then causes the proximal tubule to increase its secretion of hydrogen ions from the tubule cell into the tubule lumen so that there is an increase in the reabsorption of bicarbonate from the tubule lumen back into the plasma, and also an increase in generation of fresh bicarbonate by the tubule cells which is then secreted into the plasma. The loss of hydrogen ions in the gastric juice is therefore one cause for the rise in plasma bicarbonate.

*Chloride loss.* The loss of chloride ions lowers the plasma concentration of chloride and thus the chloride filtered at the glomerulus. If the concentration of plasma sodium has fallen to a relatively less extent, which is probable, because of the greater quantity of chloride than sodium in gastric juice, then the proportion of sodium to chloride in the tubule fluid will have risen, i.e. there will be relatively less chloride to reabsorb than sodium. This will stimulate hydrogen ion secretion from the proximal tubule cell into the lumen and so increase bicarbonate reabsorption and generation. This is another cause for the rise in plasma bicarbonate.

On the other hand, the lowered content of chloride in the tubular fluid in the proximal tubule, automatically reduces the amount of sodium that can be absorbed, for sodium reabsorption must stop as chloride and bicarbonate reabsorption become almost complete.

It follows that though the patient is sodium deficient (because of the loss of sodium in the vomit) proximal tubular reabsorption of sodium cannot be as complete as it usually is in other forms of sodium deficiency (p. 82). Sodium therefore continues to be spilled over into the distal tubule. In the distal tubule, however, sodium reabsorption is linked with an exchange for either potassium or hydrogen ions, and the relative quantities of potassium or hydrogen ions which are so exchanged depend on their intracellular concentrations. But in pyloric stenosis the patient is vomiting both hydrogen and potassium ions and the distal tubular cells will be deficient in hydrogen and potassium ions. The sodium that spills over from the proximal tubule into the distal tubule therefore is either not reabsorbed or will be reabsorbed in exchange for potassium or hydrogen ions. There is then the paradox that a patient suffering from sodium, potassium, and hydrogen ion deficiency may be excreting sodium, potassium and an acid urine (see below). The loss of sodium ions contributes to the reduction in extracellular volume and therefore to the precipitation and perpetuation of renal failure. The diminution in extracellular fluid volume increases net bicarbonate reabsorption (p. 88) and thus increases the severity of the metabolic alkalosis. The loss of potassium also contributes to the renal failure.

*Potassium loss.* The consequences of potassium loss on renal function have been described on page 324. There is some reduction in glomerular filtration rate, but the most marked feature is *polyuria* with a urine concentration which remains iso- or hypotonic. Plasma potassium is low, and to compensate for this there is a shift of potassium from the intracellular space to the plasma and extracellular space, and a reverse shift of hydrogen and sodium ions from the extracellular space into the cells. The loss of hydrogen ions from the plasma results in a rise in plasma bicarbonate, one other cause of alkalosis in pyloric obstruction.

*Sodium loss.* There is an overall sodium deficiency mainly due to the vomiting of sodium in the gastric juice, but compared with the extracellular fluid, vomit contains relatively more water than sodium so that the concentration of plasma sodium sometimes rises. Usually, however, the patient's thirst forces him to drink water, and this selective partial replacement of water to the exclusion of sodium and the rise in plasma ADH due to the lowered blood volume lower the plasma concentration of sodium below normal.

If sodium and potassium deficiency become sufficiently severe the *urine is acid*, though the plasma is becoming increasingly alkaline. This is due to the lack of available potassium on the cation exchange mechanism in the distal tubule. If sodium reabsorption is nearly complete and there is no available potassium, some of the sodium ions reabsorbed in the distal tubule will be replaced by hydrogen ions and the urine will become acid. This phenomenon must also be related to the raised concentration of hydrogen ions within the tubule cells.

*Chronic renal disease.* It is obvious that if there is some antecedent impairment of renal function the onset of pyloric obstruction and vomiting will cause a rapid deterioration of renal function.

*Alkalis and milk.* The most frequent accompaniment of pyloric obstruction is peptic ulceration, for which patients have been taking both alkalis and milk. Once glomerular filtration rate begins to fall because of dehydration or potassium deficiency, the continued administration of sodium bicarbonate is not only useless but rapidly aggravates the alkalosis. The high intake of calcium which accompanies the large ingestion of milk and certain alkalis, such as calcium carbonate, may cause hypercalcaemia or at least hypercalcuria which is an additional cause for the renal failure and also for the rise in plasma bicarbonate.

*Treatment of metabolic and renal consequences for pyloric obstruction*

Upon admission to hospital, most patients with benign pyloric obstruction cease to vomit and quickly begin to correct their electrolyte and water deficiencies almost unaided. During the first few days it is customary to wash out the stomach before meals. Water and food then pass through the pylorus and are absorbed in normal amounts; in such patients it is only necessary to make sure that they are given a mixed diet and that it is relatively low in protein until the glomerular filtration returns to normal levels.

Occasionally, however, it may be necessary to accelerate recovery by giving electrolytes and water intravenously or in additional amounts by mouth. Istonic saline is given intravenously in sufficient quantities to correct haemo-concentration, peripheral vein constriction and tachycardia. The administration of isotonic saline not only corrects the depletion of the extra-cellular fluid volume but also provides at least 40 mmol of chloride per litre to correct the chloride deficiency. (One litre of isotonic saline contains 150 mmol of sodium and 150 mmol of chloride while plasma contains 140 mmol/l of sodium and 100 mmol/l of chloride.) Once the volume of the extracellular fluid is replenished the continued administration of saline rapidly cures any remaining chloride-deficiency metabolic alkalosis, for the sodium ion is excreted while the chloride is retained. It is always important to give potassium by mouth even if plasma potassium concentration is normal, for, because of the alkalosis, there may be potassium deficiency without much change in plasma potassium. If plasma potassium concen-tration is unequivocally decreased potassium chloride should be given intra-venously in combination with isotonic saline or 5% glucose. When there is severe potassium deficiency, sodium chloride should not be given without giving potassium simultaneously, for the administration of sodium chloride may increase the urinary excretion of potassium.

It is unnecessary and perhaps harmful to use ammonium chloride for the correction of a metabolic alkalosis due to vomiting. Surgery should be avoided until renal function has recovered and there is no longer any evidence of electrolyte abnormalities.

## METABOLIC ACIDOSIS

### Metabolic acidosis with a normal 'anion gap' (p. 92) due to gastro-intestinal or urinary loss of bicarbonate (hyperchloraemic acidosis)

The commonest gastrointestinal cause of this condition is diarrhoea or small bowel, biliary and pancreatic external fistulae. Ureteric sigmoidostomy, which used to be performed in patients with pre-existing renal disease, is another gastrointestinal cause. It is described below. Renal tubular acidosis is a urinary cause of hyperchloraemic acidosis.

### Ureterosigmoidostomy

When the bladder is severely diseased it may be necessary to transplant the ureters. They can be placed so that they open either on the skin surface, into the large bowel or into an isolated segment of the small bowel. When they are placed into the sigmoid, faecal material refluxes up the ureters and causes recurrent urinary infections. In addition as the urine passes down the sigmoid the gut reabsorbs some of the urinary chloride and urea, and adds some bicarbonate. The reabsorption of urea is responsible for a rise in blood urea regardless of any change in renal function. It is distinguished from a rise in blood urea due to a depression in glomerular filtration by estimating the plasma creatinine, for creatinine is not absorbed from the bowel. The absorption of chloride from the gut and the secretion, and thus the alimentary loss, of bicarbonate causes the hyperchloraemic acidosis.

The acidosis is greatly aggravated by the simultaneous absorption of ammonium salts (p. 97) formed from the urine by urea-splitting bacteria in the urine. The steady infusion of urine into the colon can therefore be looked upon as equivalent to a continuous infusion of ammonium chloride. In addition to the acidosis the other important complications of ureterocolic anastomosis is potassium deficiency from excess loss of potassium in the faeces. It is not clear whether this is due to the inevitable pyelonephritis which accompanies this operation so that increased quantities of urinary potassium are delivered into the lumen of the bowel, or whether it is caused by the loss of large quantities of colonic mucus (which has a high concen-. tration of potassium) in the faeces due presumably to irritation of the bowel by urine.

If the patient is not to become acidotic and oedematous (from the sodium reabsorption) the kidneys have to compensate for the intestinal reabsorption by excreting increased quantities of urea, sodium chloride, hydrogen ions and particularly ammonium. After a few months the initial difference between the rates of chloride and sodium reabsorption becomes less marked and the tendency to acidosis ceases. This compensation is accompanied by marked hypertrophy of the kidneys.

Renal infections may be accompanied by partial or complete ureteric obstruction (occasionally both of these may have been present before oper-ation, due to the disease in the bladder). Both infection and ureteric obstruc-tion impair tubular function, including the ability to excrete hydrogen and ammonium, so that they may cause a rapid onset of severe acidosis. Infec-tion may also cause a urinary leak of potassium (p. 280). The nausea of acidosis diminishes the spontaneous intake of water and potassium and eventually it may cause vomiting, considerable dehydration, and contraction of the extracellular fluid volume. Dehydration, renal infection, ureteric obstruction and acidosis can each depress glomerular filtration rate; together they may rapidly cause death from acute renal failure. Alternatively, the patient may present with hypokalaemic paralysis, the symptoms of potas-sium deficiency being always more severe if there is an associated acidosis as opposed to the usual accompaniment to potassium deficiency which is an extracellular alkalosis.

These hazards are encountered most frequently immediately, or very soon, after operation. Occasionally a patient may remain well for several months and then suddenly become ill and develop an acidotic coma in a few days. It is probable that these relapses are due to an exacerbation of renal infection.

## Treatment

*Prophylactic*. Alkalis and a gut antibiotic are given during the post-oper-ative period (e.g. sodium bicarbonate 9 g/day and neomycin). Plasma elec-trolyte estimations should be made at frequent intervals and potassium given if necessary. For the first few days a catheter is kept in the rectum to shorten the time during which the urine is in contact with the mucous membrane of the bowel. Later, in order to diminish the hyperchloraemia and raise the plasma bicarbonate the supply of sodium and of chloride in the food is cut back and about 5 g of sodium bicarbonate per day is substituted. The patient is also told to allow the urine to escape from the rectum at frequent intervals.

*Curative.* If the patient subsequently complains of mild nausea, tiredness and headache, the administration of alkalis is increased (e.g. sodium bicarbonate 3 g eight-hourly), a low-salt diet is given, and a course of antibiotics should be given even if there is no overt evidence of renal infection.

When the symptoms are more severe and include vomiting, dehydration and clouding of consciousness, the rapid administration of 1/6 molar sodium bicarbonate intravenously, alternating with 5% glucose, if necessary, will usually cause a quick return of consciousness. If the renal damage is reversible the blood urea will also quickly return to normal. Antibiotics to treat the presumed urine infection are again administered together with large quantities of sodium bicarbonate by mouth until the plasma bicarbonate is normal.

## Ureteroileostomy

If the ureters are placed in an isolated segment of the ileum which empties into the bladder, most of the complications listed above can be avoided. The hazards are similar to those in ureterosigmoidostomy and for the same reasons, but they occur less frequently and are less severe. This is because the urine is only in contact with the small segment of the ileum for a shorter time. And the intraluminal pressures in this segment are much lower than in the colon so that reflux is less of a problem.

## Metabolic acidosis with an increased 'anion gap'

This condition is due to (a) increased endogenous acid production (e.g. ketoacids and lactic acid), (b) inability to excrete acid (e.g. renal failure) or (c) the ingestion of a toxic substance such as salicylates, methanol, and ethylene glycol.

## The renal disturbances of diabetic ketoacidosis

The urine in diabetic ketosis is acid and is characterised by an increased excretion of glucose, water, sodium potassium and the relatively strong acids, β-hydroxybutyric acid, acetoacetic acid and short chain fatty ketoacids. In severe cases there is metabolic acidosis, severe dehydration with a raised plasma sodium concentration, and a contraction of the extracellular fluid volume and the blood volume. The metabolic acidosis is caused principally by an accumulation of ketones due to an increased rate of ketone production, and ultimately there may also be some impairment in the kidney's ability to excrete hydrogen ions and ammonia. This impairment is due to both the sodium and potassium deficiencies which follow a prolonged osmotic glucose diuresis (Fig. 19.6). Potassium deficiency diminishes the tubule's ability to form a urine of maximum acidity which reduces the transfer of ammonia from the tubule cell to the tubule lumen. And severe sodium deficiency decreases the tubule's capacity to form ammonia. In consequence the acidosis is increased and the ketones in the urine are excreted with sodium and potassium ions, thus aggravating their deficiencies. Although there is an overall potassium deficiency there is often a shift of potassium out of the cells so that the concentration of plasma potassium tends to be raised, a phenomenon which is reversed by the administration of insulin. There is also a substantial loss of phosphate.

The loss of salt and water causes contraction of the extracellular fluid space and the blood volume; renal vasoconstriction follows and there is a reduction in renal blood flow and glomerular filtration rate, with a rise in blood urea. The fall in glomerular filtration rate also reduces the urinary excretion of ketones, and this further aggravates the metabolic acidosis. Occasionally, in very severe cases, filtration may fall to such a low rate that all the glucose *and ketones* which are filtered are reabsorbed by the tubules and none appear in the urine; this may cause considerable diagnostic confusion. The fall in glomerular filtration is also due in part to potassium deficiency, and this probably accounts for the slow recovery of renal function that sometimes follows the treatment of diabetic ketosis with only saline and insulin.

Acute renal failure with acute tubular necrosis may occur in the most severe cases.

The diagnosis of ketoacidosis may be missed because (a) the hyperglycaemia is relatively modest (e.g. below 20 mmol/l (350 mg/100 ml) (b) the plasma Acetest reaction is negative or only weekly positive because the acetoacetic acid has been converted to the β-hydroxybutyrate which the Acetest reaction does not detect, and (c) the anion gap may be normal in some patients with mild ketoacidosis.

*Treatment*

Insulin and antibiotics are given first, but to improve renal function it is essential to correct rapidly the negative sodium, water, potassium, phosphate and sometimes magnesium balances. At first large quantities of isotonic sodium chloride and sodium bicarbonate (p. 323) are administered intravenously, and when the blood glucose has begun to settle, 5% glucose is also given. It is unwise to give potassium solutions intravenously until, or unless, the urine flow is brisk, and the acute phase of the ketosis has

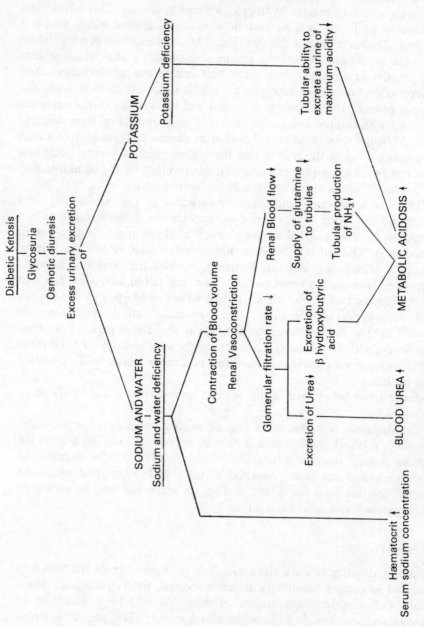

**Fig. 19.6** Renal disturbances and their consequence in diabetic ketosis.

passed, for the concentration of plasma potassium is often very high (see above).

These measures (except for potassium administration) are undertaken even in the presence of acute oliguria, for though they may be too late to prevent the development of acute tubular necrosis, their administration may limit the extent of the damage. Sometimes the blood pressure is very low, when it must be raised with blood transfusions, for a combination of renal vasoconstriction and hypotension is particularly likely to cause complete renal ischaemia and necrosis (p. 139). In most instances the blood pressure rises and the urine flow returns within a few hours of giving saline, and it becomes clear that acute tubular necrosis has not occurred.

BIBLIOGRAPHY

**Sodium**
Dirks, J H, Seely J F, Levy M 1976 Control of extracellular fluid volume and the pathophysiology of oedema formation. In: Brenner B M, Rector F C (eds) The kidney. Saunders, Philadelphia, p 495
Lipsett M B, Pearson O H 1958 Sodium depletion in adrenalectomised humans. J Clin Invest 37: 1394
Myers M G, Kearns P M, Kennedy D S et al 1978 Postural hypotension and diuretic therapy in the elderly. Canad Med Assoc J 119: 581
Schmidt R W, Bourgoignie J J, Bricker N S 1974 On the adaptation in sodium excretion in chronic uremia. The effects of a 'proportional reduction' of sodium intake. J Clin Invest 53: 1736
Thorn G W, Koepf G F, Clinton M 1944 Renal failure stimulating adrenocortical insufficiency. New Eng J Med 231: 76
Walker W G, Jost L J, Kowarski A et al 1968 Aldosterone secretion and sodium balance in salt-losing nephropathy. John Hopkins Med J 122: 45
de Wardener H E 1978 The control of sodium excretion. Amer J Physiol 235: F163
Welt L G 1959 Clinical Disorders of hydration and acid-base balance. Little Brown

**Potassium**
Brezis M, Litvin Y 1977 Syndrome of hyporeninemia and hypoaldosteronism. Study of two cases and review of the literature. Israel J Med Sci 13: 1013
Cannon P J, Ames R P, Laragh J H 1966 Relation between potassium balance and aldosterone secretion in normal subjects and in patients with hypertensive or renal tubular disease. J Clin Invest 45: 865
Elkinton J R 1952 Potassium physiologic classification, diagnosis and treatment of clinical disturbances. Advances in medicine and surgery, graduate School of Medicine, University of Pennsylvania. Saunders W B, Philadelphia.
Graeff J de, Schuurs M A M 1960 Severe potassium depletion caused by the abuse of laxatives. Acta Med Scand 166: 407
Graeff J de, Struyvenberg A, Lameijer L D F 1964 The role of chloride in hypokalaemic alkalosis. Amer J Med 37: 778
Knochel J P 1977 Role of glucoregulatory hormones in potassium homeostasis. Kidney Int 11: 443
Morgan D B, Davidson C 1980 Hypokalaemia and diuretics: an analysis of publications Brit Med J 280: 905
Stetson D L, Wade J B, Giebisch G 1980 Morphologic alterations in the rat medullary collecting duct following potassium depletion. Kidney Int 17: 45
Wallace M, Richards P, Chesser E et al 1968 Persistent alkalosis and hypokalaemia caused by surreptitious vomiting. Quart J Med 37: 577
Welt L G, Hollander W Jr, Blythe W B 1960 The consequences of potassium depletion. J Chron Dis 11: 213

**Calcium**

Adams P H 1982 Conservative management of primary hyperparathyroidism. J Roy Coll of Phys of London 16: 184

Barbour G L, Coburn J W, Slatopolsky E et al 1981 Hypercalcaemia in an anephric patient with sarcoidosis: Evidence for extrarenal generation of 1,25 dihydroxy Vitamin D. New Eng J Med 305: 440

Broadus A E, Horst R L, Lang R et al 1980 The importance of circulating 1,25-dihydroxy vitamin D in the pathogenesis of hypercalciuria and renal-stone formation in primary hyperparathyrodism. New Eng J Med 302: 421

Burnett C H, Commons R R, Albright F et al 1949 Hypercalcaemia without hypercalcuria or hypophosphataemia, calcinosis and renal insufficiency. A syndrome following prolonged intake of milk and alkali. New Eng J Med 240: 787

Epstein F H 1960 Calcium and the kidney. J Chron Dis 11: 255

Guignard J P, Jones N F, Barraclough M A 1970 Effect of brief hypercalcaemia on free water reabsorption during solute diuresis. Evidence for impairment of Na⁺ transport in Henle's loop. Clin Sci 39: 337

Leading article 1960 Idiopathic hypercalcaemia of infants. Lancet 2: 138

McQueen E G 1952 Milk poisoning and calcium gout. Lancet 2: 67

Papapoulos S E, Fraher L J, Sandler L M et al 1979 1,25 dihydroxycholecalciferol in the pathogenesis of the hypercalcaemia of sarcoidosis. Lancet i: 627

Richet G, Ardaillou R, Arneil Cl 1963 Alcalose métabolique rénale de l'hypercalémie. Actualités néphrologiques de l'hopital Necker. Ed. Médicales Flammarion Paris: p 145

Serros E R, Kirschenbaum M A 1981 Prostaglandin-dependent polyuria in hypercalcemia Amer J Physiol 241: F.224

Sherwood L M 1980 The multiple causes of hypercalcaemia in malignant disease. (Editorial) N Eng J Med 303: 1412

Shulman L E, Schoenrich E H, Harvey A M 1952 The effects of adrenocorticotropic hormone (ACTH) and cortisone on sarcoidosis. Bull John Hopk Hosp 91: 371

**Magnesium**

MacIntyre I, Hanna S, Booth C C et al 1960 Intracellular magnesium deficiency in man. Clin Sci 20: 297

Sheehan J, White A 1982 Diuretic-associated hypomagnesaemia. Brit Med J 285: 1157

Shils M E 1964 Experimental human magnesium depletion. Amer J Clin. Nutrit 15: 133

**Metabolic acidosis**

Espinel C H (1975) The influence of salt intake on the metabolic acidosis of chronic renal failure. J Clin Inves 56: 286

Garella S, Dana C L, Chazan J A 1973 Severity of metabolic acidosis as a determinant of bicarbonate requirements. New Eng J Med 289: 121

Oh M S, Carroll H J 1977 The anion gap. New Eng J Med 297: 814

**Ureteric transplant**

Annis D, Alexander M K 1952 Differential absorption of electrolytes from the large bowel in relation to uretero-sigmoid anastomosis. Lancet 2: 603

Care A D, Reed G W, Pyrah L N 1957 Changes in the reabsorption of sodium and chloride ions after uretero-colic anastomosis. Clin Sci 16: 95

Fowler D I, Cooke W T, Brooke B N et al 1959 Ileostomy and electrolyte excretion. Amer J dig Dis 4: 710

Jude J R, Harris A H, Smith R R 1959 The physiologic response to the ileal bladder. Surg Gynae and Obsttet 109: 173

Lowe K G, Stowers J M, Walker W F 1959 Electrolyte disturbances in patients with uretero-sigmoidostomy. Scot Med J 4: 473

Parsons F M, Powell F J N, Pyrah L N 1952 Chemical imbalance following ureterocolic anastomosis. Lancet 2: 599

Parsons F M, Pyrah L N, Powell F J N et al 1952 Chemical imbalance following ureterocolic anastomosis. Brit J Urol 24: 317

Pyrah L N 1954 Uretero-colic anastomosis. Ann Roy Coll Surg Eng 14: 169

Rosenberg M L 1953 Physiology of hyperchloremic acidosis following ureterosigmoidostomy: study of urinary reabsorption with radio-active isotopes. J Urol 70: Baltimore 569

Schwartz W B, Kassirer J P 1963 Effects of ureteral transplantation. In: Strauss M B, Welt L G J (eds) Diseases of the kidney. Churchill Livingstone, Edinburgh.

**Diabetic ketoacidosis**

Bernstein L M, Foley E F, Hoffman W S 1952 Renal function during and after diabetic coma. J Clin Invest 31: 711

Linton A L, Kennedy A C 1963 Diabetic ketosis complicated by acute renal failure. Postgrad Med 39: 364

McCance R A, Lawrence R D 1935 The secretion of urine in diabetic coma. Quart J Med 28: 53

Trever R W, Cluff L E 1958 The problem of increasing azotaemia during management of diabetic acidosis. Amer J Med 24: 368

**Metabolic alkalosis**

Gabow P A, Peterson L N 1980 Pathogenesis and management of metabolic acidosis and alkalosis. In: Schrier R W (ed) Renal and electrolyte disorders Little Brown and Brown and Co, Boston, p 183

Schwartz W B, Cohen J J 1978 The nature of the renal response to chronic disorders of acid-base equilibrium. Amer J Med 64: 417

**Pyloric obstruction**

Burnett C H, Burrows B A, Commons R R 1950 Studies of alkalosis: Renal function during and following alkalosis resulting from pyloric obstruction. J Clin Invest 29: 169

Burnett C H, Burrows B A, Commons R R et al 1950 Studies of alkalosis: Electrolyte abnormalities in alkalosis resulting from pyloric obstruction. J Clin Invest 29: 175

Cohen J J 1968 Correction of metabolic alkalosis by the kidney after isometric expansion of extracellular fluid. J Clin Invest 47: 1181

Graef de J, Struyvenberg A, Lameijer L D F 1964 The role of chloride in hypokalaemic alkalosis. Amer J Med 37: 778

Kassirer J P, Schwartz W B 1966 The response of normal man to selective depletion of hydrochloric acid. Amer J Med 40: 10

Kassirer J P, Schwartz W B 1966 Correction of metabolic alkalosis in man without repair of potassium deficiency. A revaluation of the role of potassium. Amer J Med 40: 19

Sanderson P H 1948 Renal failure following abdominal catastrophe and alkalosis. Clin Sci 6: 207

Seldin D W, Rector F C 1972 The generation and maintenance of metabolic alkalosis. Kidney Int 1: 306

van Goidsenhoven G M T, Gray O V, Price A V et al 1954 The effect of prolonged administration of large doses of sodium bicarbonate in man. Clin Sci 13: 383

# 20

# Tubular disorders

The most obvious and common forms of tubular disorders are those which accompany a reduction in the number of nephrons (chronic renal failure). There is, for instance, the tubule's inability to manufacture sufficient ammonium which leads to hydrogen ion retention, or the osmotic diuresis per nephron which is responsible for the inability to concentrate the urine normally. But there are, in addition, other causes of tubular disorders which occur independently of the number of nephrons and may often be accompanied with a normal glomerular filtration rate. These disorders tend to be confined either to the proximal, or the distal tubule or the collecting duct and in each site there may be one or more metabolic pathway abnormalities. The causes of these abnormalities may be congenital or acquired. On the whole the congenital causes lead to the more serious consequences.

## Functional tubular disorders of the proximal tubule

### Single metabolic pathway abnormalities

These include glycosuria, two forms of aminoaciduria, renal tubular acidosis Type II, hypercalciuria and possibly Gordon's and Bartter's syndrome, increased reabsorption of phosphate (pseudohypoparathyroidism) and increased reabsorption of calcium (familial hypocalciuric hypercalcaemia).

### Multiple metabolic pathway abnormalities (Fig. 20.1)

Fanconi was the first to draw attention to this condition. He described a syndrome consisting of a 'renal rickets,' glycosuria and phosphaturia. Since that time many other forms of metabolic bone disease associated with multiple defects of proximal tubule reabsorption have been described including not only impairment of glucose and phosphate reabsorption but also of amino acids, bicarbonate, peptides, low molecular weight proteins, uric acid, potassium and calcium. Today the term Fanconi syndrome is often applied when there are multiple defects of proximal tubule transport in the absence of bone disease. It has been suggested therefore that if the

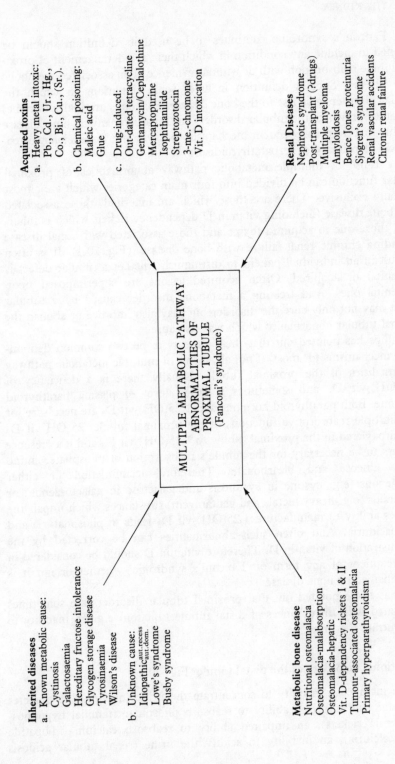

**Acquired toxins**
a. Heavy metal intoxic:
Pb, Cd, Ur, Hg,
Co, Bi, Cu, (Sr.).
b. Chemical poisoning:
Maleic acid
Glue
c. Drug-induced:
Out-dated tetracycline
Gentamycin/Cephalothine
Mercaptopurine
Isophthanilide
Streptozotocin
3-me.-chromone
Vit. D intoxication

**Renal Diseases**
Nephrotic syndrome
Post-transplant (?drugs)
Multiple myeloma
Amyloidosis
Bence Jones proteinuria
Sjogren's syndrome
Renal vascular accidents
Chronic renal failure

MULTIPLE METABOLIC PATHWAY
ABNORMALITIES OF
PROXIMAL TUBULE
(Fanconi's syndrome)

**Inherited diseases**
a. Known metabolic cause:
Cystinosis
Galactosaemia
Hereditary fructose intolerance
Glycogen storage disease
Tyrosinaemia
Wilson's disease
b. Unknown cause:
Idiopathic aut.recess
aut.dom.
Lowe's syndrome
Busby syndrome

**Metabolic bone disease**
Nutritional osteomalacia
Osteomalacia-malabsorption
Osteomalacia-hepatic
Vit. D-dependency rickets I & II
Tumour-associated osteomalacia
Primary hyperparathyroidism

**Fig. 20.1** Proximal tubule disorders.

term Fanconi's syndrome continues to be used its definition should be widened to include any condition in which there is a derangement of proximal tubule reabsorption with or without evidence of an associated metabolic bone disease. Such a definition includes some conditions in which the tubular disorders give rise to the bone disease (Fanconi's original syndrome) and others in which the tubular disorders and an accompanying bone disease are due to a third independent mechanism (e.g. vitamin D deficiency osteomalacia or primary hyperparathyroidism).

The cause of multiple metabolic pathway abnormalities of proximal tubular function can be divided into four main categories which are almost mutually exclusive. There are those which are inherited, those associated with bone disease (including vitamin D dependency rickets which is inherited), those due to acquired toxins and those associated with renal disease (including chronic renal failure with bone disease) (Fig. 20.1). It is often difficult in an individual patient to distinguish whether a tubular defect is congenital or acquired. Often acquired lesions are superimposed upon congenital ones. And treating a metabolic disorder caused by a tubular defect may not only cure the disorder but may also improve or abolish the original tubular abnormality which was its cause.

Phillips has pointed out that there appears to be two common denominator mechanisms for most, if not all, forms of multiple metabolic pathway abnormalities of the proximal tubule. Usually there is a deficiency of $1,25(OH)_2$vit $D_3$ and sometimes a raised level of plasma parathyroid hormone. Both parathyroid hormone and $1,25(OH)_2$vit $D_3$ are necessary for the multiple reabsorptive functions of the proximal tubule. 25 OH vit $D_3$ is hydroxylated in the proximal tubule to $1,25(OH)_2$vit $D_3$ and it's presence appears to be necessary for the tubule's reabsorption of phosphate, amino acids, glucose and bicarbonate. Therefore accumulation of either endogenous (e.g. cystine in cystinosis and galactose in galactosaemia) or exogenous (e.g. heavy metals and gentamycin) substances which impair the tubules ability to manufacture $1,25(OH)_2$vit $D_3$ leads to phosphaturia and aminoaciduria. And often such abnormalities can be corrected by the administration of vitamin D. Therefore vitamin D should be considered in the treatment of any form of 'Fanconi's syndrome' whether or not it is accompanied by bone disease.

It has to be pointed out that proximal tubular disorders are sometimes associated with disturbances of distal tubule function, e.g. an inability to concentrate the urine.

## Functional disorders of the distal tubule (Fig. 20.2)

These include an inability to concentrate the urine (nephrogenic diabetes insipidus), an impaired ability to reabsorb phosphate (familial hypophosphataemic rickets), an impaired ability to reabsorb calcium (idiopathic hypercalciuria), an inability to acidify the urine (renal tubular acidosis

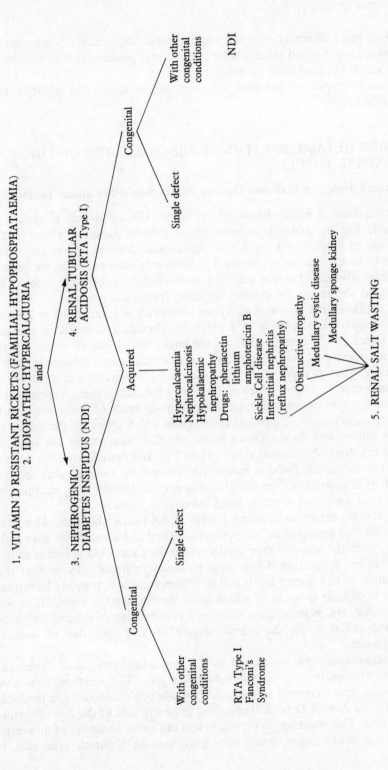

**Fig. 20.2** Distal tubular disorders.

1. VITAMIN D RESISTANT RICKETS (FAMILIAL HYPOPHOSPHATAEMIA)
2. IDIOPATHIC HYPERCALCIURIA
   and
3. NEPHROGENIC DIABETES INSIPIDUS (NDI)
4. RENAL TUBULAR ACIDOSIS (RTA Type I)
5. RENAL SALT WASTING

**Nephrogenic Diabetes Insipidus (NDI)**

Congenital — With other congenital conditions — RTA Type I, Fanconi's Syndrome

Single defect

Congenital — Single defect

Congenital — With other congenital conditions — NDI

Acquired:
Hypercalcaemia
Nephrocalcinosis
Hypokalaemic nephropathy
Drugs: phenacetin
       lithium
       amphotericin B
Sickle Cell disease
Interstitial nephritis
(reflux nephropathy)

Obstructive uropathy
Medullary cystic disease
Medullary sponge kidney

Type I) and a difficulty retaining sodium (renal salt wasting). Nephrogenic diabetes insipidus and renal tubular acidosis may be congenital or acquired. The acquired forms often co-exist.

Some examples of proximal tubule disorders single and multiple are described below.

## SINGLE METABOLIC PATHWAY ABNORMALITIES OF THE PROXIMAL TUBULE

### Impaired ability to reabsorb Cystine and certain other amino acids

This condition is usually known as cystinuria. The metabolism of cystine is normal, but an isolated abnormality of tubular function allows large amounts of cystine, and the dibasic amino acids arginine, lysine and ornithine to be excreted in the urine. The disease is inherited as an autosomal recessive disorder. Patients suffering from cystinuria also have a defect of intestinal absorption for cystine, arginine, lysine and ornthine.

In cystinuria the excretion of cystine averages 2 to 4 mmol (0.5 to 1 g per day). A solution of cystine at a pH 5 to 7 becomes saturated at around 1.25 mmol to 1.7 mmol/l (300 to 400 mg/l), and tends to come out of solution when it is acid. In patients with cystinuria it is extremely likely, therefore, that at night when the urine is both concentrated and acid it becomes supersaturated, which explains why the clinical complication of the disease is the recurrent formation of renal calculi made of cystine which are usually radio opaque. The other amino acids which appear in the urine are freely soluble and do not form calculi, nor does their excess loss seem to cause any detectable clinical abnormality. The first cystine stone commonly presents during childhood or infancy; it is rare for it to do so after the age of 30. It is a surprising feature of cystinuria that though renal calculi may recur over a number of years, renal infection is unusual.

*Treatment* consists in drinking 3 litres of fluid throughout the 24 hours, including two glasses of water upon going to bed and another two after midnight, when the first two have usually forced the patient out of bed to empty his bladder. It is claimed that such treatment will not only prevent the formation of new stones but it will also 'dissolve' those present. Nevertheless it is difficult to maintain a high urine flow during the night. If, on the other hand, this is insufficient to prevent precipitation of cystine, the urine is made alkaline by the administration of 15 g per day of sodium bicarbonate.

Cystinuria can also be treated by the oral administration of D-penicillamine at regular intervals throughout the day. The relatively insoluble cystine is then converted to the highly soluble penicillamine-cysteine-disulphide. The dose of D-penicillamine has to be adjusted to the rate of cystine excretion. This treatment is expensive and can cause a number of unwanted effects including rashes, fever, proteinuria and the nephrotic syndrome. It may sometimes be possible to combine a high intake of water during the day and a moderate dose of penicillamine during the night.

## Impaired ability to reabsorb the monoamino-mono-carboxylic amino acids (Hartnup's disease)

This disease is characterised by a pellagra-like rash after exposure to sunlight, transient attacks of cerebellar ataxia, and some accompanying emotional disturbances. The urine contains large amounts of the mono-amino-mono-carboxylic acids, alanine, valine and tryptophan, all of which share a common metabolic reabsorptive pathway in the proximal tubule. The intestinal absorption of these amino acids is also impaired. One prominent deficiency therefore is that of tryptophan so that less nicotinamide is synthethised which is the cause of the 'pellagra'. The tryptophan and other amino acids in the bowel which are not absorbed are broken down to toxic decomposition product which are absorbed and these cause the cerebral symptoms.

## Impaired ability to reabsorbed Xanthine

This condition is usually known as xanthinuria. It is due to two functional defects. First, an absence of xanthine oxidase in the liver so that the conversion of xanthine to uric acid is blocked; and, secondly, a tubular defect of xanthine reabsorption. The clearance of xanthine equals that of the glomerular filtration rate. Large quantities of xanthine therefore appear in the urine but only traces of uric acid, and the blood uric acid is exceedingly low. Occasionally, xanthine renal calculi, translucent to X-rays, may be formed. As xanthine is much more soluble in alkaline urine, treatment consists in the administration of sodium citrate or bicarbonate to those patients who are apt to form stones.

## Impaired ability to reabsorb sodium (Bartter's syndrome) (Fig. 20.3)

This syndrome is probably due to an impaired ability of either the proximal tubule or the ascending loop of Henle to reabsorb sodium or chloride. The patient persistently suffers from a shrunken extra cellular fluid volume and blood volume. There is therefore a high plasma renin activity and a high plasma aldosterone. The excess sodium reaching the distal tubule increases potassium and hydrogen ion secretion while the raised plasma aldosterone further increases urinary potassium excretion. The net effect is a hypo-kalaemic alkalosis. The raised aldosterone increases the urinary excretion of kallikrein which promotes a raised production of prostaglandin $E_2$ as does the raised level of angiotensin II and the low plasma potassium. Renal biopsy reveals grossly hypertrophied juxta glomerular apparati. All these findings stem from the persistently reduced extracellular fluid volume. They

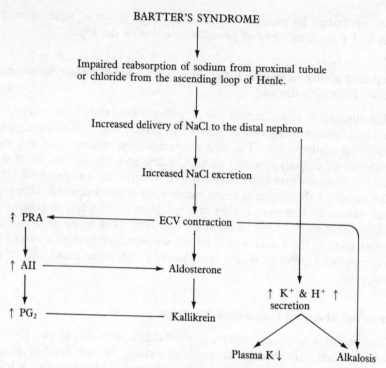

BARTTER'S SYNDROME

Impaired reabsorption of sodium from proximal tubule
or chloride from the ascending loop of Henle.

Increased delivery of NaCl to the distal nephron

Increased NaCl excretion

↑ PRA ← ECV contraction

↑ AII → Aldosterone

↑ PG₂ — Kallikrein

↑ K⁺ & H⁺ ↑
secretion

Plasma K ↓          Alkalosis

**Fig. 20.3** A proposed sequence of events in Bartter's syndrome. (Derived from Seldin 1981 In: Brenner B, Rector F C (eds) The kidney. Saunders, Philadelphia, p 17.) PRA = plasma renin activity; AII = angiotensin II; $PG_{E2}$ = prostaglandin $E_2$.

can also be induced by the continuous administration of a diuretic such as frusemide. The observation that the condition is sometimes familial, tends to occur in young male children and appears to be accompanied by abnormalities of red cell sodium transport suggest that a primary condition of unknown cause does exist but it is usually best, particularly in an adult to have the urine examined for the presence of a diuretic.

*Treatment* consists of potassium replacement and the administration of indomethacin. The latter, by abolishing the vasodilating effect of the prostaglandins appears to relieve the condition temporarily but most patients relapse within a few weeks or months.

## Excess sodium reabsorption by the proximal tubule (Gordon's syndrome)

This is characterized by hypertension, an expanded extracellular fluid volume and hyperkalaemia. Aldosterone secretion and plasma renin are low and do not rise normally upon sodium deprivation. It is possible that this syndrome is due to excess sodium reabsorption by the proximal tubule, this expands the extra-cellular fluid which raises the blood pressure and lowers the plasma renin and aldosterone secretion rate. The increase in sodium reabsorption by the proximal tubule also lowers the delivery of sodium into the distal tubule, which together with the reduced plasma aldosterone, reduces the secretion of potassium by the distal tubule. Treatment consists of a low sodium diet and diuretics.

## Impaired ability to reabsorb bicarbonate (Type II renal tubular acidosis)

If the ability of the proximal tubule to reabsorb filtered bicarbonate is impaired increased amounts of sodium bicarbonate enter the distal tubule. Hydrogen ion excretion in the distal tubule is then mainly used to reclaim the bicarbonate, the urine pH rises and net hydrogen ion excretion falls. As acidosis becomes more severe and plasma bicarbonate falls filtered bicarbonate also falls until the proximal tubule is able to reabsorb most of the filtered bicarbonate, when the distal tubule, no longer flooded with bicarbonate can now acidify the urine again. The increased delivery of sodium bicarbonate into the distal tubule may give rise to hypokalaemia which is made worse by the tendency to sodium loss and hyperaldosteronism.

The condition is rarely seen without other abnormalities of the proximal tubule. Treatment consists of the oral administration of sodium bicarbonate and potassium.

## Impaired ability to reabsorb calcium (Idiopathic hypercalciuria)

This condition is characterized by a daily urinary calcium excretion greater than 10 mmol (400 mg). It can be demonstrated that this is associated with a raised fractional excretion of calcium, an increased calcium absorption from the gut, a rise in plasma $1,25(OH)_2$vit $D_3$, a normal or raised plasma parathyroid hormone concentration and a tendency for the plasma phosphate to be low. The condition was at one time thought to be due in part to a primary increase in calcium absorption from the gut, but this has been made very unlikely by the finding that plasma $1,25(OH)_2$vit $D_3$ is raised. A possible sequence of events is outlined in Figure 20.4.

The diagnosis of idiopathic hypercalciuria is confirmed if the urinary calcium is raised in the presence of a normal plasma calcium and in the absence of hyperparathyroidism, renal tubular acidosis, malignant disease, rapidly progressive bone disease, sarcoidosis, immobilisation, Paget's disease, Cushing's disease, medullary sponge kidney, frusemide administration or self administration of vit D preparations. The disease affects 2–4 per cent of normal adults. In about 90% of individuals it causes no problems, the others tend to develop renal stones.

*Treatment.* The formation of renal stones can largely be prevented by the daily administration of a thiazide (e.g. Bendrofluazide 5mg/day). This increases distal calcium reabsorption but has no direct effects on intestinal

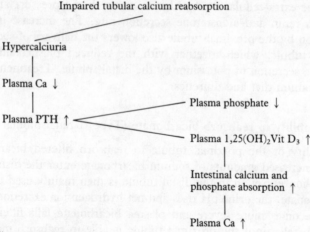

**Fig. 20.4** Idiopathic hypercalciuria.

calcium absorption. Nevertheless the diminution in urinary calcium excretion corrects the plasma calcium, which reduces plasma parathyroid hormone. This in turn lowers plasma $1,25(OH)_2$vit $D_3$ which diminishes intestinal calcium and phosphate absorption.

Dietary sodium intake and urinary output tend to be directly linked to urinary calcium excretion. It is important therefore to note the dietary intake of salt and to reduce it if it is excessive, particularly if there is some difficulty controlling the hypercalciuria.

### Excessive reabsorption of calcium (hypocalciuric familial hypercalcaemia)

This is a rare variant of a single metabolic pathway abnormality of the proximal tubule. In this benign condition there is hypercalcaemia with a relative hypocalciuria, i.e. urinary calcium excretion is within the normal range found in normal subjects with a normal plasma calcium. The fundamental functional lesion may be a generalised impaired response of the bodies tissues to ionised calcium. The main suggestive features leading to this conclusion are (1) that though plasma calcium is raised, plasma parathyroid hormone, tends to be either slightly raised or in the upper reaches of the normal range and (2) the remarkable lack of renal functional deterioration and lack of increased incidence of hypertension both of which accompany hypercalcaemia from other causes.

### Excessive reabsorption of phosphate (pseudohypoparathyroidism)

This condition like the one above does not appear to be an isolated abnormality of the proximal tubule. It is due to a failure of the receptors throughout the body to respond to parathyroid hormone with a normal increase in cyclic AMP. As a result there is an impairment in the urinary secretion of phosphate, plasma phosphate rises, plasma calcium falls and there is a compensatory rise in plasma parathyroid hormone. The unresponsiveness of the proximal tubule to the action of parathyroid hormone is also evident in that plasma $1,25(OH)_2$vit $D_3$ is low in spite of the raised plasma parathyroid hormone. And the low plasma $1,25(OH)_2$vit $D_3$ diminishes what residual effect plasma parathyroid hormone might have on bone reabsorption, for $1,25(OH)_2$vit $D_3$ is necessary for the osteoclastic action of parathyroid hormone.

Most cases are transmitted as a sex linked dominant disorder. Patients present with attacks of tetany or fits. They have characteristic round flat faces with a small bulbous nose, a thin straight mouth and strabismus; they also have short hands with stunted metacarpals. They are usually mentally retarded, of short stature and have cataracts. The diagnosis is brought to mind by the raised plasma phosphate, a low plasma calcium and confirmed by finding that the urinary excretion of cyclic AMP is not raised by an injection of parathyroid hormone.

Treatment is to raise the plasma calcium with $1,25(OH)_2$vit $D_3$ and oral calcium preparations.

## MULTIPLE METABOLIC PATHWAY ABNORMALITIES OF THE PROXIMAL TUBULE (Fig. 20.1)

### Cystinosis

This is a recessively inherited metabolic disturbance in which there is a high intracellular concentration of free cystine crystal deposition throughout the body. Their presence in the lysosomes of the proximal tubule give rise to aminoaciduria, glycosuria, phosphaturia and a bicarbonate leak. Deposition of cystine in the distal tubule leads to inability to concentrate and to acidify the urine.

The first signs of the disease appear in the first year of life with growth retardation, rickets, acidosis and hypokalaemia. There is thirst, polyuria and polydipsia. The rate of events depends on the rate of renal destruction. Glomerular filtration rate falls inexorably and death usually occurs before the age of 10 years, unless dialysed or transplanted.

### Vitamin D dependent rickets (Type I)

This is an inherited condition in which the proximal tubule has an impaired capacity to convert 25 OH vit $D_3$ to $1,25(OH)_2$vit $D_3$. It is inherited as a simple autosomal recessive trait. In contrast to vitamin D deficiency osteomalacia or rickets therefore in which plasma 25 OH vit $D_3$ is low and plasma $1,25(OH)_2$vit $D_3$ tends to be normal, in inherited vitamin D dependent rickets plasma 25 OH vit $D_3$ is normal and plasma $1,25(OH)_2$vit $D_3$ is low or undetectable. Otherwise the condition resembles that of vitamin D deficient rickets. The onset of symptoms usually occurs before the first year of life with hypotonia, weakness and failure to grow. There is mental retardation and failure to stand and walk. Some children have tetany. The characteristic signs are also present with bony deformities including bowing and thickening of the wrists and ankles. The X-rays are also typical except that the pelvis and spine are often involved in contrast to vitamin D deficient rickets.

Biochemically the hall mark of the condition is hypocalcaemia. Plasma parathyroid hormone and alkaline phosphatase are raised, faecal calcium is high and there is hypocalciuria. Plasma phosphate is normal or depressed but rarely to the levels found in familial hypophosphataemia with bone lesions. The depression of plasma phosphate is due to impaired intestinal absorption of phosphate and the tubular leak of phosptate. Aminoaciduria and bicarbonate loss also occur. It is not clear if the bone lesions which radiologically are described as those of 'rickets' are due to defect in the mineralization of the osteoid lamella lying closest to the bone trabeculae i.e. that the lesions are due to the absence of vitamin D metabolite or phosphate at the bone, or whether they are due to hyperparathyroidism. The hyperparathyroidism is caused by the hypocalcaemia which is itself due to the grossly impaired intestinal absorption of calcium. As has been stated elsewhere (p. 195) the radiological appearances of 'rickets' can be caused by both vitamin D deficiency and hyperparathyroidism.

*Treatment* consists of the administration of $1,25(OH)_2$vit $D_3$ in small 'physiological' amounts i.e. 0.5 to 1 $\mu g/24$ hr. The giving of cholecalciferol or 25 OH vit $D_3$ is irrational, but in the absence of $1,25$ OH$_2$ vit $D_3$ the administration of cholecalciferol in large amounts and raising the plasma level of $25(OH)$vit $D_3$ to very high levels will eventually increase intestinal calcium absorption and reverse the condition.

There is another condition, known as vitamin dependent rickets Type II which clinically and biochemically ressembles vitamin D dependent rickets Type I but in which the lesion is due to an end organ unresponsiveness to $1,25(OH)_2$vit $D_3$. Plasma $1,25(OH)_2$vit $D_3$ therefore is very high and plasma 25 OH vit $D_3$ is normal. The aim of treatment is to raise the plasma $1,25(OH)_2$vit $D_3$ to even higher levels with massive doses of $1,25(OH)_2$vit $D_3$ e.g. 20 $\mu g$/day or higher.

## Idiopathic childhood and adult forms of Fanconi's syndrome

The childhood form makes its appearance between 1 and 2 years of age. It is inherited by autosomal recessive transmission. Microdissection of nephrons reveals that the first part of the proximal tubule adjoining the glomerulus is thin and wasted: the so-called swan-neck deformity. There is also a decrease in the number of microvilli of the proximal tubule cells and abnormalities of the mitochondria. The condition consists of 'renal rickets', glycosuria and phosphaturia. Prognosis is relatively good in that renal failure is unusual. Treatment is symptomatic correcting the consequences of the tubular leaks if they are severe.

The idiopathic form in adults is present between the ages of 20 and 40 years. The genetic links can be autosomal dominant or autosomal recessive and the disease can occur in siblings. Bone symptoms and ill-defined lesions called adult rickets are described. The main difficulty is to make certain that the condition is truly idiopathic and not secondary to one of the known causes of Fanconi's syndrome.

## Tumourous phosphaturic osteomalacia

This is an extremely rare condition of immense interest. Patients present with phosphate depletion, histologically confirmed osteomalacia and severe hypophosphataemia associated with a tumour, which usually grows slowly and is of vascular and of mesenchymal origin situated in bone, skin or subcutaneous tissues. There is also a raised alkaline phosphatase, hyper-phosphaturia, glycosuria and aminoaciduria. Plasma calcium tends to be normal. The condition appears to be due to a substance secreted from the tumour which appears to inhibit the conversion of 25OHvit $D_3$ to $1,25(OH)_2$vit $D_3$ so that plasma $1,25(OH)_2$vit $D_3$ is low.

The patient presents with generalized bone pain with proximal myopathy. Administration of $1,25(OH)_2$vit $D_3$ induces a remission and removal of the tumour cures the condition.

## Proximal tubule lesions in chronic renal failure

Aminoaciduria (Fig. 20.5), glycosuria and bicarbonaturia from the proximal tubule occur in advanced chronic renal failure. The aminoaciduria can be reversed by the administration of $1,25(OH)_2$vit $D_3$. It has not yet been established whether the administered $1,25(OH)_2$vit $D_3$ has any effect on the glycosuria, or diminishes the bicarbonate leak which is due at least in part to the raised plasma parathyroid hormone levels.

## Proximal tubule lesions in the nephrotic syndrome

In the first few days of relapse of a nephrotic syndrome, as the proteinuria increases, there is hypocalciuria, a diminished absorption of calcium and a fall in plasma $1,25(OH)_2$vit $D_3$. Aminoaciduria and glycosuria also appear early. One has the impression that this sequence may be due to a disruption to $1,25(OH)_2$vit $D_3$ manufacture caused by the massive reabsorption and digestion, by the proximal tubule, of the proteins leaked into the tubule by the diseased glomerulus.

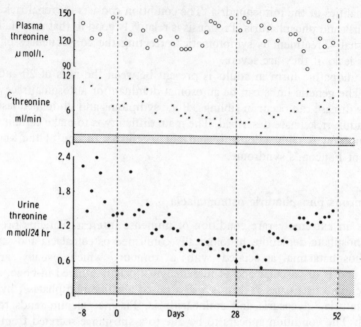

**Fig. 20.5** Aminoaciduria in chronic renal failure (creatinine clearance 12 ml/min). The clearance of threonine is raised and there is an increase of threonine in the urine. The oral administration of $1,25(OH)_2$vit $D_3$ between 0 and 28 days produced a reversible improvement without a significant change in plasma threonine. (Reproduced from Phillips 1980 CRC Crit Rev Clin Lab Sci 12: 215, with kind permission.)

## FUNCTIONAL DISORDERS OF THE DISTAL TUBULE

### Impaired ability to concentrate the urine (nephrogenic diabetes insipidus)

This condition can be congenital or acquired. The congenital form is described on page 305. The acquired form is usually a minor complication which may accompany a wide variety of conditions including hypokalaemia and the administration of lithium (Fig. 20.5). The acquired form is usually combined with some degree of inability to acidify the urine and in addition there is a group of conditions which include reflux nephropathy, obstructive uropathy, medullary cystic disease and medullary sponge kidney in which the inability to concentrate the urine is associated with some difficulty in retaining sodium (renal salt wasting).

### Impaired ability to acidify the urine (renal tubular acidosis Type I)

There is an inability to lower the urine pH below 5.3 in the presence of a relatively normal glomerular filtration rate (Fig. 20.6). The lowest pH the urine will fall to spontaneously is round 6.0 to 6.9 whereas in normal

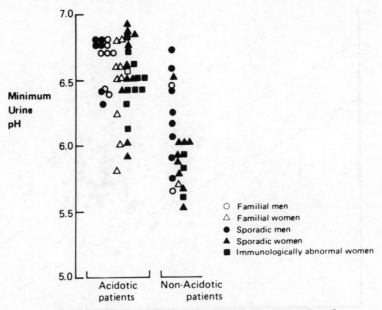

**Fig. 20.6** Minimum urine pH in 67 patients with renal tubular acidosis Type I. (Reproduced from: Feast & Wrong 1982 Jones N F, Peters D K (eds) Recent advances in renal medicine. Churchill Livingstone, Edinburgh, p 243, with kind permission.)

subjects it often falls well below 5.0. The hereditary form is familial and is usually inherited as an autosomal dominant. The syndrome may be complete or incomplete. In the complete syndrome there is hyperchloraemic acidosis, nephrocalcinosis and renal stones with osteomalacia or rickets, a tendency to lose potassium and sodium and a defect of urine concentration. In the incomplete form there is no systemic acidosis presumably because the renal disposal of hydrogen ions, although impaired, is sufficient to deal with the metabolic load of hydrogen ions. These non-acidotic cases present clinically with nephrocalcinosis, or potassium depletion. The conditions which give rise to the acquired form of renal tubular acidosis Type I (RTA Type I) are much the same as those that give rise to the acquired form of nephrogenic diabetes insipidus with one major addition. About 30% of the acquired cases of RTA Type I are linked to some autoimmune disorder in which there is an associated hyperglobulinaemia including biliary cirrhosis, thyroid disease and Sjögren's syndrome. The raised serum gamma globulin is usually IgG and is directed against smooth muscle, thyroid fraction, antinuclear factor and the Rose Waaler antibody.

*Pathophysiology*

The impaired ability of the kidney to acidify the urine is due to the tubule's inability to maintain a normal hydrogen ion gadient. Either the tubule

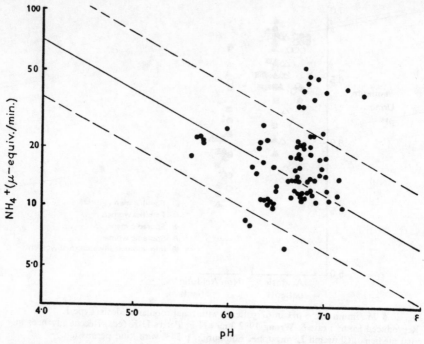

**20.7** Renal tubular acidosis. Relation between the excretion of ammonium and urine pH. The calculated regression line and 95 per cent range in normal individuals are shown. Each point represents an observation made in a patient suffering from renal tubular acidosis after the oral ingestion of a single dose of ammonium chloride. (Reproduced from Wrong & Davies 1959 Quart J Med 28: 259, with kind permission.)

cannot secrete hydrogen ions against a rising gradient or there is an increased back diffusion of hydrogen ions from the tubule cells. The functional lesion is not an impairment in the rate at which the tubule can secrete hydrogen ion. On the other hand the tubule's capacity to secrete ammonia and raise ammonium excretion does vary (Fig. 20.7), and those patients who cannot raise their rate of ammonium excretion sufficiently become acidotic. Inasmuch as patients with the same impairment in their ability to acidify can be either acidotic or not acidotic, and as the difference depends on their compensatory ability to excrete ammonium is appears that in renal tubular acidosis Type I there may be at least two functional lesions, one is an impaired ability to maintain a hydrogen ion gradient, and the other is an impaired ability to compensate for this 'first' lesion by increasing the rate of secretion of ammonia to sufficient heights.

The loss of sodium and potassium is often directly linked to the acidotic state and can be prevented by the administration of alkalis. But in some patients it appears to be a further functional abnormality of the tubule for it cannot be controlled by the administration of alkalis. In those in whom the loss of sodium and potassium appears to be primarily due to the metabolic acidosis, for it can be prevented by the administration of alkals, it is probable that the acidosis induces a diminution in sodium reabsorption in the proximal tubule, possibly as a result of a decrease in bicarbonate linked sodium reabsorption. Consequently sodium delivery into the distal tubule rises and this stimulates the exchange of potassium and hydrogen ions for the sodium. The exchange for hydrogen ions however, is limited by the 'first' functional lesion, thus the rise in potassium excretion is reciprocally greater. The overall result is one of increased sodium and potassium excretion. Sodium deficiency then stimulates aldosterone excretion which aggravates the urinary potassium loss.

The cause of the nephrocalcinosis and stone formation is unknown. Renal calculi occur in about two thirds of the patients giving rise to recurrent renal colic and haematuria. The incidence is the same in the complete and incomplete forms of the disease. The calcium in the kidney is localised to the medulla. Among the contributory factors which may determine the laying down of calcium in the kidney are the high urinary pH which decreases the solubility of calcium phosphate, the tendency for the metabolic acidosis to increase urinary calcium excretion and the increased incidence of upper urinary infection. By far the most important probable cause of the nephrocalcinosis however, is the low urinary excretion of citrate. Citrate combines with urine calcium to form soluble complexes and in normal subjects there is usually sufficient citrate in the urine to complex the total daily urinary calcium output. Furthermore the secretion of citrate by the kidney normally rises as the urine pH rises. The majority of patients with renal tubular acidosis Type 1 have a reduced urinary citrate. As it is probable that the citrate originates from the tubule cells it seems that in renal tubular acidosis there are at least three and sometimes four functional abnormalties of the tubule. The mechanism responsible for the reduced citrate excretion is not known.

The bone lesions in renal tubular acidosis are equally difficult to understand. They consist mainly of osteomalacia together with mild hyperparathyroidism. Both can be cured by the administration of alkalis and do not occur in incomplete cases i.e. those patients who suffer from the inability to acidify the urine but who are not acidotic. It appears therefore that the bone lesions are due to the acidosis. The hyperparathyroidism may just possibly be due to the tendency for hypercalciuria induced by the acidosis but the connection between persistent metabolic acidosis in RTA Type I and osteomalacia is, in the present state of knowledge, incomprehensible.

*Treatment* consists in giving patients with the complete syndrome sufficient oral alkali to raise the plasma pH to normal while patients with the incomplete syndrome are only treated if they have nephrocalcinosis. The dose of sodium bicarbonate needed to prevent acidosis is in the range of 0.5–2 mmol/kg/day though much larger amounts may be necessary in some growing infants who not only have renal tubular acidosis Type I but also have bicarbonate wasting, a combination sometimes known as Type III renal tubular acidosis.

Most of the clinical problems of renal tubular acidosis stems from the renal stones so it is wise to look for evidence of urinary infection and ureteric obstruction at frequent intervals.

*Prognosis*

Renal function is relatively well preserved and few patients develop terminal renal failure. Parenchymatous destruction of the kidney is mainly due to the chronic inflammation surrounding the calcium deposits and episodes of ureteric obstruction. Occasionally recurrent upper urinary infections may also be important, and some patients in whom the disease is associated with an autoimmune disturbance may develop renal failure from an immunologically mediated chronic intestinal nephritis

## Impaired ability to acidify the urine (renal tubular acidosis Type IV)

These patients have hyperchloraemic acidosis with *hyperkalaemia*. The condition occurs in patients with hypoaldosteronism, usually due to deficient renin production, who also have some pre-existing impairment of renal function. The functional abnormality is probably an impaired ability to exchange sodium for potassium and hydrogen ion in the distal tubule. The first is responsible for the hyperkalaemia, the second for a small distal tubular leak of bicarbonate. The administration of 9αfludrocortisone corrects the acidosis and the hyperkalaemia but large amounts are needed which may cause sodium retention and hypertension. It may then be best to give a loop diuretic to treat the hyperkalaemia and small amounts of sodium bicarbonate to correct the bicarbonate leak.

## Excess sodium reabsorption by the distal tubule (Liddle's syndrome)

This syndrome is a familial disorder affecting individuals of both sexes and of succesive generations. There is hypertension, an expanded extracellular fluid volume and hypokalaemia, with a grossly reduced aldosterone secretion rate. It has been suggested that this syndrome is due to excess sodium reabsorption by the distal tubule of unknown cause. This causes the increase in the extra-cellular fluid volume which causes the hypertension and the reduced rate of aldosterone secretion. Accordingly the low plasma potassium is due to the excessive secretion of potassium from the distal tubule due to the excess sodium reabsorption. These renal abnormalities are associated with a demonstrable abnormality of sodium transport in the erythrocytes. Treatment consists of a low sodium diet and the diuretic Triamterene which acts on the distal tubule without increasing potassium excretion.

**Impaired ability to reabsorb phosphate** (vitamin D resistant rickets, familial hypophosphataemia)

The hypophosphataemia appears to be due to a hypersensitivity of the distal tubule to the phosphaturic effect of normal concentration of plasma parathyroid hormone for if plasma parathyroid hormone is lowered by artificially raising plasma calcium, phosphate reabsorption becomes normal and the urine may become free of phosphate. In addition there is an impaired ability of the proximal tubule's $1,25(OH)_2$vit $D_3$ production to respond to the stimulus of a low plasma phosphate. Plasma $1,25(OH)_2$vit $D_3$ therefore is either normal or low. This gives rise to the diminished calcium and phosphate absorption from the gut which exacerbates the hypophosphataemia and tends to lower the plasma ionised calcium concentration. Plasma parathyroid hormone therefore tends to be either normal or raised. If it is raised other abnormalities of the proximal tubule reabsorption may become manifest (p. 352). A proposed schema of the pathogenesis of familial hypophosphataemic reckets is illustrated in Figure 20.8.

The disease is nearly always inherited as a sex-linked dominant characteristic, i.e. it appears to be placed on the X chromosome. This conclusion follows from the fact that all the daughters of the male sufferers tend to be affected but none of the sons, whereas half the sons and half the daughters of the female sufferers are affected.

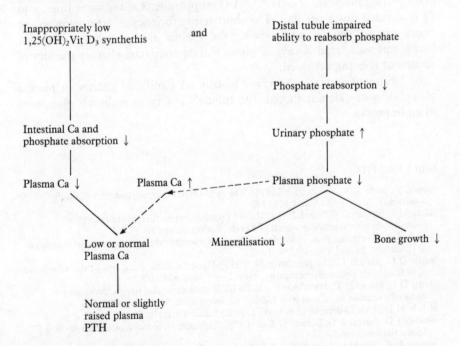

Inappropriately low $1,25(OH)_2$Vit $D_3$ synthethis

and

Distal tubule impaired ability to reabsorb phosphate

Phosphate reabsorption ↓

Intestinal Ca and phosphate absorption ↓

Urinary phosphate ↑

Plasma Ca ↓          Plasma Ca ↑ ------ Plasma phosphate ↓

Low or normal Plasma Ca          Mineralisation ↓          Bone growth ↓

Normal or slightly raised plasma PTH

**Fig. 20.8** Possible explanation for vit D resistant rickets (familial hypophosphataemic rickets).

The classical syndrome is that of dwarfism in a young boy with late 'rickets' (around the age of four to eight years), but many affected individuals, particularly women, are healthy and have no skeletal changes. Regardless of bone changes, the presence of the disease in the affected person is recognised by the low concentration of serum phosphorus and the diminished ability of the tubules to reabsorb phosphate. The tubular abnormality is detected by one or more of the several methods described earlier (p. 105). For instance, when the condition is particularly severe urinary phosphate excretion continues when the concentration of serum phosphorus is below the normal phosphate threshold of 0.7 mmol/l (2.1 mg/100 ml). Urinary calcium excretion is always low. The glomerular filtration rate is unimpaired and the concentration of serum calcium is usually normal though occasionally it is raised in the affected children (i.e. under the age of 15 years) and usually normal thereafter, and a bone biopsy shows the appearance of osteomalacia. Plasma alkaline phosphatase is raised. The impaired intestinal absorption of calcium has been demonstrated in patients with skeletal changes. There are, as yet, no reports of calcium balance studies in affected individuals with normal bones.

*Treatment.* The aim of treatment is to cure the bone lesions and accelerate growth. $1,25(OH)_2vit\ D_3$ is useful to improve the tendency for hypocalcaemia and can raise palsma phosphate if given in very large doses but this may be associated with sudden hypercalcaemic episodes. It is usual to give oral neutral phosphate ($Na_2HPO_4\ H_2O$) supplements at the same time, 1 to 4g in divided doses per day. The short term efficiency of treatment on the bones can be gauged by following the plasma alkaline phosphatase. At longer intervals serial X-rays of bones will demonstrate whether the aim of treatment is being achieved.

As treatment progresses there is usually no significant change in plasma phosphorus or calcium though the tubule's ability to reabsorb phosphate often improves.

BIBLIOGRAPHY

Abbasi V, Lowe C V, Calcagno P L 1968 The oculo-cerebro-renal syndrome (Lowe's syndrome). Amer J Dis Child 115: 145
Albright F, Burnett C H, Smith P H et al 1942 Pseudohypoparathyroidism example of Seabright-bantam syndrome; report of 3 cases. Endocrinology 30: 922
Arruda J A, Kurtzman N A 1980 Mechanisms and classification of deranged distal urinary acidification. Amer J Physiol 239: F515
Battle D C, Arruda J A L, Kurtzman N A 1981 Hyperkalaemic distal renal tubular acidosis associated with obstructive uropathy. New Eng J Med 304: 373
Battle D C, Mozes M F, Manaligod J et al 1981 The pathogenesis of hyperchloraemic metabolic acidosis associated with kidney transplantation. Amer J Med 70: 786
Bell N H 1980 Vit D-dependent rickets (Type II) Calcif Tissue Int 31: 89
Blainey J D, Adams R G, Brewer D B et al 1980 Cadmium — induced osteomalacia. Brit J Industrial Medicine 37: 278
Brewer E D, Tsai H C, Szeto K-S et al 1977 Maleic acid-induced impaired conversion of 25 OH $D_3$ to $1,25(OH)_2D_3$: Implications for Fanconi's Syndrome. Kidney Int 12: 244

Butler E A, Flynn F V 1958 The proteinuria of renal tubular disorders. Lancet 2: 978

Chase L R, Melson G L, Aurbach G D 1969 Pseudohypoparathyroidism: defective excretion of 3', 5'-AMP in response to parathyroid hormone. J Clin Invest 48: 1832

Coe F L, Favus M J 1981 Disorders of stone formation: In: Brenner B, Rector F C (eds) The kidney 37: p 1950

Coe F L, Firpo J J, Hollandsworth D L et al 1975 Effect of acute and chronic metabolic acidosis on serum immuno-reactive parathyroid hormone in man. Kidney Int 8: 262

Cochrane A M G, Tsantoulos D C, Moussouros A et al 1976 Lymphocyte cytotoxicity for kidney cells in renal tubular acidosis of autoimmune liver disease. Brit Med J 2: 276

Daniels R A, Weisenfeld I 1979 Tumourous phosphaturic osteomalacia. Report of a case associated with multiple hemangiomas of bone. Amer J Med 67: 155

Delvin E E, Glorieux F H 1981 Serum 1,25(OH)$_2$ Vitamin D concentration in hypophosphataemic Vit D resistant rickets. Calcif Tissue Int 33: 173

Eil C, Liberman U A, Rosen J F et al 1981 A cellular defect in hereditary Vit D dependent rickets Type II: defective nuclear uptake of 1,25(OH)$_2$ Vit D in cultured skin fibroblasts. New Eng J Med 304: 1588

Engelman K, Watts R W E, Klinenberg J et al 1964 Demonstration of the enzyme defect in xanthinuria. J Clin Invest 43: 1303

Fanconi G 1936 Der fruhinfantile nephrotisch-glycosurische Zwergwuchs mit hypophosphatamischer Rachitis. Jb Kinderhelk 147: 299

Feest T G, Wrong O M 1982 Renal tubular acidosis. In: Jones N F, Peters D K, (eds) Recent advances in renal medicine 2, Churchill Livingstone, Edinburgh, p 243

Gardner J D, Lapey A, Simopoulos A P et al 1971 Abnormal membrane sodium transport in Liddle's syndrome. J Clin Invest 50: 2253

Gordon R D, Geddes R A, Pawsey C G et al 1970 Hypertension and severe hyperkalaemia associated with suppression of renin and aldosterone and completely reversed by dietary sodium restriction. Australais Ann Med 4: 287

Hioco D, Ryckewaert A, Bordier P et al 1967 Le metabolisme calcique et phosphore au cours des osteomalacies vitamino-resistantes du syndrome de Fanconi et des syndromes apparentes. In: Hioco D J (ed) L'Osteomalacie. Masson et Cie, Paris

Huguenim M, Schacht R, David R 1974 Infantile rickets with severe proximal renal tubular acidosis responsive to Vitamin D. Arch Dis Childhood 49: 955

Lightwood R, Butler N 1963 Decline in primary infantile renal acidosis: aetiological implications. Brit Med J i: 855

Liddle G W, Bladsoe T, Coppage W S 1963 A familial renal disorder simulating primary aldosteronism. Trans Assoc Amer Phys 76: 199

McCurdy D K, Cornwell G G, De Pratti V J 1967 Hyperglobulinemic renal tubular acidosis: report of two cases. Ann Int Med 67: 110

McGregor M E, Rayner P H W 1964 Pink disease and primary renal tubular acidosis. Lancet 2: 1083

McSherry E, Morris R C 1978 Attainment and maintenance of normal stature with alkali therapy in infants and children with classic renal tubular acidosis. J Clin Invest 61: 509

Marx S J, Attie M F, Levine M A et al 1981 The hypocalciuric or benign variant of familial hypercalcemia: clinical and biochemical features in fifteen kindreds. Medicine 60: 397

Mason A M S, Golding P L 1970 Hyperglobulinaemic renal tubular acidosis. A report of nine cases. Brit Med J 3: 143

Milne M D 1964 Disorders of amino-acid transport. Brit Med J I: 327

Milne M D 1970 Genetic aspects of renal diseases. Progress in Medical Genetics 7: 112

Mudge G H 1958 Clinical patterns of tubular dysfunction. Amer J Med 24: 785

Muldowney F P, Freaney R, Moloney M F 1982 Importance of dietary sodium in the hypercalciuria syndrome. Kidney Int 22: 292

Phillips M E 1980 Aminoaciduria — its relationship to Vitamin D and parathyroid hormone. C R C Crit. Rev. Clin Lab Sci 12: 215

Phillips M E, Havard J, Otterud B 1980 Aminoaciduria in chronic renal failure — its relationship to Vit D and parathyroid status. Amer J Clin Nutrit 33: 1541

Pines K L, Mudge G H 1951 Renal tubular acidosis with osteomalacia: report of 3 cases. Amer J Med 11: 302

Randall R E, Taggart W H 1961 Familial renal tubular acidosis. Ann Int Med 54: 1108

Richards P, Chamberlain M J, Wrong O M 1972 Treatment of osteomalacia of renal tubular acidosis by sodium bicarbonate alone. Lancet 2: 994

Salassa R M, Jowsey J, Arnaud C D 1970 Hypophosphataemic osteomalacia associated with 'non-endocrine' tumours. New Eng J Med 283: 65

Scriver C R, Rosenberg L E 1973 Amino acid metabolism and its disorders. W B Saunders, Philadelphia

Sebastian A, Schambelan M, Lindenfeld S et al 1977 Amelioration of metabolic acidosis with fludrocortisone therapy in hyporeninaemic hypoaldosteronism. New Eng J Med 297: 576

Short E, Morris R C, Sebastian A et al 1976 Exaggerated phosphaturic response to circulating parathyroid hormone in patients with familial X-linked hypophosphataemic rickets. J Clin Invest 58: 152

Stanbury J B, Wyngaarden J B, Fredrickson D S 1978 The metabolic basis of inherited disease. McGraw-Hill Book Company, New York

Taher S M, Anderson R J, McCartney R et al 1974 Renal tubular acidosis associated with toluene 'sniffing'. New Eng J Med 290: 765

Tenenhouse H S, Scriver C R, McInnes R R et al 1978 Renal handling of phosphate in vivo and in vitro by the X-lined hypophosphataemic male mouse. Evidence for a defect in the brush border membrane. Kidney Int 14: 236

Walshe J M 1982 Treatment of Wilson's disease with Trientine (Triethylene Tetramine) dihydrochloride. Lancet i: 643

Winters R W, Graham J B, Williams T F et al 1958 A genetic study of familial hypophosphataemia and vitamin D resistant rickets with a review of the literature. Medicine 37: 97

# 21

# Immunological diseases of the kidney

The following conditions are discussed:
1. Glomerular nephritis
2. Renal disturbances in polyarteritis nodosa
3. Wegener's granulomatosis
4. Renal disturbances in disseminated lupus erythematosus
5. Renal disturbances in subacute bacterial endocarditis
6. Renal disturbances in anaphylactoid purpura
7. Shunt nephritis
8. Lung purpura with nephritis
9. Haemolytic uraemic syndrome
10. Renal disturbances in quartan malaria
11. Immunological renal disturbances in malignant disease
12. Immunological renal disturbances in liver disease

## IMMUNOLOGICAL MECHANISMS RESPONSIBLE FOR RENAL LESIONS IN MAN

Until recently it was thought that the immunological disturbances which caused renal lesions in man were either due to glomerular trapping of circulating immune complexes or to the effect of circulating antibodies directed against basement membrane. It is now apparent that the mechanisms whereby immune complexes cause renal damage are less obvious than it first seemed and that cell mediated immunological mechanisms may also cause renal lesions.

### Immune complex disease

*Circulating complexes*

When a foreign serum (the antigen) is injected into an animal it diffuses throughout the blood and extracellular fluid so that its concentration in the plasma at first falls rapidly. The plasma concentration then falls more gradually as the antigen is slowly metabolised. But at the end of 10 to 15 days there is a sudden disappearance of the antigen from the plasma, the animal develops an acute illness and circulating antibodies to the antigen make their first appearance. The disappearance of the antigen is due to the formation of a specific antibody, such as IgG or IgM to the antigen. The antibody binds on to the circulating antigen to form immune complexes. These vary in size depending on the relative concentrations of antigen and antibody. When antigen predominates in great excess the complexes are small and remain in the circulation. When antibody is in excess the complexes are very large, they are precipitated and disposed of by phagocytes in the reticulo-endothelial system. When the concentrations of plasma antigen and antibody are near equivalence the intermediate sized complexes that are formed may activate serum complement. The cascade of interaction with each of the various fractions of complement which then takes place releases a series of products which, if they are discharged into the tissues may cause a damaging inflammatory reaction.

Each successive step in the activation of complement causes the release of active split products some of which cause local damage to the capillary wall. Some cause vasodilatation and increase permeability. Others induce polymorphonuclear leucocytes to come towards the immune complexes, and yet others make the polymorphonuclear leucocytes adhere to the capillary wall. Platelets also become adherent and attach themselves to the capillary wall. The adherent leucocytes discharge their lysosomal enzymes and strip up the endothelial cell cytoplasm from the basement membrane. The clumped platelets release histamine, initiate clotting and cause the deposition of fibrin. The presence of fibrin causes both endothelial and epithelial cells to proliferate, and when it appears in Bowman's space it attracts crescentic collections of macrophages.

The administration of a single dose of foreign serum causes an acute reversible proliferation of the glomerular tufts. The daily administration of serum for several weeks produces chronic renal disease with a variety of histological changes similar to those seen in man. With fluorescein-conjugated anti-sera to, (1) the antigenic components of the foreign serum (e.g. the albumin), (2) the recipient animals' own immunoglobulins, and (3) to complement it is possible to demonstrate the presence of antigen-antibody-complement complexes bound to the glomerular tufts. The presence of fibrin can be detected in the same way. The antigen, antibody and complement are found to be distributed either in the walls of the capillary or in the mesangial areas. The pattern of distribution along the capillary walls is characteristic (p. 30). It consists of finely granular or lumpy deposits laid down on the epithelial side of the basement membrane (p. 30). The belief that it is the immune complexes in the circulation that cause renal lesions stemmed from the observation that in animal experiments the extent of the renal damage was related to the size of the complexes and therefore to their ability to penetrate the capillary wall.

*Locally produced complexes.* Nevertheless it has now been demonstrated that entrapment of pre-formed circulating immune complexes within the capillary walls is not the only mechanism whereby immune complexes can produce the histological and functional changes in glomerular tufts which occur in glomerular nephritis. Perhaps this is not surprising in that the inflammatory products produced by the activation of complement by the interaction of antigen and antibody are released where the two come together. If this occurs in the circulation there is little reason why the subsequent entrapment in the kidney of these pre-formed complexes should cause inflammation in the kidney. On the other hand those complexes that are formed where they are entrapped might cause damage. It now appears that many immune deposits within the glomerular wall, particularly those which are sub-epithelial (i.e. those which appear to have travelled right through the basement membrane) are formed in situ by the conjunction of free antibody and an antigenic constituent of the glomerular capillary wall. The antigen may be either an intrinsic glomerular antigen or it may have originated elsewhere and then been trapped in the wall. For instance if a kidney is perfused with preformed immune complexes of bovine serum albumen (BSA) and BSA antibody, only scattered mesangial deposits are seen. Whereas if free BSA and free antibody are perfused alternatively numerous in situ sub-epithelial BSA containing immune deposits are formed.

Using similar methods it is possible to produce immune deposits in the mesangium and in the sub-endothelial space. Heat aggregated IgG injected into a rabbit localises in the mesangium. If such a kidney is now transplanted into a normal rabbit which is then injected with antibody against human IgG the antibody binds to the IgG in the mesangium of the transplanted kidney and forms an immune complex in situ. No deposits form in the rabbit's own kidneys. Similarly antibodies can be demonstrated to combine with antigen within the renal interstitium to form complexes in situ which give rise to acute intestinal nephritis. The interstitial antigen may be endogenous but it may also be a derivative of a drug, such as methicillin which probably becomes bound to certain sites so that the free antibody is directed against the locally acquired hapten-host conjugate.

These observations are in keeping with the well known fact that circulating immune complexes are found in many conditions not associated with renal disease. And that immune complexes can often be demonstrated in otherwise normal kidneys obtained from patients who have died an accidental death. It follows that certain freely circulating antigens may be considerably more harmful to the kidney than are antigens contained within circulating immune complexes. And it may be, therefore, that the development of immune complex nephritis may be precipitated more by an impaired ability of the patient to clear the offending antigen by an appropriate antibody response than by the formation of circulating immune complexes.

*Inadequate disposal of antigen*

Persistence of antigen might occur because of an inadequate T or B cell response. T lymphocytic response is required for the elimination of certain viruses so that T cell deficiency could cause viral infection to persist. The antigen might persist in the face of a B cell antibody response for a variety of reasons. For instance if an antigen is repeatedly administered (penicillamine nephropathy), or an autoantigen is continuously released into the circulation as a result of allergic tissue damage (DNA nucleoprotein antigens in systemic lupus erythematosus). Alternatively a reservoir of infection might not be reached by a normal antibody response for some mechanical reason e.g. sub acute bacterial endocarditis and shunt nephritis. Glomerular nephritis is sometimes associated with chronic infection due to an easily accessible but persisting agent such as plasmodium malariae and leprosy. It is possible that nephritis could occur with infections which are not so obvious. An infection might persist in the presence of an immune response if the antibody formed was of low affinity for the antigen, or if the antibody was directed against some antigen which does not destroy the organism. Complement deficiency, which is associated with glomerular nephritis, is also involved with the disposal of immune complexes. Complement is needed to (1) solubilise immune complexes in the serum, (2) increase the rate at which complexes are taken up by the reticulo endothelial system, and (3) help antibodies destroy organisms and viruses.

It must be pointed out that the number of patients suffering from 'nephritis' in whom an antigen has been identified is small (Table 21.1). The evidence of identification ranges from a statistical association of the nephritis with a particular disease, to elution of an antigen antibody complex from the glomeruli and subsequent identification of the antigen and the antibody. The following antigens have been identified in this way, DNA, Hepatitis B, Plasmodium malariae and falciparum antigens, staphylococcus albus, salmonella typhi, treponema pallidium, toxoplasma gondii and Coxsackie B virus.

Free antigen, including macromolecular aggregates of antigen, and immune complexes of appropriate size, charge and other particular characteristic may localise in a normal glomerulus for many reasons. The concentration of antigen may remain raised because it is not cleared from the circulation due to some disorder of the complement system. An abnormality of the complement system may be either congenital or acquired (e.g. the nephritic factor in mesangiocapillary nephritis). $C_3b$ receptor sites have been found on the epithelial side of the basement membrane onto which may bind the $C_3b$ present on the surface of complexes that have activated complement. The permeability of the endothelial surface of a normal glomerular capillary is so great that it permits penetration through the endothelium of antigen aggregates, or complexes, of relatively large size. And the anionic composition of the basement membrane may interact with cationic molec-

**Table 21.1** Antigens implicated in human antigen — antibody complex mediated nephritis

| Exogenous | Endogenous |
|---|---|
| Infections | Nuclear antigens |
|   Bacteria | Thyroglobulin |
|     Streptococci | Tumour antigens |
|     Staphylococci | Immunoglobulin G |
|     Pneumococci | Brush border of renal tubules |
|     Meningococci | |
|     Salmonella typhi | |
|     Treponema pallidium | |
|     Mycobacterium leprae | |
|   Viruses | |
|     Measles | |
|     Mumps | |
|     Hepatitis B | |
|     Epstein-Barr | |
|     Mycoplasma pneumoniae | |
|     Coxiella burnetti | |
|     Coxsackie B | |
|   Parasites | |
|     Plasmodium malariae | |
|     Schistosoma | |
|     Toxoplasma | |
|   Fungi | |
|     Candida Albicans | |
|   Drugs | |
|     Penicillamine | |
|     Gold | |
|   Foreign serum | |

ules on these antigens. In addition there is the avidity and holding properties of the mesangium for many substances that pass through the endothelium.

In immune complex mediated glomerular nephritis the deposits are laid down in an irregularly sized and shaped granular or lumpy pattern.

## Anti-glomerular basement disease

Experimentally an animal is immunised with an extract of kidney tissue obtained from an animal of a different species. The antiserum is then harvested and injected into an animal of the same species as that from which the extract of kidney was obtained. The exogenous immunoglobulins contained in the antiserum bind on to the glomerular tuft and cause complement to be fixed and activated at the same site. This in turn leads to the sequence of events described above which causes tissue damage. A diffuse glomerular nephritis then develops which is usually chronic and self-perpetuating. The critical antigen in the kidney extracts used to produce anti-kidney serum is glomerular basement membrane. Therefore the active component of the antiserum is an anti-glomerular basement membrane antibody. As glomerular basement material is normally excreted in the urine, it is possible, as an alternative technique, to inoculate an animal with its own glomerular basement membrane material. This manoeuvre causes the animal to develop anti-glomerular basement membrane antibodies and a diffuse glomerular nephritis which is self-perpetuating. The perpetuation of the disease process is due to the antigenic properties of the anti-glomerular basement membrane antibody itself. This creates a vicious cycle in which the more anti-glomerular basement membrane antibody is present the more anti-glomerular basement antibody is formed.

IgG and complement are laid down along the glomerular capillary walls in a characteristic pattern. With immunofluorescence the immunoglobulin and complement are found distributed in a smooth manner along the capillary wall as if they had been painted on with one continuous stroke of a fine brush (p. 30). This is in contrast to the granular interrupted pattern seen in immune complex disease. A few minutes after the injection of anti-glomerular basement membrane antibody labelled with ferritin, electron microscopy reveals that the ferritin has been deposited between the endothelial cell cytoplasm and the basement membrane as a fine evenly distributed dust.

Anti-glomerular basement disease is a rare cause of disease in man. To demonstrate its presence unequivocally it must be shown that the immunoglobulin which is fixed in the kidney is an anti-glomerular basement membrane antibody and that there is anti-glomerular basement membrane antibody in the plasma. The former is difficult. The diagnosis is usually made therefore on the detection of anti-glomerular-basement-membrane antibody helped often, though not invariably, by finding a smooth pattern of immunoflorescence along the glomerular capillary wall. When elution studies are performed the antibody is identified by applying the eluted material from a homogenate of diseased kidney onto a frozen section of normal kidney and then demonstrating with a fluorescein labelled anti-human globulin serum, that a globulin has become fixed to the capillary wall in a smooth linear pattern. The eluted material can also be injected into monkeys in which it causes a persistent glomerular nephritis which is associated with the presence of immunoglobulin and complement laid down in a smooth linear fashion along the capillary wall.

It is now established that glomerular basement-membrane antibody reacts with the non-collagen portion of the glomerular basement membrane and also cross reacts with pulmonary alveoli and the choroid plexus. The reaction in the lung is responsible for the pulmonary haemorrhage which occurs in many, though not all, patients with Goodpasture's syndrome in whom the combination of multiple capsular crescents and rapid downward clinical course places them in that category of glomerular nephritis called rapidly progressive glomerular nephritis. Clinically the activity of the glomerular basement antibody to choroid plexus is not obvious.

The development in man of anti-GBM antibodies is associated with exposure to hydrocarbons or penicillamine and with upper respiratory tract infections, though no particular organisms have been implicated. What makes the host respond to these stimuli in this particular way is not known.

## Cell mediated disease

The recurrent presence of lymphocytes and macrophages in the kidneys of patients suffering from glomerular nephritis provides circumstantial evidence that cell mediated immunity may be involved in its cause. In some instances, such as the concentrations of lymphocytes which invade the interstitium in acute interstitial nephritis, or the accumulation of macrophages within Bowman's space which form crescents in anti-GBM nephritis, the evidence is very compelling. Experimentally it is now possible to demonstrate in many forms of glomerular nephritis that mononuclear cells can infiltrate the glomerular tuft itself, particularly into the mesangial area and that they contribute to the glomerular injury. It has also been demonstrated that an antimacrophage serum can largely prevent the lesion in experimentally induced serum sickness in rabbits. Convincing evidence of the role of cell mediated immunity in experimental nephritis has also been demonstrated by first injecting rats with small doses of rabbit anti-rat antiserum against glomerular basement membrane. Rabbit gamma globulin then becomes fixed to the rat's glomeruli but without producing detectable injury. The rats are then given lymph node cells from the rabbits which have been immunised against rat basement membrane. This induces gross histological glomerular abnormalities with segmented hypercellularity and areas of necrosis. It is probable that the few sensitised lymphocytes that are injected react with the antigen which has become fixed in the glomeruli. A local inflammatory reaction therefore occurs which mobilises a heavy concentration of monocytes as in a delayed-type hypersensitivity reaction in the skin.

In man lymphocytes from some patients with glomerular nephritis can be shown to have an in vitro reactivity against preparations of basement membrane. There is considerable evidence that lymphocytes are involved in the aetiology of 'minimal change' glomerular nephritis. In what way is not clear for there are no lymphocytes in the glomeruli of this form of nephritis. At present it would appear that the lymphocytes may act at a distance through some humoral mechanism, another form of 'cell mediated' immunological activity.

## GLOMERULAR NEPHRITIS

This disease is sometimes referred to as primary glomerular nephritis. It is a difficult disorder to define and describe. It encompasses all immunological diseases of the kidney not associated with obvious lesions in other organs. It therefore excludes such diseases as disseminated lupus erythematosus polyarteritis nodosa, sub-acute bacterial endocarditis, etc. The difficulty in describing the disease derives mainly from the lack of precise information about its aetiology and its variegated clinical and histological patterns. It is very probable that eventually it will be found to consist of several separate conditions. The several light microscopy and immunofluorescent patterns which can already be discerned support this hypothesis. The description of the disease is much influenced by whether the narrator is a clinician, a histologist, or an immunologist. In the following account glomerular nephritis is described primarily according to the many ways it may present clinically. An attempt is then made to describe which light microscopy and immunofluorescent pattern accompanies these various clinical presentations. The task is not easy for though the clinical syndromes of acute glomerular nephritis, rapidly progressive glomerular nephritis, and recurrent haematuria are each accompanied by a relatively clearcut histological and immunofluorescent pattern, these same patterns can be found in association with almost any of the other clinical presentations. Conversely, when the light microscopy appearances are normal the patient may have a nephrotic syndrome or persistent proteinuria, but either of these clinical presentations may be accompanied with several other histological patterns.

Table 21.2 illustrates the various clinical and histological combinations that are found in glomerular nephritis. The gross overlap between the many clinical syndromes and histological appearances are immediately apparent.

It is interesting to note that Richard Bright's own speculations about the aetiology of glomerular nephritis are remarkably topical: 'the structure of the kidney becomes permanently changed, either in accordance with, and in furtherance of that morbid action; *or by a deposit which is a consequence of the morbid action*'. His description of a patient with glomerular nephritis is given below. It is noticeable, that it is principally a description of acute glomerular nephritis developing into persistent glomerular nephritis; a nephrotic stage is just discernible.

## Bright's description

'A child or an adult is affected with scarlatina, or some other acute disease; or has indulged in the intemperate use of ardent spirits for a series of months or years; he is exposed to some casual cause or habitual source of suppressed perspiration: he finds the secretion of his urine greatly increased [*sic*], or he discovers that it is tinged with blood; or, without having made any such observation, he awakes in the morning with his face swollen, or his ankles puffy, or his hands oedematous. If he happens, in this condition, to fall under the care of a practitioner who suspects the nature of his disease, it is found that already his urine contains a notable quantity of albumen: his pulse is full and hard, his skin dry, he has often headache, and sometimes a sense of weight or pain across the loins. Under treatment more or less active, or sometimes without any treatment, the more obvious and distressing of these symptoms disappear; the swelling, whether casual or constant, is no longer observed; the urine ceases to evince any admixture of red particles; and, according to the degree of importance which has been attached to these symptoms, they are gradually lost sight of, or are absolutely forgotten. Nevertheless, from time to time the countenance becomes bloated; the skin is dry; headaches occur with unusual frequency; or the calls to micturition disturb the night's repose. After a time, the healthy colour of the countenance fades; a sense of weakness or pain in the loins increases; headaches, often accompanied by vomiting, add greatly to the general want of comfort; and a sense of lassitude, of weariness, and of depression, gradually steal over the bodily and mental frame. Again the assistance of medicine is sought. If the nature of the disease is suspected, the urine is carefully tested, and found, in almost every trial, to contain albumen, while the quantity of urea is gradually diminishing. If in the attempt to give relief to the oppression of the system, blood is drawn, it is often buffed, or the serum is milky and opaque; and nice analysis will frequently detect a great deficiency of albumen, and sometimes manifest indications of the presence of urea. If the disease is not suspected, the liver, the stomach or the brain divide the care of the practitioner, sometimes drawing him away entirely from the more important seat of the disease. The swelling increases and decreases; the mind grows cheerful or sad; the secretions of the kidney or the skin are augmented or diminished, sometimes in alternate ratio, sometimes without apparent relation. Again the patient is restored to tolerable health; again he enters on his active duties; or he is, perhaps, less fortunate; the swelling increases, the urine becomes scanty, the powers of life seem to yield, the lungs become oedematous, and, in a state of asphyxia or coma, he sinks into the grave; or a sudden effusion of serum into the glottis closes the passages of the air, and brings on a more sudden dissolution. Should he, however, have resumed the avocations of life, he is usually subject to constant recurrence of his symptoms; or again, almost dismissing the recollection of his ailment, he is suddenly seized with an acute attack of pericarditis, or with a still more acute attack of peritonitis, which without renewed warning, deprives him in eight and forty hours, of his life. Should he escape this danger likewise, other perils await him; his headaches have been observed to become more frequent; his stomach more deranged; his vision indistinct; his hearing depraved: he is suddenly seized with a convulsive fit, and becomes blind. He struggles through the attack; but again and again it returns; and before a day or a week has elapsed, worn out by convulsions, or overwhelmed by coma, the painful history of his disease is closed,'

## Acute glomerular nephritis

Acute glomerular nephritis is the term usually reserved for the association of an acute nephritic syndrome associated with diffuse proliferation in the glomeruli. A recognisable infection often preceeds the onset.

**Table 21.2** The clinical features, light microscopy appearances and immunofluorescence in 425 patients described by Morel-Maroger, Leathem & Richet 1972. GBM = glomerular basement membrane

| Clinical features | Light microscopy appearances | Number of patients | Type | Immunofluorescence Pattern |
|---|---|---|---|---|
| **Acute glomerular nephritis** | | | | |
| Acute nephritic syndrome | Diffuse proliferative exudative | 22 | $\beta_1C++$ IgG+ | Lumpy deposits scattered along GBM. |
| Acute renal failure | mesangial | 12 | $\beta_1C++$, IgG++ or None | Occasionally smooth linear deposits |
| **Persistent glomerular nephritis** | | | | |
| Rapidly progressive | Diffuse proliferative with crescents | 22 | Fibrinogen++ $B_1C+$ (IgA, IgM, IgG) | Coarse granular deposits of fibrin in crescents. Occasionally smooth linear deposits of immunoglobulins |
| **Chronic** | | | | |
| Recurrent macroscopic haematuria | | | | |
| Persistent proteinuria with r.b.c. | Focal proliferative | 88 | IgA++ ($\beta_1C+$, IgG+) Fibrinogen± | Diffuse in all glomeruli mainly mesangial |
| Persistent proteinuria without r.b.c. | | | | |
| Nephrotic syndrome | | | | |
| Persistent proteinuria without r.b.c. | Nil change | 96 | None | |
| Persistent proteinuria with r.b.c. | | | | |

| | | | | |
|---|---|---|---|---|
| Persistent proteinuria with and without r.b.c. | Focal proliferative | 30 | β₁C+ or None (IgM, IgG) | Diffuse, or focal granular scattered |
| Nephrotic syndrome | exudative | 6 | (see above) | (see above) |
| | Diffuse proliferative mesangial | 18 | (see above) | (see above) |
| | Diffuse proliferative with crescents | 10 | | |
| | Membranoproliferative | 33 | β₁C+ IgM and Fibrinogen | β₁C coarse granular focal or diffuse along GBM and mesangium. IgM coarse deposits — focal |
| | Focal sclerosis | 30 | IgM ± β₁C | Focal only in sclerosed areas |
| | Extra membranous | 42 | IgG+++ β₁C+++ | Diffuse finely granular along GBM *not* in mesangial areas. Occasionally smooth linear |
| Chronic renal failure | Intramembranous | 4 | β₁C++, IgM± | β₁C diffusely laid granular |
| | Advanced lesions | 12 | β₁C | Coarse granules |

## Immunological Mechanisms

Acute glomerular nephritis would appear to be at least in part an immune complex mediated disease. Deposits, containing properdin, the $\beta_1C$ globulin component of complement and less often IgG can be detected in the glomerular tufts, and immune complexes of IgG and $Cl_q$ are found in the blood together with a fall in serum $C_3$ levels. Occasionally cryoglobulin-containing IgG and $C_3$ are also found in the serum.

## Relation to infection

*Infecting organism.* In some tropical countries in which acute glomerular nephritis is still relatively common the onset is most often preceeded by an infection with a β-haemolytic streptococcus, usually types 4 and 12, though a few other strains may be involved. It is possible that the predilection of these strains to affect the kidneys is due to their having antigens in their cell walls which are the same as those in the basement membrane of the kidneys. This specificity of strain accounts for the irregular manner in which cases of acute glomerular nephritis appear. Until this was recognised, it was difficult to know why the incidence of acute glomerular nephritis varied so widely among epidemics of streptococcal infection: particularly why several members of a family should suddenly develop the disease almost simultaneously. In the western world acute glomerular nephritis occurs sporadically and the relation of the disease with organisms other than the streptococcus, is very striking e.g. pneumococcus or meningococcus.

*Site of Streptococcal infection* This is usually the throat or the skin. Typically there is such a severe sore throat that the patient has to retire to bed for several days; in children, scarlet fever was at one time a major cause of acute nephritis, but it is now less frequent, probably because of the use of penicillin. The proportion of cases in whom it is possible to obtain a satisfactory history of previous infection is about the same in children as adults.

*Interval between infection and onset.* This interval varies from 2–3 days to more than a month; it averages 14 days. It is usual for the patient to have returned to work or school before the onset of acute glomerular nephritis.

## Pathology

Characteristically, the kidneys are normal in size, shape and colour, although occasionally there may be punctate haemorrhages on the surface. Microscopically the structural changes are principally in the glomeruli, and are those of diffuse proliferative glomerular nephritis (Fig. 21.1). Often all glomeruli are equally affected, but frequently the changes vary in intensity

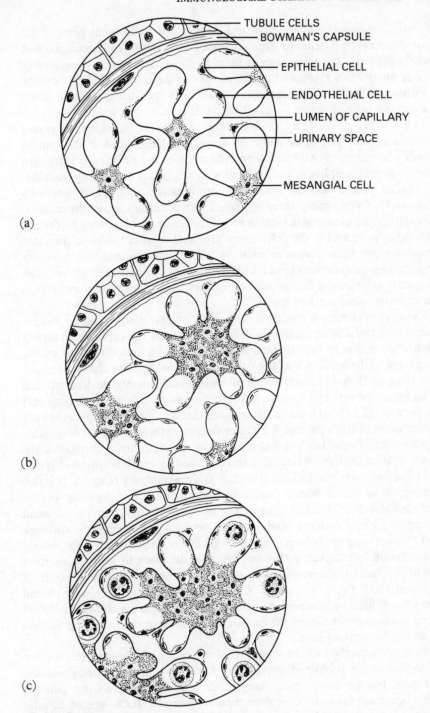

**Fig. 21.1** (a) Normal, (b) diffuse glomerular nephritis, (c) acute diffuse exudative proliferative glomerular nephritis.

not only between one glomerulus and another but in different parts of the same glomerulus. There is a great increase in the number of mesangial and endothelial cells, but what is even more striking, they have a considerably greater quantity of cytoplasm, and their nuclei are enlarged. If this change is diffuse throughout a glomerulus it then loses its normal rather delicate tracery and instead appears stuffed with nuclei and cytoplasm.

This is accentuated by a focal swelling of the capillary basement membrane, and the appearance of numerous fragmented PAS staining 'fibrils'. In some patients there is an infiltration of the glomerular tufts with numerous polymorphonuclear leucocytes. When this is seen the appearances are called acute diffuse exudative proliferative glomerular nephritis (Fig. 21.1). Occasionally there are small foci of intracapillary thrombosis. The cells of the glomerular capsule sometimes enlarge, become cuboidal and histologically resemble the cells of the proximal tubule; the loose shredded cytoplasm of these capsular cells is sometimes thought to represent precipitated protein which has leaked through the damaged glomerulus. Crescents are unusual & unequivocal evidence of inflammatory exudate in the capsular space is rarely seen.

Electron microscopy reveals that the cell proliferation is indeed mainly endothelial and mesangial in origin. The swelling of the capillary basement membrane is due in part to extensive fragmentation and shredding on the luminal or endothelial side of the basement membrane. The changes suggest that the endothelial cells are laying down basement membrane-like material at an increased rate and that the vast numbers of redundant new layers that are formed fail to bind together in a normal manner. The appearances are not unlike those of flaky pastry. With light fluorescent microscopy it is possible to show that fibrin has been deposited on the endothelial surface of the glomerular capillaries. Presumably this is secondary to the injurious effect on the basement membrane of the abnormal antigen-antibody reaction. It is this deposition of fibrin which causes the proliferation and swelling of the endothelial cells. Electron microscopy also shows the presence of small 'humps' of electron-dense material lying between the basement membrane and the overlying epithelium (Fig. 3.2). Whatever the outcome of the disease these 'humps' disappear within six weeks of the onset of acute glomerular nephritis. Immunofluorescence demonstrates granular, lumpy deposits of $\beta_1 C$ and smaller amounts of IgG scattered along the capillary walls. Small amounts of fibrinogen are seen occasionally. Very occasionally IgG is found lying as a smooth line along the capillary wall. Frequently there is no fixation of any of the antisera used.

In approximately half the cases, renal biopsies have shown the presence of focal areas of tubular degeneration. These are situated throughout the nephron, but are found most often in the distal tubules. In few patients there are focal areas of complete tubular necrosis. Each site of tubular damage is surrounded by inflammatory cells, including lymphocytes, plasma cells, eosinophils and polymorphs. Occasionally, the most severe cases show a generalised separation of the tubules by a thickening of the interstitial tissue. In the interstitial spaces there are scattered small collections of inflammatory cells, and sometimes a glomerulus may be surrounded by a band of inflammatory cells including polymorphs, eosinophils and lymphocytes. Arteriolar necroses have occasionally been seen at *post-mortem*.

In some cases of acute glomerular nephritis without proteinuria or haematuria i.e. patients who present with acute retention of salt and water and hypertension following a recent infection, there may be no structural changes except for focal areas in which the lining cells of Bowman's capsule are cuboidal.

The first lesion to resolve is the diffuse endothelial proliferation. But focal areas of mesangial proliferation remain for a considerable time thereafter, even in those patients who eventually make a complete recovery. These focal collections lie along the stalks of the glomeruli and are particularly noticeable at the periphery of a stalk. A peripheral lesion of this kind then consists of a collection of mesangial cell nuclei surrounded by a relatively large common 'eosinophilic' mass in which no cell boundaries can be discerned. Around the periphery of this lesion there lies a group of capillaries with normal walls. This residual focal mesangial proliferation is stated to be characteristic only of post-streptococcal nephritis.

The mass which surrounds the proliferated mesangial cells is composed mainly of mucopolysaccharide matrix which has been secreted in excess by mesangial cells in response to the inflammatory stimulus. The term 'lobular stalk thickening' has been coined to describe the appearances produced when this material is deposited along the long axis of the glomerular stalk.

### Clinical features

Acute glomerular nephritis is more common in males, and is seen most often below the age of 20 years; however, it is by no means confined to this age group and can be frequently seen at all ages, including the elderly. The clinical features are those of an acute nephritic syndrome (p. 240). Clinically the cardinal points are the sudden onset of oedema, gain in weight and oliguria; raised blood pressure and bradycardia; raised jugular venous pressure and dyspnoea; haematuria, proteinuria and discoloured urine. Acute glomerular nephritis is the commonest cause of acute 'heart failure' in children. It is important not to be confused by the finding that in most patients there is a high urinary white cell excretion rate, and in about a third of patients, an asymptomatic persistent bacilluria. The white cells presumably come from the acute inflammatory lesions in the kidneys which are themselves due to the deposition of antigen, etc. The organisms responsible for the bacilluria are ordinary urinary pathogens such as *E. coli*; their relevance, if any, to the primary renal lesions is unknown.

*Relationship between certain clinical and structural features*

Renal biopsy studies have shown that in acute glomerular nephritis the presence of proteinuria and haematuria is evidence of widespread and pronounced proliferative and inflammatory changes in the glomerular tufts, though the severity of these structural changes bears no relation to the extent of the proteinuria or haematuria. On the other hand *all the acute histological changes of acute diffuse glomerular nephritis can be present in the absence of proteinuria, haematuria or acute retention of salt and water.* Surprisingly, there is only an uncertain relationship between the creatinine clearance and the structural changes in the glomeruli; and the concentration of the blood urea is the poorest guide to the presence or extent of such changes. Impairment in the ability to concentrate is certain evidence of widespread focal degenerative lesions of the tubules, though these can be present without gross changes in concentrating ability; a raised erythrocyte sedimentation rate above 50 mm in the first hour (Westergren) is highly suggestive of tubular degeneration. Widespread necrosis of glomeruli is always associated with acute renal failure but otherwise there is little correlation between the presence of acute renal failure and the severity of the structural lesions.

*Course and prognosis*

In some series in children there have been no deaths, and complete recovery in almost 100%. In adults complete recovery occurs in approximately 85–95% of patients. Under 5% die within one or two weeks of acute pulmonary oedema, renal failure or hypertensive encephalopathy, while the remainder (under 10%) develop persistent glomerular nephritis. The persistent stage may either develop as a rapid deterioration during the acute phase with increasing renal failure, oedema and hypertension and death within a year, or there may be almost complete recovery, except for the continued presence of proteinuria which persists for up to 25 years before the onset of chronic renal failure. A superimposed nephrotic syndrome occurs particularly in those who develop and die of persistent glomerular nephritis within a year.

At the beginning, acute renal failure is the complication most likely to destroy the patient. Acute glomerular nephritis is one of those rare parenchymal causes of acute renal failure in which there is often complete cessation of urine flow. In adults acute renal failure due to acute glomerular nephritis nearly always causes irreversible terminal renal failure. In children, however, artificial dialysis is accompanied by recovery in most cases. Acute pulmonary oedema and hypertensive encephalopathy should respond to treatment whatever the age of the patient.

Recurrent exacerbations of haematuria and hypertension, with violent fluctuations in glomerular filtration rate and blood urea, carry an increasing risk that the patient may develop rapidly progressive persistent glomerular nephritis. Nevertheless a guarded prognosis should be given for a considerable time, for recovery may take place even if the disease has persisted in this manner for several weeks. It has been claimed that rapidly progressive glomerular nephritis never follows an attack of acute glomerular nephritis due to an infection with β-haemolytic streptococci. If the onset of acute glomerular nephritis is associated with a petechial rash, complete recovery is unusual.

The proteinuria which follows any attack of acute glomerular nephritis constitutes the most difficult prognostic problem. It is generally considered that the patient has an active renal lesion until proteinuria ceases, and that the longer this continues the more likely it is that he will develop persistent glomerular nephritis and renal failure. Complete recovery, therefore, has not taken place until proteinuria ceases. Figure 21.2, drawn from Addis's observations, illustrates how long proteinuria may continue and yet recovery occur. It can be seen that whereas in the majority proteinuria ceases within two years, there are some patients in whom it continues for six to ten years before it disappears.

It is important to note that the course of events may vary widely between various localities. There is one report from New York that 40% of patients had persistent proteinuria at nine years. Whereas in another report from Trinidad the incidence of proteinuria at 10 years was under 2%. Nevertheless both agreed that the incidence of hypertension was greater in patients who

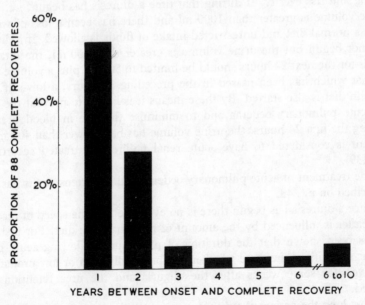

Fig. 21.2 Interval between onset and healing of acute glomerular nephritis in 88 cases who recovered completely. (After Addis, 1949.)

have had acute glomerular nephritis, *even in those in whom there is no continuing sign of activity of the nephritis.*

### Treatment

*Prophylactic.* It is reasonable to try and eradicate the β-haemolytic streptococcus from a small community (i.e. a family), in which a case of acute glomerular nephritis has occurred. The organism is highly sensitive and easily removed by one injection of long-acting penicillin.

*Curative.* There is no known way of preventing acute glomerular nephritis developing into persistent glomerular nephritis. Accordingly, treatment is directed solely at saving the patient's life and shortening the duration of the acute attack.

An attempt should be made to isolate the β-haemolytic streptococci immediately on the day of admission. Penicillin administration is begun on the same day and continued for a considerable time thereafter. Opinions differ, but some authorities consider that penicillin should be continued until proteinuria disappears, however long that may be.

Bed rest is essential, for it is remarkable how often a diuresis and recovery will begin within a few hours of the patient's retiring to bed, irrespective of the duration of the illness up to that time. Rest in bed also diminishes the risk of acute pulmonary oedema and hypertensive crises. For the first 24 hours it is well to allow only 500 ml of sweetened fruit juice by mouth and nothing else. This allows time to observe the direction the illness is taking and its severity. If during that time a diuresis has begun, i.e. if the urine volume is greater than 1000 ml and there has been a loss of weight, then a normal diet and unrestricted intake of fluids is allowed. If a diuresis has not begun but the urine volume is greater than 400 ml, the intake of fluids for the next 24 hours should be limited to 500 ml plus a volume equal to that which has been passed in the preceding 24 hours; a low-salt, low-protein diet is also started. By these means it is hoped to prevent the onset of acute pulmonary oedema and to minimise the rise in blood urea. If, during the first 24 hours, the urine volume has been lower than 400 ml the patient is considered to have acute renal failure and treated accordingly (p. 139).

The treatment of acute pulmonary oedema and hypertensive fits has been described on p. 243.

Once a diuresis has begun there is no evidence that the speed of recovery thereafter is influenced by the amount of protein in the diet. For instance, it has been shown that the duration of proteinuria following acute glomerular nephritis is the same whether an abnormally high or low protein diet is given for some weeks after the oliguria and the urea retention have ceased.

How long the patient should remain in bed once the oedema, the raised jugular venous pressure, hypertension and raised blood urea have disappeared is sometimes determined by the number of red cells or the amount of protein being excreted in the urine. Progress is best guided by the red cell excretion. The aim is to allow the patient to get up once the red cell excretion, *though still raised*, has reached a relative plateau. The excretory rate should have fallen to somewhere near 1 000 000/hour. Usually, however, progress is judged by the extent of the proteinuria, and again it should reach a steady level before the patient is allowed to get up. As a rough approximation, it should fall below 1 g/24 hours, or be no greater than + in a sample of urine with specific gravity above 1.016.

It is clearly a useless and unwarrantable interference with the patient's liberty to keep him in bed until proteinuria disappears, for (1) proteinuria will persist for over a year in about half of the patients who eventually make a complete recovery (Fig. 21.2), and (2) in those in whom the disease remains active proteinuria may persist as the only abnormality for 25 years. There is no evidence that the duration of rest in bed influences the eventual course of the disease.

## Differential diagnosis

The onset of acute glomerular nephritis is sometimes indistinguishable from that of several other conditions which give rise to an acute nephritic syndrome. The history of recent infection, the low level of serum complement and the identification of the streptococcus, and an antistreptolysin titre greater than 1 in 300 are useful distinguishing points. Occasionally a patient may present with acute renal failure following the use of a sulphonamide for a streptococcal infection. It may then be extremely difficult to decide whether the patient has acute glomerular nephritis or acute tubular necrosis. In such cases it is essential that the ureters be catheterised to make certain that they are not plugged with crystals of sulphonamide and tubular débris (p. 139).

The two conditions which cause most confusion are some cases of polyarteritis nodosa, and disseminated lupus erythematosus; often the correct diagnosis is only made retrospectively. A pyrexia for longer than the first two to three days, or the continued presence of macroscopic haematuria are highly suggestive of a diagnosis of polyarteritis nodosa.

## Persistent glomerular nephritis

Clinically, persistent glomerular nephritis either (1) follows an attack of acute glomerular nephritis in a clinically recognisable manner, or (2) more commonly it presents without any previous known history or evidence of renal disease.

## Presenting renal syndromes

Persistent glomerular nephritis may present as a rapidly progressive renal failure, recurrent haematuria (usually with persistent proteinuria), persistent proteinuria, a nephrotic syndrome, or chronic renal failure.

## Rapidly progressive glomerular nephritis (acute crescentic rapidly progressive glomerular nephritis)

Clinically, rapidly progressive glomerular nephritis is a form of primary glomerular nephritis which ends in death from renal failure within a few weeks or months. As so often happens with the vocabulary of renal disease, the term has also been used by histologists to define a certain pathological appearance characterized by the presence of numerous and voluminous crescents. One form of clinically rapidly progressive glomerular nephritis is that of Goodpasture's syndrome (glomerular nephritis + pulmonary haemorrhage), thus some authorities tend to think that all patients with rapidly progressive glomerular nephritis have Goodpasture's syndrome whether or not there are pulmonary haemorrhages. Others use the term *rapidly progressive glomerular nephritis* when there is evidence of anti glomerular basement antibodies regardless of the clinical course. The subject is a semantic jungle where the innocent should be on their guard against making ambiguous assumptions. The term acute crescentic rapidly progressive glomerular nephritis defines a small important group which is described here.

### Immunological mechanisms

There is evidence for both immune complex mediated, and anti glomerular basement membrane, disease. But in some patients no deposits can be found. There is also a heavy interstitial infiltration with inflammatory cells so that a cell mediated mechanism may play a part.

### Pathology

At autopsy it is unusual for there to be more than some cortical narrowing to be seen with the naked eye. The macroscopical appearances of the kidney in patients dying during a nephrotic syndrome may either resemble those found in patients dying of persistent glomerular nephritis with chronic renal failure, or both kidneys are pale, smooth and enlarged. Death from chronic renal failure is associated with bilateral, symmetrical, shrunken, irregular and firm kidneys, the surfaces of which are pitted from contraction of underlying fibrous tissue, and raised by areas of hypertrophied nephrons.

The outstanding histological lesion on light microscopy is the presence of numerous thick and enveloping capsular crescents which appear to encompass the glomerular tufts (Fig. 21.3). The crescents consist of macrophages bound together by fibrin. They do not consist of a proliferation of the parietal epithelial cells of Bowman's capsule, as was once thought. Electron microscopy suggests that these crescentic collections of macrophages may be a response to local areas of glomerular capillary rupture due to necrosis which allow blood to leak directly into the capsular space. Alternatively the macrophages may have invaded the capsular space through small ruptures of Bowman's capsule itself. These occur relatively frequently and tend to be overlooked. Light microscopy evidence of necrosis of the glomerular tuft is unusual. The glomerular tufts, apart from being compressed, often look remarkably normal though a few may show mild focal proliferation of the mesangium. As the disease progresses there are an increasing number of sclerosed glomeruli. The tubules are invariably widely separated by a marked increase in interstitial material which is heavily infiltrated with chronic inflammatory cells. As in acute glomerular nephritis there are often scattered foci of tubular necrosis.

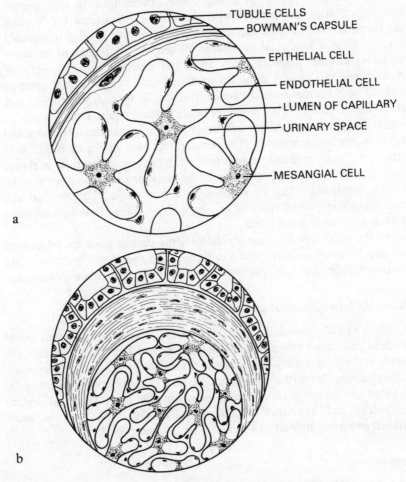

Fig. 21.3 (a) Normal, (b) acute crescentic glomerular nephritis.

The outstanding immunofluorescent finding is the presence of fibrinogen in the crescents, in the necrotic areas within the tuft and in intramembranous deposits. $\beta_1 C$ is also seen in coarse irregular deposits in the capillary walls and in the mesangial areas. IgA, IgG and IgM is found in various combinations in a coarse, irregular and globular pattern along the capillary wall, and in the mesangium. Occasionally IgG is found in a smooth intensely fluorescent line along the capillary wall. It is very important to note that acute, crescentic rapidly progressive glomerular nephritis is seldom associated with anti GBM disease. Electron microscopy reveals the focal discontinuities of the capillary walls, mentioned above, and intramembranous deposits.

### Clinical features

The disease tends to occur in young adults, in contrast to polyarteritis nodosa, which also may present with the same clinical features. It often begins abruptly with an acute nephritic syndrome or may develop insidiously with or without a nephrotic syndrome. When it is a sequel to an acute nephritic syndrome there is often an initial diuresis and the signs of pulmonary oedema usually diminish or disappear, but the patient remains severely ill with lassitude, headache and malaise. Some oedema remains and there is much pallor. The blood pressure remains raised and tends to continue rising, the erythrocyte sedimentation rate is considerably raised and there is a persistent anaemia. Glomerular filtration rate and blood urea fluctuate, but both gradually deteriorate; the ability to concentrate is always grossly impaired from the beginning. Proteinuria may increase greatly and a nephrotic syndrome often develops after a few weeks. Urinary red cell excretion is always raised to extremely high levels. From time to time there may be macroscopic haematuria.

When the condition develops insidiously, the patient presents because of increasing lethargy, malaise and headache. The signs and symptoms are those just described except that there is no evidence of pulmonary oedema.

### Relationship between clinical and structural features

Clinically a rapidly downhill progressive course can occur with many other conditions than acute crescentic disease (see below). But when crescents are present in large numbers the patient tends to present in the manner described above. Nevertheless, the glomerular changes give little information about the extent of functional impairment. On the other hand, extensive tubular and interstitial lesions correlate well with the creatinine clearance and gross inability to concentrate the urine (p. 33).

### Prognosis

If less than 50% of the glomeruli contain crescents the disease is unlikely to be fatal within the next few years whereas if they are present in more than 80% of glomeruli death from renal failure with severe hypertension can be expected within two years. The finding of anti-GBM antibodies is of far less prognostic importance for the disease may be rapidly fatal in their absence, or linger on with little continued deterioration of renal function in its presence. Intercurrent infections may precipitate an acute deterioration. The likelihood of their occurrence is increased when the patient's renal failure has to be treated by haemodialysis because of the vulnerability to infection of the arteriovenous shunt.

## Treatment

Several methods have been tried but as the nature of the disease is such that it has been impossible to organise a control trial it is difficult to know how effective they are. Plasmapheresis can sometimes cause an acute improvement in renal function but it must be started before glomerular filtration rate is below 10 ml/min. It is usual to accompany this treatment with some form of immunosuppression such as cyclophosphamide and prednisone. Others have used very high doses of prednisone (100 mg/day) including the intravenous administration of 1 to 3 g of methylprednisone per day (given over 20 min) for three successive days. Dypiridamole and heparin have also been given.

## Differential Diagnosis

Polyarteritis and disseminated lupus erythematosus are the two conditions with which the rapidly progressive form of persistent primary glomerular nephritis may be most often confused. Occasionally when the onset is gradual and the patient is middle aged or older the condition may have to be distinguished from subacute endocarditis, amyloid disease or myelomatosis. A renal biopsy is the only way to make certain of the diagnosis. Other conditions which may cause confusion are Goodpasture's syndrome, haemolytic uraemic syndrome and malignant hypertension.

## Recurrent macroscopic haematuria including some cases of persistent proteinuria with microscopic haematuria, and others with persistent proteinuria without haematuria

This group is brought together by the histological appearances of focal proliferative glomerular nephritis.

## Immunological Mechanisms

The histological appearances are those of immune complex disease. IgA and other complexes are found in the mesangium and can also be detected in the blood.

*Pathology*

Often all the glomeruli look normal. When lesions are evident they are in the glomeruli and are both focal and segmental, i.e. only some glomeruli are involved and initially only a portion of a glomerulus is affected. (Fig. 21.4). The lesions consist of mesangial cell proliferation with intercapillary eosinophilic deposits, capsular adhesions, focal areas of glomerular fibrosis and very occasionally partial necrosis of the tuft.

The main immunodeposit is IgA which is present in the mesangium in irregular shaped clumps together with $C_3$ and properdin. In striking contrast to the light microscopy abnormalities, however, which are focal and segmental, mesangial IgA is present in *all* the glomeruli, whether or/not they appear normal on light microscopy, and it is scattered diffusely within each tuft. This is of the greatest interest for it emphasises the fact that immu-

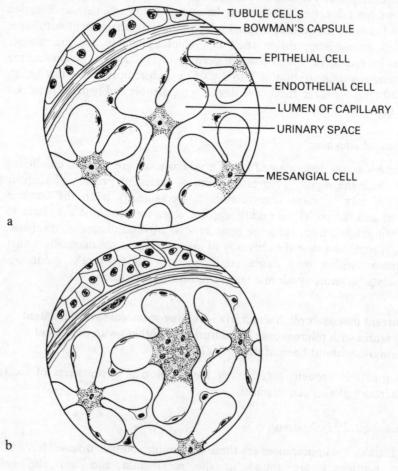

TUBULE CELLS
BOWMAN'S CAPSULE
EPITHELIAL CELL
ENDOTHELIAL CELL
LUMEN OF CAPILLARY
URINARY SPACE
MESANGIAL CELL

a

b

**Fig. 21.4** (a) Normal, (b) focal proliferative glomerular nephritis.

noglobulin can be fixed to the capillary wall without producing a recognisable light-microscopy change in the capillary wall. Sometimes the mesangium contains, in addition small amounts of IgG and fibrinogen.

When there are IgA deposits there may be a wide variety of other deposits. Frequently there are diffuse, focal, granular scattered deposits of $C_3$ together with occasionally small deposits of IgM, IgG or fibrin. In a third of those patients who have recurrent haematuria no deposits can be detected. It has been claimed that, in women, this disease is mainly seen in those on the contraceptive pill. The tubules and renal interstitium are normal. Deposits of IgA and $C_3$ are also present in the skin.

## Clinical features

Recurrent haematuria in glomerular nephritis is sometimes known as recurrent 'focal' nephritis. It occurs most commonly in young or adolescent males. Often each attack is associated with a sore throat or 'cold' and a general feeling of malaise out of proportion to the upper respiratory symptoms. These are not due to infection with β-haemolytic streptococci. It has been claimed, but not proven, that a virus is sometimes responsible. Haematuria begins at the same time or within one to three days of the onset of sore throat and it may last several weeks. As it settles the patient's general symptoms also improve. During the attack there may be some transient mild impairment of renal function but no oedema or hypertension. In between the attacks the patient feels well. Eventually most patients have persistent proteinuria though it may not become persistent until they have had several relapses. A raised urinary red cell excretion accompanies the persistent proteinuria. Some patients with the pathological lesions described above have never suffered from macroscopic haematuria. Either they have persistent proteinuria with microscopic haematuria or persistent proteinuria without haematuria.

The geographical incidence of 'focal nephritis' particularly that associated with deposits of IgA varies considerably being relatively rare in Great Britain and much more frequent in Singapore and South Australia where the prognosis also appears to be considerably worse.

## Course and prognosis

At one time it was considered that when macroscopic haematuria and a sore throat developed simultaneously the renal condition was benign and transient. It is probable that with a single episode this is a justifiable conclusion. When there are recurrent attacks, however, the long-term prognosis is not so good. Some patients have been known to have recurrent attacks for 25 years without any marked deterioration. But others with perhaps more frequent attacks eventually die of renal failure and hypertension. In an unknown number the attacks cease and there appears to be a full recovery. As in all immunological diseases of the kidney children have the best prognosis and and often do well even though they have multiple attacks.

## Treatment

There is no consistently effective treatment. It seems reasonable to keep the patient in bed until he feels better, and it is convenient that the duration of this period usually coincides with the duration of macroscopic haematuria. Some authorities give prophylactic oral penicillin to avoid a superimposed β-haemolytic streptococcal infection. In some patients prednisone may produce a quick remission, but in others it only makes things worse.

*Differential diagnosis.* This syndrome is quite easily separated clinically and histologically from the rapidly progressive form of persistent glomerular nephritis or acute glomerular nephritis. The combination of recurrent painless haematuria and a sore throat should exclude local structural conditions of the kidney though the condition has been confused with recurrent urinary infections or renal stones. The first attack is the most difficult to distinguish with any certainty. It can easily be confused with the onset of polyarteritis nodosa, Henoch-Schönlein's purpura or of some 'bleeding' disorder.

## Nephrotic syndrome, or persistent proteinuria with or without haematuria, associated with either no light microscopy changes or with equivocal changes

This group of patients either have a nephrotic syndrome, which is indistinguishable from that which occurs in patients who have marked histological abnormalities. Or the patient may present with asymptomatic proteinuria sometimes with microscopical haematuria.

## Immunological mechanism

The immunological basis for this condition continues to be even more puzzling than for the other forms of glomerular nephritis. On the one hand the disease is the only form of glomerular nephritis which consistently responds to steroids and immuno-suppressive drugs such as cyclophosphamide. On the other hand there are no immune deposits or signs of inflammation in the kidney. Recently it has become evident that there is a disturbance in lymphocyte function. This can be demonstrated by: (1) a diminished capacity of the patient's lymphocytes to be stimulated *in vitro* by mitogens, which is due to the presence of some substance in the plasma (2) a cytoxicity of some of the lymphocytes to human kidney tissue *in vitro* and (3) and alteration in suppressor cell activity. The relevance of these abnormalities to the functional lesion in the glomerular basement membrane which makes it more permeable to serum protein is not perceptible.

*Pathology*

The light microscopy appearances are either normal (nil change) or there is an equivocal increase in the number of mesangial cells (minimal change). Electron microscopy, however, usually shows fusion of the epithelial foot processes and very occasionally electron dense deposits in or near the glomerular basement membrane. Electron microscopy also demonstrates very small amounts of fibrin in the glomerular wall which are too small to be detected with immunofluorescence. Antisera specific for IgG, IgA, IgM, $\beta_1$C globulin and fibrinogen fail to demonstrate any fixation of these materials on the glomerulus.

*Course and prognosis*

These patients have an excellent prognosis and eventually have a complete remission of activity. They may remit permanently after the first attack of a nephrotic syndrome or they may have several relapses and remissions. Prednisone often hastens recovery, and cyclophosphamide may produce a long remission if the patient is prednisone dependent (p. 172).

*Treatment*

This is described in the section on the nephrotic syndrome (p. 171).

*Differential diagnosis*

Persistent proteinuria with or without haematuria in the presence of a nephrotic syndrome and a normal renal biopsy including immunofluorescence is diagnostic. The most difficult differential diagnosis is that of focal glomerular sclerosis (see below) which may be overlooked in the first biopsy because the early sclerotic lesions are small and few and far between, and, most important, they begin in the glomeruli which are near the medulla. It is also possible to miss an early extra membranous glomerular nephritis if the biopsy is only examined with a light microscope, before the capillary walls have thickened. With silver stains and immunofluorescence however the distinction is easily made. Systemic lupus erythematosus may sometimes present as a nephrotic syndrome with a normal renal biopsy on light microscopy but immunofluorescence demonstrates widespread deposition of immunoglobulin. Minimal change nephrotic syndrome may also accompany Hodgkins disease. But persistent proteinuria with haematuria without a nephrotic syndrome (perhaps during a remission of the disease) should promote a thorough examination of the urinary tract for a neoplasm.

**Patients with persistent proteinuria with and without microscopical haematuria, or a nephrotic syndrome or chronic renal failure who do not fit into the four groups described above**

The pathological findings in this group include *all* those histological changes that accompany glomerular nephritis, other than 'nil change'. Three have already been described. They are the diffuse proliferative, and focal proliferative lesions, and capsular crescents which accompany the clinical syndromes of acute glomerular nephritis, rapidly progressive glomerular nephritis and recurrent macroscopic haematuria. But these pathological changes are also found in some patients with persistent proteinuria with or without microscopical haematuria, or in others who have a nephrotic syndrome or chronic renal failure. These clinical syndromes are also accompanied by five additional pathological appearances in the glomeruli. They are: extra membranous; membrano-proliferative; focal sclerosis, intramembranous; and advanced lesions, the origin of which is no longer distinguishable.

*Immunological mechanism*

There is no doubt that this condition is in part mediated by the deposition of immune complexes. Because the immune deposits are situated furthest away from the capillary lumen it is unlikely that they are preformed in the circulation. It is more probable that they are formed *in situ*. A conclusion which is re-enforced by the fact that when there is no obvious antigenic association (see below) circulating immune complexes are rarely found.

**Extra membranous**

There is a diffuse even thickening of the capillary wall which electron microscopy demonstrates to be due to deposits located on the epithelial side of the glomerular basement membrane (Fig. 21.5). With haematoxylin and eosin these deposits are faintly eosinophilic and indistinguishable, from the other components of the capillary wall. With silver stains, however, which pick out the basement membrane it is often possible to demonstrate that the basement membrane sends up spiky projections between the extra membranous deposits. This gives the glomerular wall, when stained with silver, the appearance of a black stumpy, rather irregular comb (Fig. 3.3). At first before these argyrophyllic spikes have been formed the presence of the extramembranous deposits may be overlooked by light microscopy. Conversely, at a later stage the deposits may become surrounded by fusion of the tips of the spikes so that the deposits are surrounded by a layer of argyrophyllic basement membrane material. Proliferation of the tufts is unusual and never more than mild. Immuno-fluorescence always demonstrates a diffuse (i.e. in all parts of all glomeruli) fixation of IgG along the capillary wall but not in the mesangial area. This appearance is present before and after the characteristic argyrophyllic spiky projections are discernible. The IgG is usually laid down in a finely granular pattern but occasionally it has been found as a smooth linear deposit (as in rapidly progressive glomerular nephritis). In most biopsies $C_3$ is detected in the same pattern as the IgG and in the same location, though in smaller amounts. Occasionally small focal granular deposits of IgA, IgM and fibrinogen can also be detected. When the light microscopy appearances are normal (see above) the finely granular fixation of the anti IgG in a regular manner in all the glomerular capillaries permits the lesion of extra membranous glomerular nephritis to be detected nevertheless.

(There is a variant of extra membranous glomerular nephritis, sometimes called 'mixed deposit' disease, in which, in addition to the sub-epithelial deposits there are also sub-endothelial and intramembranous deposits yet these patients do not have and do not develop systemic lupus erythematosus.)

## Clinical course and prognosis

Patients with extra membranous glomerular nephritis who present with

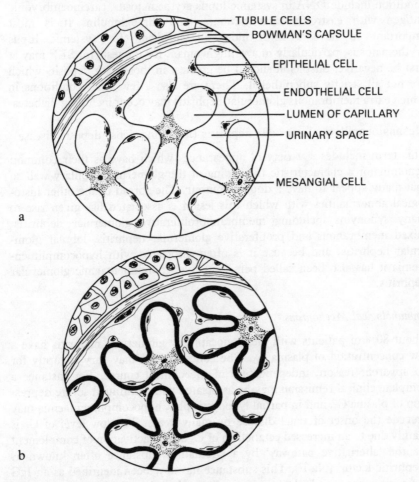

a

b

**Fig. 21.5** (a) Normal, (b) extra membranous glomerular nephritis.

persistent proteinuria in the absence of a nephrotic syndrome do remarkably well. In some, the disease does not appear to progress and in a few there is complete recovery. In the others (the majority) there is, on the whole, a slow deterioration of renal function. In one series 75% of the patients were alive at 10 years, with complete recovery in about 25%. In some however, the rate of deterioration is much more rapid. As usual children do best even if their nephrotic syndrome is accompanied by haematuria.

*Treatment.* No specific treatment is known. Steroids do not help.

*Differential Diagnosis.* There are many forms of secondary extra membranous glomerular nephritis which must be sedulously excluded. For instance the following extrinsic antigens are closely connected with the histological appearance of extra membranous glomerular nephritis, Hepatitis B (particularly among heroin addicts), gold, penicillamine, tridione, filariasis and mercury. Identifiable intrinsic antigens which may also give rise to the same condition include DNA in systemic lupus erythematosus, carcinoembryonic antigen with gastrointestinal tumours, and thryoglobulin. It is most important to have a high index of suspicion for systemic lupus erythematosus, particularly in a young woman, for the tests for SLE may at first be negative. Suspicion should be greatest in those with deposits which are not all strictly subepithelial. There are also a few other conditions in which extra membranous glomerular nephritis may occur including diabetes.

## Mesangiocapillary glomerular nephritis (including dense deposit disease)

This term includes a variety of appearances which have as their common denominator a characteristic thickening of the glomerular capillary wall so that many appear to have a double contour. The spread of the other histological abnormalities with which this lesion is associated has given rise to many synonyms including membranoproliferative glomerular nephritis, mixed membranous and proliferative glomerular nephritis, lobular glomerular nephritis, and because it is often associated with hypocomplimentaemia it has also been called persistent hypocomplimentaemic glomerular nephritis.

### Immunological Mechanisms

About 80% of patients with mesangiocapillary glomerular nephritis have a low concentration of plasma $C_3$. The concentration may vary abruptly for no apparent reason, independently of the clinical course. For instance a complete clinical remission may be associated with continued severe depression of plasma $C_3$, and in partial lypodystrophy, hypocomplimentaemia may precede the onset of renal disease by many years. The low level of $C_3$ is mainly due to an increased catabolism of $C_3$ due to activation of complement via the 'alternative pathway' by a circulating substance often known as 'nephritic factor' (Ne F). This substance has now been identified as an IgG molecule whose antibody activity is directed against $C_3bBb$ moiety of the alternate pathway $C_3$ convertase. Once the $C_3$ convertase is bound to antibody it is protected from the usual mechanisms which are involved in it's destruction. Thus what would under physiological circumstances be a trivial labile alternative pathway convertase, instead becomes a persistent $C_3$ convertase causing massive $C_3$ break-down in plasma. It does not appear, therefore, that this abnormality is responsible for the renal lesion. It is a marker of a genetic predisposition to develop mesangio-capillary glomerular nephritis by some other means.

*Pathology*

There is a combination of mesangial cell proliferation, an increase in mesangial cell cytoplasm and matrix, with grossly irregular thickening of the capillary walls (Fig. 21.6). Sometimes the large accumulation of mesangial cytoplasm and matrix gives the glomerular tuft a lobular appearance (Fig. 21.6). In a substantial number of patients (approximately 10–20%) there may be an important (30 to 100%) number of capsular crescents. And neutrophil polymorphs are often found in the glomerular tuft. Electron microscopy demonstrates that the capillary wall thickening is due to extensions of mesangial cell cytoplasm penetrating and extending between the glomerular basement membrane and the endothelium. With silver stains this gives the glomerular capillary wall where this has happened, the appearance of two argyrophyllic parallel lines separated by an empty space sometimes known as 'double contors' (Fig. 3.1).

Electron microscopy reveals the presence of two types of deposits. One is finely granular and lies beneath the endothelium of the capillary wall, and in the mesangium including the extensions mentioned above. The other deposits are very dense and, though irregular in size and shape they lie in a continuous ribbon like manner occupying most of the central area of the capillary basement membrane which they tend to thicken, leaving only a thin clear line of normal basement membrane on either side. This appearance which is known as dense deposit disease can usually be recognised in a thin section by light microscopy. Dense deposits are also found in the mesangium and the basement membrane of Bowman's capsule and of some tubules.

Immunofluorescence demonstrates a coarse, irregular granular deposition of $C_3$, mainly in the capillary walls, and to a lesser extent in the mesangial areas. Sometimes this is diffuse, occasionally focal. Usually there are also focal coarse intramembranous deposits of IgM and fibrinogen, occasionally granular, irregular, diffuse deposits of IgG are found. IgA is not found. Very occasionally there is only $C_3$ unaccompanied by the presence of any immunoglobulin. In the biopsies showing a lobular pattern the $C_3$ is located only in the periphery of each lobule, never in the centre.

There are focal areas of interstitial nephritis, their number reflecting the severity of the glomerular lesion.

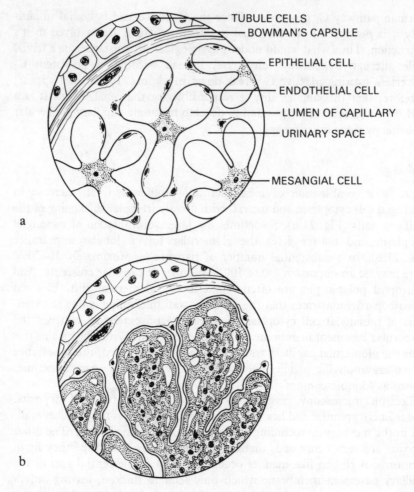

TUBULE CELLS
BOWMAN'S CAPSULE
EPITHELIAL CELL
ENDOTHELIAL CELL
LUMEN OF CAPILLARY
URINARY SPACE
MESANGIAL CELL

a

b

**Fig. 21.6** (a) Normal, (b) mesangio capillary glomerular nephritis.

## Clinical course and prognosis

In a third of patients the clinical manifestation of the disease are preceded by an acute respiratory infection. The disease is relatively common in children and is seen as often in girls and women as in boys and men, which is unusual for in the other forms of glomerular nephritis men usually predominate. Children fare better than adults but overall the prognosis is death from renal failure sooner or later. Approximately 50% of patients survive 10 years. Clinical remissions, with absence of proteinuria, can occur but the histological lesions remain. Relapses usually recur within a few years. The prognosis like that of rapidly progressive glomerular nephritis is particularly related to the incidence of capsular crescents, with death from renal failure within two years when more than 80% of the glomeruli contain crescents. In the absence of crescents renal function may remain normal for many years but when deterioration does occur it tends to be rapid. The presence of the electron dense deposits does not appear to effect the outcome. The prognosis is worse in the presence of a nephrotic syndrome and best in those who have had a remission.

## Treatment

There is no specific treatment. The effect of prednisone is often more lethal than helpful.

## Differential Diagnosis

The lobular pattern of mesangial proliferation with thickened glomerular walls can be seen in systemic lupus erythematosus. Superficially this has a striking resemblence to lobular mesangiocapillary glomerular nephritis but the characteristic double contour lesion of the capillary wall does not occur.

## Focal sclerosing glomerular nephritis

### Immunological mechanisms

None have been identified. Its relation to other forms of glomerular nephritis and the fact that it recurs in a transplanted kidney (as so many other forms of glomerular nephritis) suggest that the condition is due to an immunological disturbance.

### Pathology

At first the lesions are focal and they are characteristically segmental. Initially the lesions tend to be predominantly in the deepest glomeruli (those furthest from the cortex) so that a biopsy that does not penetrate the cortico medullary region may fail to reveal their presence. The lesions consist of a segmental skrinkage of the glomerular tuft which at this point adheres to a capsule (Fig. 21.7). The lesion contains eosinophilous deposits, hyaline capillary thrombi and fatty deposits. In most biopsies focal collections of IgM and $C_3$ can be demonstrated, confined to the sclerosed areas. Focal areas of tubular atrophy are always present. Their number is in proportion to the number of glomeruli which are affected.

Sometimes the glomerular lesions appear during the 'healing' phase of focal glomerulonephritis when residual areas of focal proliferation can be seen.

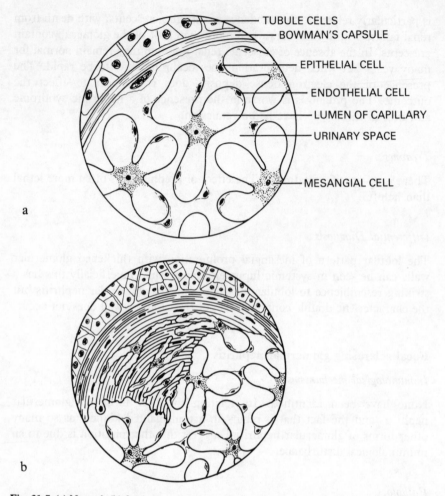

TUBULE CELLS
BOWMAN'S CAPSULE
EPITHELIAL CELL
ENDOTHELIAL CELL
LUMEN OF CAPILLARY
URINARY SPACE
MESANGIAL CELL

a

b

**Fig. 21.7** (a) Normal, (b) focal sclerosing glomerular nephritis.

## Course and prognosis

Focal sclerosis may accompany a nephrotic syndrome or persistent protein-uria from the beginning or it may be superimposed on what at first appeared to be minimal change glomerular nephritis. Characteristically a nephrotic syndrome associated with focal sclerosis does not respond to steroids though it may do so at the beginning of the illness. The prognosis is poor, most patients eventually dying of renal failure. When the lesion is associated with proliferative or other varieties of renal pathology the prognosis tends to follow that of the associated lesion.

## Treatment

There is no known treatment.

*Differential diagnosis*

In the absence of proliferation the lesion is not found in association with any other histological abnormality. The main concern is that what appears at first to be a minimal change glomerular nephritis with a good prognosis, may eventually turn out to be focal sclerosing glomerular nephritis. A useful distinguishing feature is the presence of tubular atrophy. This is not seen in minimal change glomerular nephritis.

## Advanced lesions

Beyond a certain stage in glomerular nephritis from any cause the normal structural layout of the kidney is completely shattered and it becomes unrecognisable. There is a large amount of fibrous tissue interspersed with nephrons which are either hypertrophied or in various stages of disintegration. Glomeruli are scarce, scarred and sclerosed, and contain few nuclei. In some glomeruli there are coarse granular focal deposits of $\beta_1C$, globulin on the remnants of the glomerular basement membrane. In others there is no fixation of antisera. It is clear that at this stage immunofluorescence is now as useless as light microscopy in identifying the

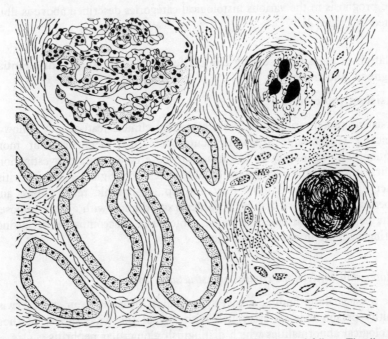

**Fig. 21.8** Schema of persistent glomerular nephritis with chronic renal failure. The diagram emphasises the following points: the gross generalised disturbance with a hypertrophied glomerulus and tubule, surrounded by a matting of connective and fibrous tissue in which are embedded atrophic tubules, disintegrating glomeruli and some chronic inflammatory cells. One glomerulus is completely fibrosed (depicted as solid black) while the third shows a crescent and deposits of an eosin staining material in the tuft.

original lesion. Most of the tubules which remain are insignificant, atrophic, and have flattened epithelium and narrow lumens. Hypertrophied tubules are easily identified by their large glomeruli and exceedingly wide tubules; it is in these large nephrons that the 'broad' casts of chronic renal failure originate (Fig. 21.8).

In all varieties of persistent glomerular nephritis there may be changes in the arteries; including atheroma, intimal and medial thickening, endarteritis obliterans and arteriolar necroses. These in turn will produce varying degrees of ischaemic changes in the renal parenchyma (p. 261) in addition to those just described.

There is increasing evidence from serial biopsies in individual patients that the histological appearances in the glomeruli rarely change from one variety of 'histological' glomerular nephritis to another, i.e. a patient with no definite abnormality or 'membranous' change will not subsequently develop 'proliferative' changes and vice versa. This is in contrast to the tubules which may suddenly become severely affected having previously been intact.

## Overall prognosis

The prognosis in the various histological categories described above is illustrated in Figure 21.9.

## Relation of certain presenting clinical features to prognosis, differential diagnosis and treatment

### Persistent proteinuria

Persistent proteinuria, as the only abnormal clinical feature may follow a clinically recognisable attack of acute glomerular nephritis, but more frequently it does not do so. It is usually discovered on routine investigation. At first it may be the only indication of the presence of glomerular nephritis. Later a nephrotic syndrome may develop, or chronic renal failure and hypertension, or there may be a sudden exacerbation with a superimposed acute nephritic syndrome. Often the proteinuria is accompanied by a fluctuating increase in red cell excretion.

### Relationship between the clinical and structural features

The most striking finding is that symptomless proteinuria in an otherwise healthy person may be associated with any of the wide variety of those histological abnormalities which distinguish glomerular nephritis.

### Course and prognosis

The most important point is that persistent proteinuria carries an uncertain

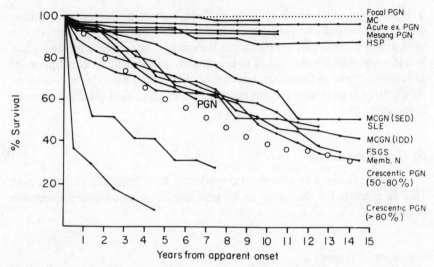

**Fig. 21.9** The survival of patients with various types of histopathologic patterns of glomerular nephritis found in renal biopsies. The curves have been calculated by the method of Cutler and Ederer. The data are drawn from a total of over 2500 patients.
(Reproduced from Cameron 1979 in: Black D, Jones N F (eds) Renal disease. Blackwell Scientific, 329, with kind permission.)

Key: Focal PGN      Focal proliferative glomerular nephritis
MC              Minimal change
Acute ex. PGN   Acute exudative proliferative glomerular nephritis
Mesang. PGN     Mesangial proliferative glomerular nephritis (lobular stalk thickening)
HSP             Henoch-Schönlein purpura nephritis
MCGN (SED)      Mesangiocapillary glomerular nephritis with subendothelial deposits
SLE             Systemic lupus erythematosus nephritis
MCGN (IDD)      Mesangiocapillary glomerular nephritis with intra-membranous dense deposits (dense deposit disease)
FSGS            Focal and segmental glomerulosclerosis
Memb.n.         Membranous nephropathy
Crescentic      Crescentic (extracapillary) proliferative glomerular nephritis with
PGN (50–80%)    between 50 to 80% of glomeruli involved by crescents
Crescentic      Crescentic (extracapillary) proliferative glomerular nephritis but with
PGN (>80%)      more than 80% of glomeruli with cresents

The *open circles* represent the survival of patients with stage I and II carcinoma of the breast. It is apparent that the prognosis given for focal proliferative glomerular nephritis is more favourable than that described in the text. It is probable that this is due to a preponderance in this series of children in whom the disease is relatively frequent and milder.

prognosis whatever the histological appearance, and that the longer it has persisted the poorer the outlook. As can be seen in Figure 21.9 a renal biopsy does permit some rough prediction about mean survival but individual variations are very great.

*Differential diagnosis*

As nearly all renal disease presents with proteinuria the differential diagnosis is a wide one. The first step is to exclude orthostatic proteinuria. Subsequently an extensive investigation is necessary, including an intravenous pyelogram, a renal biopsy, urinary cell excretion rate, creatinine clearance, and in some patients the ability to concentrate and to acidify. It is important to remember not to forget the possibility of subacute bacterial endocarditis, particularly in an elderly patient in whom the usual clinical manifestations are inconspicuous.

**Nephrotic syndrome**

The clinical features of a nephrotic syndrome have been described on page 162. It is usual for the onset to be gradual, but a rapid onset sometimes occurs.

*Course and Prognosis*

The course and prognosis will vary according to the histological appearances. The oedema and heavy proteinuria may fluctuate with complete remissions interspersed with relapses. An exacerbation or relapse of oedema and proteinuria is sometimes heralded by the onset of an acute nephritic syndrome. When renal failure supervenes generalised oedema often persists though there is less proteinuria. Before the introduction of antibiotics the commonest cause of death in patients with a nephrotic syndrome was infection.

As death is due either to renal failure or hypertension it is clear that as long as there is no evidence of either, the immediate and short-term prognosis is good. But even when these ominous signs do appear the prognosis is not necessarily poor, for sometimes, after an anxious few weeks, renal function may improve, haematuria ceases and the blood pressure returns to normal. Occasionally glomerular filtration rate may remain around 40–60 ml/min for many years even though there may be intermittent periods of transient deterioration (in two cases for up to 20 years). In some instances the blood pressure rises gradually but there is no marked deterioration in renal function. The earlier in the disease that hypertension and renal failure occur the worse the prognosis, particularly in children; it is also a bad sign when there is massive oedema which is difficult to remove.

*Differential diagnosis*

The other conditions in which the nephrotic syndrome may appear are given on p. 162. Cases due to myelomatosis, diabetes, anaphylactoid purpura and irradiation of the kidneys are relatively easy to distinguish. Amyloid disease of the kidney may be inferred from the clinical history and confirmed by biopsy; occasionally a renal biopsy shows amyloidosis when the clinical history is unhelpful or misleading and a liver biopsy negative. Thrombosis of the renal vein is suspected if there is evidence of inferior vena caval thrombosis, recurrent pulmonary emboli from an unknown site, or the patient is known to have only one kidney, or amyloidosis. It is important to keep in mind the association of a nephrotic syndrome with neoplasia (Hodgkins in the young, and carcinoma of colon in the elderly) and the administration of certain exogenous substances such as trioxidone, gold and penicillamine.

To distinguish a nephrotic syndrome due to primary glomerular nephritis from oedema to polyarteritis nodosa and systemic lupus erythematosis (SLE) may be difficult. Polyarteritis as a cause of the nephrotic syndrome is unusual; at the onset it may be very difficult to distinguish from glomerular nephritis; renal biopsy is rarely helpful. The diagnosis is made when some more characteristic features of polyarteritis nodosa become evident (peripheral neuritis, fever, tachycardia, muscle pains, etc.) and is confirmed by muscle biopsy. SLE is the most difficult condition to distinguish from glomerular nephritis, for sometimes there are no firm clinical reasons for suspecting the diagnosis. And the histological changes in SLE overlap those of glomerular nephritis. In the last resort the distinction between the two diseases has to be made on the presence of the clinical features, of SLE cells in the peripheral blood or bone marrow, and evidence of nuclear antigenic material in the peripheral blood. The search should be repeated from time to time for the renal manifestations of SLE may precede the systemic signs of the disease by some months.

*Treatment.*

Treatment is either symptomatic or it attempts to be curative. Persistent proteinuria does not need symptomatic treatment and the symptomatic treatment of the nephrotic syndrome is described on p. 71. Prednisone and cytotoxic drugs have no effect on the course of glomerular nephritis when it is accompanied by any of the light microscopy changes described. There is some evidence that, on the contrary, the use of prednisone or cytotoxic drugs in such patients, particularly adults, may shorten survival because of their serious side effects.

## Chronic renal failure

The clinical features of chronic renal failure have been described in Chapter 13. This is the final stage through which pass most patients who eventually succumb to persistent glomerular nephritis. In a few cases it is already known that the patient suffers from persistent glomerular nephritis. In most patients the symptoms of advanced chronic renal failure, hypertensive cardiac failure, or malignant hypertension are the first indication of its presence.

*Relationship between the histological and structural features*

The individual lesions are the same as those described in patients with persistent proteinuria, recurrent haematuria or the nephrotic syndrome. The main difference is that the lesions are now more extensive, particularly those involving the tubules and interstitial spaces.

Renal function and the duration of survival are only poorly correlated with the extent of the histological findings.

*Course and prognosis*

The rate of renal destruction varies very greatly; it may fluctuate with quiescent periods and acute exacerbations. The duration of the disease, from beginning to end, may extend to 30 years, but, once glomerular filtration rate has begun to fall and the blood urea to rise, there is a tendency for the advance of chronic renal failure to be fairly rapid an inexorable. As a very rough approximation once the blood urea is greater than 15 mmol/l (100 mg/100 ml) the prognosis is not likely to be greater than 3–5 years, and when it is over 30 mmol/l (200 mg/100 ml) it is less than 1–2 years. These figures relate to the concentration of blood urea when the patient is on an unrestricted diet, has not had a recent haemorrhage or attack of diarrhoea and vomiting, is free from cardiac failure, and is not suffering from an acute exacerbation of the disease process as evidenced by the development of an acute nephritic syndrome or haematuria. It has already been stressed repeatedly how circulatory insufficiency exacerbates renal failure and tends to give an erroneous impression of the extent of any underlying renal structural damage. Such an exacerbation may cause death from acute renal failure at a time when there is only a moderate amount of renal structural damage.

Hypertension shortens the duration of survival, particularly if it is difficult to treat.

*Differential diagnosis*

Unless there is a suggestive past history, it is almost impossible to be certain of a diagnosis of persistent glomerular nephritis as a cause of chronic renal failure without a renal biopsy.

Persistent glomerular nephritis has to be distinguished from the other causes of chronic renal failure (p. 181). It is important that there should be no confusion with chronic renal failure due to *chronic urinary obstruction*; the distinction is not particularly difficult.

The most common cause of confusion is nephrosclerosis (i.e. renal destruction directly due to hypertension (p. 260)). The distinction is often impossible without a renal biopsy. Statistically the more severe the renal failure the more certain the diagnosis of persistent glomerular nephritis becomes, for 'non-malignant' hypertension only rarely causes advanced renal failure. Again, if a patient is found to have malignant hypertension and there is no previous history of renal disease, it may be impossible to determine whether there exists an underlying chronic structural lesion such as persistent glomerular nephritis. Malignant hypertension is more likely to be a complication of preexisting renal disease of the kidneys are small, or the renal failure is advanced when the diagnosis is first made.

Treatment is that of chronic renal failure (p. 212). It aims at minimising or controlling certain functional impairments. It is doubtful if any method slows the rate of renal structural disintegration, except the control of hypertension and possibly some reduction in protein intake.

## GOODPASTURE'S SYNDROME (lung purpura with nephritis)

### Clinical features

The prototype of this rare condition is a young man between 18 and 25 year who becomes ill during a pandemic of influenza. Following an upper respiratory or gastric type of influenzal illness there is a sudden onset of profuse haemoptysis which lowers the haemoglobin within a few days. Serial chest X-rays demonstrate the presence of fluctuating pulmonary shadows due to blood in the pulmonary alveoli. The presence of glomerular nephritis is usually detected a few days after the onset of the haemoptysis. There is proteinuria, haematuria (sometimes macroscopic) and renal failure. Death usually occurs within a few months from renal failure: occasionally there is acute renal failure.

In the past few years it has become apparent that the disease can present in a much milder form with alternate relapses and remissions and a relatively slow deterioration of renal function. In some patients the disease has predominantly affected the lungs while renal function has remained normal except for proteinuria. In others renal failure has followed some months after the first haemoptysis.

### Pathology

The condition represents a form of anti-glomerular basement disease in which anti-glomerular basement antibodies can be detected in the blood and IgG and $C_3$ are laid down in a smooth linear pattern in the capillary walls of the glomeruli, the tubules and the alveoli. The renal lesion is one of rapidly progressive glomerular nephritis with numerous capsular crescents and a tendency to have segmental areas of necrosis in the same glomeruli. The lungs contain collections of haemosiderin in the alveoli and alveolar walls, with many histiocytes; both these changes are presumably consequent upon the haemorrhage.

## Treatment

The most promising form of treatment appears to be plasma exchanges to lower the circulating concentration of anti-glomerular-basement membrane antibody, together with prednisone, and cyclophosphamide or azathioprine (Fig. 21.10). But treatment must start before glomerular filtration rate has fallen below 10 ml/min. Great care must also be taken to avoid intercurrent infections for they give rise to sudden and alarming deteriorations of renal function, often when the condition appears to be improving. Nevertheless it must be pointed out that control trials of therapy have not been carried out and spontaneous recoveries, even after the onset of anuria, have been reported. Some patients, in whom the disease has not been arrested have subsequently survived on maintenance haemodialysis. Renal transplantation must not be performed until anti-glomerular-basement-membrane antibodies have disappeared from the plasma, for otherwise the transplanted kidney is rapidly destroyed. As might be anticipated bilateral nephrectomy appears to hasten the disappearance of the anti-glomerular-basement-membrane antibodies.

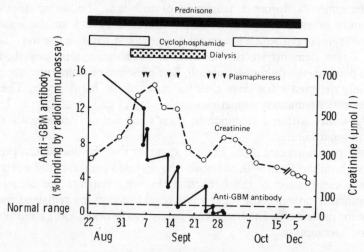

Fig. 21.10 Successful treatment of Goodpasture's syndrome with plasma exchange, prednisone, cyclophosphamide and haemodialysis. Conversion: Traditional to SI units approx 6.0 mg/100 ml. = creatinine 500 μmol/l (Reproduced from Lockwood, Boulton-Jones, Lowenthal et al 1975 Brit Med J 2: 252, with kind permission.)

## HENOCH-SCHONLEIN'S SYNDROME (Anaphylactoid purpura)

### Clinical features

Anaphylactoid purpura is characterised by a purpuric rash, abdominal pains, polyarthritis and haematuria; these usually occur in the young and follow a well-recognised infection such as tonsillitis, or occasionally they may be precipitated by the ingestion or administration of some substance to which the patient is subsequently found to be sensitive, e.g. tomatoes.

About 10–20% of all cases of anaphylactoid purpura have haematuria and proteinuria; an acute nephritic syndrome may also be present. In the majority of patients there is subsequently a rapid and complete recovery, while a few continue to excrete protein and red cells. In most of these proteinuria eventually disappears, but in the remainder it persists, chronic renal failure develops, and death occurs in one to five years. Recurrent attacks of macroscopical haematuria are a characteristic feature of this last group; they may also develop transient acute nephritic syndromes, and on occasion a nephrotic syndrome.

Approximately 10 per cent of those who have haematuria and proteinuria at the onset of an attack of anaphylactoid purpura die of chronic renal failure subsequently. As always the presence of numerous capsular crescents carries a poor prognosis.

*Immunological Mechanism*

The condition is a form of IgA nephritis. Immune complexes containing IgA, and others with IgG, are found in the circulation, and occasionally during the acute phase, circulating cryoglobulins can also be detected. Immunoglobulins are found in the renal lesions.

The removal of circulating complexes with plasma exchange does not appear to stop the deterioration of renal function (Fig. 21.11).

*Pathology*

The renal lesions consist of focal and segmental proliferative glomerular nephritis with diffuse granular deposits of IgA, IgG, $C_3$ and properdin in the glomerular capillary walls. The presence of properdin is an indication of alternative activation of complement. Capsular crescents may be present. The importance of the circulating complexes to the renal damage is problematical (Fig. 21.11). There are even larger deposits of fibrin diffusely distributed in all the glomeruli particularly in the mesangial areas. Focal collections of chronic inflammatory cells are present in the interstitial tissues, particularly around the abnormal glomeruli and there are areas of tubular atrophy. Electron microscopy reveals the presence of deposits in or near the mesangium either sub-endothelial or sub-epithelial. Deposits of IgA and $C_3$ are also found in the skin.

*Treatment*

It is doubtful if any treatment influences the course of the renal lesions; nevertheless, it is reasonable, in the acute attack, to treat any residual infection with antibiotics. In some, instances when there are recurrent

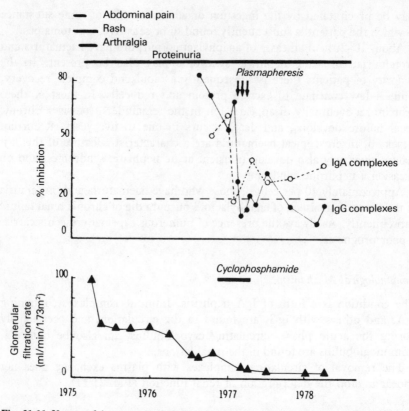

**Fig. 21.11** Unsuccesful treatment of Henoch-Schönlein's syndrome and nephritis with plasma exchanges and cyclophosphamide though the concentration of immune complex containing IgA and IgG in the plasma was lowered. IgA and IgG complexes expressed as per cent inhibition of agglutination. (Reproduced from Levinsky & Barratt 1979 Lancet 2: 1100, with kind permission.)

relapses due to β-haemolytic streptococcal infections, it may be necessary to give prophylactic penicillin.

Treatment of the advanced renal disturbances is unrewarding, though occasionally a patient may respond dramaticaly to ACTH or adrenal steroids; there are even some reports of complete cure. More often, however, adrenal steroids only produce a rapid rise in blood pressure, jugular venous pressure and blood urea, and treatment must be discontinued.

## RENAL POLYARTERITIS NODOSA

Polyarteritis nodosa produces generalised disturbances (such as fever), and focal vascular lesions. The kidneys are involved in about 80% of cases, either alone or in combination with other organs.

## Immunological Mechanism

There is little to suggest the underlying nature of the disease. Immune complexes are only rarely found in the plasma and only scanty deposits of IgG, IgM and $C_3$ are occasionally found in the glomeruli.

## Pathology

The characteristic vascular lesions in the kidney may occur in the glomerular capillaries, the arterioles, or the small and medium sized arteries. In renal biopsies, however, the overall changes are difficult to distinguish from those of glomerular nephritis. The arterial lesions are scattered and difficult to find.

The characteristic glomerular lesion is a focal necrotising capillaritis in the midst of an acute inflammatory reaction; occasionally the entire glomerulus is necrosed. The arterioles may either show arteriolar necrosis with perivascular inflammatory cell reaction, or endarteritis obliterans (i.e. the same lesions as in malignant hypertension, except for the perivascular inflammation). The medium and small sized arteries show the diagnostic lesion of polyarteritis nodosa; that is focal areas of acute segmental necrosis of a part or the whole of the arterial wall, together with an acute inflammatory reaction which invades and surrounds the necrotic area.

All these lesions occlude the lumen of the affected vessels and therefore the changes in the renal parenchyma (and the clinical features) largely depend on which vessels are involved. When the glomerular capillaries and the arterioles are affected the glomeruli show exudative and proliferative changes.

When the small and medium sized arteries are affected there will be wedge-shaped areas of infarction in which the glomeruli will at first only appear 'coagulated' or 'clumped' and then fibrosed and structureless, while the tubules, particularly the proximal tubules, become atrophied at an early stage. Relatively normal renal tissue may surround the infarcts.

Sometimes when the larger vessels are affected, the glomeruli may appear relatively normal but there are widespread tubular changes throughout the renal parenchyma, including tubular separation, changes in the nuclei, flattening of the tubular cells, and increase in size of their lumens. It is possible that these lesions are due to partial occlusions of the arcuate arteries.

Immunofluorescence demonstrates the presence of large amounts of fibrin deposits. These are focal in the glomeruli and in some vessels. Electron dense deposits are seen only very infrequently.

When the vascular lesions heal there are focal areas of marked intimal fibrosis which contain capillaries (the sites of recanalised thrombi); focal ruptures of the internal elastic lamina; and areas of focal fibrosis of the arterial walls extending into the surrounding tissues.

*Clinical features*

The wide variety of pathological changes accounts for the extensive range of clinical features. Renal polyarteritis nodosa may present as acute renal failure, chronic renal failure, an acute nephritic syndrome, or a nephrotic syndrome; the predominant abnormality may be proteinuria or severe haematuria, or tubular inability to control electrolyte excretion. The blood pressure tends to rise after the renal symptoms have appeared, and may continue to rise until there is malignant hypertension. The disease is more common in men than women and is more easily diagnosed in the young than in the elderly.

Acute renal failure occurs if there are extensive necrotic lesions in the glomeruli, while proteinuria, chronic renal failure and severe hypertension are more likely if the lesions are in the small and medium sized arteries and there are multiple infarcts.

One of the most frequent ways in which renal polyarteritis presents is as an acute nephritic syndrome. For a few weeks the diagnosis is usually confused with acute glomerular nephritis, but eventually the slow rate of recovery, or the stormy course of the syndrome, together with the appearance of some other non-renal clinical feature of polyarteritis nodosa, suggests the proper diagnosis. There may be attacks of severe unexplained central abdominal pain, fever, tachycardia, leucocytosis and eosinophilia, peripheral neuritis, pulmonary symptoms and radiological opacities in the lungs, skin rashes and nodules, or muscle pains and tenderness. The most characteristic features of active renal polyarteritis are (1) recurrent, irregularly spaced, sharp attacks, of unremitting, unilateral loin pain of sudden onset, usually lasting less than an hour, which are followed by an increased rate of red cell excretion in the urine. These probably occur at the moment of, or shortly after, the formation of small renal infarcts; occasionally the pain radiates to, or may be situated entirely in, the flanks and front of the abdomen; and (2) long continued excretion of fluctuating quantities of *macroscopic* haematuria is also a feature. Selective renal arteriogram may reveal a very characteristic appearance. This consists of small rounded opacities less than 1 mm diameter lying irregularly in the cortex.

The ability of the kidney to concentrate the urine is often impaired to a far greater extent than is the glomerular filtration rate.

*Course and prognosis*

The natural clinical course is often one of remissions and relapses, and occasionally evidence of such fluctuations can be found at autopsy, when both healed and active lesions of polyarteritis are seen. At any moment acute activity may cease. Ultimate recovery then depends on the extent of the vascular lesions, for healed lesions may continue to produce harmful effects, such as malignant hypertension or chronic renal failure.

Death may occur from lesions in other sites, but renal failure is the commonest cause of death in polyarteritis. Many cases develop renal failure fairly rapidly and die within a few months; those who begin with acute renal failure die within a few days.

Nevertheless some cases do recover; their number is not known, for unless there is positive histological evidence the diagnosis is uncertain, and it is obvious that such evidence is obtained less often in those patients who recover than in those who succumb.

*Treatment*

Before the use of cortisone the majority of cases of renal polyarteritis nodosa died of renal failure or hypertensive cardiac failure within one or two years of the onset of the disease. Steroids, however, often produce a remarkable and immediate remission of the acute symptoms, and in some cases they indubitably prolong life. The dose should be large (e.g. 40–100 mg prednisone per day), and it is essential that once a favourable effect has been produced the quantity should be continued uninterruptedly at a high level for several weeks. If the dose of adrenal steroids is lowered too rapidly there is often a relapse of symptoms, which for some inexplicable reason then no longer responds to adrenal steroids, or only does so when they are given in very large and potentially dangerous amounts (150 mg of predisone per day). Treatment with adrenal steroids should be continued for at least a year, the dose being lowered very gradually at monthly intervals during that time (e.g. by 1–2 mg each month); if signs of activity persist (e.g. raised ESR) treatment should be continued for longer.

The complications of adrenal steroid therapy have been mentioned (p. 173). The most important risk in the treatment of polyarteritis nodosa is retention and accumulation of salt and water, which may precipitate cardiac failure or a further rise in blood pressure. Initially, therefore, it is essential to measure the patient's weight and blood pressure and observe his jugular venous pressure each day. If necessary salt and water retention can be controlled by diuretics, and if the blood pressure begins to rise, it should be lowered by hypotensive drugs (p. 222). In some cases in which the blood pressure is very high at the onset it may be advisable for it to be lowered before beginning treatment with adrenal steroids.

*Differential diagnosis*

The renal disturbance caused by polyarteritis may suggest almost any form or renal disease. A renal biopsy is of some help in diagnosis, but unless a necrosed arteriole or artery is seen, surrounded by an intense inflammatory reaction, the precise diagnosis remains in doubt; and the chance of finding such a lesion in the small amount of tissue removed by biopsy is remote. Immunofluorescent studies make it relatively easy to distinguish the renal lesions of disseminated lupus erythematosus and most cases of primary glomerular nephritis.

A useful clinical point in difficult cases is the presence of fever, however mild. If blood cultures are negative, there are no lupus erythematosus cells, antinuclear factor or DNA antibodies in the peripheral blood, and the urine is sterile, renal disease associated with a pyrexia is due to polyarteritis nodosa until it is proved to the contrary. When polyarteritis is responsible for a nephrotic syndrome it is characteristic that the 24-hour urinary excretion of protein and the decrease in plasma proteins are more moderate than the extent of the oedema would suggest. Intermittent cardiac failure of uncertain origin and associated with only mild hypertension is another tenuous indication of polyarteritis.

## WEGENER'S GRANULOMATOSIS

A necrotising granulomatous condition of unknown cause mainly seen in older men. It usually affects the nasopharynx, the sinuses and lungs before the kidneys. There are recurrent nose bleeds and a purulent nasal discharge sometimes leading to a saddle nose deformity from destruction of bone. Renal involvement is often heralded by haematuria and is followed by a relentless rapid deterioration of renal function. As in polyarteritis nodosa, there is usually a fever and generalised symptoms such as weight loss and arthralgia.

The renal glomerular lesions are identical to the microscopical lesions of ployarteritis nodosa. At first there are focal areas of glomerular necrosis, later focal proliferation and crescents appear. It is one of the conditions in which there may be numerous glomerular crescents. Immunofluorescence techniques may demonstrate almost any pattern from nothing, to glomerular deposits of IgG and $C_3$, or $C_3$ fibrinogen, and even IgA, usually along the glomerular capillary wall and occasionally in the mesangial area. Fibrinogen is always found in the crescents.

The diagnosis is made by biopsy of a lesion in the upper respiratory tract. It is supported but not confirmed by the renal biopsy appearances described above. Without treatment, death occurs within a few months of the diagnosis being made though often there may have been a preceeding history of some nasal problem for many months or years. Treatment with steroids and cyclophosphamide may control the condition but usually treatment has to be continued indefinitely. Plasma exchange is excellent for controlling acute exacerbations.

## RENAL LUPUS ERYTHEMATOSUS

Systematised lupus erythematosus (SLE) resembles polyarteritis nodosa in that it also produces generalised disturbances and affects a wide variety of organs including, particularly, the kidney.

*Immunological and other aetiological factors* (Fig. 21.12)

SLE is the outstanding example of a soluble immune complex disease. Antigens and their respective antibodies have been identified in the circulation and in the tissues. As it is now well established that the course of the disease bears no consistent relationship with the presence of circulating immune complexes, it is possible that the harm is done by the formation of complexes in situ. The disease in man closely resembles a similar disturbance in a strain of New Zealand mice which become infected in utero with Concornavirus. It is thought that the human disease might be initiated by the same virus. The lymphocytes from patients with active SLE express coded material for concornavirus genetic material, and SLE can sometimes

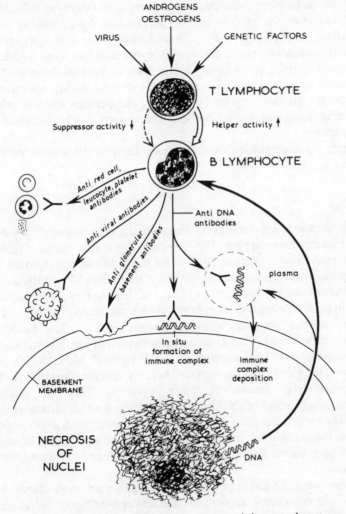

Fig. 21.12 Some possible aetiological mechanisms in systemic lupus erythematosus.

occur in small outbreaks within a family. In two such families the family dog also developed lupus. In addition there is evidence that genetic and humoral factors are also important. The disease tends to be familial. Identical twins have a 60% concordance for SLE even when apart. SLE is associated with inborn $C_2$ deficiency, the HLA-B8 haplotype and also with the DRW2 and DRW3 antigen. Androgens protect and oestrogens exacerbate the disease which probably accounts for the tenfold greater incidence of SLE in women.

Once the disease is established the principal immunological abnormality is one of B cell overactivity with antibodies being formed against a variety of tissues but principally against nuclear material, such as DNA. Hence the antinuclear factor (ANF) test for SLE; the antibody against doublestranded DNA being specific for the disease. The initiating step may be the release of nuclear material into the circulation from cells destroyed by viral infection. Thereafter the process can be perpetuated by circulating cytotoxic antibodies. Antibodies are also directed against virus antigen, red cells, polymorphoneuclear leucocytes, lymphocytes, and basement membrane. B cell hyperactivity appears to be due at least in part to diminished T cell suppressor activity which may in turn be due to inadequate information from the B cells that they are hyperactive, and perhaps also from the presence of lymphocytotoxic antibodies. There may also be increased T cell helper activity.

During an exacerbation of the disease there is a transient decrease in plasma $C_3$.

*Pathology*

The glomerular lesions include nil change on light microscopy (approx 30%), extra membranous (approx 15%), focal proliferative (approx 25%) and diffuse proliferative (approx 30%). The term diffuse proliferative is used when proliferative lesions of the tuft affect more than 50% of the glomeruli. The light microscopy appearances of each of these lesions are similar to those found in primary glomerular nephritis, with sometimes certain characteristic differences. For instance, extremely rarely, structureless haematoxylin 'bodies' can be found. They consist of aggregation of breakdown products of disintegrating nuclei circulating in the peripheral blood which become trapped in the glomerular capillaries. There are also the classical, very hard to find, 'wire loop' lesions of lupus nephritis. They are eosinophilic homogeneously staining thickened areas of the wall of certain glomerular loops. They are due to focal areas of voluminous electron dense deposits lying between the endothelial cell cytoplasm and the basement membrane. Focal areas of necrosis are also more common in SLE than in primary glomerular nephritis.

In many ways the EM appearances in the kidney are more diagnostic than are the light microscopy appearance. Dense deposits can be found on either side of the basement membrane, within the membrane and in the mesangial area. The large size of the endothelial deposits and the presence of intramembranous deposits are very characteristic of lupus nephritis. Immunofluorescence shows mainly deposits of IgG laid out in a granular pattern along the glomerular wall. Focal and diffuse proliferation may be associated with varying involvement of the tubules and collections of interstitial inflammatory cells.

In a substantial number of patients the histological appearances alter with time. Focal proliferative may change to diffuse proliferative or very occasionally to extra membranous. Deaths from an accelerated form of renal functional deterioration may take place before there has been much disintegration and absorption of nephrons. In such cases the kidneys macroscopically are of normal size, or enlarged, while histologically there is a striking proliferation of both the glomerular capsule and the tufts, thickening and granularity of the capillary walls, exudates, haemorrhages, and even necrosis in the tufts. If, on the other hand, the changes have occurred more slowly, particularly when they have been retarded by prednisone, the kidneys will be smaller and the histological changes will resemble more closely those of advanced primary glomerular nephritis.

Vascular changes may not be particularly pronounced, though sometimes the lesions of polyarteritis nodosa, or fibrinoid necrosis of arterioles, may be present.

## Clinical features

Renal lupus erythematosus presents with proteinuria, a nephrotic syndrome, chronic renal failure or occasionally as an acute nephritic syndrome.

Proteinuria and a nephrotic syndrome are the two most frequent presentations. Usually the correct diagnosis is not suspected until some other more characteristic feature of lupus erythematosus becomes manifest, e.g. skin lesions, fever, pleural effusion, pericarditis, arthritis, leucopenia, or a high erythrocyte sedimentation.

The diagnosis is sometimes suspected from the low plasma $C_3$, or the finding of anti-nuclear-antibody (ANF). Tests of varying specificity are then used such as the presence of antibodies to double stranded DNA.

## Course and Prognosis with SLE

Sometimes a patient may develop a nephrotic syndrome without a raised blood cholesterol. By the time chronic renal failure occurs the diagnosis is easier to make. It is characteristic that the blood pressure rises less frequently and much later than in other causes of renal failure, and that malignant hypertension is exceptional.

## Relation between the clinical and structural features

In keeping with most other renal diseases there is little correlation between the clinical picture and the histological changes, except that when there is some degree of renal failure there are lesions in the interstitium and tubules as well as in the glomeruli. But in the absence of renal failure, proteinuria may be present with either no histological abnormality, or with well-defined lesions in both the glomeruli, the interstitial space and the tubules.

### Course and prognosis

Follow-up studies with serial renal biopsies have shown that it is most unusual for patients with systemic lupus erythematosus, who initially have no renal lesions on light microscopy to develop lesions at a later date. Similarly, it is uncommon for a patient whose renal lesions are confined to the glomeruli to develop tubular and interstitial lesions subsequently, though it can happen.

Without treatment with steroids and immunosuppressive drugs, the prognosis is much worse for those patients with diffuse proliferative lesions. With treatment, however, this difference tends to disappear (Fig. 21.13).

As usual the young do better than the less young and the prognosis tends to be less good if the disease begins with a nephrotic syndrome. Persistent hypertension and renal failure with a blood urea greater than 20 mmol/l

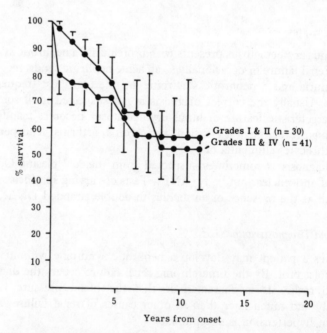

Fig. 21.13 Survival of patients with lupus nephritis. Grade I and II minimal change and focal proliferative; Grade III and IV diffuse proliferative and membranous. There is no statistical difference between the two curves. (Reproduced from Cameron, Turner, Ogg et al 1979 Quart J Med XLVIII: 1, with kind permission.)

(120 mg/100 ml) also carry a poor prognosis. Transient rises of blood pressure however, during acute exacerbation of SLE are not important.

In the absence of hypertension or renal failure, pregnancy does not appear to influence the progress of the disease though there is often a flare up of activity. Contraception is difficult, for oral contraceptives are associated with an increased risk of thrombophlebitis and hypertension, and intrauterine devices give rise to infection, endometritis, dysmenorrhea and haemorrhage.

In many patients with SLE nephritis especially those with local and diffuse proliferative lesions, a relapse follows a preliminary increase in anti DNA antibodies and fall in serum complement. Renal failure is now a relatively rare cause of death in SLE and accounts for only half the deaths in patients with lupus nephritis. The other deaths are due to sepsis, cerebrovascular lupus and myocardial disease.

## Treatment

There is no doubt that steroids are very effective against the systemic and other non renal manifestations of SLE such as fever and arthritis. And it is generally considered that the deterioration in renal function associated with the more florid lesions in diffuse proliferative lupus nephritis (such as focal necrosis and severe interstitial damage) also respond to large doses of steroids. But a controlled trial of the use of steroids in diffuse proliferative lupus nephritis has not been carried out. Treatment starts with 100 mg/day of prednisone for one week diminishing by 20 mg/day in the second and third week. 60 mg/day is then continued for about 3–4 months when the dose is gradually reduced over the next year until the required maintenance dose of around 10 mg/day (if necessary) is reached. Renal function, proteinuria, microscopic haematurie, ESR and symptoms are monitored at frequent intervals. It is problematical whether, in view of their good prognosis, any treatment is necessary to try and influence the course of events in patients with other histological renal lesions of SLE.

Some control trials have been performed to find out if the addition of azathioprine or cyclophosphamide to steroid therapy can help prevent the progression of diffuse proliferative lupus nephritis. Their addition to prednisone in the treatment of the SLE in the New Zealand mice does produce a greater amelioration than the use of prednisone alone. Both drugs seem to help but the sepsis and bladder problems associated with cyclophosphamide has deterred many from using it.

Plasma exchange has been used. Its efficiency is capricious and is unrelated to the presence of immune complexes. Its use now seems to be restricted to certain patients who show continued deterioration in spite of high doses of immune therapy.

It is most important to note that renal function in patients with SLE, particularly those with lupus nephritis, appears to be even more susceptible to inhibition of prostaglandin synthethase than in normal subjects. The use of aspirin, indomethacin, meclofenamate and other forms of prostaglandin synthethase inhibitors such as naproxen, ibuprofen and fenoprofen therefore, which are very likely to be used in the treatment of arthritis in SLE may produce an acute deterioration of renal function which may be attributed to a flare up of the nephritis. It is probable that the use of such drugs in patients with advanced renal failure can precipitate an irreversible shut down of renal function. Conversely their inadvertent discontinuation may induce a miraculous recovery of renal function which is then attributed to whatever treatment is specifically being given to control the renal lesion.

Patients with any form of SLE should try to avoid factors which may cause an acute exacerbation of the process e.g. infections, sun bathing, drugs such as penicillin, certain cosmetics, hair dyes and certain household and garden chemicals.

### Differential diagnosis

The diagnosis of SLE is made from the overall clinical features plus the information derived from several laboratory measurements some of which are more specific than others. Without the latter it may be impossible to distinguish with certainty renal lupus erythematosus from other causes of renal disorders such as glomerular nephritis, renal polyarteritis nodosa and the renal lesions which accompany sub-acute bacterial endocarditis. A skin biopsy can be helpful. Granular deposits of IgG, IgM, $C_1q/$ or $C_3$ are seen at the dermal epidermal junction, as a band of fluorescence, in 70–90% of patients with SLE. This appearance is found equally in 'sun exposed' or 'shaded' skin. It is a reasonably sensitive and specific test for the diagnosis of SLE though it is not helpful in assessing the type and extent of any associated renal involvement.

## RENAL DISTURBANCES IN SUB-ACUTE BACTERIAL ENDOCARDITIS (focal embolic nephritis)

These lesions are due to emboli and to an immunological disturbance.

### Pathology

Macroscopically the kidney may appear normal, but if a considerable number of glomeruli are undergoing acute changes it may be swollen and covered with numerous petechial haemorrhages, as in acute glomerular nephritis, malignant hypertension and diffuse lupus erythematosus. Before the advent of antibiotics fresh or healed infarcts could be detected macroscopically in about half the cases. The size of the lesions suggested obstruction of arcuate or large interlobular arteries. The presence of infarcts was confirmed on microscopy and showed a great variety in age.

The characteristic microscopical lesion is an area of acute necrosis of a part or the whole of a glomerulus, surrounded by varying quantities of acute inflammatory cells, and in the midst of which there may be intracapillary thrombi. These lesions are usually scattered in widely seperated glomeruli but sometimes they are present in the majority. They are very similar to the changes seen in the glomeruli in polyarteritis nodosa. It is usual for these lesions to be accompanied by focal proliferation. Subsequently these lesions appear to sclerose. Fibrous or hyalin material can be found situated at the periphery of a portion of an otherwise normal glomerulus, often adhering to the capsule. Occasionally the appearances are mainly those of diffuse proliferative glomerular nephritis. Mesangiocapillary glomerular nephritis has also been described. Areas of severe interstitial inflammation are often found with focal necrosis of tubules and these areas tend to be associated with endarteritis and arterolar sclerosis.

Immunofluorescence demonstrates diffuse granular deposition of $C_3$ along the glomerular capillary walls of all glomeruli whatever the light microscopy appearances. IgG and IgM are found, less often, in the mesangium. Electron microscopy shows deposits in the mesangium, occasionally of very large size.

The purpuric skin lesions are due to a vasculitis in which are deposited IgG and complement.

### Immunological and other aetiological mechanisms

There is no doubt that the large infarcts are mainly due to embolisation. The nature of the glomerular lesion is less obvious. It has been pointed out that the same appearances can be seen at the edge of a renal infarct in areas of partial ischaemia. Furthermore injections of an autolysed muscle into a renal artery can induce focal fibrinoid glomerular lesions. On the other hand there is also little doubt that most of the glomerular lesions are due to immune complex disease. The glomerular lesions are rarely seen until the infection has been present for at least six weeks, at a time when it is difficult to obtain a positive blood culture. Circulating immune complexes can be detected in the serum of most patients and the concentration increases with the duration of symptoms (Fig. 21.14). At the same time there is a fall in serum $C_3$. And as has been pointed out above complement and immune globulins can be demonstrated scattered throughout the glomeruli whether the light microscopy lesions are focal or diffuse.

### Clinical features

Frequently the patient is thought to be suffering from sub-acute bacterial endocarditis, and routine examination of the urine shows occasional showers of red cells, or frank haematuria; such findings then help to establish the correct diagnosis.

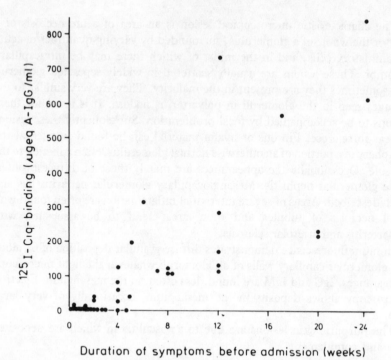

Fig. 21.14 Significant positive correlation between the peak level of circulating immune complex and the duration of symptoms before admission in 40 patients with infective endocarditis. Immune complexes measured by $^{125}$I-Clq binding assay. (Reproduced from Kauffman, Thompson, Valentijn et al 1981 Amer J Med 71: 17, with kind permission.)

Sometimes the diagnosis of endocarditis has bot been considered or has been rejected because pyrexia and cardiac murmurs have been absent, or repeated blood cultures have been sterile. In these patients the significance of the proteinuria and the excretion of a few red cells may not be properly appreciated. This occurs particularly in the elderly, who may then die of renal failure. On the whole, however, renal failure in subacute bacterial endocarditis is unusual and terminal renal failure very rare.

### Diagnosis

A positive blood culture settles the diagnosis. When blood cultures are sterile, renal and skin biopsies are helpful.

### Treatment

This consists in identifying the organism, determing its sensitivity to various antibiotics, and then giving the appropriate one in suitable doses for a period of six weeks or longer depending on when the blood cultures become sterile. If renal failure does not improve immediately large doses of prednisone, given for a short time, with the antibiotic will usually produce a rapid improvement.

In early cases treatment successfully prevents the further development of renal disturbances, but in cases with advanced renal failure such treatment is unlikely to save life.

## RENAL DISTURBANCES IN DISSEMINATED INTRAVASCULAR COAGULATION, THROMBOTIC THROMBOCYTOPENIC PURPURA AND HAEMOLYTIC URAEMIC SYNDROME

The many similarities shared by these three conditions are much more striking than their differences. And certainly, when they are considered from a renal angle, they seem to form one continuum. At the risk therefore of oversimplifying a confused and confusing subject the following schema, based partly on certain findings and partly on hypothesis is put forward as an introduction to understanding.

### Pathogenesis

It has been proposed that the initiating abnormality is a lack of a plasma substance (antithrombin III) which normally stimulates production of prostacyclin from the vascular endothelium. The mechanism which initiates this deficiency is not understood but it appears to be linked to many associated factors such as infection. Prostacyclin is a potent endogenous inhibitor of platelet aggregation on the luminal surface of blood vessels. Its absence leads to widespread intravascular coagulation. The speed of events and the localisation of the main lesions then determine the clinical course. If the process is a fulminating one the picture is one of disseminated intravascular coagulation with thrombocytopenia and purpura without anaemia. Widespread thrombotic occlusive lesions of arterioles may acutely affect the function of certain organs, particularly the brain (fits), kidney (acute renal failure) and the adrenals (acute hypoadrenalism). Or internal haemorrhages into the peritoneum or plasma may cause a sudden hypovolaemic hypotensive death.

If the patient survives this cataclysmic onset or more probably if the process is more gradual the mural intravascular thrombi become organised. The resultant roughening of the luminal surface causes haemolysis (microangiopathic anaemia) with a rapid fall in haemoglobin, the appearance of fragmented red cells, a raised reticulocyte count and plasma bilirubin and a fall in plasma haptoglobin. The platelet count now tends to be normal or even raised. The incorporation of the mural thrombi into the arteriolar walls causes severe occlusion of many arterioles. These lesions are particularly pronounced and widespread in the kidney where they cause acute renal failure with salt and water retention together with extremely high levels of plasma renin activity. A combination which, as pointed out in Chapter

16, always gives rise to the most damaging and uncontrollable form of hypertension.

The role of immune mechanism in these conditions is not very clear for circulating immune complexes are rarely found nor are there any important deposition of immunoglobulin in the kidney. On the other hand patients with the haemolytic uraemic syndrome have low levels of serum complement.

## Clinical course

*Acute disseminated intravascular coagulation.* The patient presents with acute renal failure following a sudden unsuspected devastating fall in blood pressure. There may be some relatively minor preceding event such as a dilatation and curretage or something more serious such as a clinically evident septicaemia. There is severe thrombocytopenia, purpura and a tendency to haemorrhage either internally into the peritoneum or pleura, or externally. The thrombin time is abnormal and the concentration of serum fibrin degradation products is raised though fibrinogen levels are not a useful guide to the condition.

The renal lesions consist of thrombi containing fibrin throughout the vasculature of the kidney including glomerular capillaries, arteries and arterioles. There are also many areas of tubular necrosis. Fresh intravascular thrombi are found in other organs particularly the lungs, pancreas and spleen. The adrenals may be completely infarcted.

This is a fulminating condition which often leads to death from haemorrhage.

*Thrombotic thrombocytopenic purpura.* This condition is probably a variant of disseminated intravascular coagulation but there remains some doubt because the thrombin time and serum fibrin degradation products tend to be normal.

The onset of the condition is more gradual than that of acute disseminated intravascular coagulation and is always associated with fever. It occurs predominantly between the ages of 10 and 40. The characteristic clinical feature is that the cerebral vessels are the ones most severely affected. The presenting symptoms are therefore severe headaches, mental changes, fits, hemiparesis, etc. The kidneys show various degrees of functional deterioration. There is also (as the name implies) purpura, thrombocytopenia and a microangiopathic anaemia.

The renal lesions are the same but less severe, as those described below in the adult haemolytic uraemic syndrome.

Death usually occurs within a few months of the onset. It is rarely due to renal failure.

*Haemolytic-uraemic syndrome in children under the age of two years.* There is usually a prodromal phase characterised by acute transient gastro-intestinal or respiratory symptoms, or general malaise. There is then a rapid onset of haemolytic anaemia (microangiopathic anaemia) with acute renal failure or an acute nephritic syndrome. There may also be thrombocytopenia and purpura.

Renal biopsy demonstrates areas of cortical necrosis and a specific glomerular lesion consisting of a thickening of the glomerular capillary walls due both to the deposition of a fluffy finely fibrillar material, and to a marked swelling of the endothelium. The capillary lumina may also contain aggregations of platelets and disintegrating red cells. These lesions appear to occlude blood flow through the tufts. There is also some mesangial thickening. Occlusive lesions of the intrarenal arteries and arterioles (see below) are not prominent. Immunofluorescent findings are similar to those described in the adult form of haemolytic uraemic syndrome (see below).

*Haemolytic uraemic syndrome in adults and older children.* In adults this syndrome can follow a variety of presumed causative or associated factors including pregnancy, the contraceptive pill (oestrogen), septicaemia, drugs (phenylbutazone), viral infections and dysentry. The patient usually presents with acute renal failure, severe hypertension and micro-angiopathic anaemia. There may be thrombocytopenia and purpura or the platelet count is normal or even raised. There is usually a leucocytosis.

Renal biopsy shows two forms of glomerular lesions. The first is the one that has been described above in young children with this syndrome. The other consists of ischaemic glomeruli with thickening and wrinkling of the glomerular basement membrane with atrophy of the tuft and disappearance of most of the nuclei. These are due to widespread occlusive lesions of the arteries and arterioles by fibroblastic internal proliferation of the intima. A reaction which has presumably been induced by the preceding thrombotic process (Fig. 21.15). This vascular lesion is the same as that seen in malignant hypertension, scleroderma and some cases of SLE.

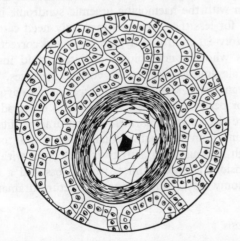

Fig. 21.15 Obstruction of an artery by intimal proliferation in a patient with haemolytic uraemic syndrome of pregnancy.

Immunofluorescence shows no immunoglobulins in the glomeruli. Most arterial walls however, contain IgM and $C_3$, an unspecific finding. The outstanding abnormality is the presence of large amounts of fibrinogen in the sub-endothelial space of the glomerular capillaries and in the glomerular thrombi. Fibrinogen is also present in the thickened intima and media of some of the arteries.

## Prognosis

In the right hands the prognosis in very young children tends to be excellent. It is interesting that the incidence of this condition in children tends to fluctuate with the occurrence of small epidemics, in each of which the disease tends to have a particular course and prognosis.

In adults the prognosis is poor. Most patients either dying of renal failure or having to be placed onto maintenance haemodialysis. The prognosis is particularly bad in those who show extensive changes in the intrarenal arteries.

## Treatment

The basic treatment is the administration of either prostacyclin ($PGI_2$), antithrombin III or fresh plasma, and when there is hypovolaemia, fresh whole blood. Aspirin and dipyridamole can also be given to control platelet aggregation. At the same time full supportive therapy for the various manifestations of these syndromes must be used. Severe hypertension hypovolaemia, profound electrolyte abnormalities and fits must be controlled. If possible it is preferable to use peritoneal dialysis instead of haemodialysis to control renal failure, for the administration of heparin which is necessary for the performance of the haemodialysis is dangerous.

Young children with the haemolytic uraemic syndrome in whom anuria has been present for less than 24 hours may only need careful monitoring of fluid and electrolytes, control of hypertension and correction of aciduria. In those patients who are not volume depleted, fluid intake should be limited to insensible fluid loss until urine volume increases. Unless anaemia is severe blood transfusion should be given sparingly to avoid overloading. The indication for peritoneal dialysis include fluid overload, rapidly rising blood urea, severe electrolyte abnormalities and uraemic fits.

In some adults in whom the renal vascular lesions appear to be irreversible, and the very high plasma renin activity is associated with severe uncontrollable hypertension, anorexia, thirst, weight loss and a mental change, bilateral nephrectomy may change the whole picture dramatically.

## Differential diagnosis

The sudden onset of acute renal failure or an acute nephritic syndrome with severe progressive Coomb-negative haemolytic anaemia narrows the choice.

The main concern is to find out if there is an underlying renal disease, such as scleroderma, SLE or pre-existing nephrosclerosis. A renal biopsy should be performed. A skin biopsy is also useful, particularly to distinguish whether purpura is due to a vasculitis.

## SHUNT NEPHRITIS

A diffuse proliferative glomerular nephritis with many infiltrating leucocytes which occurs in children with an infected (coagulase-negative staphylo-coccus) ventriculo-atrial shunt. Complement and IgM are found along the capillary walls. When the shunt is removed the renal lesions rapidly resolve and disappear. The condition would appear to be due to immune complex nephritis.

## RENAL DISTURBANCES IN MALIGNANT DISEASE

Occasionally a patient with a carcinoma, chronic lymphatic leukaemia or Hodgkin's disease, may develop a nephrotic syndrome. In those with a carcinoma or chronic lymphatic leukaemia the renal lesion is membranous glomerular nephritis with IgG immunofluorescent deposits. In one patient the immunoglobulin eluted from the glomeruli reacted specifically with the surface plasma membrane antigens of the neoplastic tumour cells. Removal of a tumour may cause a rapid diminution of proteinuria and temporary recovery.

In Hodgkin's disease the renal biopsy findings are usually nil or minimal with no deposition of immunoglobulin. The abnormalities of lymphocyte function which are found in patients with minimal change glomerular nephritis who do not have Hodgkin's disease are also found in patients who do have Hodgkin's disease.

## RENAL DISTURBANCES IN QUARTAN MALARIA

Large numbers of children infected with quartan malaria, particularly in East Africa, develop a nephrotic syndrome or sometimes an acute nephritic syndrome. The renal lesions consist of focal and segmental glomerular proliferation. Glomerular capsular crescents, and interstitial and tubular changes are rare. IgG, IgA and IgM and $\beta_1 C$ can be demonstrated in a granu-lar pattern mainly distributed along the walls of the capillaries. Occasion-ally the fluorescence can be smooth and linear. Malarial antigens have been demonstrated both in the serum and fixed onto the glomerular capillaries. Treatment with cyclophosphamide in a control trial has been found to diminish the proteinuria. Otherwise intensive treatment of the malaria gradually eradicates the disease.

## RENAL LESIONS IN LIVER DISEASE

A mild impairment of renal function in cirrhosis of the liver is well recognised. It is often overlooked because the diminished dietary intake of protein in chronic alcoholism, or the diminished urea production in liver failure causes the plasma urea level to remain normal in spite of a diminution of glomerular filtration rate. Occasionally there may be a nephrotic syndrome, or only proteinuria. The outstanding lesion histologically is an intercapillary thickening associated with lumpy mesangial deposits of IgG, IgA and complement. Occasionally there is focal mesangial proliferation. The glomerular capillary walls are unaffected. There is no correlation between the severity of the renal lesion and the severity of the liver disease but there may be some relation between the accumulation of mesangial immunoglobulins and the raised plasma gammaglobulin.

REFERENCES

**General**
Couser W G 1981 What are circulating immune complexes doing in glomerulonephritis? New Eng J Med 304: 1230
Denman A M 1978 Lymphocyte function and disease. Brit Med J 2: 980
Levinsky R J 1981 Role of circulating immune complexes in renal diseases. J Clin Path 34: 1214
McCluskey R T, Bhan A K 1982 Cell-mediated mechanisms in renal diseases. Kidney Int 21 (Suppl 11): S6
Peters D K, Lachman P J 1974 Immunity deficiency in pathogenesis of glomerulonephritis. Lancet 1: 58
Rocklin R E, Lewis E J, David J R In vitro evidence for cellular hypersensitivity to glomerular-basement-membrane antigens in human glomerulonephritis. New Eng J Med 283: 497
Solling J, Olsen S 1981 Circulating immune complexes in glomerulonephritis. Clin Nephrol 16: 63
Sugisaki T, Yoshida T, McCluskey R T et al 1980 Autoimmune cell-mediated tubulointestinal nephritis induced in Lewis rats by renal antigens. Clin Immunol Immunopathol 15: 33
Sutherland J C, Markham R V, Mardiney M R 1974 Subclinical immune complexes in the glomeruli of kidneys post-mortem. Amer J Med 57: 536
Williams D G 1981 New ideas in the pathogenesis of nephritis. J Clin Path 34: 1223
Williams R C 1981 Immune complexes: A clinical perspective. Amer J Med 71: 743
Wilson C B, Brewer B M, Stein J H 1979 Immunologic mechanisms of renal disease. Churchill Livingstone, Edinburgh
**Aetiological mechanisms**
Couser W G 1981 What are circulating immune complexes doing in glomerulonephritis? New Eng J Med 304: 1230
Couser W G, Salant D J 1980 In situ immune complex formation and glomerular injury. Kidney Int 17: 1
Denman A M 1978 Lymphocyte function and disease. Brit Med J 2: 980
Fleuren G, Grond J, Hoedemaeker P J 1980. In situ formation of subepithelial glomerular immune complexes in passive serum sickness. Kidney Int 17: 631
Germuth F G, Rodriguez E 1973 Immunopathology of the renal glomerulus. Immune complex deposit and anti-basement membrane disease. Little Brown and Company, Boston
Glynn L E, Holborow E J 1952 Conversion of tissue polysaccharides to autoantigens by group-A Beta-haemolytic streptococci. Lancet 2: 449

Humphrey J H 1982 The value of immunological concepts in medicine. J Roy Coll Phys 16: 141

Levinsky R J 1981 Role of circulating immune complexes in renal diseases. J Clin Path 34: 1214

McCluskey R T, Bhan A K 1982 Cell mediated mechanisms in renal diseases. Kidney Int 21, Suppl 11: S6

Mallick N P, McFarlane H, Taylor G et al 1972 Cell-mediated immunity in nephrotic syndrome. Lancet i: 507

Naruse T, Miyakawa Y, Kitamura K 1974 Membranous glomerulonephritis mediated by renal tubular epithelial antigen-antibody complex. J Aller Clin Immunol 54: 311

Ooi B S, Ooi Y M, Hsu A et al 1980 Diminished synthesis of immunoglobulin by peripheral lymphocytes of patients with idiopathic membranous glomerulonephropathy. J Clin Invest 65: 789

Peters D K, Lachmann P J 1974 Immunity deficiency in pathogenesis of glomerulonephritis. Lancet i: 58

Solling J, Olsen S 1981 Circulating immune complexes in glomerulonephritis. Clin Nephrol 16: 63

Sutherland J C, Markham R V, Mardiney M R 1974 Subclinical immune complexes in the glomeruli of kidneys post-mortem. Amer J Med 57: 536

Taube D, Chapman S, Brown Z et al D G 1981 Depression of normal lymphocyte transformation by sera of patients with minimal change nephropathy and other forms of nephrotic syndrome. Clin Nephrol 15: 286

Williams D G 1981 New ideas in the pathogenesis of nephritis. J Clin Path 34: 1223

Wilson C B 1980 Specific renal diseases. Immunologic considerations In: Stein J H (ed) Nephrology. Grune and Stratton, New York p 275

Wilson C B, Dixon F J 1981 The renal response to immunological injury. In: Brenner B M, Rector F C (eds) The kidney, Saunders W B Philadelphia, p 1237

Zabriskie J B 1971 The role of streptococci in human glomerulonephritis. J Exper Med 134: 180

### Glomerular nephritis

Atkins R C, Glasgow E F, Holdsworth S R et al 1976 The macrophage in human rapidly progressive glomerulonephritis. Lancet i: 830

Black D A K, Rose G, Brewer D B 1970 Controlled trial of prednisone in adult patients with the nephrotic syndrome. Brit Med J 3: 421

Bright R 1836 Cases and observations, illustrative of renal disease accompanied with the secretion of albuminous urine, Guy's Hosp Rep i: 338

Cameron J S 1979 The natural history of glomerulonephritis. In: Black D, Jones N F (eds) Renal disease. Blackwell Scientific Pub. Oxford, p 329

Cameron J S 1979 Pathogenesis and treatment of membranous nephropathy. Kidney Int 15: 88

Chamberlain M J, Pringle A, Wrong O M 1966 Oliguric renal failure in the nephrotic syndrome. Quart J Med N S 35: 215

Coggins C H 1979 A controlled study of short-term prednisone treatment in adults with membranous nephropathy. A collaborative study of the adult idiopathic nephrotic syndrome. New Eng J Med 301: 1301

Editorial 1979 Poststreptococcal glomerulo nephritis. Brit Med J 2: 1243

Habib R, Gubler M C, Loirat C et al 1975 Dense deposit disease: A variant of membranoproliferative glomerulonephritis. Kidney Int 7: 204

Habib R, Kleinknecht C, Gubler M C et al 1973 Idiopathic membrano-proliferative glomerulonephritis in children. Report of 105 cases. Clin Nephrol i: 194

Heptinstall R H 1983 Pathology of the kidney. Little, Brown and Company, Boston

Hood S A Velosa J A, Holley K E et al 1981 IgA — IgG nephropathy: predictive indices of progressive disease. Clin Nephrol 16: 55

Hutt M S R, Pinniger J L, de Wardener H E 1958 The relationship between the clinical and histological features in acute glomerular nephritis based on a study of renal biopsy material. Quart J Med N S 27: 265

McPhaul J J, Mullins J D 1976 Glomerulonephritis mediated by antibody to glomerular basement membrane. J Clin Invest 57: 351

Morel-Maroger L, Leathem A, Richet G 1972 Glomerular abnormalities in non-systemic diseases: Relationship between findings by light microscopy and immunofluorescence in 433 renal biopsy specimens. Amer J Med 53: 170

Morrin P A F, Hinglais N, Nabarra B et al 1978 Rapidly progressive glomerulonephritis (29 cases). Amer J Med 65: 446

M R C 1971 Controlled trial of azathioprine and prednisone in chronic renal disease. Brit Med J 2: 239

Nissenson A R, Mayon-White R, Potter E V et al 1979 Continued absence of clinical renal disease seven to 12 years after post-streptococcal acute glomerulonephritis in Trinidad. Amer J Med 67: 255

Papper S 1978 Clinical Nephrology. Little Brown and Company, Boston

Rodriguez-Iturbe B, Carr R I, Garcia R et al 1980 Circulating immune complexes and serum immunoglobulins in acute post-streptococal glomerulonephritis. Clin Nephrol 13: 1

Sissons J G P, Woodrow D F, Curtis J R et al 1975 Isolated glomerulonephritis with mesangial IgA deposits. Brit Med J 3: 611

Spitzer A 1977 Ten years of activity. A report for the International Study of Kidney Disease in Children. In: Kluthe R, Vogt A, Batsford S R (eds) Glomerulonephritis. John Wiley and Sons, New York

Werra P de, Morel-Maroger L, Leroux-Robert C et al 1973 Glomerulities à dépôts d'IgA diffus dans le mésangium. Schweiz Med Wschr 1: 3761

**Goodpasture's syndrome**

Bergrem H, Jerwell J, Brodwall E K et al 1980 Goodpasture's syndrome. A report of seven patients including long-term follow-up of three who received a kidney transplant. Amer J Med 68: 54

Zimmerman S W, Varanasi U R, Hoff B 1979 Goodpasture's Syndrome with normal renal function. Amer J Med 66: 163

**Henoch-Schönlein's syndrome**

Counahan R, Winterborn M H, White R H R et al 1977 Prognosis of Henoch-Schönlein nephritis in children. Brit Med J 2: 11

**Polyarteritis nodosa and Wegener's granulomatosis**

Ahlstrom C G, Liedholm K, Truedsson E 1953 Respirato-renal type of polyarteritis nodosa. Acta Med Scand 144: 323

Davson J, Ball J, Platt R 1948 Kidney in periarteritis nodosa. Quart J Med N S 17: 175

Fauci A S, Wolff S M 1973 Wegener's granulomatosis: Studies in eighteen patients and a review of the literature. Medicine 52: 535

Rose G A, Spencer H 1957 Polyarteritis nodosa. Quart J Med N S 26: 43

**Systemic lupus erythematosus**

Cameron J S, Turner D R, Ogg C S et al 1979 Systemic lupus with nephritis: A long term study. Quart J Med N S 48: 1

Donaldio J V, Holley K E, Ferguson R H et al 1978 Treatment of diffuse proliferative lupus nephritis with prednisone and combined prednisone and cyclophosphamide. New Eng J Med 299: 1151

Glassock R J 1981 Glomerulonephritis in systemic lupus erythematosus. Amer J Nephrol 1: 53

Kimberley R P 1978 Renal prostaglandins in systemic lupus erythematosus. Lancet ii: 553–555

Lambert P H, Dixon F J 1968 Pathogenesis of the glomerulonephritis of NZB/W urine. J Exp Med 127: 507

**Sub-acute bacterial endocarditis**

Boulton-Jones J M, Sissons J G P, Evans D J et al 1974 Renal lesions of sub-acute infective endocarditis. Brit Med J 2: 11–14

Gutman R A, Striker G E, Gilliland B C et al 1972 The immune complex glomerulonephritis of bacterial endocarditis. Medicine 51: 1–25

Kauffmann R H, Thompson J, Valentijn R M et al 1981 The clinical implications and the pathogenetic significance of circulating immune complexes in infective endocarditis. Amer J Med 71: 17

Morel-Maroger L, Straer J-D, Harreman G et al P 1972 Kidney in sub-acute endocarditis. Arch Path 94: 205

**Haemolytic-uraemic syndrome etc.**

Goldstein M H, Chung J, Strauss L et al 1979 Hemolytic-uremic syndrome. Nephron 23: 263

Hauglustaine D, Van Damme B, Vanrenterghem Y et al 1981 Recurrent hemolytic uremic syndrome during oral contraception. Clin Nephrol 15: 148

Morel-Maroger L 1980 Adult hemolytic-uremic syndrome. Kidney Int 18: 125

Remuzzi G, Marcesi D, Mecca G et al 1978 Haemolytic-uraemic syndrome: deficiency of plasma factor(s) regulating prostacyclin activity? Lancet ii: 871

Segonds A, Louradour N, Suc J M et al 1979 Postpartum hemolytic uremic syndrome: a study of three cases with a review of the literature. Clin Nephrol 12: 229

Webster J, Rees A J, Lewis P J et al 1980 Prostacyclin deficiency in haemolytic-uraemic syndrome. Brit Med J 281

**Shunt nephrits**

Stickler G B, Shin M H, Burke E C et al 1968 Diffuse glomerulonephritis associated with infected ventriculoatrial shunt. New Eng J Med 279: 1077

**Renal disturbances in quartan malaria**

Allison A C, Hendrickse R G, Edington G M et al 1969 Immune complexes in the nephrotic syndrome of African children. Lancet i: 1232

Voller A, Draper C C, Shwe T et al 1971 Nephrotic syndrome in monkey infected with human quartan malaria. Brit Med J 4: 208

Ward P A, Kibukamusoke J W 1969 Evidence for soluble immune complexes in the pathogenesis of glomerulo nephritis of quartan malaria. Lancet i: 283

**Renal disturbances in malignant disease**

Cantrell E G 1969 Nephrotic syndrome cured by removal of gastric carcinoma. Brit Med J 2: 739

Dathan J R E, Heyworth M F, Maciver A G 1974 Nephrotic syndrome in chronic lymphocytic leukaemia. Brit Med J 3: 655

Ghosh L, Muehrcke R C 1970 The nephrotic syndrome. A prodrome to lymphoma. Ann intern Med 72: 379

Lewis M G, Loughridge L W, Phillips T M 1971 Immunological studies in nephrotic syndrome associated with extrarenal malignant disease. Lancet ii: 134

Loughridge L, Lewis M G 1971 Nephrotic syndrome in malignant disease of non-renal origin. Lancet i: 256

**Immunological renal disturbances in liver disease**

Fisher E R, Perez-Stable E 1968 Cirrhotic lobular glomerulonephritis. Correlation of ultrastructural and clinical features. Amer J Pathol 52: 869

Manigand G, Morel-Maroger L, Simon J et al 1970 Lésions rénales glomérulaires et cirrhose du foie. Rev Europ Etud Clin Biol 15: 989

Sakaguchi H, Dachs S, Grishman E et al 1965 Hepatic glomerulosclerosis. An electronic microscopic study of renal biopsies in liver diseases. Lab Invest 14: 533

# 22

# Infection of the urine and associated conditions

The nomenclature in which this subject is embedded is confusing. In this section infection of the urine and the conditions with which it may be associated can be divided into:
1. Infection of the urine
2. Symptoms and signs associated with urinary infection
3. Infections of the lower urinary tract
   a. asymptomatic bacteriuria
   b. cystitis
   c. urethritis
   d. prostatitis
4. Infections of the upper urinary tract
   a. acute pyelonephritis
   b. reflux nephropathy
   c. interstitial nephritis in the absence of renal scarring
5. Differential diagnosis of chronic or recurrent renal infections
   a. phenacetin nephropathy
   b. loin pain and haematuria syndrome
   c. obstructive uropathy.

## INFECTION OF THE URINE

### Diagnosis

Because of the risk of infection it is no longer justifiable to catheterise the bladder routinely to obtain urine for culture. Urine is therefore obtained either by a mid stream sample (MSU) or by suprapubic aspiration.

*MSU.* Using this technique the urine sample is often contaminated by organisms which reside in the urethra and the vulva. It is imperative therefore that cultures from mid stream samples of urine should be quantitated. It is then possible to distinguish whether the organisms found in the urine are likely to be contaminants or whether they were present and multiplying in the bladder before micturition. If the urine is carefully collected (see below) and either cultured immediately or kept cold until it is cultured, then a bacterial count greater than 100 000/ml has an 85% probability of being due to true infection of the urine; a count of less than 10 000/ml is due to contamination. Two consecutive cultures with counts greater than 100 000/ml increase the probability that there is an infection to 99%. In a well run establishment counts between 10 000/ml and 100 000/ml should occur in less than 10% of all urine cultures. If they occur more frequently the urine is not being collected with sufficient care. When the count is between 10 000/ml and 100 000/ml it should be repeated. Pure cultures with only one type of organism support the probability that the organisms are multiplying in the bladder. These interpretations of the significance of quantitative bacterial cultures do not hold if the patient is on antibiotics. The uselessness of culturing the urine in a non-quantitative manner is well illustrated in Figure 22.1 where a non-quantitative and a quantitative technique are compared. It can be seen that a report of 'growth' from a non-quantitative culture gives no indication whether the urine is infected or contaminated.

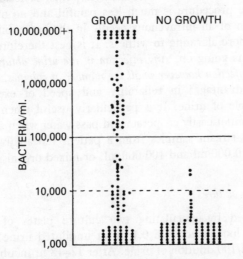

**Fig. 22.1** Routine urine culture report of 'growth' and 'no growth' compared with the number of organisms found on quantitative culture. Each dot represents one urine. The interrupted horizontal line is at 10 000 organisms/ml and the continuous horizontal line is at 100 000/ml. The block of dots at the bottom of the figure represent counts of from less than 100/ml to 2000/ml and at the top of the figure the block indicates counts greater than 10 000 000/ml. (Reproduced from Bradley & Little 1963 Brit Med J 2: 361, with kind permission.)

Urine is collected from a woman after swabbing the perineum with soap and water, rinsing with sterile water and drying with a sterile swab. It is unwise to use a disinfectant for a drop may fall into the urine that is being collected and sterilise it. The labia are then held open and the patient is asked to micturate. The whole volume of urine is collected, the first 10–15 ml into one container and the remainder into a wide-mouthed autoclaved honey jar. Urine is obtained from a man in a similar way, after cleaning the urethral meatus with benzalkonium chloride 1/1000. The urine in the autoclaved jar is cultured. There are a variety of ways to perform quantitative cultures. For routine purposes it is only necessary to distinguish whether the count is greater than 100 000/ml or less than 10 000/ml. Culturing the urine not only establishes whether or not the urine is infected but it also permits the sensitivity of the organism to various antibiotics to be established.

### Suprapubic aspiration

The bladder is allowed to fill either after the administration of several glasses of water or after the administration of 20 mg of frusemide. When the bladder is palpable, *and not before*, a sample of urine is obtained by inserting into the bladder a number 1 needle in the mid line of the anterior surface of the abdomen 1 inch above the symphysi pubis. A local anaesthetic is unnecessary. The procedure is much less painful and no more dangerous than the insertion of an intravenous needle in the antecubital fossa but it is considerably more alarming to witness. It is best therefore if the patient cannot see what is going on. *Any infection in the urine obtained in this way represents a true infection however small the number of colonies.* The technique has enormous advantages in reliability and speed of execution over a mid stream sample of urine. It is particularly useful when the patient is obese, dirty or cannot easily cooperate and pass water when asked. It is also useful when mid stream samples from a patient repeatedly give bacterial counts between 10 000/ml and 100 000/ml, or mixed organisms.

### Quantitative urine culture

This is performed by inoculating two culture plates of MacConkey's medium. One is inoculated with 0.1 ml of undiluted urine and the other with 0.1 ml of a 1/100 dilution of urine. After 12–18 hr incubation the presence of less than 100 colonies on the first plate indicates a urinary bacterial count of less than 1000 organisms per ml, while more than 100 colonies on the other plate indicates a urinary bacterial count of more than 100 000 organisms per ml.

A semi quantitative assessment can be obtained with a platinum loop or preferably, but more expensively, with a 'dip slide' method. Both techniques are standardised against the quantitative method just described. The volume of urine taken up by a platinum loop must be the same each time. Therefore the loop must not change its shape with wear and tear, and the method of withdrawal of the loop from the urine must be rigidly standardised. The commercially available dip-slides consist of a glass or plastic slide on which the culture medium has been affixed (different mediums can be applied to the two sides). The slide is dipped into the urine and withdrawn.

It is then placed in a sterile screw top container. After incubation the density of growth on the slide is proportional to the bacterial count of the urine specimen. This method has enormous advantages in general practice in that once the slide is in the container it may be transported at leisure, or sent through the post to the laboratory, without, in contrast to the original urine, it affecting the density of the growth on the slide.

Some well recognised pathogens of the urinary tract may require unusual conditions for their growth (e.g. a raised osmolarity or a high concentration of $CO_2$). These are known as fastidious organisms. They are easy to miss and it is laborious to look for them.

*Infecting organisms*

The usual route of infection is from below, up the urethra. It is not surprising, therefore, that the organisms most commonly found in the urine are faecal, e.g. E. coli, Proteus spp, and Pseudomonas spp. Nevertheless Streptococcus saprophyticus is now the second commonest urinary pathogen in young women (15 to 35%), and infections with Staphylococcus aureus also occur.

*Some of the organisms which cause urinary infections*

| Linnaean name | Comment |
| --- | --- |
| Escherichia coli | The most frequent cause of acute urinary infections |
| Staphylococcus aureus (Coag +ve) | Occasionally found in structurally abnormal urinary tracts |
| Streptococcus saprophyticus | Causes up to 35% of all urinary infections |
| Klebsiella pneumoniae | Usually in mixed infections and when there are structural deformities of the urinary tract |
| Pseudomonas pyocyanea | Frequently after antibiotic therapy and indwelling catheter |
| Proteus vulgaris Streptotoccus faecalis | Often follows catheterisation in women and occurs with stones |
| Haemophilus influenzae | Rarely found |

Mixed growth of organisms, particularly if they include Lactobacillus spp and Cornybacterium spp (normal inhabitants of lower urethra and vagina), are very suggestive of contamination. A pure culture of any organism, even if the bacterial count is less than 100 000 per ml is likely to be due to a true infection. If in doubt a suprapubic aspiration of urine may be performed. A true infection with Proteus spp, which is a slow growing organism, sometimes yields a urine bacterial count below 100 000 ml.

*Localisation of urinary infection*

Sometimes it is important to know whether the urinary organisms are confined to the bladder or whether they are also multiplying in the upper urinary tract. This can be ascertained either by inserting ureteric catheters, which is an invasive technique which is not without hazard and which can occupy much valuable 'urological' time, or by an ingenious technique devised by Fairley. The patient is encouraged to drink a large quantity of fluids. A catheter is placed in the bladder. The urine is collected and the bladder then filled with a solution containing neomycin and 'elase' (a combination of fibrinolysin and desoxyribonuclease). After an hour the bladder is emptied and washed out with several litres of sterile water to remove all the neomycin. The catheter is now lying in a sterile bladder and if the urine that emerges from the catheter is infected then the organisms have come from the upper urinary tract. On the other hand if the urine is sterile then the organisms that were present before the bladder was washed out were confined to the lower urinary tract.

There are other less precise techniques which attempt to localise the site of infection. One is to quantitate the proportion of antibody coated bacteria present in the urine. Washed urine sediment is mixed with fluorescein–conjugated antihuman globulin and incubated at 37°C for 30 min. The antibody coated bacteria can then be seen to fluoresce. It was originally claimed that if the proportion of such bacteria exceeded 25%, the organisms came from the kidney. Unfortunately the specificity of the assay appears to be only 77%, the predictive value of a positive assay 81%, and the predictive values for a negative assay 79%. The predictive value for a positive assay is greater the longer the infection has lasted before the assay is performed. It is not known why this test is of little value in children.

The serum antibody titre and the ability of the kidney to concentrate the urine have also been used to localise the site of the infection. The antibody titre is only reliable in those patients in whom there is, on other grounds, little doubt that they are suffering from a severe attack of acute pyelonephritis. On the other hand an impairment in the patient's ability to concentrate the urine can be a useful early indication of an upper urinary infection particularly in difficult cases, and the diagnosis is re-enforced if the ability to concentrate rises after treatment with antibiotics.

## Examination of the urine for evidence of inflammation

An infection of the urine is often accompanied by an excess number of white cells in the urine. Such an excess may therefore be useful corroborative evidence that there is a true infection of the urine. But it is important to stress that whereas a positive urine culture is evidence of infection (with the provisos mentioned above), an increased number of white cells in the urine is only evidence of inflammation. It does not follow automatically that this inflammation is due to an infection with pyogenic organisms.

The methods used to determine the white cell content of the urine accurately are described on page 51. It is necessary to mention that some reactionary routine laboratories refuse to culture a urine unless it contains more than a normal number of white cells. Conversely some clinicians are apt to ignore a positive urine culture if the number of white cells in the urine is not raised. Both practices are to be deplored. It is well established that the urine may be heavily infected without its content of white cells being raised, particularly in patients with chronic upper urinary infection and in symptomless bacteruria. 'Sterile' pyuria classically occurs in renal tuberculosis when it is strictly inaccurate to say that the urine is sterile. It also occurs in many other conditions including phenacetin nephropathy, acute glomerular nephritis, renal stones, and after renal vein thrombosis. Sterile pyuria can also occur following an active renal infection with pyogenic organisms, for instance during recovery from an attack of acute pyelonephritis treated with antibiotics.

Sometimes the presence of an active inflammatory focus in the renal tract is *not* accompanied by an excess number of white cells in the urine. If, nevertheless, it is suspected that such a focus exists, its presence may be revealed by giving the patient 40 mg of prednisolone phosphate intravenously, when there may be a prompt increase in the number of white cells in the urine. This test is particularly useful in investigating patients who have been given antibiotics for an alleged attack of acute pyelonephritis before the urine has been examined. Later when the patient feels better and the urine is sterile, and contains a normal number of white cells the diagnosis of a recent urinary infection may be difficult to uphold. The prednisolone test is also useful in a patient with recurrent renal infections which appears to be in an inactive stage (Fig. 22.2). It is not known how prenisolone produces this effect. If the white cell excretion rate is raised without giving prednisolone there is clearly little point in doing a prednisolone test.

## Defences against the urine becoming infected

It is remarkable that a baby girl wearing a nappy may have faeces teeming with E. coli and other gram negative organisms plastered against her external urethral orifice for several hours each day while the bladder urine, an excellent culture medium maintained at 37°C, remains sterile less than 1 cm away. The main defence against bacterial invasion up to the lumen of the urethra is probably the urethra's potent bactericidal environment which is due, in part at least, to the ability of the mucosa to secrete secretory IgA. Bladder mucosa is also bactericidal for the same reason. An additional defence mechanism is the washout effect of micturition which is most efficient the higher the urine flow and the greater the frequency of bladder emptying. The composition of the urine itself, aside from its content of secretory IgA, influences bacterial growth. The lower the urine pH, or the higher the urine osmolality and urea the slower the growth.

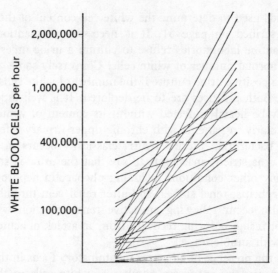

**Fig. 22.2** White cell excretion rate before and after the administration of 40 mg prednisolone phosphate intravenously to 25 patients with radiological evidence of reflux nephropathy, but in whom the urine was uninfected and the white cell content of the urine was normal. In about half of the patients there was a brisk rise in white cell excretion to a rate above 400 000/hr indicating that though these patients' urine was normal before the prenisone injection an active focus of inflammation was still present adjoining the lumen of the renal tract. (Reproduced from Little 1965 J Clin Path 18: 556, with kind permission.)

## Aetiology and prevention of urinary infection

When organisms are introduced into a normal bladder which can empty completely it is usual for the bacteria to be evacuated. Persistent bacteriuria does not develop. On the other hand if bacteria gain access to the bladder of an individual who suffers from some deformity of the renal tract including lesions which cause some residual urine to be present after voiding (e.g. prostatic hypertrophy, vaginal prolapse) the chances of developing persistent bacteruria are very great.

Bacteria are most likely to gain access to the bladder during catheterisation and urological investigations. The incidence of bacteriuria following these manoeuvres can be reduced by the introduction into the bladder of an antiseptic or antibiotic at the end of the procedure. It is also wise to culture the urine of patients with known abnormalities of the renal tract from time to time. Another way in which organisms commonly enter a woman's bladder for the first time is at the beginning of active sexual life. There is much to be said for giving all virgins 50 mg of nitrofurantoin to take at night for the first two or three weeks after they cease to be virgins. The urine may also become infected as a result of poor perineal hygiene or alternatively the use of a strong antiseptic which causes irritation, pruritus and local infections. Masturbation and insufficient lubrication during sexual intercourse may also be responsible for some urinary infections.

## SYMPTOMS AND SIGNS ASSOCIATED WITH INFECTED URINE

There may be no symptoms, when the condition is known as asymptomatic bacteriuria. When there are symptoms and signs the urine is often offensive and there may be haematuria. The *symptoms* may be localised to the lower urinary tract, the kidney areas, or they may be systemic. Lower urinary tract symptoms include suprapubic discomfort and tenderness, nocturia, frequency of micturition, urgency and dysuria. Most commonly the dysuria is present during micturition and is relieved as it ceases, but it may be most pronounced at the end of micturition and become incapacitating for 10 to 15 min thereafter. This symptom is sometimes referred to as strangury. Dysuria which is most severe during micturition is more likely to be due to trigonitis while strangury is more probably due to urethritis. Sometimes there is persistent urethral discomfort when a vaginal examination reveals the presence of a thickened tender urethra which can be rolled against the back of the symphysis pubis.

Upper urinary symptoms and signs include loin pain and tenderness. The patient tends to lean towards the side of the pain and may prefer to keep the hip flexed to relax the muscles upon which the inflammed kidney is lying.

Systemic signs include fever, and rigors, nausea and vomiting (particularly in pregnancy), tiredness, sweating and loss of weight. These are most usually due to renal infections.

It must be stressed, however, that the patient's complaints may be an unreliable guide to the site from which the organisms are originating (Table 22.1) particularly if the symptoms are not severe. For instance loin pain is about as common in upper urinary infections as it is in infections confined to the lower urinary tract. On the other hand a rigor, or a temperature greater than 101°F and loin tenderness are almost always due to a renal infection.

**Table 22.1** Symptoms in relation to the site of the infection (Fairley test)

|  |  | Localisation of infection | |
|---|---|---|---|
|  |  | Upper urinary tract | Lower urinary tract |
| Symptomatic patients | 43 | 21 (49%) | 22 (51%) |
| Frequency | 32 | 18 (56%) | 14 (44%) |
| Dysuria | 35 | 18 (51%) | 17 (49%) |
| Loin pain | 31 | 15 (48%) | 16 (52%) |
| Temp. >101°F/38°C | 19 | 13 (68%) | 6 (32%) |
| Haematuria | 6 | 3 (50%) | 3 (50%) |

### Gram negative septicaemia

Approximately half all gram negative septicaemias originate from organisms growing in the urine. Most often their presence in the urine is unsuspected until the septicaemia declares itself following instrumentation or other operative interference of the urinary tract. The death rate is high (25–60%) and is due to the release of endotoxin into the circulation. This causes rigors, hypotension, rapid respiration due to 'shock lung' and other evidence of a disseminated intravascular coagulation which diminishes the blood flow to all organs.

These disasters could be avoided if urine cultures were routinely performed on all patients in whom it is proposed to perform some urological manipulation. Gram negative septicaemia occurs more frequently in patients on immunosuppressive treatment or who suffer from certain diseases (e.g. Hodgkins) in which the normal immunological defences are impaired.

## INFECTIONS OF THE LOWER URINARY TRACT

These include:
a. Asymptomatic bacteriuria
b. Cystitis
c. Urethritis
d. Prostatitis.

### Asymptomatic bacteriuria

The incidence of asymptomatic bacteruria in women changes with age. In schoolgirls it is about 1 to 2% in contrast to schoolboys in whom it is 0.03%. Immediately after puberty the incidence in girls rises to about 10%, it then falls to about 5% until the age of 60–70 years when it rises again to 20–30% in elderly women. The rise after puberty is due to sexual activity, for the incidence of asymptomatic bacteriuria in nuns is the same as in schoolgirls before puberty. The incidence of bacteriuria also rises with parity. It appears that each year approximately one quarter of adult women with asymptomatic bacteriuria revert to having a normal uninfected urine while an equal number become infected.

Radiological investigations of asymptomatic bacteriuria in schoolgirls reveals that about 40% have a radiological abnormality of whom about half have scarred kidneys with ureteric reflux. Radiological investigation of asymptomatic bacteriuria in adult women, whether pregnant or not, shows that about 18% have some renal abnormality, as compared to 6% in a matched uninfected control group.

It is not clear whether routine screening of schoolgirls for the presence of asymptomatic bacteruria is economically worthwhile for it is now obvious that most of the important renal scarring takes place before the age of five. On the other hand there is evidence that in those with renal scars, particularly if they have ureteric reflux, control of the bacteriuria does reduce the incidence of further scarring. As a compromise it would seem best to have a very low threshold for culturing a child's urine and to thoroughly investigate any individual found to have an infected urine.

There is no doubt that routine screening of pregnant women for the presence of bacteria is worthwhile for unless the bacteriuria is controlled 20–25% will develop acute pyelonephritis (p. 502). The routine screening of non-pregnant adult asymptomatic women is now thought to be a waste of money. Surprisingly there is little evidence that the treatment of bacteriuria even in women with symptoms has much effect on the rate of progress of renal damage in patients with scarred kidneys (see below).

## Cystitis

This term is used whether or not the urine is infected to describe the symptoms of dysuria and frequency of micturition. If the urine is then found to be uninfected, the term urethral syndrome is apt to be used. When the urine is infected one of the following microbial agents are given for 3–5 days. For E. coli and micrococcal infections, co-trimoxozole 2 tab. b.d.; trimethoprin 100 mg b.d.; amoxycillin 500 mg t.d.s.; nitrofurantoin 50 mg q.d.s.; ampicillin 500 mg q.d.s. As an alternative a single large dose of an antibiotic (e.g. ampicillin 3 g) has been found useful if there is a fair certainty that the upper urinary tract is not infected. For mycoplasma and chlamydial infections tetracycline 500 mg q.d.s. for one week, and for fastidious organisms amoxycillin or erythromycin, should be given.

## Urethritis (Urethral syndrome)

The symptoms resemble those of cystitis except that there is apt to be agonising *post* micturition pain in the urethra, a continuous dragging feeling in the urethra, dyspareunia and little suprapubic pain. It is often difficult to culture an organism from the urine with conventional culturing techniques. Gonococcal and chlamydial infections should be excluded. A *pure* growth of corynebacteria, a fastidious streptococcus or lactobacillus suggest that they may be the cause of the inflammation. There may or may not be pyuria and even when present the urine may be sterile with routine culture methods.

## Prostatitis

In some patients with prostatitis organisms can be isolated from the urine by conventional techniques and pus cells can be demonstrated in prostatic secretions which have been obtained after prostatic massage with a finger in the rectum. In other patients pus cells can be demonstrated in this way but the urine is sterile. Some patients have dysuria, frequency, some pain on defaecation and a mildly tender prostate and yet they have a sterile urine and there are no pus cells in the urine. In the absence of organisms a course of tetracycline in relatively high doses is often useful. Trimethoprim may also be of benefit because it is still effective in the alkaline medium of the prostatic fluid.

## INFECTIONS OF THE UPPER URINARY TRACT

### Acute pyelitis, acute pyelonephritis and acute necrotising papillitis

*Pathology*

The appearances of the kidneys depend largely on whether any underlying renal deformity was present before the onset of the acute infection. The following descriptions only refer to changes produced by infection. They are divided into three groups depending on their severity: (1) acute pyelitis; (2) acute pyelonephritis; and (3) acute necrotising papillitis.

*Acute pyelitis.* This is the term which pathologists give to an acute infection confined to the lining membrane of the renal pelvis, that is an infection which does not involve the renal parenchyma. At *post-mortem* such a limited distribution is found extremely rarely; it does not follow that it is equally infrequent in life. It is usually bilateral.

*Acute pyelonephritis.* This is nearly always bilateral. Macroscopically the kidneys are usually enlarged and occasionally small abscesses show through the capsule. The surface may be discoloured by areas of pallor and congestion. On section, greyish wedge-shaped areas can be seen extending upwards from the pyramids into the cortex; there are also yellow streaks radiating from the medulla. The pelvis is red and covered with pus.

The pelvis microscopically is covered with an inflammatory exudate which penetrates within the pelvic wall; sometimes there are also areas of superficial necrosis. The renal parenchymatous lesions are more numerous in the pyramids and medulla. The tubules contain and are surrounded by leucocytes, though occasionally these are confined to the interstitial tissues. There are similar collections of neutrophils in the interstitial tissues of the cortex, in addition, some glomeruli become selectively invested by a thick concentration of acute inflammatory cells. In a few, the capsule is breached and leucocytes can be seen invading the glomerular space. In some sites an inflammatory destruction of tubules may cause a crowding together of glomeruli which are then separated only by granulation tissue. A varying number of small abscesses may be disseminated throughout the renal parenchyma and, before the use of antibiotics, bacteria were also found in large numbers.

The vascular lesions are of particular importance, and in this connection it should be recalled that the renal pelvis extends as far upwards as the cortico-medullary junction (p. 9). It is not surprising, therefore, to find that sometimes the acute inflammatory process involves some of the larger arteries and veins. Dense infiltrations with leucocytes may be localised in the arterial wall, leading to destruction of the muscle and elastic tissues; occasionally this process leads to occlusion of the lumen by a thrombus, and complete infarction of wedge-shaped areas of cortex. Other large arteries may show moderate degrees of narrowing of the arterial lumen by endarteritis. In the areas of acute inflammation thrombosis of arterioles is relatively frequent.

*Acute necrotising papillitis.* This consists of an acute pyelonephritis of such severity that there is a focal suppurative necrosis of one or more renal pyramids. The process begins at the apices of the pyramids and extends upwards into the medulla, but does not involve the cortex. Microscopically there is a dense purulent exudate throughout the affected area which is sharply demarcated from the viable parenchyma.

## Infecting organisms, route of infection and associated conditions

There is increasing evidence that the strains of organisms that cause acute infections of the upper urinary tract are often specifically adapted to do so. Either they are immune to the bactericidal activity of plasma or they have some other particular property that distinguishes them from other strains, e.g. they haemolyse red blood cells. In a large proportion of cases the bacteria having ascended the ureter and invaded the highly vascular parenchyma, then spill into the blood and cause a bacteraemia and septicaemia. In some instances the bacterial invasion of the renal parenchyma is associated with a rise in serum antibody titre to the infecting organism.

The infecting organism may be conveyed to the kidney in (1) the blood stream, (2) the urine, from the bladder, up to the lumen of the ureters, or (3) the lymphatics alongside the ureters. Observations in human infection suggest that the organisms nearly always travel up the ureters. Acute upper urinary infections in previously normal kidneys occur predominantly in women whose urine has contained large numbers of organisms for considerable periods before the onset of symptoms. There is no doubt, however, that a transient bacteraemia can also cause pyelonephritis. Occasionally (e.g. after routine catheterisation) the two mechanisms occur together; the bladder urine is first infected by the catheter, the organisms then multiply in the bladder and after an interval there is a simultaneous bacteraemia and acute pyelonephritis. In animal experiments organisms have been introduced into the bladder after tying one ureter. It has been found that the kidney with a patent ureter becomes infected while the other kidney remains intact, unless there is an associated bacteraemia. The lesions in both human and animal infections are often most pronounced in the medulla. In animals it has been shown that the medulla's ability to restrain bacterial growth is relatively poor. This is due to the hypertonicity of the medulla which inhibits (1) the natural bactericidal activity of plasma, (2) the mobilisation of white cells towards an injured area, and (3) the phagocytic capacity of the white cells.

Most infections occur in kidneys with normal urinary tracts, nearly always in women. A few infections occur during a widespread and easily recognised dissemination of organisms from a primary focus, such as malignant endocarditis, osteomyelitis, empyema, etc.; the renal lesion thus caused is sometimes known as a 'pyaemic kidney' but, as it is indistinguishable from severe acute pyelonephritis from other causes, it is included here. Some infections are superimposed on a pre-existing lesion such as a renal scar or an obstructive lesion. Lesions which obstruct the urinary tract include certain abnormalities of the renal parenchyma which deform the calcyes, such as hypoplasia, polycystic kidneys, and scarring from previous infections (including tuberculosis). Other causes are congenital abnormalities of the pelvis, ureter and urethra; aberrant renal arteries; renal and ureteric calculi; pregnancy; 'neurogenic bladders'; pelvic tumours; prostatic enlargement and urethral strictures. Calculi and pregnancy are the two most frequent causes of obstruction.

Infections frequently complicate other parenchymal renal diseases; for instance, acute pyelonephritis may develop in a patient known to be suffering from renal polyarteritis nodosa. In this connection it is interesting to note that animal experiments have shown that the intravenous administration of large numbers of Gram-negative organisms only causes acute pyelonephritis if the ureters are temporarily occluded or the kidneys are already scarred from previous infections. It has also been shown in animals that an increased susceptibility to infection can be produced by a period of potassium deficiency or hypertension.

*Clinical features*

The most important paradox to remember is that many patients with acute pyelonephritis have severe constitutional symptoms such as fever and rigors and feel extremely ill without having any localising symptoms or signs either in the loins, abdomen or bladder, i.e. they do not have loin pain, abdominal tenderness, frequency or dysuria. Others with acute pyelonephritis do have tender loins and flanks, and may also have lower urinary symptoms. Frequently there is much nausea and vomiting particularly in pregnancy. The urine always contains a large number of white cells and bacteria, and sometimes there is gross macroscopical haematuria; proteinuria is rarely greater than +. The clinical features give no clue to the identity of the infecting organism.

As it is clinically difficult, particularly at the onset, to differentiate between acute pyelitis and pyelonephritis, and as renal biopsies show that a substantial number of clinically mild cases may show inflammatory lesions in the cortex, it is best to consider that all upper urinary infections involve the renal parenchyma, i.e. that all such infections are due to acute pyelonephritis.

The extent of the parenchymatous involvement depends mainly on the presence of urinary tract obstruction or reflux; the greater the obstruction or reflux the more extensive the infection. Obstructions are often found in patients of either sex who have recurrent infection; they underlie most upper urinary infections that occur in men, whereas women mostly have recurrent infections without any abnormality of the urinary tract.

Renal function in upper urinary infections may be unaffected, or it may be so severely impaired that the patient dies from acute renal failure. Characteristically renal function returns to its previous level as the infection subsides. The magnitude of this transient impairment is probably of some value in assessing the amount of parenchyma that has been invaded in the acute inflammatory process. Proper appraisal may be difficult if some degree of renal failure preceded the infection; at such times renal function should be re-examined a few weeks after the infection has been controlled.

*Acute necrotising papillitis.* This occurs most often in elderly diabetics, most of whom have suffered from previous upper urinary infections. In addition to the usual features of a severe acute upper urinary infection, haematuria occurs frequently and, if the lesion is bilateral, there is a sudden reduction in urine flow with the onset of acute renal failure. Sometimes pieces of necrosed papillae appear in the urine. If the patient recovers, the loss of part of one or more papillae may be defined in an I.V.P. or retrograde pyelogram.

Necrosis of papillae also occurs in phenacetin nephropathy (p. 465) and sickle cell anaemia. There have also been reports of patients on continuous sulphonamide therapy for chronic urinary infection who have developed renal colic or ureteric obstruction due to the necrosis of a papilla without any evidence of an associated acute infection. More recently non-steroidal anti-inflammatory drugs such as indomethacin have been found to cause papillary necrosis.

## Relationship between clinical and structural features

Renal biopsy studies have shown that in acute pyelonephritis there is a striking lack of correlation between the severity of the constitutional symptoms and impairment of renal function on the one hand, and histological appearances on the other. The main reason for this discrepancy is probably the focal nature of the disease.

The most important observation is that severe acute pyelonephritic lesions of the cortex, with inflammatory cell replacement of the tubules, can be found in patients who, clinically, have suffered only from a mild 'pyelitis'. In one series, such lesions were found in one quarter of a group of patients with clinical signs and symptoms of an acute upper urinary infection. As autopsy findings have shown that, on the whole, pyelonephritic lesions are focal, and more advanced in the medulla, such biopsy findings suggest that nearly all patients with an upper urinary infection have destructive lesions of the cortex and medulla.

It is interesting to note that it is unusual for these acute destructive lesions to be associated with any recognisable change in the intravenous pyelogram at the time of the infection. The abnormalities which do occur include a diminished density of the radio-opaque medium on the most affected side, localised renal swelling, and compression and elongation of one calyx. The difference in density is not a helpful finding, while the other two abnormalities are rare.

*Sequelae of acute pyelonephritis*

If the pyelogram is repeated a few months to a few years later, changes will be evident, the nature of which will depend on the patient's age. In children serial pyelograms often reveal the development of fresh cortical scarring with clubbing or distortion of one or more calyces. In adults, cortical scarring and clubbing and distortion of calyces rarely develop, but the kidneys show a reduction in length of 0.6 to 6.0 cm, which confirms the renal biopsy findings that clinical acute pyelonephritis in adults is usually associated with some destruction of the parenchyma. The radiological appearances of cortical scarring with distortion and clubbing of calyces are referred to as those of reflux nephropathy (see below). Usually these appearances are found in a child or adult who has never suffered from an overt attack of acute pyelonephritis. It must be stressed that they rarely *develop* after childhood.

*Prognosis*

An acute infection of the renal parenchyma may cause death if it is sufficiently extensive, or if it is superimposed upon pre-existing chronic renal disease.

Once the acute infection has been controlled, the risk of further attacks and the development of chronic pyelonephritis depends a great deal on whether or not there is permanent deformity of the renal tract such as bladder diverticulum, prostatic hypertrophy, or ureteric reflux (p. 455). Usually such deformities precede infections, but the changes produced in the renal parenchyma and pelvis by sufficiently severe or recurrent infections may themselves perpetuate the tendency to infection. Even when the renal tract is radiologically normal the rate of recurrent bateriuria following an attack of acute pyelonephritis is 50% at six months, and 80% at 18 months.

It is essential to remember that a patient suffering from advanced renal failure secondary to an acute renal infection may rapidly recover once the infection is controlled; it is unwise, therefore, to give a prognosis during the acute phase of the infection.

*Differential diagnosis*

Fever, particularly with rigors, tenderness and pain in one or both loins suggest, and the finding of pus and organisms in the urine tend to confirm, the diagnosis of acute pyelonephritis. The higher the fever and the greater the loin tenderness the more likely is the urinary infection to be in the kidneys, but otherwise there is remarkably little correlation between the patient's symptoms and the site of the infection (see Table 22.1). A recent impairment in renal function, particularly an impaired ability to concentrate the urine, and the presence of an abnormal intravenous pyelogram also increase the likelihood of the infection being in the kidney. Occasionally when local symptoms and signs are absent, the diagnosis only becomes apparent after a routine examination and culture of the urine. The finding of a high serum antibody titre to the bacterium present in the urine is presumptive evidence that the organism has invaded the parenchyma. An acute urinary infection should always be kept in mind when the patient is known to suffer from some other chronic parenchymal renal disease.

*Treatment*

Patients used to recover from acute upper urinary infections before antibiotics were available. It is probably true, therefore, that many infections would recover if treatment were limited to the administration of large quantities of water. In practice it is best to give an antibiotic in all upper urinary infections, for if the inflammatory process has penetrated into the renal parenchyma it is reasonable to suppose that quick control of the infection will lessen the residual damage.

An antibiotic is usually administered without first identifying the organism responsible for the infection. The repeated success of this blind manoeuvre ensures its continuity, but there is no doubt that it is more satisfactory to culture the urine and determine the sensitivity of the organism. When there are recurrent infections it is imperative that this be done. Antibiotics are excreted in the urine at varying rates, but in all instances their urinary concentration is greater than their simultaneous concentration in body fluids. Contrary to original expectations it is only necessary to give sufficient antibiotics to obtain an effective urinary antibacterial level. The administration of antibiotics should be continued for at least three weeks, and certainly *for some days after all trace of tenderness in the loins has disappeared.*

When there has been evidence of extensive parenchymal invasion, that is, if renal function has been depressed by the infection, it is advisable to continue treatment for two to three months.

The choice of antibiotic is determined by the sensitivity of the infecting organism, but if the diagnosis is clear cut it is unnecessary to wait 24 hours for the results of urine culture; treatment is started immediately with either co-trimoxazole, ampicillin or cephalexin after some urine has been obtained

**Table 22.2** Antibacterial agents used to treat urinary infection

| Agent | Normal dose | Route of administration | Relevant anti bacterial spectrum | Comment | Use in renal failure |
|---|---|---|---|---|---|
| Co-trimoxazole | 2 tab. b.d. | Oral or Parenteral | Gram-ve bacilli except pseudomonas Staphylococci some Streptococci | Few side effects Hypersensitivity to sulphonamide | Modified dosage |
| Trimethoprim | 200 mg b.d. | Oral | Same as co-trimoxazole | Useful in patients with known sulphonamide intolerance | Modified dosage in severe renal failure |
| Sulphadimidine | 3 g loading dose 1 g 6 hrly | Oral or Parenteral | Gram-ve bacilli except pseudomonas Staphylococci some Streptococci | Hypersensitivity | Modified dosage in severe renal failure |
| Penicillin V | 500 mg q.d.s. | Oral or Parenteral | v. wide range at this dosage because of extremely high urine concentrations | Toxicity minimal except for Hypersensitivity | Useful in renal failure |
| Ampicillin/ amoxycillin | 500 mg 8 hrly | Oral or Parenteral | Gram-ve bacilli except Klebsiella spp pseudomonas Streptococci some Staphylococci Lactobacilli | Rashes Candida infections | Modified dosage |
| Flucloxacillin | 250 mg t.d.s. | Oral | Gram +ve cocci | Loss of nails with massive doses in renal failure | None |
| Mecillinam | | Oral | Effective against some gram-ve species which are resistant to ampicillin e.g. Proteus | Ineffective against Gram +ve organisms and pseudomonas | Modified dosage |
| Colistin | 120 mg 8hrly | Parenteral | Gram-ve bacilli useful against pseudomonas spp | Ototoxic nephrotoxic | Modified dosage |
| Carbenicillin | 5 g 6 hrly | Parenteral | Gram-ve bacilli useful against pseudomonas spp | In combination with tobramycin for treatment of severe infection with pseudomonas spp | Modified dosage |

| Drug | Dose | Route | Spectrum / Comments | Renal failure |
|---|---|---|---|---|
| Carfecillin (phenyl ester of carbenicillin) | 0.58–1 g 6 hrly | Oral | Same as carbenicillin | Resistance apt to develop. Useful for treatment of pseudomonas at home | Modified dosage |
| Ticarcillin | 5 g 6 hrly | Parenteral | Effective against pseudomonas at lower doses and at longer intervals between doses than carbenicillin | In combination with tobramycin for severe pseudomonas spp infection | Modified dosage |
| Tobramycin | 100 mg 8 hrly | Parenteral | Gram-ve bacilli +ve organisms useful against pseudomonas | Ototoxic Nephrotoxic but ? less than gentamycin | Modified dosage |
| Nitrofurantoin | 50 mg 6 hrly | Oral | Gram-ve bacilli except pseudomonas and proteus Staphylococci Streptococci | Nausea with higher doses Acute lung reactions Rashes | Contra-indicated |
| Nalidixic acid | 1 g 6 hrly | Oral | Gram-ve bacilli except pseudomonas good for proteus | Nausea Rashes CNS disturbances Phototoxic reactions | Unchanged dose until GFR <10 then avoid |
| Cephalexin | 500 mg tds | Oral or Parenteral | Wide spectrum | Relatively non toxic Cross allergenicity with penicillin | Useful in renal failure with modified dose |
| Erythromycin | 500 mg qds | Oral | Streptococci Lactobacilli Staphylococci L. Forms | Non toxic Elimination of gram+ve commensals. Predisposes to infection with gram-ve species | Unchanged dose |
| Tetracycline | 250 mg 6 hrly | Oral or Parenteral | Wide spectrum good for proteus | Contraindicated in pregnancy and children Useful for prostatitis | AVOID |
| Doxycycline | 100 mg o.d. | Oral | Same as for tetracycline | Same as tetracycline | Can be used in normal doses in advanced renal failure |
| Metronidazole | 400 mg 8 hrly | Oral | Anaerobic organisms | Nausea, drowsiness | Reduce dose |

for culture. If the patient is severely ill with septicaemia, an aminoglycoside such as tobramycin should also be used. Other antibiotics are listed in Table 22.2.

During a course of treatment the urine should be cultured at least once to make certain that the antibiotic is effective. When the course of antibiotic is finished the urine should be cultured approximately 7, 14 and 30 days later and then at monthly intervals. The treatment and prevention of further attacks is discussed below.

*Precautions in patients with renal failure.* Most drugs are excreted in large amounts in the urine so that their plasma and urine concentrations are closely related to the state of renal function. When renal function is impaired the plasma level of such drugs may rise to toxic levels (e.g. strep-tomycin and nitrofurantoin) while conversely their concentration in the urine may fall to such low levels that the concentration is insufficient to sterilise the urine, even if the organism is sensitive. Cephalexin, doxycycline and penicillin are the safest drugs to use in the presence of severe renal impairment.

*It is imperative that, with the exception of doxycycline, all other forms of tetracycline should be recognised to be highly poisonous for patients with renal failure. They cause a brisk rise in blood urea, with vomiting and a rapid deterioration of renal function.*

*Prevention of further attacks.* The prevention of recurrence is sometimes a surgical procedure, with the repair or removal of a structural deformity or ureteric reflux. Otherwise the prevention of further attacks depends on keeping the urine sterile. This can be done in one of three ways. The first consists of giving a short course of an appropriate antibiotic in normal doses, each time the urine is found to be infected *or* symptoms recur. In order that treatment should be prompt the patient keeps a supply of one of the wide spectrum oral antibiotics at home. Urine cultures are performed at regular intervals. Alternatively urinary sterility can be maintained by giving long courses of a simple urinary antibiotic in small propylactic doses. The antibiotic is given once in the 24 hours and is best taken at night on retiring. During the night the concentration of the urine is at its highest so that the concentration of the antibiotic which it contains is also at its highest, this urine remains in the bladder for some considerable time, and the bladder at this time is therefore in an advantageous position to repel any bacterial invasion introduced during sexual intercourse. Nitrofurantoin 50 mg, cephalexin 125 mg, and trimethoprim 20 mg/sulphamethoxazole 100 mg (Paediatric) have each been found useful, particularly nitrofuran-toin. Side effects on such small doses are most unusual.

Occasionally none of these methods prevents frequent reinfections of the urine but the patient does not develop overt clinical symptoms. This may happen if the patient has some residual urine which it is not possible to treat, or a renal stone. The administration of antibiotics presumably keeps the population of organisms below a critical number necessary to produce symptoms. In such a situation it is best to continue whichever treatment is being given and to watch and wait.

**Reflux nephropathy** (chronic atrophic pyelonephritis)

This condition *can only be diagnosed radiologically*, and at post mortem. The radiological appearances are those of focal areas of parenchymal scarring (shrinkage). On an intravenous pyelogram such an area should be recognised because (1) the thickness of the parenchyma is measurably diminished and (2) the calyx of the papilla which adjoins the shrunken piece of parenchyma seems to have been turned inside out (i.e. it has become clubbed) (Fig. 22.3).

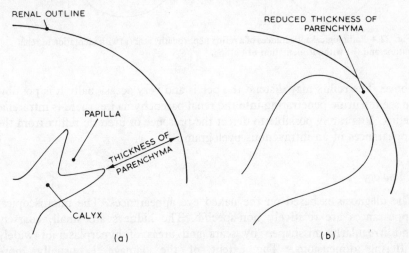

**Fig. 22.3** Diagram to explain (a) normal calyx, papilla, and overlying renal parenchyma and (b) reflux nephropathy scar.

Sometimes the scars indent the outline of the kidney but often they do not so (Fig. 22.4). The absence of an indentation at the site of a scar is liable to lull the unwary into overlooking gross focal parenchymal shrinking. In order to detect the presence of parenchymal scarring it is useful to measure the distance between the renal outline and an imaginary line drawn through the outermost points of each calyx.

The distribution of the scars is asymmetrical within a single kidney and between the two kidneys. There may be several scars in one kidney and none in the other. The scars are mainly situated at the poles while the unaffected areas tend to hypertrophy. A single scar most commonly occurs at the right upper pole. An affected kidney is always shorter than normal.

A micturating cystogram will demonstrate ureteric reflux of varying severity in a proportion of patients who have the type of scars described

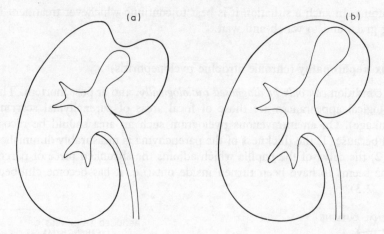

**Fig. 22.4** Radiological appearances of a reflux nephropathy scar (a) with identation of renal outline and (b) without identation of outline.

above. The reflux may distend the pelvis and very occasionally it is possible to see the urine penetrating into the renal parenchyma i.e. there is intrarenal reflux. It is rarely possible to detect the presence of ureteric reflux from the appearances of an intravenous pyelogram.

*Pathology*

The diagnosis is based on the naked eye appearances. The microscopical appearances are relatively non-specific. The kidneys are small, coarsely and irregularly misshapen by scars and areas of hyperplasia of widely differing dimensions. The extent of the damage is usually more pronounced on one side than on the other and is sometimes entirely unilat-

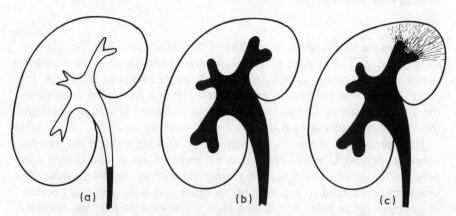

**Fig. 22.5** Radiological reflux. (a) Moderate, (b) gross, and (c) intrarenal reflux demonstrated radiologically during micturition.

eral. The cut surfaces show dilatation of some calyces with gross reduction of the thickness of the overlying parenchyma while other calyces are normal and surrounded by hypertrophied parenchyma. Fibrous scars extending from the pelvis to the capsule can also be seen.

The microscopical appearances consist of patches of intense infiltration with lymphocytes and plasma cells; these areas are distributed in a haphazard manner, but concentrated more in the medulla than in the cortex. The tubules in these sites are either small and atrophic, or dilated with flattened epithelium and contain collections of a homogeneous eosin staining material ('thyroid areas'). The glomeruli resist the inflammatory invasion better than the tubules; some may appear almost unchanged while others have normal tufts, though they are surrounded by a thick collar of fibrous tissue (Fig. 23.3); the remainder, however, show varying degrees of change in the tufts, including fibrosis and atrophy. Frequently the changes of acute pyelonephritis are found interspersed and superimposed in the relatively normal areas between the scars. The scarring due to reflux consists principally of wedge-shaped areas of inflammation, but there may also be similar shaped areas of ischaemic infarction; often the two are histologically inseparable. The characteristic lesion caused by the reflux is a parenchymal scar adherent to a clubbed calyx. The papilla is no longer present. An ischaemic scar may be situated at any site but even when situated near a papilla it is unusual for the calyx to be clubbed. The extent of vascular abnormalities varies but in patients who have had severe hypertension changes can be demonstrated in both the larger arteries as well as in the arterioles. The arcuate, interlobar and interlobular arteries show gross thickening of focal areas of the external elastic lamina with fibrous replacement of varying amounts of the arterial walls, including the elastic and muscle coats; they may also show extensive fibrocellular proliferation of the intima. These changes which in the larger arteries are presumably due to the parenchymal scar in which they are situated may produce extreme narrowing of the lumen, though complete occlusion is rare. The arterioles show the changes associated with either malignant or non-malignant hypertension. Whenever there are malignant hypertensive changes there are also widespread and severe changes in the larger arteries.

*Aetiology*

The renal lesions are due to a reflux of urine from the bladder up the ureters and into the renal parenchyma. Reflux may occur because of some obstructive lesion or because of a neuropathic bladder (e.g. spinal injury, poliomyelitis). More commonly it is due to a genetic abnormality of the lower ureter which instead of travelling very obliquely through the thick bladder wall tends to have a shorter more direct passage. This prevents the lower ureter from being occluded by the bladder musculature during micturition. Therefore, as the bladder contracts urine travels up the ureter as well as through the urethra. And sometimes in some patients the intra pelvic pressure rises sufficiently for the urine to reflux directly into the renal parenchyma. It is the intrarenal reflux which causes the parenchymal scarring, and the amount of damage that this causes is considerably greater if the urine is infected.

Reflux scars tend to be at the poles of the kidney because, as the intra pelvic pressure rises, the uriniferous ducts opening onto the surface of the papillae of the calyces which are situated at the two poles have openings which remain open and allow urine to flow upwards, whereas the ducts of the papillae in the calyces in the middle portion of the kidney are occluded by the rising pressure and do not allow retrograde flow. On the other hand it has been demonstrated that when the pelvic urine is heavily infected the openings of the ducts of the papillae in the middle of the kidney become patulous. A rise in pelvic pressure now causes retrograde flow into the parenchyma. This probably explains why in some instances all the calyces of a kidney are affected and the whole kidney atrophies. It is most unusual to find scars confined to the mid portion of the kidney.

Ureteric reflux probably begins in utero. It can certainly be demonstrated in the first few weeks after birth and the evidence suggests that most of the scarring takes place in the first year of life. Reflux tends to diminish and may dissapear with age though this process is delayed by the presence of a persistently infected urine. For instance 25% of infants with reflux have gross reflux which distends the pelvis and calyces, whereas reflux of this severity occurs in less than 5% of adults with reflux. It is this form of reflux which is associated with loin pain which comes on immediately before and persists during the initial act of micturition. Nevertheless some degree of reflux tends to persist. In adults ureteric reflux can be demonstrated in 35% of patients with unilateral scars and in 50% of those with bilateral scars.

Intrarenal reflux not only produces scars but also slows the growth of the kidney (Fig. 22.6).

Aged 4 years                                    Aged 11 years

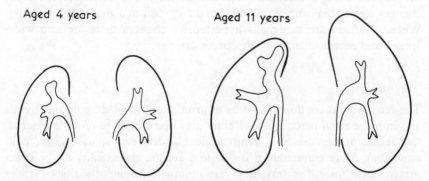

Fig. 22.6 Tracing of outline of pelves and kidneys at age 4 years and 11 years of a child with a unilateral scar demonstrating the progress of the scar and the retardation of renal growth. (Reproduced from Hodson 1967 Radiology 88: 857, with kind permission.)

*Clinical features*

In infancy the presence of ureteric reflux and renal scar formation is often unsuspected unless there are gross systemic disturbances. During childhood recurrent fevers, loin pain and an offensive urine may draw attention to the kidneys. But it is clear that in many patients after the initial damage has been created the urine spontaneously becomes sterile and there may be a quiescent period lasting many years.

In adults reflux nephropathy is often a symptomless condition only revealed when the urine becomes infected. If the kidneys become infected the commonest symptom is loin pain and tenderness with or without febrile episodes. Sometimes these attacks have been present for many years and usually they have *not* been accompanied by any lower urinary symptoms. It is customary for the loin pain to have been ignored first by the patient and then by her doctor. Many patients will admit to intermittent spells of tiredness, headache and loss of appetite for no obvious reason in recent years. Occasionally there is a history of acute pyelonephritis but it is very rare to obtain, from an adult, a history suggestive of urinary infection in childhood. A few patients first present with either hypertension or with lower urinary symptoms such as frequency and dysuria but with no upper urinary symptoms. Very rarely the presentation is one of asymptomatic proteinuria.

Characteristically, when there are symptoms, the urine is infected (i.e. there are more than 100 000 organisms/ml of urine), and contains an excess number of white cells (i.e. more than 10 mm³ or more than 40 000/hr). In addition proteinuria is usually present though it is seldom greater than 5 g/24 hours. Some patients with persistent active upper urinary tract infection have high antibody titres to the infecting organism. The absence of these abnormalities does not exclude the presence of chronic renal infection. Urinary infection may be revealed to be due to fastidious organisms which need special culturing conditions, and an injection of prednisolone phosphate intravenously may provoke a sudden rise in white cell excretion (p. 441) which demonstrates that there is a site of active inflammation some where along the urinary tract.

It must be stressed that the radiological appearances of reflux nephropathy are no proof that the patient is suffering from an active renal infection even if the urine is infected and there is pyuria. Some patients with the radiological appearances of reflux nephropathy have a urinary infection which is confined to the bladder. The only way a diagnosis of renal infection can be confirmed is to establish that organisms are descending the ureters from one or both kidneys. Statistically however if the urine from a patient with reflux nephropathy is infected it is usually found that the organisms arise from the upper urinary tract. In keeping with the focal nature of the chronic reflux nephropathy it is characteristic that there is often a marked difference in renal function between the two kidneys. This information can often be inferred from the inequality in renal size but it is only accurately obtained from an estimation of total renal function such as a 24 hr creatinine clearance, and a non-invasive radio nuclide investigation which determines the relative contribution of each kidney to total function. In this way an assessment can be made of the likelihood of the remaining larger kidney being able to sustain life if the smaller is removed.

In general the pattern of renal functional impairment is the same as that described in the section on chronic renal failure (p. 181). The presence of an active urinary infection, however, significantly reduces the ability to concentrate more than the glomerular filtration rate. But with antibiotic treatment this discrepancy disappears and it becomes apparent that persistent impairment in renal function is associated with parallel changes in glomerular filtration and in the ability to concentrate. The ability to acidify usually remains normal though occasionally a patient will present with a low plasma pH and plasma bicarbonate and a raised plasma chloride due to an inability to acidfy.

In some patients with prolonged severe upper urinary tract infection there may be a considerable increase in the plasma concentration of gamma globulins together with a high erythrocyte sedimentation rate. A finding such as this in a patient in whom the presence of reflux nephropathy is not known may cause some confusion. The renal impairment and abnormal electrophoretic pattern may suggest a diagnosis of myelomatosis. After treatment with antibiotics the erythrocyte sedimentation rate and the plasma protein pattern gradually return to normal.

## Relationship between clinical and structural features

There is little correlation between the amount of renal parenchyma involved, as gauged by radiology, and renal function. It is possible to find patients with reflux nephropathy who have had a nephrectomy on one side and a hemiphrectomy on the other with a normal blood urea, and a plasma creatinine below 1.2 mg/100 ml. Often renal function deteriorates without any further measurable change in the radiological appearances.

## Course and prognosis

In children, if the urine remains sterile, the disease may remain quiescent and undetected unless hypertension or advanced renal failure develop. If the urine is infected it may not only give rise to ill health but, particularly in those with persisting reflux, there may be new scar formation and further retardation of renal growth.

In adults it is characteristic that, whether or not the urine is infected, renal function remains unchanged for 10–20 years. Very rarely, however, in a patient with chronic renal failure an acute fulminating untreated superimposed acute pyelonephritis can cause death from acute renal failure. It is equally characteristic that, although, in a patient with some pre-existing impairment of renal function, an acute upper urinary infection may cause an almost terminal state of renal failure, an unexpected recovery may take place. For these reasons it is impossible to gauge the prognosis in an individual case until renal failure is advanced or malignant hypertension is superimposed.

In the past the main obvious cause of a gradual deterioration of renal function in reflux nephropathy was either an associated surreptitious ingestion of phenacetin or bilateral severe reflux. Recurrent asymptomatic bacteria rarely seems to affects renal function. It is even difficult to detect a persistent impairment of function in patients who have had several unequivocal clinical upper urinary infections with fever and rigors.

It has been claimed that the renal function of a very small number of patients with either persistent sterile pyuria, or in whom a small number of organisms are found only intermittently, will deteriorate. In some of these it has been claimed that the deterioration of renal function is due to the presence of fastidious organisms.

Approximately half the patients with reflux nephropathy have a normal blood pressure but it is nevertheless the renal disease which most often gives rise to malignant hypertension. Established hypertension is often aggravated by a clinically obvious phase of infection.

## Incidence of reflux nephropathy

Reflux nephropathy (often referred to as chronic pyelonephritis) is an uncommon cause of death from renal failure in adults. This is best gauged by the proportion of patients with reflux nephropathy who are placed onto maintenance haemodialysis. In our unit, where a diagnosis of reflux nephropathy or chronic pyelonephritis is not made unless the characteristic radiological appearances are present, less than 5% of the women and 2% of the men coming to dialysis have had reflux nephropathy. It is true that the yearly European Dialysis and Transplant Association report gives a much higher incidence and that some authors have claimed that it is about 40%. It is probable that this discrepancy is due in part to less stringent diagnostic criteria. In some units it is the practice to diagnose 'chronic pyelonephritis' when the cause of the renal failure is unknown. In some countries such as Switzerland, it may also be due to the greater incidence of phenacetin nephropathy for the radiological appearances of reflux nephropathy and those of phenacetin nephropathy overlap.

## Treatment

Gross ureteric reflux which *distends* the pelvis and calyces should be treated surgically. Less severe reflux may influence the efficacy of antibiotic treatment for it prevents total evacuation of the urine at each micturition. If antibiotics are unable to control the infection, it may be necessary to operate. On the other hand every effort should be made to avoid surgery. There are now many reports that reflux, particularly in children, has disappeared following the prolonged administration of antibiotics.

Once it has been established that the urine of a patient with the radiological appearances of reflux nephropathy is infected every attempt should be made to suppress the infection, and then to prevent its recurrence. In children, if this is successful, it will prevent much morbidity, further destruction of renal parenchyma and will allow the kidneys to grow. In adults, treatment certainly diminishes morbidity and it also diminishes the possibilities of an acute fulminating pyelonephritis. It is best to begin with a full course of the appropriate antibiotics. Subsequently continuous and prolonged attention should be maintained by the patient and her doctor to detect any minor change in general condition, and the urine should be examined frequently. If the patient experiences similar symptoms to those she has had with previous attacks or if there is fever, pains in the loins, dysuria or a sudden increase in white cell excretion, antibiotics should be started at once, whether or not the urine contains organisms. If the patient is intelligent she can be given some antibiotic to keep at home and to take at the first sign of a recurrence. If there are frequent recurrences they can sometimes be controlled by the administration of one small dose of a single antibiotic each night, e.g. 50 mg of nitrofurantoin or 125 mg cephalexin (see above). The urine must be cultured at regular intervals during treatment to check on the sensitivity of the organism. During pregnancy a woman known to suffer from reflux nephropathy should be given prophylactic antibiotics until two weeks after delivery.

If the disease has extensively involved one kidney and the other is sound it may be wise to remove the diseased kidney, for if the blood pressure is not raised preoperatively, the operation will prevent its rising; and, if it is already raised, the operation may cause it to return towards normal. Nevertheless, if the kidney is not causing any symptoms, the urine is uninfected and the blood pressure is normal, it may occasionally be justifiable to do nothing except keep the patient under observation.

Stones should be removed for otherwise the patient will either have recurrent infections or it will be necessary to continue antibiotics indefinitely. It is difficult to predict which patients with hypertension will have a fall of blood pressure following a unilateral nephrectomy (p. 274). Many of the successful operations have been in patients who had an acute and accelerated form of hypertension. The functional integrity of the other kidney should be assessed before operation. If one kidney is smaller than the other, the other should be larger than normal. If it isn't it is itself diseased.

## Interstitial nephritis due to chronic infection in the absence of renal scarring

Clinically this condition can only be diagnosed with any confidence if the patient has recurrent upper urinary tract infections, a 'normal' intravenous pyelogram and a gradual deterioration of renal function. One's impression is that such patients are rare but there is a strong possibility that they are missed. For instance if is agreed that one attack of acute pyelonephritis can reduce the length of a kidney by several centimetres without altering the renal outline or the appearance of the pelvis it is possible that chronic infection might do the same. But gradual overall shrinkage of this nature is most unlikely to be noticed, for, to be aware of what is going on it is necessary to monitor a series of intravenous pyelograms obtained over some years in a patient whose intravenous pyelograms appear normal throughout.

Furthermore it is alleged that the organisms responsible for interstitial nephritis may only appear in the urine intermittently and may be difficult to culture with routine methods. For instance the infection may be due to protoplasts. These are conventional organisms without their capsules. In this state they can only exist in hypertonic media. As the renal medulla is the only persistently hypertonic area in the body and as it is particularly susceptible to infection, (p. 447) it is possible that continuing destruction of the kidneys in patients with 'sterile' urine is sometimes due to a persisting infection with such organisms. In such patients a sterile pyuria may be the only evidence that there is an inflammatory process somewhere along the urinary tract. And in some patients the pyuria is only evident if a provocative injection of prednisone is given intravenously.

It has been suggested that active persistent infection may not be necessary for parenchymal destruction to continue after a renal infection. In animal experiments there is some suggestion that bacterial antigens may remain in the kidneys after the death of the bacteria and cause a continuing inflammatory reaction. It has been claimed that it has been possible to identify the presence of antigenic bacterial remnants in the renal parenchyma in some patients with sterile urines who have died of renal failure of unknown cause. It is not clear however, what significance to place on this finding for it is very possible that bacteria may become lodged in pre-existing scars. Antikidney antibodies cannot be found in recurrent upper urinary tract infection either circulating or deposited in the kidney. The only evidence that an immunological process may be involved in bacterial infection of the kidney is the demonstration of a suppressor cell population and a serum factor both capable of depressing cell mediated mechanisms in experimental renal infection in animals.

The diagnosis of chronic renal infection is not much advanced by a renal biopsy, for the changes which take place (interstitial nephritis) are not specific of infection. The wide range of possible causes of interstitial nephritis is listed in Table 22.3. It is not exhaustive. For instance it does not include viruses such as cytomegalic virus which are known to invade the kidney.

On the whole therefore the histological changes associated with 'pyelonephritis' have been more of a hindrance than a help. There used to be a general

**Table 22.3** Some causes of interstitial nephritis

| | |
|---|---|
| Ageing | Potassium depletion |
| Hypertension | Hyperphosphataemia |
| Nephrosclerosis | Irradiation |
| Immunological reaction | Lead and cadnium poisoning |
| Obstruction | Acute tubular necrosis |
| Analgesic nephropathy | Medullary cystic disease |
| Diabetes mellitus | Leptosporosis |
| Drugs | Sickle cell anaemia |
| Crystal nephropathy — calcium | Hereditary nephropathies |
| uric acid | Diffuse intravascular coagulation |

tendency to ascribe a cause for the histological appearances of interstitial nephritis where none was evident histologically; the choice having been influenced by the clinical history, the blood pressure, the biochemical findings or the urine culture. If no obvious choice was available, the inflammation of the interstitial spaces (interstitial nephritis) was assumed to be due to infection. This remarkable habit was responsible for the ludicrous disparity reported between the various estimates of the incidence of renal infection in kidneys examined at autopsy (from 10–80%!).

*Conclusion*

The diagnosis of interstitial nephritis due to chronic infection is a most difficult one. Clearly if the patient suffers from recurrent vague loin pain with occasional tenderness in the renal angle, has unexplained mild fevers and an excess of white cells in the urine, a normal intravenous pyelogram with focal areas of inflammation in a renal biopsy, and the condition settles upon being given an antibiotic, there is some justification for proposing that the symptoms may have been due to chronic infections in the kidneys. If, in addition, the urine is found to be infected and the infection is *repeatedly* traced to originate from the upper urinary tract the diagnosis of chronic renal infection is confirmed. Many of these points are difficult to pin down and to try do so it is sometimes necessary to have a certain tenacity of purpose which may seem out of proportion to the poor yield.

## DIFFERENTIAL DIAGNOSIS OF CHRONIC OR RECURRENT RENAL INFECTIONS

Probably the commonest cause of pain in the loins is constipation. A diagnosis of 'chronic pyelonephritis' is often made if a constipated woman is found to have an infected urine. Another source of confusion, particularly in a patient who has not been examined thoroughly, is pain from the lower thoracic spine. Other conditions with which reflux nephropathy or recurrent renal infection with a normal pyelogram may be confused include phenacetin nephropathy, the loin pain and haematuria syndrome and, obstructive uropathy.

**Phenacetin nephropathy**

The association between the consumption of phenacetin and papillary necrosis in man was first described in 1953. By 1966 most pharmaceutical firms in Great Britain had decided to remove phenacetin from their proprietary products. But they continued to include phenacetin in the BP and BPC preparations which they were under contract to manufacture. In 1966 approximately 540 000 kg of phenacetin was being consumed in Great Britain in combination with some other analgesic, usually aspirin. In 1974 the sale of phenacetin across the counter without a precription was prohibited but it could still be prescribed by prescription. In 1980 the drug was finally banned from use.

It was estimated that when phenacetin was freely available there was a yearly incidence of approximately 600 new cases of phenacetin nephropathy. The world incidence was not known but the disease was much commoner in many other countries including South Africa, Australia Switzerland, Norway and Sweden, in some of which phenacetin nephropathy was the commonest cause of terminal renal failure. Presumably therefore the yearly world wide incidence of phenacetin nephropathy must have been several thousand. In 1967, 3 000 000 kg of aspirin was being consumed per year in Great Britain, 2 000 000 kg of which was in preparations which did not contain phenacetin. It is remarkable therefore that aspirin which inhibits prostaglandin synthethase in the renal medulla, diminishes renal blood flow and sometimes causes acute renal failure in patients with a pre-existing impairment of renal function does not appear to be an important cause of papillary necrosis in man. From 1963 to 1982 the total world literature only revealed 150 patients in whom it was claimed that aspirin (in the absence of phenacetin) might have caused papillary necrosis. It has also been proposed that the papillary damage was due to the combination of phenacetin and aspirin. This is unlikely for (1) in some countries with a high incidence of phenacetin nephropathy the phenacetin was combined with other drugs many of which are not known to be nephrotoxic, and (2) in those countries in which phenacetin has been banned, the incidence of new cases of 'analgesic' papillary necrosis appears to have fallen, though the consumption of aspirin continues. These observation apply to man. Rats and rabbits are different. They appear particularly susceptible to the administration of aspirin and can be made to develop papillary necrosis with aspirin as well as with phenacetin. This difference in species susceptibility has thoroughly confused some authorities who, on the basis of the animal studies, claim that aspirin is as responsible as phenacetin in causing papillary necrosis in man. In the absence of these observations on animals, phenacetin would have been banned far earlier.

*Pathology*

The macroscopic appearances are the most characteristic and are due to the multiple loss of papillae. Some papillae are green, others are black and leathery with the tip slightly twisted away from its normal position. Other papillae are absent. The calyces are then clubbed but tend to be narrowed as they travel towards the pelvis. The overlying parenchyma is reduced in size but the gross asymmetrical distortions found in reflux nephropathy do not occur. Microscopically the lesion consists of a chronic inflammation of the interstitial spaces which is particularly marked in the medulla and papillae. Tubules are eventually destroyed while the glomeruli tend to remain intact.

## Clinical findings

Several groups of individuals were liable to take phenacetin in large amounts. The majority were women in whom the diagnosis was first made around the age of 50 years. The most understandable group consisted of persons who suffered from some chronic painful disease, such as rheumatoid arthritis, for which analgesics offer some relief. Another group consisted of workers such as watchmakers who were liable to headaches. In some Swiss factories it used to be customary for the firm to distribute phenacetin free of charge to its workers. A third group were compulsive analgesic consumers. They had no pain or headache and they obtained no over-whelming pleasure from the ingestion of phenacetin. Their habit usually started for some trivial reason and they could be induced to stop without much effort. Others were chronically neurotic with inadequate personalities or suffered from reactive depression; often they were alcoholic. They tended to claim that the tablets were for their headache.

A remarkable group was first described from Sweden; it provided the first conclusive evidence of the toxicity of phenacetin. A whole village became addicted to phenacetin. The drug became a symbol of friendliness and sociability. When a few people gathered together they would offer each other a phenacetin tablet as a preliminary to conversation, while those who were invited out to dinner would take their hosts a 'gift wrapped' packet of phenacetin.

Patients often presented for some vague complaint, or there might be renal colic with haematuria, or chronic renal failure and hypertension. The renal colic was caused by the passage of necrosed papillae which could some-times be recognised in the urine. Persistent proteinuria was an early sign.

The correct diagnosis was made by asking the right questions. It was characteristic of patients with this condition that they lied about their intake of analgesic and it might take some time before the truth emerged. There-fore the use of questionnaires to determine the prevalence of phenacetin nephropathy were misleading and useless. Apart from the history the most characteristic findings were a sterile pyuria and radiological evidence of loss of papillae.

*Radiological appearances*

The main distinctions from reflux nephropathy are (1) the disease is always bilateral, (2) and though it is focally distributed in that some papillae are more affected than others, there are no gross focal areas of parenchymatous destruction with compensating hypertrophy of the remaining areas such as is seen in reflux nephropathy. The characteristic appearance is one of bilaterally small kidneys with several abnormal calyces on both sides. These calyces are long and narrow and seen to stretch out towards the outer border of the kidney, in a slightly sigmoid fashion, known in France as 'langue de chat'. Patchy calcification often occurs, sometimes it lies on the surface of a devitalised papilla and thus appears as ring shadow. Occasionally another type of ring shadow is seen when contrast medium surrounds a separated papilla lying free in the calyx. Sometimes a papilla may be only partially separated so that the contrast around it gives it an 'egg in cup' appearance.

*Functional and urinary changes*

Phenacetin nephropathy causes severe impairment of the ability to concentrate long before there is any impairment in glomerular filtration rate, e.g. a maximum osmolality of 400 mosmol/kg with a plasma creatinine of 100 $\mu$mol/l (1.0 mg/100 ml). Almost as often there is an impairment in the ability to acidify. There may also be a sodium leak, and such patients rarely have hypertension; or may have had hypertension earlier which no longer needs treating as the disease progresses. They are therefore very susceptible to dehydration, vomiting and diarrhoea (see below). The urine often contains an increased number of white cells in the absence of infection though infection does occur from time to time.

*Prognosis*

The continued consumption of large amounts of phenacetin in a patient who has developed papillary necrosis leads to death. On the other hand, if the patient stops taking phenacetin, renal function nearly always stops deteriorating and often improves slightly. This makes the search for the disease particularly imperative. Surgical operations are dangerous for they may precipitate wide-spread necrosis of surviving papillae and a sudden deterioration in renal function. This is probably due to the routine dehydration, and the other multiple anaesthetic and surgical causes of renal ischaemia superimposed upon pre-existing damaged papillae. If surgery cannot be avoided it is best to use a local or spinal anaesthetic and to make certain that there is no dehydration by giving large amounts of intravenous saline before, during and after the operation (p. 217). Ureteric strictures and uroepithelial malignancy are other complication of phenacetin nephropathy.

*Treatment*

All cases are due to self-administration. Many patients will readily stop taking tablets containing phenacetin if they are told of the damage it causes. Patients who are in pain, however, must be advised that other analgesics are available; the censure implied by the term 'analgesic abuse' to such patients is inappropriate and indefensible. If instead of taking phenacetin-containing tablets the patients are allowed to consume up to six tablets of aspirin or paracetomol per day for several years there is no further deterioration in renal function and sometimes there is some recovery.

Patients with phenacetin nephropathy do not do well on maintenance haemodialysis or after a renal transplantation because of (1) their peculiar mental state which includes some degree of dementia due to cerebral atrophy, and (2) ill defined disturbances of their immunological systems.

## Loin pain and haematuria syndrome

Clinically this syndrome causes much diagnostic confusion. It occurs mainly in young women who have some medical connection. The patient complains of severe bouts of loin pain which usually affects only one kidney at a time. It is most unusual for the pain to be present in both kidneys simultaneously. From time to time there is macroscopic haematuria, sometimes coinciding with a severe bout of pain. The urine is uninfected, the intravenous phelogram normal, and the patient therefore tends to be referred from one specialist to another including general physicians, urologists, general surgeons, gynaecologists, orthopaedic surgeons and occasionally to psychiatrists. Some patients are so anxious to persuade their medical attendants that they are physically ill that they will resort to various deceptions such as artificially raising the temperature of the clinical thermometer. When these subterfuges are discovered they have the opposite effect to that which the patient wishes in as much as the doctor is now convinced that there can be little physically wrong with the patient. In addition the same type of patient seems to derive some peculiar satisfaction from the pain, and more particularly from the observation that the doctor is baffled. Not all patients behave in this way.

The diagnosis is made by selective angiography which reveals focal areas of irregularities and increased tortuosity of the smaller arteries in the cortex. Renal biopsies are often negative but about half show partial occlusions of some of the small vessels. In addition there is one report from a group who performed several nephrectomies for the relief of the pain. Examination of the kidneys that were removed revealed multiple small infarcts with partial occlusions of some of the medium sized renal arteries. The cause of the disease is unknown and why the lesions cause pain and haematuria, particularly the pain, is unknown. There are many other conditions associated with acute arterial occlusions which do not cause loin pain or macroscopic haematuria. Occasionally the condition seems to have been precipitated by oral contraceptives, particularly those with a high oestrogen content, and it has been reported in men receiving oestrogen therapy for cancer of the prostate. It has also been demonstrated that the platelets show increased stickiness.

Treatment with renal denervation gives a few months respite from pain. Otherwise there is nothing but encouragement and analgesics. It is unwise to remove a kidney for, as stated above the condition can recur in the remaining kidney. There are some claims that dipyridamole and aspirin may help. The natural history of the condition is obscure.

## Obstructive uropathy

This condition may be associated with upper urinary infections. The radiological changes however, though superficially similar to those of reflux nephropathy can usually be distinguished without difficulty. There is a uniform dilatation of all the calyces with no *focal* loss of parenchymal thickness. Sometimes there may be severe blunting of the renal papillae particularly before the obstruction is relieved. Persistent obstruction leads to an overall reduction of kidney size and a uniform reduction in parenchyma thickness. In children renal growth is impaired and continues to be impaired after the obstruction is relieved (Fig. 22.7).

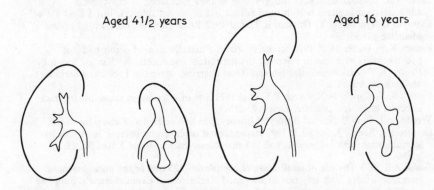

Aged 4 1/2 years        Aged 16 years

Fig. 22.7 Obstructive uropathy of the left kidney due to ureteric calculus (passed at 4½ years). Tracings of the subsequent pyelograms show an overall decrease in the rate of growth on the left side over the next 11½ years compared with hypertrophy of the right kidney. (Reproduced from Hodson 1967 Radiology 88: 857, with kind permission.)

BIBLIOGRAPHY

Acquatella H, Little P J, de Wardener H E et al 1967 The effect of urine osmolality and pH on the bactericidal activity of plasma. Clin Sci 33: 471
Anderson R J, Gambertoglio J G, Schrier R W 1976 Clinical use of drugs in renal failure. Thomas, Springfield

Andriole V T 1966 Acceleration of the inflammatory response of the renal medulla by water diuresis. J Clin Invest 45: 847

Andriole V T, Epstein F H 1965 Prevention of pyelonephritis by water diuresis; evidence for the role of medullary hypertonicity in promoting renal infection. J Clin Invest 44: 73

Angell M E, Relman A S, Robbins S L 1968 Active chronic pyelonephritis without evidence of bacterial infection. New Eng J Med 278: 1303

Aoki S, Imamura S, Aoki M et al 1969 Abacterial and bacterial pyelonephritis. Immunofluorescent localization of bacterial antigen. New Eng J Med 281: 1375

Asscher A W, Brumfitt W (eds) 1975 Urinary tract infection. A symposium. Kidney Int Suppl No 4

Asscher A W 1980 The challenge of urinary tract infections. Academic Press, London

Bailey R R, Gower P E, Roberts A P et al 1971 Prevention of urinary-tract infection with low-dose nitrofurantoin. Lancet 2: 1112

Bailey R R, Gower P E, Roberts A·P et al 1973 Urinary-tract infection in non-pregnant women. Lancet 2: 275

Bell D, Kerr D N S, Swinney J et al 1969 Analgesic nephropathy. Clinical course after withdrawal of phenacetin. Brit Med J 3: 378

Birch D F, Fairley K F, Pavillard R E 1981 Unconventional bacteria in urinary tract disease: Ureaplasma urealyticum. Kidney Int 19: 58

Braude A I, Siemienski J S, Jacobs I 1961 Protoplast formation in human urine. Trans Assoc Amer Phys 74: 234

Burden R P, Booth L J, Ockenden B G et al 1975 Intrarenal vascular changes in adult patients with recurrent haematuria and loin pain — A clinical, histological and angiographic study. Quart J Med 44: 433

Burry A F 1967 The evolution of analgesic nephropathy. Nephron 5: 185

Burry A F 1970 The pathology and pathogenesis of renal papillary necrosis. In: Kincaid Smith P, Faireley K F (ed) Renal infection and Renal Scarring. Mercedes Publishing Services, Melbourne, Australia

Curtis J R, Koutsaimanis K G, Buggey D et al 1973 Evaluation of doxycycline administration in patients with renal failure and in normal subjects. Brit J Urol 45: 445

Eknoyan G, Qunibi W Y, Grissom R T et al 1982 Renal papillary necrosis: an update. Medicine 61: 55

Fairley K F, Butler H M 1970 Sterile pyuria as a manifestation of occult bacterial pyelonephritis with special reference to intermittent bacteriuria. In: Kincaid-Smith P, Fairley K F (eds) Renal infection and Renal Scarring. Mercedes Publishing Services, Melbourne, Australia

Fairley K F, Carson N E, Gutch R C et al 1971 Site of infection in acute urinary tract infection in general practice. Lancet 2: 615

Freedman L R 1975 Natural history of urinary infection in adults. Kidney Int 8: S96

Goldstein I, Renais J, Scebat L 1980 Experimental nephropathy induced in rabbits by immunization with Escherichia coli 055 lipopolysaccharide. Israel J Med Sci 16: p 566

Gower P E 1975 The use of small doses of cephalexin (125 mg) in the management of recurrent urinary tract infection in women. J Antimicrobial Chemotherapy i: Suppl 93

Gower P E 1976 A propsective study of patients with radiological pyelonephritis, papillary necrosis and obstructive atrophy. Quart J Med N S XLV, No 178, p 315

Gower P E 1979 Analgesic nephropathy. In: Black D, Jones N F (eds) Renal disease. Blackwell Scientific Publishers, Oxford, p 640

Gower P E, Marshall M J, Dash C H 1975 Clinical, pharmocokinetic and laboratory study of penicillin V in the treatment of acute urinary infection. J Antimicrobial Chemotherapy i: 187

Grimlund K 1963 Phenacetin and renal damage at a Swedish factory. Acta Med Scand 174 suppl 405

Gruneberg R N, Leigh D A, Brumfitt W 1969 Relationship of bacteriuria in pregnancy to acute pyelonephritis, prematurity and fetal mortality. Lancet 2: 1

Hallett R J, Pead L, Maskell R 1976 Urinary infection in boys. Lancet 2: 1107

Heptinstall R H 1966 Pathology of the kidney. Little, Brown and Co, Boston, Mass

Hodson C J 1967 The radiological contribution toward the diagnosis of chronic pyelonephritis. Radiology 88: 857

Hodson C J 1970 Differential diagnosis between atrophic pyelonephritis and analgesic nephropathy. In: Kincaid-Smith P and Fairley K F (eds) Renal infection and renal scarring. Mercedes Publishing Services, Melbourne, Australia

Hodson C J, Craven J D 1966 The radiology of obstructive atrophy of the kidney. Clin Radiol 17: 305

Hodson C J, Maling T M, McManamon P J et al 1975 The pathogenesis of reflux nephropathy (chronic atrophic pyelonephritis). Brit J Radiol, Suppl No 13

Hutt M S R, Chalbers J A, MacDonald J S et al 1961 Pyelonephritis: observations on the relation between various diagnostic procedures. Lancet i: 351

Itatani H, Koide T, Okuyama A et al 1977 Development of the ureterovesical junction in human fetus. In consideration of the vesicoureteral reflux. Invest Urol 15: 232

Kalmanson G M, Glassock R J, Harwick H J et al 1975 Cellular immunity in experimental pyelonephritis. Kidney Int 8: S35

Kass E H 1957 Bacteriuria and the diagnosis of infections of the urinary tract. Arch Intern Med 100: 709

Kincaid-Smith P 1978 Analgesic Nephropathy Symposium. Kidney Int 13: 1

Koutsaimanis K G, de Wardener H E 1970 Phenacetin nephropathy with particular reference to the effect of surgery. Brit Med J 4: 131

Little P J 1966 The incidence of urinary infection in 5000 pregnant women. Lancet 2: 925

Little P J, de Wardener H E 1966 Acute pyelonephritis. The incidence of re-infection of 100 patients. Lancet 2: 1277

Little P J, McPherson D R, de Wardener H E 1965 The appearance of the intravenous pyelogram during and after acute pyelonephritis. Lancet i: 1186

Little P J, Sloper J S, de Wardener H E 1967 A syndrome of loin pain and haematuria associated with disease of the peripheral renal artery. Quart J Med 36: 253

Maskell R 1982 Urinary tract infection. Edward Arnold, London Mihatsch M J, Knusli C 1982 Phenacetin abuse and malignant tumours. An autopsy study covering 24 years (1953–1977) Klin Woch 60: 1339

Mihindukulasuriya J C L, Maskell R, Polak A 1980 A study of fifty eight patients with renal scarring associated with urinary tract infection. Quart J Med N S, XLIX, No 194 p 165

Miller T, North D 1979 Immunolobiologic factors in the pathogenesis of renal infection. Kidney Int 16: 665

Mundt K, Polk B F 1979 Indentification of site of urinary-tract infections by antibody-coated bacteria assay, Lancet 2: 1172

Murray R M, Lawson D H, Linton A L 1971 Analgesic nephropathy: Clinical syndrome and prognosis. Brit Med J i: 479

Murray R M, Timbury G C, Linton A L 1970 Analgesic abuse in psychiatric patients. Lancet i: 1303

Riedasch G, Ritz E, Mohring K et al 1978 Antibody coating of urinary bacteria: relation to site of infection and invasion of uroepithelium. Clin Nephrol 10: 239

Roberts A P, Phillips R 1979 Bacteria causing symptomatic urinary tract infection or asymptomatic bacteriuria J Clin Path 32: 492

Rolleston G L, Shannon F T, Utley W L F 1970 Relationship of infantile vesicoureteric reflux to renal damage. Brit Med J i: 460

Shand D G, Nimmon C C, O'Grady F et al 1970 Relation between residual urine volume and response to treatment of urinary infection. Lancet i: 1305

Shouval D, Ligumsky M, Ben-Ishay D 1978 Effect of cotrimoxazole on normal creatinine clearance. Lancet i: 244

Smeets F, Gower P E 1973 The site of infection in 133 patients with bacteriuria Clin. Nephrol i: 290

Smellie J M, Katz G, Gruneberg R N 1978 Controlled trial of prophylactic treatment of childhood urinary tract infection. Lancet 2: 175

Smellie J M, Normand I C S, Katz G 1981 Children with urinary infection: A comparison of those with and those without vesicoureteric reflux. Kidney Int 20: 717

Stamey T A, Govan D E, Palmer J M 1965 The localisation and treatment of urinary tract infections: The role of bactericidal urine levels as opposed to serum levels. Medicine 44: 1

Thomas V L, Forland M 1982 Antibody-coated bacteria in urinary tract infection. Kidney Int 21: 1

Torres V E, Moore S B, Kurtz S B et al 1980 In search of a marker for genetic susceptibility to reflux nephropathy. Clin Nephrol 14: 217

Vivaldi E, Cortan R, Zangwill D P et al 1959 Ascending infection as a mechanism in pathogenesis of experimental non-obstructive pyelonephritis. Proc Soc Exp Biol N Y 102: 242

Whitworth J A, Fairley K F, O'Keefe C M et al 1975 Immunogenicity of Escherichia Coli O antigen in upper urinary tract infection. Kidney Int 8: 316

# 23

# The kidney, glycosuria and diabetes mellitus

## GLYCOSURIA

It has been pointed out in Section 6 that the quantity of glucose which passes through a glomerulus in one minute is the product of the filtration rate and the plasma glucose, and that normally the urine is free from glucose because this filtered glucose is reabsorbed in the proximal tubule. The rate at which glucose can be reabsorbed, however, is limited, and at normal glomerular filtration rates many of the tubules cannot reabsorb a greater amount than that which is delivered to them when the plasma glucose is about 170 mg per 100 ml. The appearance of glucose in the urine therefore denotes that either: (1) a normal tubular reabsorbing capacity for glucose has been exceeded by an increased rate of delivery through the glomerulus; or (2) a reduced reabsorbing capacity of some, or most, of the tubules has been exceeded, though the rate of delivery is normal.

Glycosuria is never due to an increased glomerular filtration rate, so that when the tubular capacity to reabsorb glucose is normal the appearance of glucose in the urine is due to hyperglycaemia, as in diabetes, thyrotoxicosis and Cushing's disease, or following a gastroenterostomy when there is an excessively rapid intestinal absorption of glucose.

Glycosuria associated with a diminished tubular reabsorptive capacity and a normal blood glucose is often a benign familial condition which is known as *renal glycosuria* (the condition is also known as 'renal diabetes' and 'pseudo-renal diabetes', names which only confuse). If the reabsorbing capacity of only a few of the tubules is abnormal an estimation of the total capacity of the kidneys to reabsorb glucose (Tmg) may be within normal limits; but when more tubules are involved the total capacity to reabsorb glucose is reduced; familial renal glycosuria may be associated with either of these findings.

It is clear that when there is glycosuria the simplest way to differentiate between hyperglycaemic glycosuria, and renal glycosuria is to estimate the concentration of blood glucose. The blood should be taken at the midpoint of a short urine collection period, perferably during a fast. If this test is not decisive a glucose tolerance test should be done.

There are three other variations on this theme of glomerular supply and tubular reabsorption of glucose which are clinically important.

1. If, in a patient suffering from diabetes *and* renal glycosuria, insulin dosage is being adjusted according to the output of glucose in the urine, hypoglycaemia may be induced. This often occurs in pregnant diabetics.

2. Very occasionally, contraction of the extracellular fluid space in diabetic acidosis may cause such severe renal vasoconstriction and fall in glomerular filtration rate that, though there is hyperglycaemia, the amount of glucose being delivered to the tubule may still be within its reabsorbing capacity, and no glucose appears in the urine.

3. Finally, there are those rare cases of glycosuria associated with a normal blood sugar in which diminished tubular capacity to reabsorb glucose is not an isolated, benign functional lesion, but is only one of many similar but more serious abnormalities of tubular function, i.e. Fanconi's syndrome.

## DIABETES MELLITUS

The renal complications of diabetes mellitus are:
1. Diabetic nephropathy of the glomerulus
    a. diffuse intercapillary glomerulosclerosis
    b. nodular intercapillary glomerulosclerosis
    c. microaneurysms
    d. exudative deposits
2. Vascular
    a. nephrosclerosis
    b. atherosclerosis
3. Infections
    a. acute pylonephritis
    b. papillary necrosis
    c. renal carbuncle
    d. xanthogranulomatous pyelonephritis
4. Neurological. Atonic bladder (hydronephrosis).

**Diabetic nephropathy**

10% of diabetics need insulin to survive. Insulin dependent diabetics tend to be younger than those who do not need insulin, and in the United States, approximately half of them die of renal failure after they have been on insulin for about 20 years. Among the older patients who do not need insulin only 5 per cent die of renal failure. The majority succumb to coronary thrombosis, hypertensive cardiac failure and cerebrovascular accidents before the renal lesions are sufficiently advanced to produce any substantial change in renal function.

*Pathology*

There are several distinct lesions. In the most benign form of diabetic nephropathy there is a diffuse thickening of the mesangial areas of the glomeruli due to an excess laying down of a basement membrane-like material (Fig. 23.1). This is caused by an anabolic increase in protein metabolism and is accompanied by an increase in kidney size and weight. Electron microscopy shows that the basement membrane is enormously thickened and that, at first, globular masses of basement membrane material lie in the endothelial cells. The epithelial cells often have disorganised foot processes; sometimes these are no longer distinct and instead are converted into large islets of cytoplasm covering the outer surface of the capillary. This diffuse form of intercapillary glomerulosclerosis tends to be the only glomerular lesion which occurs in the older insulin-independent diabetics in whom renal functional deterioration is slow and terminal renal failure is unusual. Very rarely the appearances and the basement membrane changes are identical to those of membranous glomerular nephritis with a diffuse thickening of the glomerular capillary walls.

In young insulin-dependent diabetics an accelerated form of diabetic nephropathy tends to be superimposed on the diffuse process. Three additional lesions now make their appearance; so-called exudative deposits;

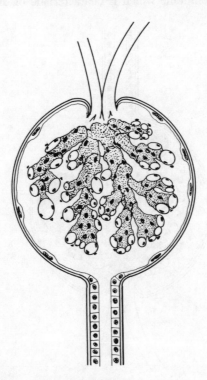

**Fig. 22.1** Diffuse intercapillary glomerulosclerosis.

microaneurysms and nodular intercapillary glomerulosclerosis. The exudative lesions consist of homogeneous 'drops' lying within or in close apposition to Bowman's capsule (Fig. 23.2). They are more easily detected by electron microscopy, and contain some immunoglobulin G. The microaneurysms are situated at the periphery of the glomerulus (Fig. 23.3). They consist of a focal ballooning of a damaged capillary loop, as if it had come adrift from its attachment to the mesangium. At first the lumen of the aneurysm is filled with red cells and platelets. Subsequently it tends to silt up from the centre outwards with a laminated eosinophilic material which comes from the blood or from the increased anabolism of the mesangial cells. The microaneurysm finally becomes the peripheral rounded eosinophilic nodular masses which were first described by Kimmelstiel and Wilson (Fig. 23.4). It is unusual however, for the microaneurysm to be totally occluded. Each nodule may occupy up to one quarter of the glomerulus so that three to five will destroy the glomerulus.

The cause of the focal capillary damage which leads to the formation of microaneurysms is not known. Microaneurysms are not only found in the glomerulus, they also occur in the retina and peripheral nerves giving rise to diabetic retinopathy and neuropathy, and these invariably accompany the deterioration of renal function. It has been pointed out that the thickened capillary basement membrane which is characteristic of diabetes occurs in

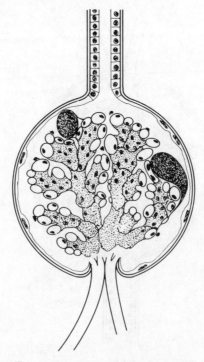

**Fig. 22.2** Diffuse intercapillary glomerulosclerosis with two exudative lesions.

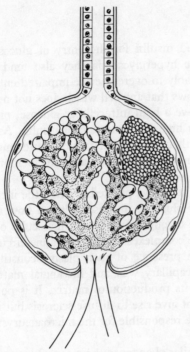

**Fig. 22.3** Diffuse intercapillary glomerulosclerosis with microaneurysm filled with red cells.

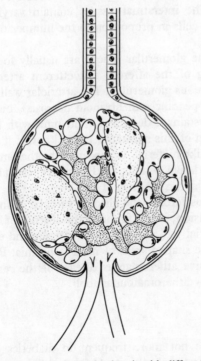

**Fig. 22.4** Nodular intercapillary glomerulosclerosis with diffuse inter-capillary glomerulosclerosis.

cells which do not need insulin for the entry of glucose, and that most diabetics not only have hyperglycaemia they also tend to have a raised plasma insulin, presumably to overcome the impaired entry of glucose into most other cells. It follows that any cell which does not need insulin for the entry of glucose will have a high intracellular glucose, providing an ample source of energy, and a high concentration of insulin. As insulin increases anabolism it is possible that this combination of events might be responsible for the increased protein synthethis and basement membrane accumulation by certain capillaries in diabetes.

On the other hand others have pointed out that the increased glomerular permeability to protein plus the increased plasma flow and filtration rate probably lead to a large through-put of macromolecules of various proteins including some immune complexes and non immune circulating aggregates. It is suggested that the presence of such plasma constituents continually being handled by the capillary wall and mesangial matrix stimulates the mesangium to increase its production of matrix. It is possible to envisage that such a process might give rise to diffuse sclerosis but it is more difficult to accept that it could be responsible for the microaneurysms or the nodular lesions.

The tubules show similar changes to those found in persistent glomerular nephritis, and very occasionally the proximal tubules contain large quantities of glycogen. The interstitial tissues contain varying collections of chronic inflammatory cells in proportion to the number of glomeruli which are seriously affected.

*Vascular lesions.* The glomerular lesions are usually found in association with gross thickening of the afferent and efferent arterioles (mainly the afferent) of the contiguous glomerulus. The arteriolar walls keep their sharp outline (unlike the appearances in fibrinoid necrosis), but are widened by some material which stains a deep and vivid pink with haematoxylin and eosin; the composition of this substance is not known; it is not collagen or basement membrane-like material. It appears to be the same material as that which is in the exudative lesions in Bowman's capsule; a protein-like substance containing high quantities of fat.

In diabetics, nephrosclerosis, the chronic vascular lesion which typically accompanies hypertension, is also found in the absence of hypertension. The narrowing of the arterial tree with fibroelastic tissue and eosinophilic material causes large wedge shaped areas of renal ischaemia. Renal ischaemia is also caused by extensive atheromatous disease of the renal artery and its major branches and by atheromatous emboli.

### Infection

Urinary infections are not more frequent in diabetics than in an aged matched population of normal subjects. On the other hand when diabetics do have an upper urinary infection it tends to run a fulminating course.

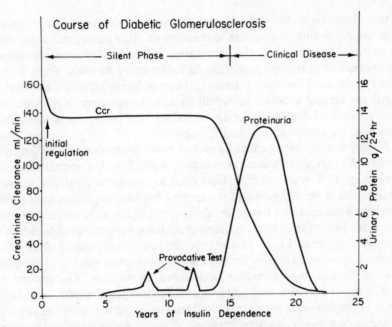

**Fig. 23.5** Composite drawing showing course of diabetic nephropathy. Exercise and other stress will cause intermittent proteinuria before a sustained protein leak which may lead to a nephrotic syndrome. Initial regulation = start of insulin. (Reproduced from Friedman & Shieh 1980 In: Friedman E A, L'Esperance F A (eds) Diabetic renal-retinal syndrome. Grune & Stratton, New York, p 135, with kind permission.)

Diabetes is the only condition in which a urinary infection may cause papillary necrosis, usually with acute renal failure.

### The natural history of diabetic nephropathy in insulin-dependent diabetics

The following succinct summary and Figure 23.5 are by Friedman and Shieh.*

"Anatomic and functional abnormalities in the diabetic kidney are detectable a decade or more before any clinical evidence of renal disease. Insulin-dependent diabetics at the onset of hyperglycemia have large kidneys, big glomeruli, an increased glomerular surface area and supernormal glomerular filtration rate (GFR). After beginning insulin treatment, a fall in both renal size and GFR occurs, though still to above normal values. For about the next 10 to 15 years a high GFR continues, though without clinical consequences.

Persistent proteinuria is usually the first clinical finding in long term diabetics. While kidney biopsies from asymptomatic diabetics will show

* Friedman E A, Shieh S D 1980 Clinical management of diabetic nephropathy. In: Friedman E A, L'Esperance F A (eds) Diabetic renal-retinal syndrome. Grune & Stratton, New York, p 135

glomerulosclerosis after only three to five years, proteinuria before the 10th year usually occurs in response to exercise, or other stress, and is transient. A continuous increase in the proportion of diabetics who are proteinuric occurs year by year, with more than half affected by 20 years. From the time when proteinuria becomes sustained, the renal lesion gradually becomes the dominant clinical problem in overall patient management. Nephrotic range proteinuria (>3.5 g/24 hr), often exceeding 10 g/24 hr, leads to hypoproteinemia, leg swelling, and finally, anasarca.

Within one to three years of onset of heavy proteinuria, GFR begins to decline. The serum creatinine rises exponentially from the normal range after a mean of 17.3 years. Each patient's fall in creatinine clearance follows a straight line if the reciprocal of the serum creatinine is plotted against time. During this accelerated loss of renal function, which occurs over two to five years, the patient may seem to disintegrate from vigorous good health to the marginal existence of an invalid. At the same time that kidney failure becomes apparent, vitreous hemorrhages may obscure vision and peripheral vascular disease may endanger both lower extremities. The patient who previously had been a well compensated functioning diabetic, now faces a series of progressively worse catastrophies which cost the vitality of key organ systems. Not every insulin-dependent diabetic follows the sad course of such a renal-retinal syndrome leading to blindness and uremia in the 20th year. Some diabetics may survive 40 years without nephropathy. What has been detailed is the characteristic course of the approximately half of insulin-dependent diabetics who become uremic within 20 years, as summarized in Figure 23.5.

*Relationship between clinical and structural features*

Electron microscopy studies on renal biopsies from diabetic patients are beginning to show that the changes in the glomerular basement membrane probably precede the onset of proteinuria by several years. It has also been established that electron microscopy abnormalities appear about five years after the clinical onset of diabetes, whereas light microscopy changes begin to be obvious after 10 years. The histological changes are the same whether the diabetes follows pancreatitis or haemochromatosis.

The extent of the proteinuria is greatest with severe structural changes, but it has to be pointed out that some authorities do not agree that it is possible to predict the pathological lesions from the clinical course. They point out that Kimmelstiel — Wilson lesions may be found in patients who have never had proteinuria or other evidence of renal disease and that some patients dying of renal failure subsequent to a nephrotic syndrome may not show the characteristic nodular lesions though all will have the diffuse lesions. When light microscopy lesions are evident it is usual to be able to discern diabetic retinal lesions with an ophthalmoscope. This relationship is so close that the finding of retinal changes is a good indication that renal changes are present whether or not there is proteinuria.

*Other disturbances of renal function*

The osmotic diuresis provoked by the glycosuria causes many of the characteristic features of diabetes mellitus, for it is responsible for the high urinary excretion of water, sodium and potassium, which gives rise to polyuria, thirst and lassitude.

As glucose is a dense molecule, urine that contains glucose will tend to have a higher specific gravity than its colour would suggest, i.e. a pale urine may be found to have a specific gravity of 1.026.

The glycosuria of diabetes is secondary to hyperglycaemia. But its extent may give a misleading impression of the height of the blood glucose, for patients with diabetes often have renal glycosuria, and glycosuria may therefore be present when the blood glucose is normal. Paradoxically the glucose Tm is *raised* in diabetes; the cause of this teleologically reasonable phenomenon is not known; it tends to subside after the administration of insulin. The simultaneous presence of renal glycosuria and a raised glucose Tm is presumably due to a splaying out of the individual nephrons capacity to reabsorb glucose.

Chronic renal failure associated with the classical lesions of diabetes has been found in patients who have never had glycosuria and in whom the diagnosis of diabetes has not been made. It is probable that in some of these patients, owing to a combination of a low glomerular filtration rate and a greatly increased ability to reabsorb glucose, there was no glycosuria, though there may have been hyperglycaemia. In a few patients the blood glucose has been measured and found to be normal, though at post-mortem there is, in addition to the characteristic diabetic renal lesions, widespread hyalinisation of the islets of Langerhans.

A few diabetic patients require less insulin as they develop chronic renal failure. This may be due to the gradual obliteration of the kidney's ability to catabolise insulin (p. 245). On the other hand some diabetic patients may need more insulin, and it is well known that non-diabetic persons who develop chronic renal failure have a diabetic-type glucose tolerance curve. Both these observations are possibly due to the uraemia impairing hepatic function. Normally as plasma glucose rises, there is a rise in plasma insulin which inhibits further release of glucose from the liver into the blood. If normal liver slices are incubated in uraemic plasma however this response to insulin is less pronounced. It is inferred that the diabetic glucose tolerance curve of patients with chronic renal failure may be due to the liver continuing to supply glucose into the blood as glucose is being absorbed from the gut.

*Dangers in the use of contrast media in radiological investigations*

The use of radiological contrast materials to perform an intravenous pyelogram or an arteriogram in diabetic patients is liable to cause an acute deterioration of renal function. Some reports state that this occurs in 60 per cent of patients and that of these 22% develop acute renal failure of such severity that they will require dialysis. Usually the episode of acute renal failure is transitory with a return of renal function within a week. But some patients take longer and in others the damage is irreversible (Fig. 23.6).

This hazard is greatest in the elderly with pre-existing renal failure especially if there is widespread vascular disease and some impairment of liver function. It is probable that diabetic patients are particularly at risk because radiological investigations are performed when they are already dessicated by hyperglycaemia and glycosuria, and are then further dried out by the thoughtless use of a routine preparation for a pyelogram which may include a ritual period of prolonged fluid deprivation and purgation. Contrast agents should be used with some care in diabetic patients and if possible the investigation should be performed by an alternative method such as ultrasound, radionuclides or with a computerized scanner. It is possible that the prophylactive use of I.V. saline might be as helpful in preventing this problem as it is in preventing the deterioration of renal function in patients with chronic renal failure who have a surgical operation.

*Treatment*

It is to be hoped that one or more of the methods which are at the moment being investigated to keep the blood glucose within normal limits will prevent the development of diabetic nephropathy. These include some method of continuous administration of insulin controlled by the blood sugar (a 'bionic pancreas'), pancreatic transplantation, combined pancreatic and renal transplantation and the injection of Islets of Langerhan.

In the meantime it is generally considered that much can be achieved to delay the onset of diabetic nephropathy by careful, repeated monitoring of the patient's progress so as to obtain the best control possible of the blood sugar concentration with the conventional means of treatment at present available. It is important to remember not to use phenformin after the onset of renal failure for it may lead to severe metabolic acidosis from excess lactic acid production. It is claimed that careful control of the blood pressure with antihypertensive therapy will also slow down the deterioration in renal function. The use of a cardioselective β-blocker such as metopropol may cause less problems from hyperglycaemia than propranolol.

Until recently the prognosis was very depressing. Overall the vascular complications of diabetes in the heart, brain, eye and peripheral vessels limited rehabilitation during treatment with dialysis or transplantation. Survival was shortened or associated with incapacitating complications, though in about 80% of patients, after starting maintenance haemodialysis or being transplanted, vision remained stable or improved. There was a tendency to try and transplant the patient or place him onto maintenance haemodialysis before the onset of severe retinopathy, when the glomerular

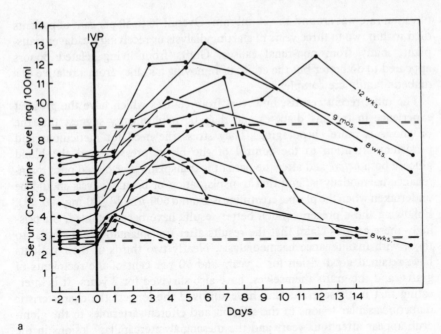

a

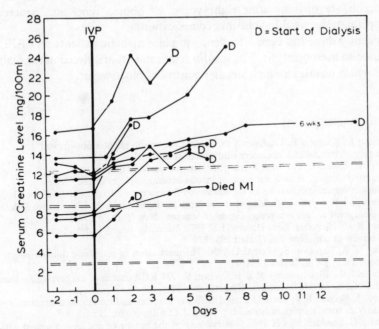

b

**Fig. 23.6** Serum creatinine plotted before and after an intravenous pyelogram in 22 diabetic patients (a) 13 individuals who developed reversible renal failure and (b) 9 who developed irreversible renal failure. M I = myocardial infarction. Conversion: Traditional to S I units — creatinine 10 mg/100 ml = 880 μmol/l. (Reproduced from Harkonen & Kjellstrand 1977 Amer J Med 63: 939, with kind permission.)

filtration rate was around 15–20 ml/min. Overall 40 to 50 per cent of patients died within two to three years of starting dialysis or receiving a cadaver transplant, many from non-renal causes. Grafts from living related donors appeared to do better but the ethics of removing a kidney from a relative in a diabetic family are complex.

The most recent results, however, from centres which have the greatest experience in treating diabetes and diabetic nephropathy suggest that the prognosis is more encouraging. They stress the need for meticulous and persistent attention to the control of the blood pressure and the blood glucose both *before* and after the patient is transplanted or placed onto maintenance haemodialysis, and that transplantation or haemodialysis should be undertaken when the plasma creatinine is around 600 μmol/l (7.0 mg/100 ml). Following these precepts much better results have been obtained. Surprisingly these centres claim that the results after transplantation are similar to those with maintenance haemodialysis. Nearly two thirds of their patients have retained good vision for 2 years and 90 per cent of the recipients of grafts, and the grafts themselves, have also survived for 2 years. It is interesting that in those grafts that have survived the longest the characteristic diabetic vascular lesions in the afferent and efferent arterioles to the glomeruli appear after four years and the mesangial intercapillary lesions in the glomeruli are obvious after eight years. Combined renal and pancreatic transplantations would avoid this complication.

Recently there has been a tendency to place diabetic patients on CAPD as opposed to haemodialysis. The insulin requirements are placed in the dialysis fluid which ensures a much steadier control of blood sugar.

BIBLIOGRAPHY

Bengtsson K, Karlberg B, Lindgren S 1972 Lactic acidosis in phenformin–treated diabetics. A clinical and laboratory study. Acta Med Scand 191: 203
Berns A W, Owens C T, Hirata Y et al 1962 The pathogenesis of diabetic glomerulosclerosis. A demonstration of insulin-binding capacity of the various histopathological components of the disease by fluorescence microscopy. Diabetes 11: 308
Bloodworth J M B 1980 Pathology of the kidney. In: Friedman E A, L'Esperance F A (eds) Diabetic renal retinal syndrome. Grune & Stratton, New York, p 159
Brenner B M, Hostetter T H, Humes H D 1978 Molecular basis of proteinuria of glomerular origin. New Eng J Med 298: 826
Brodsky W A, Rapoport S, West C D 1950 The mechanism of glycosuric diuresis in diabetic man. J Clin Invest 29: 1021
Engerman R L, Bloodworth J M B Jr, Nelson S 1977 Relationship of microvascular disease in diabetes to metabolic control. Diabetes 26: 760
Farber S J, Berger, E Y, Earle D P 1951 Effect of diabetes and insulin on maximum capacity of renal tubules to reabsorb glucose. J Clin Invest 30: 125
Farrant P C, Shedden W I H 1965 Observations on the uptake of insulin conjugated with fluorescein isothiocyanate by diabetic kidney tissue. Diabetes 14: 274
Freedman L R 1957 Inapparent diabetes mellitus as a cause of renal insufficiency due to Kimmelstiel-Wilson lesions. John Hopk Hosp Bull 100: 132
Friedman E A, Shieh S D 1980 Clinical management of diabetic nephropathy. In: Friedman E A L'Esperance F A (eds) Diabetic renal-retinal syndrome. Grune and Stratton, New York, p 135

Goetz F C 1982 Recent progress in the management of end-stage diabetic nephropathy. Clinics Endocrinol and Metabol 11: 579

Harkonen S, Kjellstrand C M 1977 Exacerbation of diabetic renal failure following intravenous pyelography. Amer J Med 63: 939

Heptinstall R H 1983 Pathology of the kidney Diabetes mellitus and gout. Little Brown, Boston, 929

Horsfield G I, Lannigan R 1965 Exudative lesions in diabetes mellitus. J Clin Path 18: 47

Hostetter T H, Rennke H G, Brenner B M 1982 The case for intrarenal hypertension in the initiation and progression of diabetic and other glomerulopathies. Amer J Med 72: 375

Jonasson O 1980 Transplantation of pancreatic islets. In: Friedman E A, L'Esperance F A (ed) Diabetic renal retinal syndrome. Grune and Stratton, New York, p 413

Keen H, Viberti G C 1981 Genesis and evolution of diabetic nephropathy. J Clin Path 34: 1261

Kimmelstiel P, Wilson C 1936 Intercapillary lesions in glomeruli of kidney. Amer J Path 12: 83

Mauer S M, Barbosa J, Vernier R L et al 1976 Development of diabetic vascular lesions in normal kidneys transplanted into patients with diabetes mellitus. N Eng J Med 295: 916

Mogensen C E 1982 Long-term antihypertensive treatment inhibiting progression of diabetic nephropathy. Brit Med J 285: 685

Monasterio G, Oliver, J Muiesan G et al 1964 Renal diabetes as a congenital tubular dysplasia. Amer J Med 37: 44

Rogers J, Robbins S L, Jeghers H 1952 Intercapillary glomerulosclerosis. A clinical and pathologic study. Amer J Med 12: 692, 700

Taft H P, Finckh E S, Joske R A 1954 Biopsy study of kidney in diabetes mellitus. Aust Ann Med 3: 189

Traeger J, Dubernard J M, Touraine J et al 1980 Technical and clinical aspects of segmented pancreatic transplantation in man. In: Friedman E A, L'Esperance F A (eds) Diabetic Renal-Retinal Syndrome, Grune and Stratton, New York, p 403

Viberti G C 1979 Early functional and morphological changes in diabetic nephropathy. Clin Nephro 12: p 47

Bradley S E, Bradley G P, Tyson C J et al 1950 Renal function in renal diseases. Amer J Med 9: 766

Govaerts P 1952 The physiopathology of glucose excretion by the human kidney. Brit Med J 2: 175

Reubi F C 1954 Glucose titration in renal glycosuria. Ciba Foundation Symposium on the Kidney. J and A Churchill, London

Smith H W 1951 The Kidney. Structure and Function in Health and Disease. Oxford University Press, New York

Starling E H, Verney E B 1925 The secretion of urine as studied on the isolated kidney. Proc Roy Soc B 97: 321

Steinitz K 1940 Studies on the condition of glucose excretion in man. J Clin Invest 19: 299

# 24

# Renal disturbances in pregnancy

1. Physiological changes:
    Renal blood flow and glomerular filtration rate
    Lactosuria and glycosuria
    Orthostatic proteinuria
    Aminoaciduria
    Uric acid excretion
    Acid base metabolism
    Water metabolism
    Hormonal changes
    Sodium and water retention, hypotension and vascular reactivity
    Blood pressure
    Ureteric and pelvic dilatation
2. Mechanisms responsible for hypertension, proteinuria and oedema
3. Pregnancy induced nephropathy and renal vascular abnormalities
4. Pre-eclampsia
5. Acute renal failure
6. Pregnancy and pre-existing renal disease
7. Renal infections
8. The incidence of other renal diseases during pregnancy.

## PHYSIOLOGICAL CHANGES

*Renal blood flow and glomerular filtration rate*

By the fourth month of pregnancy renal blood flow has increased by about 50% and glomerular filtration rate by about 30%. The rise is associated with a 1 cm increase in the length of the kidneys and may be related to the increasing concentration of circulating placental lactogen which has a growth hormone like effect. There is an associated doubling of the plasma volume and 20% increase in extracellular fluid volume with widespread arterial and venous vasodilatation (see below). These changes tend to revert to normal by the end of pregnancy. Patients with pre-existing essential hypertension without severe nephrosclerosis, or patients with glomerular nephritis but with only mild impairment in renal function also demonstrate a rise in renal blood flow and glomerular filtration rate in the early months of pregnancy.

The increase in glomerular filtration rate together with the diminished protein breakdown of pregnancy cause the blood urea to be considerably lower than normal, e.g. 2.5 mmol/l (15 mg/100 ml). Unless this increase in glomerular filtration rate and fall in blood urea is appreciated, a false impression of renal functional efficiency during pregnancy may be held. Either an underlying renal disease is unsuspected because the filtration rate and blood urea are within normal (i.e. non-pregnant) limits, or a sudden deterioration in renal function after pregnancy is erroneously considered to be evidence that pregnancy has injured the kidneys. If during pregnancy the glomerular filtration rate is lower than the 'non-pregnant' normal rate, or the blood urea is raised above the normal 'non-pregnant' concentration, it is evidence of considerable impairment of renal function, and perhaps extensive structural damage.

## Glycosuria and lactosuria

Most women during pregnancy excrete an increased quantity of both glucose and lactose. Glycosuria is due to a lowered renal threshold for glucose reabsorption. (At one time glycosuria after the oral ingestion of glucose was suggested as a test of pregnancy.) Lactosuria is simply related to the presence of lactose in the mother's blood; as it is not reabsorbed by the tubules, all that is filtered through the glomerulus appears in the urine.

After delivery glycosuria rapidly disappears and there is an increase in both the incidence of lactosuria and the amount that is excreted.

## Orthostatic proteinuria

The incidence of orthostatic proteinuria varies considerably; some reports state that it is as high as 20%. It is probably caused by (1) an exaggeration of the normal mechanism for orthostatic proteinuria, i.e. a lordosis which rotates the liver forwards, thus compressing the inferior vena cava and causing a rise in renal venous pressure; and (2) uterine compression of the left renal vein as it crosses the midline. The first mechanism causes protein to be excreted through both ureters, whereas with the second, proteinuria is present only on the left side. In order, therefore, to distinguish orthostatic from other causes of proteinuria, the urine should be tested for protein, after the patient has been lying on her side.

## Aminoaciduria

The urinary excretion of amino acids is raised with substantial losses of histidine, threonine, serine, glycine and alanine. The cause is probably the combination of a raised plasma parathyroid hormone concentration and the raised glomerular filtration rate. The first depresses amino acid tubular reabsorption while the second increases markedly the amount to be reabsorbed.

## Uric acid

Uric acid clearance increases and plasma uric acid falls during the early part of pregnancy and returns to normal during the last three months.

## Acid base metabolism

Pregnant women hyperventilate. As a result arterial pH is around 7.44 and $P_{CO_2}$ and plasma bicarbonate are reduced. The ability to excrete an acid load and to acidify the urine are normal.

## Water metabolism

By the end of pregnancy, due to sodium retention, the average woman has retained about 6–8 litres of water — most of it in the last three months. This is accompanied with a modest reduction of plasma osmolality, perhaps due to increased baroreceptor activity; for the kidney's ability to dilute the urine is normal. It is important that this test is performed with a woman on her side for if she lies on her back the weight of the uterus on the inferior vena cava tends to pool the blood in the legs and lower abdomen which causes a sudden fall in 'effective' circulating blood volume.

## Some hormonal changes

Plasma prolactin, cortisol, oestrogen, prostaglandin E and parathyroid hormone are high as is the concentration of placental lactogen. Plasma renin activity, renin concentration, renin substrate, angiotensin II and aldosterone are also elevated. The cause of the rise in this second group is not certain. There are several possibilities: (a) the increased level of plasma oestrogen which increases renin substrate production and renin activity, (b) the contribution of angiotensin II secreted from the pregnant uterus and feto-placental unit, and (c) a compensatory phenomenon to counteract the natriuretic effect of the raised plasma progesterone and, less importantly, the raised glomerular filtration rate.

## Salt and water retention, hypotension and vascular reactivity

During a normal pregnancy there is a gradual retention of 500 to 900 mmol of sodium. The bulk of this is sequestered into the uterus and its content. The mechanism responsible for this retention is not known. It is associated with a definite increase in extracellular fluid volume and blood volume which in the majority of women is sufficient to become evident as oedema. Though plasma angiotensin II and aldosterone are raised the aldosterone 'escape' mechanism should prevent such a large retention of sodium. But in spite of the salt and water retention, the raised blood volume and plasma angiotensin II and aldosterone, a normal pregnancy is associated with a *fall* in blood pressure. A possible explanation is that the marked generalised vasodilatation of pregnancy, the cause of which is unknown, redistributes the blood volume away from the thorax. It is well established that *vasoconstriction* does the opposite, it redistributes the blood from the periphery towards the centre. It is possible therefore that overall vasodilatation by diminishing the intrathoracic volume lowers intrathoracic vascular pressures so that, though the total blood volume is increased, the volume receptors in the thorax signal a *fall* in blood volume. By analogy with what occurs with an increase in intrathoracic pressure it is very likely that a diminution in pressure will depress the natriuretic and sodium transport inhibiting properties of the blood. A reduction in the plasma concentration of the sodium transport inhibitor could account for the extreme resistance to the pressor effects of infused angiotensin II which is such a prominent feature of a normal pregnancy (Fig. 24.1).

This hypothesis, outlined above, which tries to explain how in pregnancy a large blood volume and a raised plasma angiotensin II are associated with

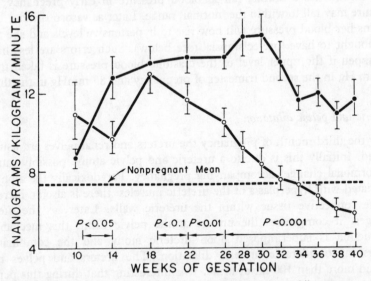

**Fig. 24.1** Comparison of the mean angiotensin II dose (nanograms per kilogram per minute) required to raise the diastolic blood pressure 20 mmHg in 120 primigravidas who remained normotensive (black circles) and 72 who ultimately developed toxemia (open circles). A higher dose is required in normotensive pregnancies than in nonpregnant females (broken line), suggesting resistance to the effect of angiotensin II. However, women who developed toxemia showed a progressive fall in angiotensin II resistance (which was significant after the twenty-third week), eventually becoming more sensitive to angiotensin II than normal women. (Reproduced from Grant, Daley, Chand et al 1973 J Clin Invest 52: 2682, by copyright permission of The American Society for Clinical Investigation.)

a fall in blood pressure is in keeping with it's converse which has been put forward earlier (p. 260) to explain how in essential hypertension a normal or low blood volume and a low plasma renin are associated with a rise in arterial pressure. In the latter, however, there is some evidence that the hypothesis may be true in that the plasma of patients with essential hypertension has been found to contain a raised concentration of a circulating sodium transport inhibitor. The plasma content of sodium transport inhibitor in normal pregnancy has not yet been measured.

### Blood pressure

Mean blood pressure starts to decrease early in pregnancy. The mean diastolic levels in mid pregnancy averaging 10 mmHg less than after delivery. As pregnancy advances the blood pressure rises again towards the mother's normal pressure. The early fall in arterial pressure is due to a fall in vascular reactivity and peripheral vascular resistance, and the return of the arterial pressure towards normal near term is due to a return of vasoconstrictor reactivity.

It is important to be aware of these changes otherwise mistakes of interpretation are made. For instance, in a woman with mild essential hypertension who has a normal fall in blood pressure in early pregnancy, the pressure may fall to within the 'normal' range. Later as vasoconstrictor tone returns her blood pressure will now rise to hypertensive levels and she may be thought to have 'pre-eclampsia' (see below). Such errors are less liable to happen if the upper level of the diastolic blood pressure is taken to be 75 mm Hg in the second trimester of pregnancy and 85 mmHg in the third.

### Ureteric and pelvic dilatation

After the third month of pregnancy the ureters and renal pelves are usually dilated. Initially this is due to a ureteric and pelvic atony, possibly caused by hormonal changes accompanying pregnancy. Paradoxically the atony is associated with hyperplasia of the ureteric muscles; there is also an increase in the connective tissue within the ureteric walls. Later, as the uterus enlarges, it compresses the ureters at the pelvic brim; this mechanical obstruction is superimposed upon ureteric atony and the combination results in considerable ureteric dilatation. The ureters and pelves may contain more than 100 ml of urine. It is interesting that during this period of ureteric dilatation there is no vesico ureteric reflux. Normally the uterus is tilted towards the right side and, in consequence, it is usual to find the ureteric dilatation on the right to be greater than on the left. After delivery ureteric dilatation gradually subsides in about three months. These changes are more marked in primigravidae than in multiparae. They are probably due to the increased concentrations of circulating oestrogens. Male rats given diethylstilboestrol develop similar changes in their ureters to those seen in pregnant female rats, and at the same time their susceptibility to renal infection also rises.

## HYPERTENSION AND PROTEINURIA INCLUDING PRE-ECLAMPSIA

Hypertension may precede pregnancy or it may develop at any time during it's course. Hypertension may be accompanied by proteinuria, often a sign that there is shortly going to be an accelerating rise in blood pressure and a deterioration of renal function.

In the absence of pre-existing renal disease hypertension in pregnancy can be conveniently divided into the following categories:

1. Hypertension and proteinuria
   a. coming on in the first six months
   b. coming on in the last three months (pre-eclampsia)
2. Hypertension without proteinuria
   a. coming on in the first six months
   b. coming on in the last three months
3. Hypertension known to precede pregnancy and to continue thereafter
4. Hypertension which has recurred in each repeated pregnancy.

Hypertension is always a danger to the fetus and may be so to the mother. The most investigated form of hypertension is that which develops in the last three months, and is accompanied by proteinuria. It is known as pre-eclampsia or toxaemia of pregnancy. This syndrome most often occurs in primigravidae. It may rapidly lead to oliguria, renal failure and hypertensive encephalopathy (eclampsia).

The onset of hypertension in pre-eclampsia is preceded, over several months, by a gradual increase in vascular reactivity from the 'normal' blunted levels which are usual in pregnancy to levels which are found in the non-pregnant state, and then to a reactivity which is greater than normal (Fig. 24.1). At the same time plasma angiotensin II rises and there is a good correlation between the diastolic pressure and plasma angiotensin II (Fig. 24.2). These changes are associated with some evidence of intravascular coagulation with thrombocytopenia, a gross suppression of fibrinolytic activity and a tendency for platelets to sequester in the kidney.

The sequence of events which gives rise to this syndrome is indubitably linked to a diminished uterine blood flow and the continued presence of the fetus and placenta within the uterus. There is evidence of placental underperfusion and the syndrome is immediately reversed if the uterus is emptied of it's contents. Uterine blood flow may be inadequate because of vascular disease (as in pre-existing essential hypertension) or because of an increased demand for blood as in a twin pregnancy, both conditions in which the incidence of pre-eclampsia is raised. In primiparae uterine blood flow may be less adequate than in multiparae because the uterine vascular system

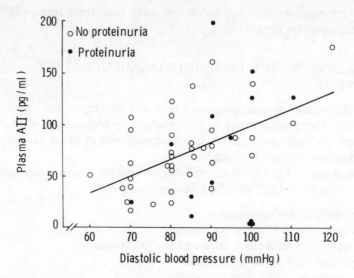

**Fig. 24.2** Relationship between diastolic blood pressure and stimultaneously measured venous angiotensin II levels in 50 primigravidae at term. (Reproduced from Symonds & Broughton Pipkin 1978 Amer J Obstet Gynecol 132: 473, with kind permission.)

is less well developed. There is also evidence that in patients who develop pre-eclampsia the usual trophoblastic erosion by the placenta of the uterine spiral arteries is deficient.

Reduction of uterine and therefore placental blood flow has certain local hormonal consequences which eventually intensify the placental ischaemia (Fig. 24.3). Acute reductions of uterine blood flow in animals increases the secretion of angiotensin II and of prostaglandin E-like substances from the uterus and placenta. The net effect is one of placental vasodilatation which compensates for the fall in uterine blood flow. But with chronic reduction of uterine flow, though the angiotensin II production continues to be stimulated, the production of prostaglandins is *reduced* and the vasoconstrictor effect of the angiotensin II on the placenta is allowed free rein.

It is probable that it is this spiral of vasoconstriction which causes the focal areas of placental degeneration which are such a prominent feature of pre-eclampsia. And there is much evidence that it is the thromboplastin released from these areas into the circulation which induces widespread vascular lesions throughout the body, particularly in the kidneys. Experimentally the renal lesions of pre-eclampsia can be reproduced in an animal by a continuous intravenous infusion of thromboplastin. Moreover the reason why the kidneys are so seriously affected in pre-eclampsia is that in pregnancy the normally intense fibrinolytic properties of the glomerular capillaries is depressed. Presumably it is the fibrin deposits in the glomeruli that cause the proteinuria, and it is the intense renal ischaemia caused by

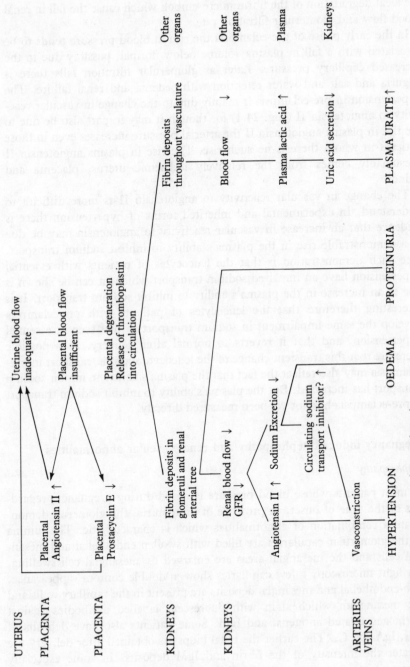

Fig. 24.3 Possible sequence of events in pre-eclampsia.

the local degradation of the fibrin micro-emboli which cause the fall in renal blood flow and glomerular filtration rate.

In the early phase of pre-eclampsia the rise in blood pressure tends to be associated with a fall in plasma volume below normal, possibly due to the increased capillary pressure. Later as glomerular filtration falls there is oliguria and salt and water retention with oedema and renal failure. The hypertension in pre-eclampsia is mainly due to the change in vascular reactivity to angiotensin II (Fig. 24.1) for though it may in part also be due to the rise in plasma angiotensin II the arterial pressure increases even in those patients in whom there is no such rise. The rise in plasma angiotensin II presumably comes from the relatively ischaemic uterus, placenta and kidney.

The change in vascular reactivity to angiotensin II is more difficult to understand. In experimental and inherited forms of hypertension there is evidence that an increase in vascular reactivity to angiotensin may be due to a demonstrable rise in the plasma's ability to inhibit sodium transport. One such demonstration is that the leucocytes of patients with essential hypertension have an impaired sodium transport which, it can be shown is due to an increase in the plasma's ability to inhibit sodium transport. It is interesting therefore that the leucocytes of patients with pre-eclampsia develop the same impairment in sodium transport as that seen in essential hypertension, and that it reverts to normal after delivery. It is possible therefore that this transient change of the leucocyte sodium transport in pre-eclampsia may also reflect the fact that the plasma's ability to inhibit sodium transport has increased. But the plasma's ability to inhibit sodium transport in pre-eclampsia has not yet been measured directly.

## Pregnancy induced nephropathy and renal vascular abnormalities

### Nephropathy

In most patients whose blood pressure is raised during pregnancy, regardless of the time of onset, or presence of proteinuria, the glomeruli demonstrate a combination of abnormalities which is characteristic. The lumina of the glomerular capillaries are filled with swollen endothelial and mesangial cells and the mesangial areas are enlarged by mesangial cell swelling. On light microscopy a few capillaries show a 'double contour' appearance. Sub-endothelial and mesangial deposits are present in the capillary walls and the mesangium which stain with fluorescent labelled antibodies against fibrinogen related antigens, and IgM. Some patients also have deposits of IgG, IgA and $C_3$. The earlier the renal biopsy is obtained after delivery the greater the intensity of the fibrin and IgM deposits. In some especially severe cases occlusive masses of fibrin are found in the glomerular capillaries, which may lead to cortical necrosis. The cell swelling is presumably due to the deposition and subsequent absorbtion of fibrin from the surface of the cells.

In a few patients the renal biopsy also reveals the presence of oedema, inflammatory exudates and fibrosis of the interstitial spaces. And in some there are arteriosclerotic changes and fibrinoid deposits in the arterioles.

## Vascular abnormalities

Selective renal angiography 1 to 24 months after a history of pre-eclampsia has demonstrated the presence of persisting residual structural and haemodynamic abnormalities of the intrarenal circulation in a high proportion of patients. The lobar, interlobar and arcuate arteries show tortuosity and irregularity of the lumina which give rise to zig-zag or corkscrew contours, or a beaded appearance. Some arteries associated with areas of cortical ischaemia are completely occluded. These are the same appearances as those found in the loin pain and haematuria syndrome which it is known can be precipitated by the administration of oestrogens, and in which it has been shown, in nephrectomised kidneys, that the radiological appearances are due to fibrin deposition in the pre-arteriolar arteries. In addition angiography also demonstrates disturbances of intrarenal blood flow with asynchronous arterial filling, segments of arterial stasis, and focal areas of abnormal cortical perfusion.

## Relation between the clinical and the renal biopsy findings in hypertension in pregnancy

The characteristic glomerular lesions described above can be found in any patient who has had hypertension during pregnancy whether or not they also had proteinuria, and they can be discerned super-imposed on a pre-existing nephropathy from some other cause such as the nephrosclerosis that accompanies essential hypertension. The lesions are not thought to be due to the rise in arterial pressure per se for they can develop in patients whose blood pressure has been carefully controlled. Neither is the extent and severity of the lesions correlated with the severity of the clinical picture. The histological changes in mild pre-eclampsia are often identical to those in eclampsia. There is however, a good correlation between the glomerular changes and plasma uric acid. A rise in plasma uric acid therefore is an indication that the process of thromboplastin release and fibrin deposition has now caused swelling of the endothelial and mesangial cells.

The vascular lesions of the larger renal vessels demonstrated on angiography after pregnancy are not related to the extent of arteriolar damage as assessed in a renal biopsy. It is not known whether the radiological lesions precede the pregnancy, and are aggravated by the pre-eclamptic episode, or whether they are entirely due to the pregnancy. It has been demonstrated that after pregnancy these patients have abnormalities of urinary sodium excretion which resemble those found in patients with essential hypertension, and it is possible therefore that the vascular lesions may predispose the patient to persistent hypertension later in life.

## Pre-eclampsia

### Renal function

It is a remarkable fact that the renal blood flow in pre-eclampsia is frequently within normal limits, though there is wide variation both above and below normal. The commonest abnormality is a fall in glomerular filtration rate; it may fall to 50 ml/min without a decrease in renal blood flow. It is possible that the depression in glomerular filtration rate is due to the cytoplasmic swelling of the cells lining the glomerular tufts. The fall in filtration rate often bears no relation to the clinical severity of the toxaemia. After delivery there is a sudden rise in filtration rate and for a short time it may reach 250 ml/min; there is an accompanying diuresis and urine volumes up to 550 ml an hour have been described.

In severe eclampsia there is a generalised peripheral vasoconstriction, and as in all clinical conditions associated with generalised vasoconstriction it is particularly marked in the kidney. Renal ischaemia may be sufficiently prolonged and extensive to cause acute tubular necrosis and acute renal failure.

### Clinical features

Pre-eclampsia occurs most frequently in primigravidae and in women who have a persistent rise in blood pressure before the start of pregnancy.

The disease is characterised by hypertension, oedema and proteinuria. It is not an acute nephritic syndrome, for the jugular venous and right auricular pressure are usually normal, i.e. pulmonary venous congestion does not occur, except very occasionally in the terminal phase of eclampsia. Nor does it fit within the definition of a nephrotic syndrome, for again, with the exception of very severe cases, the plasma protein concentrations are relatively normal or are altered to only a minor extent, and proteinuria is never greater than 5 g 24 hours.

The onset takes place after the first twenty weeks of pregnancy and is most common in the last six. It can be predicted to a certain extent, for it occurs in those women who have put on weight too rapidly, though 50 per cent of these will have a normal pregnancy. The first symptoms may be headache or dizziness due to the rise in blood pressure, or there may be oedema, or the patient may have symptomless proteinuria. The rise in blood pressure may precede the onset of oedema, or proteinuria, by many weeks. As the blood pressure rises there may be visual disturbances from vascular changes in the retinae; hypertensive encephalopathy (eclampsia) is preceded by intense, boring frontal headache. In some cases there may be epigastric pain, sometimes of great severity. From the initial symptom to the first convulsion the syndrome may be telescoped into a matter of hours; fortunately the development of symptoms is usually slower. There is always some degree of oliguria. With the convulsions there may be temporary anuria, and very occasionally acute renal failure develops. Unless there is acute renal failure the specific gravity of the urine during a period of oliguria is high.

After delivery the symptoms and signs usually subside rapidly, though in exceptional cases the most prominent features of the disease may occur in the first two or three days of the puerperium.

## Differential diagnosis

It is essential to exclude contamination of the urine by protein from vaginal discharge. The most common causes of proteinuria in the first six months of pregnancy are orthostatic proteinuria and chronic renal disease. Excluding acute pyelonephritis, which is not difficult to diagnose, other acute renal diseases are very rare during pregnancy. Other causes of proteinuria include cardiac failure, severe anaemia and renal tuberculosis. If the urine has not been examined before the twentieth week, and proteinuria is found subsequently, all these causes of proteinuria must be considered as well as the probability of pre-eclampsia.

Not many patients with pre-eclampsia have a urinary infection. On the other hand a large proportion of women with reflux nephropathy develop pre-eclampsia.

## Prognosis

The immediate prognosis of pre-eclampsia is excellent, unless there are fits; the mortality of eclampsia varies between 10–40 per cent, one of the causes of death being acute renal failure.

The ultimate prognosis is difficult to assess. Following pre-eclampsia some women develop a persistent rise in blood pressure, and their prognosis is then that of hypertension, including its effects on the kidney. This would seem to indicate that pre-eclampsia may cause persistent hypertension. Nevertheless statistical evidence shows that the incidence of hypertensive vascular disease in women is the same whether or not they have borne children. The conclusion, which is generally accepted, is that persistent hypertension following pre-eclampsia only develops in women who were inevitably bound to have a rise in blood pressure later, and that the pre-eclampsia has only accelerated its onset. The situation is complicated further by the fact that in a few patients it has been demonstrated that persistent hypertension following pre-eclampsia has been due to renal artery stenosis. It is clear that persistent hypertension following pre-eclampsia should always be thoroughly investigated.

There is no published evidence whether pre-eclampsia gives rise to chronic renal disease other than that which may accompany the subsequent development of hypertension. Occasionally, however, a patient who has had pre-eclampsia whose urine is known to have been protein-free before pregnancy develops persistent proteinuria without hypertension after pregnancy. Biopsies of such patients several years later show persisting structural alterations in the glomeruli, particularly of the basement membrane. The prognosis in these patients is not known.

When a woman has had pre-eclampsia in her first pregnancy the incidence of pre-eclampsia in the second pregnancy is about 30%. If a multiparous woman has pre-eclampsia the incidence of a recurrence with a subsequent pregnancy is about 60%. These figures are slightly less following eclampsia, and greater in women with persistent hypertension between pregnancies.

*Treatment*

The presence of hypertension at any time during pregnancy, should be treated. The administration of methyl-dopa, and old standby, should be discontinued for it is inefficient and depresses the patient. The use of beta-blockers, which have been demonstrated not to prejudice fetal development are preferable. In addition to hypotensive drugs, the best treatment, once pre-eclampsia has declared itself is bed rest.

Infection of the urine should be looked for and treated vigorously. Pregnancy must be terminated if the blood pressure continues to rise with increasing proteinuria, the development of retinal changes and uncontrollable deterioration. The treatment of hypertensive encephalopathy consists of sedation, lowering the blood pressure and termination of pregnancy.

Whatever the state of the patient or the development of the fetus, if plasma uric acid rises in the last three months of pregnancy the patient should be promptly admitted to hospital. The rise in uric acid is due to a simultaneous rise in plasma lactic acid which diminishes tubular secretion of uric acid and thus diminishes uric acid excretion (p. 508). The cause of the rise in lactic acid is obscure; it may be related to the laying down of fibrin and it's ischaemic consequences, throughout the vascular tree (Fig. 24.3).

It is important to keep in mind that acute renal failure may develop, in order that its treatment may not be delayed.

## ACUTE RENAL FAILURE DURING PREGNANCY

Acute renal failure either occurs early in pregnancy when it is usually a complication of abortion, or it occurs at the end of pregnancy, when it is a complication of pre-eclampsia, accidental haemorrhage, or post-partum haemorrhage.

### Acute renal failure complicating abortion

This used to be a common cause of acute renal failure. The cause was loss of blood, reduction in blood volume, intense renal ischaemia and sepsis.

The massive blood loss, the prolonged period of renal ischaemia and the sepsis were due to the abortion having been procured illegally and the patient was therefore trying to conceal the abortion for as long as possible. Death used to occur in approximately half the cases and was nearly always due to sepsis with Cl welchii or Staph aureus. 'Cortical necrosis' (see below) was nearly always related to sepsis.

## Acute renal failure in late pregnancy

Again the cause of the renal lesion is renal ischaemia resulting from haemorrhage and intravascular coagulation. It is possible that in addition there may be a direct nervous vasoconstricting stimulus from the uterus to the kidneys.

Acute tubular necrosis is much more common with accidental haemorrhage (approximately 12% of all cases) than following postpartum haemorrhage, and yet the blood pressure remains unchanged or rises in the former and tends to fall in the latter. Possibly the compensatory renal vasoconstriction which accompanies the reduction in circulating blood volume following postpartum haemorrhage is not so great or so prolonged as in accidental haemorrhage. It is more likely however that the main factor is the increased intravascular coagulation which takes place in accidental haemorrhage. It is sometimes associated with microangiopathic haemolytic anaemia.

Occasionally eclampsia may cause acute renal failure because of widespread arteriolonecrotic lesions, similar in all respects to those found in malignant hypertension.

Death occurs in an uncertain number and is usually due to irreversible renal failure associated with extensive cortical necrosis.

### Pathology

The ischaemic tubular necrosis may be focal as described on page 140, or may be so extensive that the entire cortex is involved, when the condition is known as 'cortical necrosis'. In the more severe and extensive lesions the arteries are also necrosed and contain thrombi.

### Clinical features, course and treatment

Diagnosis is often delayed because the focus of concern is initially on the poor circulatory state of the patient. The clinical features and treatment of acute renal failure have been described on page 143.

One of the aims of treatment is to prevent the development of acute renal failure. In eclampsia the use of hypotensive drugs or caudal anaesthesia to produce a widespread vasodilatation will not only lower the blood pressure and control the convulsions, but will diminish the renal vasoconstriction and prevent tubular necrosis. Often the quantity of blood that has been lost is underestimated for the clinical signs of blood loss may be trivial. If uterine stretch is considered to be an important factor in the acute renal failure of accidental haemorrhage it would seem reasonable to rupture the membranes as soon as the diagnosis of accidental haemorrhage is made.

The importance of infection in acute renal failure following abortion is such that all these patients should be given large doses of penicillin, ampicillin and metronidozole on admission (i.e. immediately after a high vaginal swab has been obtained for culture). Neither pelvic infection early in pregnancy nor an enlarge uterus late in pregnancy is a contraindication to peritoneal dialysis provided the catheter is inserted high in the abdomen.

## Acute renal failure developing a few weeks after delivery

This disastrous condition which strikes without warning two to five weeks after a normal pregnancy and delivery, is a form of haemolytic uraemic syndrome in which there is often an associated cardiomyopathy. Death from cardiac failure may occur in spite of maintenance haemodialysis. Or the patient survives only to remain on dialysis. A few survive with advanced irreversible chronic renal failure.

# PREGNANCY IN RELATION TO PRE-EXISTING CHRONIC RENAL DISEASE

Opinions vary. Addis, after a long experience, stated that 'There is no instance in which we can be sure that the renal lesion interfered with pregnancy. There is no evidence that any of them have been harmed by pregnancy.' Other authors are less sanguine.

## Effect of pregnancy on chronic renal disease

*In patients without renal failure*

In the absence of hypertension pregnancy rarely if ever causes a deterioration of renal function in patients with glomerular nephritis. In the presence of hypertension, however, about half the patients will develop a persistent deterioration of renal function. It is not clear whether this is due to inadequate control of the blood pressure. The proteinuria of diabetic nephropathy often increases during pregnancy but improves after delivery.

*In patients with renal failure*

With glomerular nephritis the issue is relatively clear cut. Either there is a sudden deterioration in renal function, with increased proteinuria and a rise in blood pressure before the twentieth week, or pregnancy causes no harm. When there is an exacerbation of the renal disease some permanent additional impairment of function remains thereafter.

With other renal diseases, such as reflux nephropathy or polycystic disease, the prognosis depends more directly and less mysteriously on whether or not renal infections are allowed to develop.

*Management*

If a woman with chronic renal disease is anxious to have a child and is aware of the risks involved, it is reasonable that she should try and become pregnant only if her blood pressure is normal and renal function is not less than 50% of normal. Once pregnancy has begun, renal infections should be prevented (p. 454), and renal function, the urine deposit, the extent of proteinuria and the height of the blood pressure carefully watched. Pregnancy is discontinued at once if there is evidence of a deterioration of renal function.

Some women with hypertension without renal failure, with or without renal disease may insist on becoming pregnant. The outcome is unpredictable. In some of these women the blood pressure during pregnancy may become normal without hypotensive therapy and they have an uneventful delivery with a live infant at term. The majority of women however continue to have hypertension which becomes more pronounced. Such women either abort or have a miscarriage and the fetus dies. Nevertheless with obsessional attention to treatment it is possible to obtain live births even in this group in whom the blood pressure is raised. The blood pressure has to be lowered and kept below a diastolic of 90 mmHg. One of the most useful drugs is propranolol together with a diuretic. The patient must be seen at least once a week in the first six months and twice a week thereafter. If the blood pressure starts to rise in spite of treatment the patients should be put to bed, monitored at least twice a day and hypotensive treatment rapidly adjusted accordingly. The patient may have to stay in bed during the last two months of pregnancy. Labour should be induced as soon as possible.

Women with chronic renal disease and moderately well advanced renal failure (blood urea 17 mmol/l (100 mg/100 ml) or more) should not become pregnant, for any further deterioration in renal function may be crippling. Pregnancies should be terminated if they occur.

Occasionally a pregnant woman presents with advanced renal failure and refuses to have the pregnancy terminated. A few such patients have been successfully managed with conservative treatment. Others have been haemodialysed until the birth of a live infant.

## EFFECT OF CHRONIC RENAL DISEASE ON PREGNANCY

*In patients without renal failure*

This group includes women with proteinuria of varying severity with or without hypertension, mainly suffering from glomerular nephritis. A third will develop 'pre-eclampsia', and in a third of these the fetus will not survive. Because of the dangers of accidental haemorrhage it is usual to terminate pregnancy, if the fetus is sufficiently large, at about the thirty-third week.

### In patients with renal failure

Such women tend to be sterile. If the blood urea is raised above 9 mmol/l (60 mg/100 ml) in the first few months of pregnancy it is unlikely that there will be a live birth. The patients either abort early or develop accidental haemorrhage later. Eclampsia is uncommon.

## Unilateral kidney

When there is only one kidney pregnancy should not be attempted until the functional and structural state of the kidney has been examined; it should be remembered that a nephrectomy is often performed for a renal disease which may be bilateral.

## Ectopic kidney

If both kidneys are ectopic the fetus should be delivered by Caesarean section. If there is one ectopic kidney and the other kidney is in the normal place it is worth attempting a normal birth, but if there are likely to be any complications such as a breech presentation, it is best to do a Caesarean section.

## RENAL INFECTIONS

Acute pyelonephritis* is the most common complication of pregnancy. It occurs in about 2% of all pregnancies and is responsible for a great deal of discomfort and distress, and a few immediate deaths both of the mother and the fetus.

### Aetiology

About three-quarters of all cases of acute pyelonephritis of pregnancy occur in the 5–8% of women who have *persistent* bacteriuria throughout preg-

---

* At one time obstetricians sometimes called the usual type of acute upper urinary infection in pregnancy an acute pyelitis, and reserve the term acute pyelonephritis for those extremely severe infections with gross impairment of renal function which are usually due to a staphylococcal organism. This is a misleading use of language.

nancy. Unfortunately it is not possible to identify this group by any other means than performing a quantitative urine culture. Nearly all are asymptomatic, nor is the presence of bacteriuria related to previous catheterisation, past symptoms of urinary tract disease, or white cell excretion rate, and it occurs equally among women with or without anaemia. The incidence of acute pyelonephritis in women with previously sterile urine often follows catheterisation of the bladder during or shortly after delivery.

The remarkable severity and persistence of pyelonephritis in pregnancy is probably due to the dilatation, atony and compression of the ureters (see above).

*Clinical features*

The incidence of acute pyelonephritis begins at the fourth month and continues well into the puerperium. Much of the incidence in the puerperium is due to catheterisation. About 15% of women have some difficulty in initiating micturation in the first few days of the puerperium because of episiotomies, prolonged labour, etc. They are liable to be catheterised in order to relieve overdistention of the bladder. Symptomatically the infection is either bilateral or, when unilateral, it is usually on the right side. The physical signs and symptoms have been described on page 448. Mild cases only complain of backache; they may admit to occasional feverish symptoms or pain on passing water with some reluctance, considering that such symptoms are normal in pregnancy. Some attacks may be associated with such severe vomiting that the patient is thought to be suffering from hyperemesis gravidarum.

As in all forms of renal infection the most helpful diagnostic features are rigors, fever, tenderness in the costo-vertebral angles, an increased number of urinary white cells and a significant number of organisms in the urine.

Intravenous pyelogram should only rarely be performed and then the number of films should be strictly limited, for there is evidence to suggest that acute leukaemia in children may follow fetal exposure to diagnostic X-rays. In pregnancy, other non-invasive forms of investigation, are more appropriate. A unilateral *left-sided* infection is particularly likely to be due to some additional disturbance of the renal tract, such as a calculus. It is also important to spot the presence and position of ectopic kidneys.

*Differential diagnosis*

It is remarkable that often in acute pyelonephritis of pregnancy there are no lower urinary symptoms. If therefore a pregnant woman has an unexplained fever the urine should be cultured immediately. On the other hand it is now well established that over 70% of pregnant women who do complain of lower urinary symptoms have a sterile urine.

*Treatment*

*Prophylactic.* It is possible, by routinely culturing the urine of all patients at the beginning of pregnancy, to identify those among whom most of the attacks of acute pyelonephritis will occur. A week's course of a suitable antibiotic (e.g. co-trimoxazole) will abolish the bacteriuria for the rest of the pregnancy in the majority of bacteriuric women. In about 15% of such women, however, the urine will either remain infected or become rein-fected. Recurrent reinfection can usually be treated with nitrofurantoin 50 mg in the evening until the end of pregnancy. Those in whom the urine cannot be made sterile with one antibiotic should be given another or a combination of antibiotics until the urine is sterile, and then placed on to nitrofurantoin 50 mg in the evening until delivery. With these measures the incidence of disabling attacks of acute pyelonephritis can be considerably reduced. The administration of antibiotics does not harm the fetus or give rise to an increased incidence of neonatal jaundice.

It has been proposed that this prophylactic manoeuvre should be under-taken as a routine antenatal service, for it has been claimed that it not only lowers the incidence of acute pyelonephritis but that it also substantially diminishes the incidence of pre-eclampsia and the peri-natal mortality rate. There is no doubt that at one time this was true in certain underdeveloped parts of Boston, Mass., and the West Indies which contained an impover-ished population in which the overall incidence of pre-eclampsia and prematurity were extrememly high; and in those women who had persistent bacteriuria it was even higher. In other parts of the world, however, such as London and Aberdeen, the incidence of toxaemia and prematurity is much lower and is no greater in untreated bacteriuric women than in women with sterile urine. Sterilising the urine of women with bacteriuria in London and Aberdeen therefore cannot lower the incidence of toxaemia or the prematurity rate. In Melbourne the overall incidence of prematurity is low and yet it is considerably greater among the bacteriuric women, neverthe-less, sterilising the urine of bacteriuric women does not lower the incidence of prematurity. It is probable that the high prematurity rate of bacteriuric women in Australia is due to the high incidence of structural damage of the kidneys among such women (see below). And that this in turn is due to the high consumption of phenacetin prevalent in Australia. There is no evidence that bacteriuria of pregnancy increases the incidence of abortion early in pregnancy. The incidence of bacteriuria in women who do abort is no greater than in women who do not abort.

It now appears therefore that unless the overall incidence of pre-eclampsia prematurity is high, such as in Boston, Mass., or the West Indies the only benefit to be obtained from treating asymptomatic bacteriuria of pregnancy is to reduce the incidence of acute pyelonephritis. Some authorities consider that this is not a sufficient return for the expense and inconvenience involved in culturing the urine of all pregnant women. They point out that nowadays acute pyelonephritis is easily treated and rarely leads to protracted admission to hospital. Others point out that (1) the expense and inconvenience of culturing the urine can be reduced by certain simplifications; (2) that acute pyelonephritis is sometimes followed by recurrent ill health for some months after delivery; and (3) that if acute pyelonephritis is not prevented, it has to be treated, and to do this effectively it is necessary to have efficient bacteriological facilities for following up the patients. It is suggested that such facilities are better used to prevent the attacks of acute pyelonephritis. Whatever the result of these deliberations there is no doubt that pregnant women who are known to suffer from a pre-existing renal disease should always have their urine cultured. Many of the objections raised are no longer relevant if one of the commercially available dip slides or filter paper techniques for culturing the urine are used. The whole procedure can be carried out in the antenatal clinic and only samples which are suspicious need be looked at by a bacteriologist.

*Curative.* The treatment of acute pyelonephritis has been discussed on page 451. The liability for the urine to become reinfected is particularly great in pregnancy (80% within six months), and treatment with antibiotics should be continued until delivery and for one month thereafter. Very occasionally antibiotic treatment is unavailing, the patient's condition deteriorates rapidly and pregnancy has to be terminated.

*Prognosis*

Intravenous pyelograms performed after delivery show that in England 35% of bacteriuric women who developed acute pyelonephritis during or immediately after pregnancy have some structural renal abnormality including scarring and clubbing of calyces. Similar lesions are found in 14% of bacteriuric women who have not developed acute pyelonephritis. There is now little doubt, that most if not all these abnormalities precede the acute attack of pyelonephritis. It is probable that most of the claims that acute pyelonephritis of pregnancy causes extensive renal damage, followed eventually by chronic renal failure, hypertension and death have been based on patients with reflux nephropathy (p. 455) who happen to have had acute pyelonephritis during pregnancy.

*Geographical differences*

It is interesting to note that the incidence of radiological abnormalities of the kidneys in bacteriuric women differs considerably from one place to another. In London it is 18% whereas in Melbourne it is 57%. The whole subject of renal infection in pregnancy presents striking regional differences. These should be kept in mind when discussing the subject.

## INCIDENCE OF OTHER RENAL DISEASES IN PREGNANCY

Excluding renal infections, the onset of a new renal disease during pregnancy is very rare. Acute glomerular nephritis is the most common. There is no difficulty in diagnosis if attention is paid to the jugular venous pressure and the urinary deposit. The sudden onset of pulmonary congestion and rise in blood pressure excludes other causes of proteinuria and oedema. If the acute phase of the disease is safely negotiated pregnancy may continue normally with no subsequent deterioration of renal function.

Very occasionally nephrotic glomerular nephritis may develop for the first time during pregnancy. The massive proteinuria, the normal blood pressure and jugular venous pressure distinguish the diagnosis. Such patients have occasionally been successfully treated with prednisone and had a normal pregnancy.

BIBLIOGRAPHY

Aber G M 1982 The kidney in pregnancy. In: Jones N F, Peters D K (eds) Recent advances in renal medicine. Churchill Livingstone, Edinburgh, p 177

Andriole V T, Cohn G L 1964 The effect of diethylstilboestrol on the susceptibility of rats to haematogenous pyelonephritis. J Clin Invest 43: 1136

Bailey R R 1969 Asymptomatic bacteriuria in 200 women undergoing uterine curettage following abortion. New Zealand Med J 70 (446): 13

Bucht H 1951 Studies on renal function in man with special reference to glomerular filtration and renal plasma flow in pregnancy. Scand J Clin Lab Invest 3: suppl 3

Chesley L C, Cosgrove R A 1955 A continuing follow-up study of eclamptic women. Obstet Gynaec (N Y) 5: 697

Ferris T F 1979 The kidney and pregnancy. In: Strauss M B, Welt L G (eds) Diseases of the kidney. Little Brown, Boston, Ch 39, p 1321

Flynn F V, Harper C, De Mayo P 1953 Lactosuria and glycosuria in pregnancy and the puerperium. Lancet 2: 698

Forrester T E Alleyne G A O 1980 Leucocyte electrolytes and sodium efflux rate constants in the hypertension of pre-eclampsia. Clin Sci 59: 199S

Goldsmith H J, De Boer C H, Menzies D N et al 1971 Delivery of healthy infant after five weeks' dialysis treatment for fulminating toxaemia of pregnancy. Lancet 2: 738

Gower P E, Haswell B, Sidaway M E et al 1968 Follow-up of 164 patients with bacteriuria of pregnancy. Lancet 1: 990

Herwig K R, Merrill J P, Jackson R L et al 1965 Chronic renal disease and pregnancy. Am J Obst and Gynec 92: 1117

Hytten F E, Thompson A M 1968 Maternal physiological adjustments. In: Assali N S (ed) Biology of gestation. The maternal organism. Academic Press, New York, vol 1, Chap 8, p 449

Katz A I, Davison J M, Hayslett J P et al 1980 Pregnancy in women with kidney disease. Kidney Int 18: 192

Kenney R A, Lawrence R F, Miller D H 1950 Haemodynamic changes in the kidney in 'toxaemia of late pregnancy'. J Obstet Gynaec Brit Emp 57: 17

The kidney in pregnancy 1968 In: Nettles J B (ed) Clinical obstetrics and gynaecology II, No 2. Hoeber, USA, p 459

Lindheimer M D, Katz A I, Nolten W E et al 1977 Sodium and mineralocorticoids in normal and abnormal pregnancy. Advances in Nephrology 7: p 33

Little P J 1966 The incidence of urinary infection in 5,000 pregnant women. Lancet 2: 925

Nochy D, Birembaut P, Hinglais N et al 1980 Renal lesions in the hypertensive syndromes of pregnancy. Immunomorphological and ultrastructural studies in 114 cases. Clin Nephrol 13: 155

Redman C W G, Beilin L J, Denson K W E et al 1977 Factor-VIII consumption in pre-eclampsia. Lancet 2: 1249

Robson J S, Martin A M, Ruckley V A et al 1968 Irreversible post-partum renal failure. Quart J Med 37: 423

Rodbard S (editor) 1964 Supplement on hypertension, blood pressure and toxaemia of pregnancy. Circulation 30: suppl 2

Seymour A E, Petrucco O M, Clarkson A R 1976 Morphological and immunological evidence of coagulopathy in renal complication of pregnancy. In Lindheimer M D (ed) Hypertension in pregnancy, John Wiley and Sons Inc p 139

Sheehan H L, Moore H C 1953 Renal cortical necrosis and the kidney of concealed accidental haemorrhage. Blackwell Scientific Pub Oxford

Sims E A H 1971 The kidney in pregnancy. In: Strauss M B, Welt L G (eds) Diseases of the kidney Little Brown and Company, Boston, Chapter 32, p 1155

Sims E A 1965 Kidney disease in pregnancy. Ann Rev Med 16: 221

Smith K, McClure Browne J C, Shackman R et al 1968 Renal failure of obstetric origin. Brit Med Bull 24: 49

Soler N G, Malins J M 1971 Prevalence of glycosuria in normal pregnancy. A quantitative study. Lancet i: 619

Stirrat G M, Redman C W G, Levinsky R J 1978 Circulating immune complexes in pre-eclampsia. Brit Med J 1: 1450

Studd J W W, Blainey J D 1969 Pregnancy and the nephrotic syndrome. Brit Med J 1: 276

Symonds E M 1981 The renin-angiotensin system in pregnancy. In: Wynn R M (ed) Obstetrics and gynaecology annual. Appleton-Century-Crofts, p 45

Symonds E M, Broughton Pipkin F 1978 Pregnancy hypertension, parity, and the renin-angiotensin system. Amer J Obstet and Gynaec 132: 473

Vassalli P, McCluskey R T 1965 The coagulation process and glomerular disease. Amer J Med 39: 179

# 25

# The kidney, gout and uric acid

Abnormalities of uric acid metabolism which give rise to an increase in plasma urate can cause chronic or acute renal failure. On the other hand abnormalities in renal function can cause a rise or fall in plasma urate.

## Structural changes associated with hyperuricaemia

*Acute hyperuricaemia* can cause acute renal failure. This is due to precipitation of urates in the lumen of the tubules, calyces and ureters. It only occurs with extremely high plasma concentrations of urate.

*Chronic hyperuricaemia* (Fig. 25.1) can cause chronic renal failure; the following changes are seen:

a. Very occasionally there is an easily demonstrable deposition of urates within the renal parenchyma
b. Interstitial nephritis
c. Nephrosclerosis
d. Uric acid stones.

Urates are found in the interstitial spaces. They cause necrosis of the tubules in the immediate vicinity of the deposits, and are surrounded by focal concentrations of inflammatory cells. Very rarely the deposits can become sufficiently large to be macroscopically recognisable tophi, particularly in the tips of the pyramids. Whether or not urates are seen, the predominant histological abnormality is one of interstitial nephritis. The vascular lesions are those sclerotic changes found in chronic hypertensive vascular disease, but hypertension is *not* essential for their presence. Uric acid stones contribute to the destruction of the kidneys by causing obstruction and predisposing to infection.

## Effect of acute hyperuricaemia on renal function

In man, a brief intravenous infusion of urates sufficient to cause a transient rise of plasma urate can cause a reversible depression of glomerular filtration. A relatively acute rise in plasma urate occurs in leukaemia, polycy-

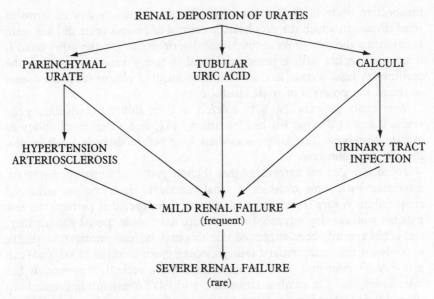

**Fig. 25.1** Aetiology of structural changes associated with the renal deposition of urates. (Derived from Emmerson BT 1976 Med J Aust 1: 403 with kind permission).

thaemia, congenital haemolytic anaemia, myelomatosis, and lymphosarcoma when it is due to the high turnover of cells containing large nuclei. The patient usually succumbs before the rise in plasma urate causes any detectable impairment in renal function. Occasionally, however, acute renal failure may be precipitated by treatment. This follows either the administration of cytotoxic drugs, or the beginning of radiotherapy. There is then an enormous rise in plasma urate (e.g. up to 3000 $\mu$mmol/l (50 mg/100 ml) because of the widespread destruction of cells; the large quantities of filtered uric acid precipitate in the tubules causing acute obstruction. Very rarely a previously healthy person, not on any treatment, may present with a rapid onset of renal failure due to a spontaneously high plasma urate occurring at the onset of leukaemia.

*Effect of chronic hyperuricaemia on renal function*

Until recently it was generally assumed that persistent hyperuricaemia inevitably caused progressive renal failure. It is now apparent that either this was a gross oversimplification or that over the years things have improved. Nevertheless the position is still obscure. Recent retrospective studies in patients with gout or asymptomatic hyperuricaemia suggests that renal functional deterioration due to hyperuricaemia is of no great moment until plasma urate is greater than about 800 $\mu$mmol/l (13 mg/100 ml) in man, and 600 $\mu$mmol/l (10 mg/100 ml) in women. This conclusion is in line with one prospective study in patients with hyperuricaemia due to various forms of renal disease in which the prophylactic control of plasma urate did not seem to influence the rate of renal functional deterioration. On the other hand it is not in keeping with a prospective trial in gouty subjects in which the preliminary results seem to show that the control of plasma urate does seem to retard the progress of renal insufficiency.

Most gouty patients also have a defect in their ability to concentrate the urine, a loss of diurnal rhythm for urinary pH, and a depressed ability to excrete ammonia. The latter is evident long before there is a fall in glomerular filtration rate.

There is a general agreement that though gout and hyperuricaemia are associated with some measure of renal functional deterioration, advanced renal failure is rare. It has been suggested, therefore, that perhaps the few patients who develop advanced renal failure have some special abnormality, and it has recently been suggested that this may be lead intoxication. There is no doubt that symptomatic lead poisoning (with elevated blood lead) can give rise to gout and 'lead' nephropathy. More recently however, it has been found that the administration of 2 g of EDTA/day intramuscularly in three divided doses for three days to a group of patients with 'primary' gout, in whom the blood concentration of lead was normal, induced a rise in the urinary excretion of lead which was about double that obtained in a group of patients suffering from other renal diseases and in a group of normal controls.

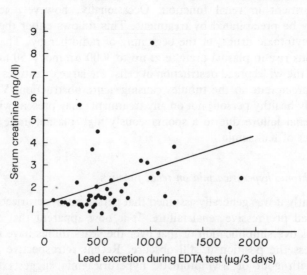

CREATININE VS MOBILIZABLE LEAD

**Fig. 25.2** Relation between serum creatinine and urinary lead excretion in 44 patients with gout. Conversion: traditional to SI units — creatinine. 1 mg/100 ml = 88 $\mu$mol/l: lead 1000 $\mu$g/3 days = 4.8 $\mu$mol/3 days. (Reproduced from Batuman, Maesaka, Hadded et al 1981 New Eng J Med 304: 520, with kind permission.)

In the patients with gout there was also a loose but significant correlation between serum creatinine and the result of the EDTA test suggesting that patients with gout who develop severe renal failure are those who have been most exposed to lead.

Another group of gouty patients who develop terminal renal failure is that of young women in whom the disease is familial. It is a rare condition of great importance because if it is diagnosed early it appears possible to control the advance of renal functional deterioration. It appears to be due to an excessive production of uric acid of unknown cause. Advanced renal failure may develop before the age of 10 years but usually the pace of events is slower. The renal failure precedes the arthritis. The characteristic faetures are proteinuria, a raised plasma urate (when compared to children of the same age and sex), a remarkable inability to concentrate the urine which appears very early in the disease, and the appearances in a renal biopsy of patchy interstitial nephritis with marked thickening of the basement membrane in the distal and collecting tubules. The histological appearances are remarkably similar to those associated with nephrosclerosis due either to age or hypertension, but in these girls the vessels are normal. This supports the conclusion that the lesions which are found so frequently in gouty-middle-aged patients, are not necessarily due to the patient's age or accompanying hypertension.

### Effect of renal function on plasma urate

In some patients with persistent hyperuricaemia the rise in plasma urate is due to a selective impairment of the kidney to excrete uric acid. Initially the glomerular filtration rate is normal. Many of these patients also have an increased production of uric acid and have therefore considerable rises in their plasma concentration of urate. This group includes patients with acute arthritis and others with familial hyperuricaemia without arthritis.

A similar selective impairment in the ability to excrete uric acid, but without overproduction of uric acid, occurs in a number of other conditions where it may cause a mild rise in plasma urate. It is probable that in all these conditions the kidney's inability to excrete uric acid is due to a raised plasma lactate which is a known inhibitor of uric acid excretion. This phenomenon occurs in a proportion of patients with 'essential' hypertension, myxoedema, toxaemia of pregnancy, glycogen-storage disease, ketotic conditions such as starvation and following the ingestion of alcohol. Hypercalcaemia and overt lead poisoning will also cause hyperuricaemia.

The ingestion of pyrazinamide, pempidine, mecamylamine and many diuretics, including particularly chlorothiazide and frusemide also directly inhibit tubular secretion of uric acid and may cause quite brisk rises in plasma uric acid.

The advent of renal functional deterioration in a person who already has an impaired ability to excrete uric acid will aggravate the uric acid retention

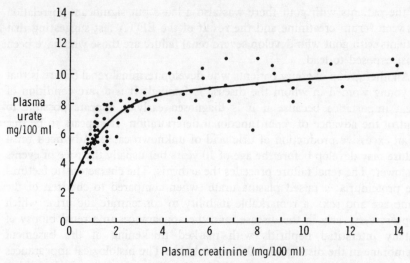

**Fig. 25.3** Relationship between glomerular filtration rate and plasma urate in non gouty patients with renal disease. Computer drawn curve. (Reproduced from Hatfield & Simmonds 1974 Guy's Hospital Reports 123: 271, with kind permission.)

and cause the rise in plasma urate to be more pronounced. The development of renal failure in persons with no previous impairment in the ability to excrete uric acid causes a rise in plasma urate. But the rise is much less than that predicted from the fall in glomerular filtration rate. This is mainly due to an increase in urate excretion per nephron secondary to varying combinations of reduced urate reabsorption and increased tubular secretion. The mechanisms responsible for this remarkable adjustment are not known. The slow rise in plasma urate in renal failure is also due in part to a diminished production of uric acid which is demonstrated by the fact that though the plasma urate remains normal the urinary excretions of urate falls progressively as the renal failure gets worse (Fig. 25.4).

On rare occasions there may be a congenital or acquired defect in the proximal tubule's capacity to reabsorb uric acid. The urinary leak of urates then leads to a fall in plasma urate.

### Clinical features of hyperuricaemia

If a patient is known to have a persistent rise in plasma uric acid, renal disturbances should be anticipated. The main difficulty is the variety of ways in which a patient with hyperuricaemia may present for the first time. There may be the typical arthritis of gout, or multiple aches and pains which are shrugged off as 'rheumatism'. The young with familial hyperuricaemia may have hypertension which is first discovered either at a routine medical examination or as a sequel to toxaemia of pregnancy. Sometimes asymptomatic proteinuria is the first abnormality to be noticed, or the patient first

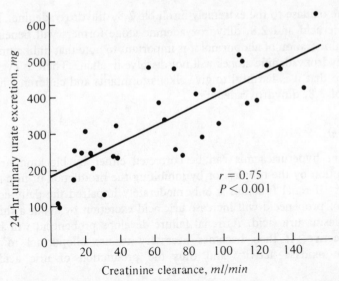

**Fig. 25.4** The fall in the renal excretion of urate which occurs with reduction in renal glomerular excretory function. Conversion: traditional to SI units — urate 250 mg = 1.5 mmol. (Reproduced from Emmerson & Row 1975 Kidney Int 8: 65, with kind permission.)

presents with acute pyelonephritis. A few patients will present with uric acid stones.

It is an excellent rule to measure the concentration of uric acid in the plasma of all patients suffering from proteinuria or any other renal disturbance, hypertension, arthritis or vague aches and pains.

*Uric acid stones* may occur in any patient with hyperuricaemia due to overproduction of uric acid. The stones are formed because of the increased quantity of uric acid being excreted in the urine. The majority of uric acid stones, however, occur in patients with a normal plasma urate who are not excreting an excess amount of uric acid in the urine. In these patients the stones are formed because the urine is persistently acid. Whereas in a normal individual the urinary pH rises to 6 or higher during the day, the urinary pH of these patients remains below 6, or more usually below 5.5 throughout the 24 hours. The cause of this functional disturbance is not clear. It is associated with a moderate impairment in the ability to excrete ammonia which must contribute to the persistent acidity.

The formation of stones is associated with renal colic, haematuria, proteinuria, pyelonephritis and urinary obstruction.

'Uric acid' stones may occasionally not be made of uric acid. The usual methods used to measure uric acid do not distinguish between uric acid and adenine. Very occasionally the uric acid stones turn out to be due to crystals of 2,8, dihydroxyadenine due to a congenital defect of the adenine salvage enzyme adenine phosphoribosyl transferase. In its absence the only alternative route of disposal of the relatively soluble adenine is by oxidation by xanthine oxidase to the extremely insoluble 2,8, dihydroxyadenine. Though both uric acid and 2,8, dihydroxyadenine stone formers will benefit from the administration of allopurinol it is important to note that unlike uric acid, 2,8, dihydroxyadenine stones will not dissolve in alkali. There is even some evidence that it is harmful to give alkalis to infants and children who form stones of 2,8, dihydroxyadenine.

*Treatment*

Persistent hyperuricaemia can be corrected either by blocking uric acid reabsorption by the tubules, or by inhibiting the production of uric acid by the liver. If renal function is only moderately impaired the daily administration of probenecid will increase uric acid excretion by about a third and lower plasma uric acid. As renal failure develops probenecid will become less effective. It then becomes necessary to use allopurinol to inhibit xanthine oxidase activity and thus the production of uric acid from xanthine.

Inasmuch as renal function in occupational lead nephropathy will improve if the patients are given 1 g of EDTA three times a week for up to four years, it has been suggested that patients with severe gouty nephropathy might be treated in the same way.

A sudden rise in plasma urate with precipitation in the tubules, such as that which may complicate the treatment of leukaemia with chemotherapy can be avoided by the administration of allopurinol. Attempts should be made to prevent vomiting and dehydration which often accompanies this form of treatment.

It is very important to remember that most diuretics, and severe weight reducing diets, may cause a rise in plasma urate. In some patients this may precipitate gout or some deterioration of renal function. In a patient with some pre-existing impairment of renal function this risk should be prevented by the administration of allopurinol as soon as the plasma urate begins to rise. In a patient with normal renal function the plasma urate can be controlled if necessary with probenecid.

Uric acid stones associated with a persistently acid urine are best treated with an increased intake of fluid and 50–100 mmol of sodium bicarbonate per day. Elderly subjects, in whom it is important to avoid precipitating pulmonary congestion, can be given acetazolamide in the evening which increases sodium excretion and keeps the urine alkaline during the night.

BIBLIOGRAPHY

Batuman V, Maesaka J K, Haddad B et al 1981 The role of lead in gout nephropathy. New Eng J Med 304: 520
Berger L, Yu T 1975 Renal function in gout IV. An analysis of 524 gouty subjects including long term follow-up studies. Amer J Med 59: 605

Berkowitz D, Glassman S 1965 Effects of hypertriglyceridemia on urinary uric acid outputs. Circulation 32 (suppl ii): 2

Bluestine R, Kippen I, Klinenberg J R 1969 Effect of drugs on urate binding to plasma proteins. Brit Med J 4: 590

Boss G R, Seegmiller J E 1979 Hyperuricaemia and gout. New Eng J Med 300: 1459

Duncan H, Dixon A StJ 1960 Gout, familial hyperuricaemia, and renal disease. Quart J Med N S 29: 127

Elion G B, Benezra F M, Beardmore T D et al 1980 Studies with allopurinol in patients with impaired renal function. Adv Exp Med Biol 122A: 263

Emmerson B T 1976 Gout, uric acid and renal disease. Med J Aust i: 403

Emmerson B T 1963 Chronic lead nephropathy: the diagnostic use of calcium EDTA and the association with gout. Aust Ann Med 12: 310

Emmerson B T, Row P G 1975 An evaluation of the pathogenesis of the gouty kidney. Kidney Int 8: 65

Fessel W J 1979 Renal outcomes of gout and hyperuricaemia. Amer J Med 67: 74

Fineberg S K, Altschul A 1956 The nephropathy of gout. Ann Intern Med 44: 1182

Handler J S 1960 The role of lactic acid in the reduced excretion of uric acid in toxaemia of pregancy. J Clin Invest 39: 1526

Hatfield P J, Simmonds H A 1974 Uric acid and the kidney. Guy's Hospital Reports 123: 271

Holmes E W, Kelley W N, Wyngaarden J B 1972 The kidney and uric acid excretion in man. Kidney Int 2: 115

Kritzler R A 1958 Anuria complicating the treatment of leukaemia. Amer J Med 25: 532

Lieber C S, Jones D P, Losowsky M S et al 1962 Inter-relation of uric acid and ethanol metabolism in man. J Clin Invest 41: 1863

Maurice P F, Hennemanm P H 1961 Medical aspects of renal stones. Medicine 40: 315

Mikkelsen W M, Dodge H J, Valkenburg H 1965 The distribution of serum uric acid values in a population unselected as to gout and hyperuricaemia. Amer J Med 39: 242

Nugent C A, Macdiarmid W D, Tyler F H 1964 Renal excretion of urate in patients with gout. Arch Int Med 113: 115

Nugent C A, Tyler F H 1959 The renal excretion of uric acid in patients with gout and in non-gouty subjects. J Clin Invest 38: 1890

Pak Poy R K 1965 Urinary pH in gout. Austral J Med 14: 35

Pearce J, Aziz H 1969 Uric acid and plasma lipids in cerebrovascular disease. Part I/ Prevalence of hyperuricaemia. Brit Med J 4: 78

Praetorius E, Kirk J E 1950 Hypouricaemia with evidence for tubular elimination of uric acid. J Lab Clin Med 35: 865

Scott J T 1980 Long term management of gout and hyperuricaemia. Brit Med J 281: 1164

Seegmiller J E, Grayzel A I, Howell R R et al 1962 The renal excretion of uric acid in gout. J Clin Invest 41: 1094

Simmonds H A, Sahota A, Potter C F et al 1978 Adenine phosphoribosyltransferase deficiency presenting with supposed 'uric acid' stones: pitfalls of diagnosis. J Roy Soc Med 71: 791

Simmonds H A, Warren D J, Cameron J S et al 1980 Familial gout and renal failure in young women. Clin Nephrol 14: 176

Snaith M L, Scott J T 1971 Uric acid clearance in patients with gout and normal subjects. Ann Rheum Dis 30: 285

Steele T H, Rieselbach R E 1967 The contribution of residual nephrons within the chronically diseased kidney to urate homeostasis. Amer J Med 43: 876

Videbaek A 1950 Polycythaemia vera. Acta med Scand 138: 179

Wedeen R P, Malik D K, Batuman V 1979 Detection and treatment of occupational lead nephropathy. Arch Int Med 139: 53

Yu T F, Gutman A B 1964 Effect of allopurinol (4 hydroxypyrazolo (3,4d) pyrimidine) serum and urinary uric acid in primary and secondary gout. Amer J Med 37: 885

# 26

# Renal disturbances in monoclonal gammopathies

Monoclonal gammopathy is the term given to the unrestrained proliferation of a single abnormal B cell clone. Normal, and abnormally proliferating B cells manufacture only one type of immunoglobulin. An abnormally proliferating clone, in addition to making an excess of a single type of immunoglobulin, may manufacture the molecule in a faulty manner. A B cell normally manufactures heavy and light chains in the right proportions so that, as the complete immunoglobulins are assembled, no excess residue of free chains of either type remains. Abnormal clones, however, may manufacture an excess of heavy or light chains, more commonly the latter. Heavy chains do not harm the kidney, but light chains, both κ and λ are nephrotoxic. Free light chains are best known as Bence-Jones protein.

Complete immunoglobulins are too large to pass through the glomerular filter so that in a monoclonal gammopathy (e.g. myelomatosis) the plasma concentration of the excessively produced immunoglobulin is raised while little of it appears in the urine. On the other hand light chains which have a molecular weight of 22 000 daltons pass through the glomerular capillaries with ease so that their concentration in the plasma is low while they are present in large amounts in the urine. It is also characteristic of monoclonal gammopathies that the plasma concentrations of those immunoglobulins which are not manufactured by the abnormal clone are depressed.

Electrophoresis of normal plasma reveals that each of the various bands in which IgG, IgA, IgM etc are situated is relatively wide because each band is made up of a multiplicity of antibodies. When however, an abnormal clone manufactures large amounts of an immunoglobulin, it appears electrophorectically, as a thin narrow intensely concentrated band within one of the wider bands, reflecting the fact that it is composed of a single antibody. The term paraprotein has been used in the past to describe the presence in the plasma of such a band, and the word also includes an excess of heavy or light chains. Usually the presence of a paraprotein can be shown histologically to be accompanied by an overt proliferation of some form of B cell. When such a proliferation cannot be demonstrated the patient is said to be suffering from a 'benign gammopathy'.

## Waldenström's macroglobulinaemia

The main clinical features of this disease are unrelated to the kidney. Renal disturbances are due either to the high concentrations of IgM which are produced by the lymphocytes or to amyloidosis. IgM is a large molecule which may materially increase the viscosity of the plasma. It is characteristically found precipitated in round amorphous eosinophilic plugs in the lumina of glomerular capillaries. Presumably this is one cause for the associated fall in glomerular filtration rate. It is also possible that the deterioration of renal function is due in part, to the extraordinary rise in plasma viscosity that must take place in the efferent arteriole when the glomerular filtrates has been removed from the plasma.

Occasionally IgM molecules may either aggregate with one another, or with normal IgG, when they may form antigenic, complement fixing, immune complexes which may cause membranous or proliferative glomerular nephritis. When such aggregates can be precipitated by a fall in temperature they are then known as cryoglobulins. Nevertheless the deleterious effect of these immune complexes on the kidney does not appear to be related to their thermal characteristics. Death from renal failure in Waldenström's macroglobulinaemia is unusual.

## Diffuse myelomatosis

The paraproteins in this condition are formed by a clone of plasma cells. They consist of IgG, IgA and IgD, and usually there is also an excess of light chains, both λ and K. At first the main clinical features, are unrelated to the kidney. Eventually, however, renal disturbances are very common. They are due to the presence of light chains, hypercalcaemia, hyperuricaemia and amyloidosis.

The characteristic pathological appearances are (1) the precipitation of obstructive casts of light chains, together with various other proteins, in the lumina of the distal and collecting ducts and (2) tubule cell damage, with intracellular crystallization, due to the reabsorption of light chains.

Myelomatosis casts are often surrounded by a macrophagic reaction which is difficult to explain. The casts themselves are often fractured by the microtome into several irregular rod shaped fragments lying parallel to each other within the lumen of the tubule. In the glomeruli mesangial deposits of κ light chains cause a nodular glomerulosclerosis which resembles diabetic nephropathy. The proteinuria of myelomatosis nearly always contains albumin whether or not Bence–Jones' protein is also present. Occasionally, however, Bence-Jones' protein is the only protein present; it is important to remember that Bence-Jones' protein cannot be detected with Albustix. The most accurate way to detect the presence of Bence-Jones' protein is to examine the urine immuno-electrophoretically. It can also be identified by warming the urine; the protein at first comes out of solution and appears as a white precipitate, but as the urine becomes warmer the precipitate redissolves and the urine becomes clear. If, however, other proteins are present, the persistent precipitate which they form on heating obscures the presence of Bence-Jones' protein. To establish the presence of Bence-Jones' protein when other proteins are present it is therefore necessary to filter the urine immediately after it has been brought to the boil. The precipitated albumin and globulins will then be separated from the Bence-Jones' protein which remains in the clear filtrate. This filtrate is observed as it cools and Bence-Jones' protein will appear when the temperatures falls to 70° C. It is important that the warmed urine should not be allowed to cool before it has passed through the filter, for otherwise the Bence-Jones' protein is precipitated on the wrong side of the filter and does not appear in the filtrate. To keep the urine warm it is best to filter small amounts at a time, to reheat the urine at frequent intervals, and to place the filter paper upon a warm funnel. It is characteristic of multiple myelomatosis that if Bence-Jones' protein is present, it appears in large quantities; Bence-Jones' proteinuria is sometimes found in other conditions but only in small amounts.

The rate of deterioration in renal function varies from acute renal failure to a modest impairment which remains static. Acute renal failure often follows an intravenous urogram which has been performed in the usual manner (which includes a ritual period of fluid deprivation) in a patient in whom the diagnosis of myelomatosis had not yet been suspected. The prescence of the contrast medium in the concentrated tubule fluid causes the precipitation of widespread tubular casts.

The low plasma concentrations of all the immunoglobulins not manufactured by the proliferating clone of cells is probably the cause of the patient's increased susceptibility to infection.

*Hypercalcaemia, hyperuricaemia and amyloidosis*

Renal failure in diffuse myelomatosis can also be caused by the hypercalcaemia which sometimes accompanies the massive bone resorption induced by the lesions in the bone marrow. In these lesions there is also a high turnover of nucleo-proteins and therefore an increased production of uric acid. This may cause a sufficient rise in plasma urate to be responsible for a rapid deterioration of renal function (p. 512). Sometimes treatment which destroys the myeloma cells releases large amounts of nucleo-protein and causes a brisk rise in plasma urate. Amyloidosis occurs in 10 per cent of patients with myelomatosis and may also contribute to the renal functional impairment. It is most often seen in patients with Bence-Jones' proteinuria. If a patient with multiple myelomatosis develops a nephrotic syndrome it is nearly always due to amyloidosis.

## Treatment

Death is frequently due to renal failure. Often this is precipitated by dehydration and the consequent precipitation of protein in the tubules. The patient should therefore be encouraged to drink large volumes of fluids. When the daily excretion of Bence-Jones' protein is high the fluid intake should amount to about 4 litres a day. The rate of excretion of Bence-Jones' protein can sometimes be controlled by the administration of melphalan or cyclophosphamide. Hypercalcaemia can sometimes be controlled in the same way, or with prednisone. This acts in part by inhibiting the multiplication of the myeloma cells. It is also helpful to avoid bed rest. Hyperuricaemia can be avoided or controlled by the administration of allopurinol (p. 514). If the plasma viscosity rises to dangerous levels it can be lowered quickly by plasmapheresis. This often has to be done as an emergency because of a rapid deterioration of renal function.

In order to try to prevent renal failure in myelomatosis therefore, it is imperative to measure the rate of Bence-Jones' protein excretion, and the plasma concentrations of calcium and uric acid at frequent intervals.

## Prognosis

50% of all patients with myelomatosis who present with a blood urea greater than 13 mmol/l (80 mg/100 ml) die within the next 10 weeks in spite of treatment. Other poor prognostic signs are a Bence-Jones' protein concentration in the blood greater than 2 g/l, a plasma albumin of less than 30 g/l and a haemoglobin of less than 7.5 g/100 ml. IgA myelomatosis is sometimes associated with a rapid deterioration of renal function of unknown cause.

BIBLIOGRAPHY

Argani I, Kipkie G F 1964 Macroglobulinaemic nephropathy: acute renal failure in macroglobuli naemia of Waldenstrom. Amer J Med 36: 151

Armstrong J B 1950 A study of renal function in patients with multiple myeloma. Amer J Med Sci 219: 488

Beaufils M, Morel-Maroger L 1978 Pathogenesis of renal disease in monoclonal gammopathies: current concepts. Nephron 20: 125

Bentzel C J, Carbone P P, Rosenberg L 1964 The effect of prednisone on calcium metabolism and Ca⁴⁷ kinetics in patients with multiple myeloma and hypercalcaemia. J Clin Invest 43: 2132

Clyne D H, Brendstrup L, First M R et al 1974 Renal effects of intraperitoneal kappa chain injection. Induction of crystals in renal tubular cells. Lab Invest 31: 131

Falconer-Smith J F, Van Hegan R I, Esnouf M P et al 1979 Characteristics of renal handling of human immunoglobulin light chain by the perfused rat kidney. Clin Sci 57: 113

Feizi T, Gitlin N 1969 Immune-complex disease of the kidney associated with chronic hepatitis and cryoglobulinaemia. Lancet 2: 873

Gamble C N, Ruggles SW 1978 The immunopathogenesis of glomerulo-nephritis associated with mixed cryoglobulinaemia. New Eng J Med 299: 81

Hobbs J R 1971 Immunocytoma. O' mice an' men. Brit Med J 2: 67

MacAlister C L O, Addison N V 1961 Renal aspects of myelomatosis. Brit J Urol 33: 141

Mallick N P, Dosa S, Acheson I W et al 1978 Detection, significance and treatment of paraprotein in patients presenting with 'idiopathic' proteinuria without myeloma. Quart J Med 47: 145

Morel-Maroger L, Basch A, Danon F et al 1970 Pathology of the kidney in Waldenstrom's macroglobulinaemia. New Eng J Med 283: 123

Myeloma Workshop 1971 Brit Med J 2: 319

Putnam F 1962 Structural relationships among normal human y-globulin, myeloma globulins and Bence-Jones proteins. Biochem Biophys Acta 63: 539

Tubbs R R, Gephardt G N, McMahon J T et al, 1981 Light chain nephropathy Amer J Med 71: 263

Verroust P, Mery J-P, Morel-Maroger L et al 1971 Glomerular lesions in monoclonal gammopathies and mixed essential cryoglobulinaemia IgG-IgM. Adv Nephrol I: 161

# 27

# Renal amyloid

Histologically amyloid is an eosinophilic substance which appears structureless on light microscopy but which has a characteristic fibrillary pattern on electron microscopy. It may be distributed throughout all the organs of the body. The fibrils which are 10 nm in width contain, either AL protein which consists of fractions of light chains (either κ or λ) derived from myeloma cells, or lymphocytes, or AA protein the origin of which is unknown but which is totally unrelated to AL protein. The AL protein fibrils can be harvested in vitro from cultures of plasma cells (or lymphocytes) and macrophages. The plasma cells and lymphocytes make fractions of light chains. These are then phagocytosed by the macrophages and turned into the final protein units which are polymerised into fibrils. Both AL and AA fibrils are bound together by a globulin called 'P component' which is arranged in a rod like manner between the fibrils. The AA protein is an acid soluble fraction of amyloid, it is a polypeptide, insoluble in water with a molecular weight of 8500 daltons.

Normal plasma contains a material which binds to antibody raised against AA. This material is known as Serum AA or SAA. In the serum it may be polymerised AA, or AA bound to a carrier molecule. The concentration of SAA in a normal person rises with inflammation and with age, particularly after the age of 70–75 years. In vitro, normal plasma can 'clear' added SAA and there is an impression that those individuals whose plasma can clear added SAA most quickly are less likely to develop amyloidosis. There is close connection between amyloidosis and myelomatosis: (1) as stated above, the AL protein consists of light chains, (2) the bone marrow of patients with amyloidosis often contains an excess of plasma cells and (3) 10% of patients with myelomatosis develop amyloidosis.

*Pathology*

The kidneys are usually smooth, resilient and enlarged. The cut surface shows that both the cortex and medulla are broader than normal and the demarcation between them is sharp; the glomeruli can be identified as small translucent deposits which stain dark brown upon the addition of iodine.

Occasionally there is considerable disorganisation, the kidneys are small and scarred and the cortex and medulla difficult to recognise.

Under the microscope amyloid material is found in the walls of all vessels, including the glomerular capillaries and the peritubular venous capillaries. The changes also include lobular stalk thickening, and nodular masses of amyloid deposits in the mesangium. Later it is characteristic that the glomeruli may appear to be almost entirely replaced by amyloid material at a time when the glomerular filtration rate may be only moderately impaired. Apart from the characteristic staining reactions, the appearances are often much the same as those found in glomerular nephritis and diabetes. Electron microscopy reveals that the basement membrane may be normal; the deposits of amyloid lying on either side. In other sites the amyloid material invades and thickens the basement membrane so that it merges into a nearby mass of amyloid. At autopsy the glomeruli mostly consist of solid, structureless, compact masses of amyloid of about the same size as a normal glomerulus. The amyloid material, which is laid in the peritubular venous capillaries, may be very thick but does not invade the tubule cells.

The tubule cells show the characteristic changes found in nephrotic glomerular nephritis, i.e. those changes found with heavy proteinuria, with intracellular deposits of lipoid, and collections of an eosin-staining material of uncertain origin. Tubular atrophy is also present. The distribution of amyloid is important. If it is predominantly in the glomeruli the prognosis is much better than if it is widespread in the interstitium and vessels.

Without the use of special stains it is easy to confuse renal amyloidosis with diabetic nephropathy and, particularly, persistent glomerular nephritis. But even special stains may mislead. Amyloidosis can sometimes be demonstrated on electron microscopy when all special stains are negative. Both AL and AA proteins are polymerised in the same layered zig-zag manner to form the amyloid fibrils. It is this common pattern which gives these two dissimilar proteins their similar electron microscopy properties and birefrigence.

*Clinical features*

There are many forms of amyloidosis in all of which amyloid may be laid down in the kidney.

**Primary amyloidosis**

Primary amyloidosis in which the amyloid material is AL in type occurs with myelomatosis and certain lymphocyte disturbances. The urine usually contains light chains. In some patients there is little or no evidence of myelomatosis and the urine does not appear to contain light chains; such cases are the true 'primary' amyloidosis. It is more probable however, that the absence of light chains in the urine is due to the urine not having been examined sufficiently often or that the methods used have not been sufficiently sensitive. This form of amyloidosis is difficult to treat and seems to run a rapid course to terminal renal failure, often within six months of diagnosis.

## Reactive systemic amyloidosis

Reactive systemic amyloidosis in which the amyloid material is AA in type is associated with chronic sepsis such as tuberculosis, chronic osteomylitis or recurrent upper urinary infections in paraplegic patients. It also occurs in association with rheumatoid arthritis and in Crohn's disease but not in ulcerative colitis. The natural history of this form of renal amyloidosis extends over several years. The rate of events can sometimes be modified by successful treatment of the associated condition, particularly if there is sepsis. Often the renal amyloid seems to progress to a certain point and then remains static. In a very few patients the amyloid deposits in serial renal biopsies are reported to have regressed.

## Hereditary amyloidosis

Hereditary amyloidosis in which the amyloid material is also AA can occur either as a familial condition characterised by polyneuropathy, cardiomyopathy, splenomegally and minimal renal involvement or as a complication of mediterranean recurrent fever (MRF). The latter is a relatively common condition in the countries which border on the eastern mediterranean and the Black Sea. It occurs in patients whose origins are in Asia Minor and it is transmitted in an autosomal recessive fashion. About 50% of those who suffer from mediterranean recurrent fever develop amyloidosis. The deposits of amyloid predominate in the kidney and the deposition of amyloid at other sites rarely produce any clinically obvious changes before renal failure is well advanced. The disease is characterised by recurrent attacks of abdominal pain associated with a fever lasting a few days to weeks. The number of such clinically overt attacks is unrelated to the development of renal amyloid.

Amyloid can be discerned in the renal arterial tree before there is proteinuria. When there is proteinuria focal and local glomerular lesions are present. Later there is usually a nephrotic syndrome, during the course of which renal vein thrombosis often occurs. It is thought that renal vein thrombosis is often precipitated by treating the oedema too vigorously with diuretics. The nephrotic syndrome, which may occur in any form of amyloidosis is particularly severe, for the hypoproteinaemia may not only be due to the proteinuria but also to a decreased rate of protein synthethis as a consequence of hepatic amyloidosis, and also to an impaired absorption of amino-acids because of the amyloid deposits in the small bowel. Finally as the patient becomes uraemic, the proteinuria tends to continue unabated.

Terminal renal failure occurs within one to three years of the onset of the nephrotic syndrome.

## Senile amyloidosis

Senile amyloidosis in which the amyloid material may be some substance other than AL or AA is mainly deposited in the heart and rarely gives rise to any clinical renal disturbance.

### Differential diagnosis of renal amyloidosis

If the diagnosis is suspected, a renal biopsy should settle the diagnosis. It is unlikely to be overlooked if all biopsies which show any deposits of eosinophilic material are stained for amyloid. When performing a renal biopsy the rubbery consistency of the kidney increases the risk of bleeding. If the diagnosis is suspected therefore it is preferable to try and make the diagnosis on a rectal biopsy. But it is important to note that a rectal biopsy is only useful if it contains a few vessels. A 'negative' report in the absence of vessels is most misleading.

Occasionally any form of renal amyloidosis can present as acute renal failure due to a renal vein thrombosis. The thrombosis begins in the intra-renal vessels and extends medially.

There is an impression that hypertension occurs less often, comes on later and is less severe in renal amyloid than in other forms of renal failure. This is probably due to a few patients who have amyloid deposits in their sympathetic chains. This may eventually cause hypotension. 'In chronic renal failure, the persistence of postural hypotension, in spite of the administration of large amounts of salt, is amyloid' is a useful aphorism. In a few patients a heavy deposit of amyloid around the collecting duct has caused difficulty in reabsorbing water and the patients have suffered from severe polyuria and polydipsia for many years.

### Treatment

The treatment of the amyloidosis is primarily the treatment of the associated condition when this is known and possible. In experimental casein loaded animals the administration of colchicine prevents the accumulation of amyloid. For this reason colchicine has been given to patients with amyloidosis, particularly those with mediterranean recurrent fever. The effect of colchicine on the amyloid deposits is debatable but its beneficial effects on the disabling bouts of abdominal pain, the proteinuria and nephrotic syndrome, have been startling. The painful crises have disappeared and proteinuria has often diminished considerably with resolution of the nephrotic syndrome. It is doubtful if the renal deposits have regressed but there is a strong impression that the colchicine slows the rate of progression and may sometimes halt deterioration. The dose starts at 0.5 mg daily and is raised slowly to 1 mg t.d.s. Children appear to need the *same* dose without adjustment for weight. The main side effects are diarrhoea and a reversible azoospermia. 10% of patients are resistant to the beneficial effects of colchicine.

Amyloid fibrils in vitro can be denatured by dimethyl suphoxide (DMSO) and in experimental animals amyloid deposits have been shown to 'move' from the liver and spleen to the kidney. DMSO has therefore been tried in human amyloid and claims have been made that this resulted in an increase in the urinary excretion of AA fibrils. It is unlikely, however, that DMSO will ever be used extensively unless the patient, and his near ones, are anosmic. One dose of DMSO gives the breath a repulsive odour for one week, due to the exhalation of methyl sulphide.

Serial renal biopsies from adult patients with rheumatoid arthritis suggest that once renal amyloidosis is sufficiently severe to cause some impairment in renal function, the renal lesions are irreversible. Treatment with adrenal steroids may produce a remission of symptoms, and proteinuria may cease, but the renal lesions remain.

In general patients with amyloidsois do not do well on haemodialysis because of the difficulties with hypotension and vascular access into arteries and veins containing amyloid. Grafts develop amyloid deposits within a few months. On the other hand some authorities have claimed that as long as the heart is not clinically involved and the urinary excretion of light chains can be controlled the prognosis with maintenance haemodialysis and transplantation is similar to that of other patients. One's own small experience has been less fortunate. It is interesting that in mediterranean recurrent fever maintenance haemodialysis seems to prevent the painful crises, but that they recur when the patient receives a transplant.

BIBLIOGRAPHY

Barclay G P T, Cameron H MacD, Loughridge L W 1960 Amyloid disease of the kidney and renal vein thrombosis. Quart J Med N S 29: 137
Beer de F C, Fagan E A, Hughes G R V et al 1983 Serum amyloid A protein concentration in inflammatory diseases and its relationship to the incidence of reactive systemic amyloidosis. Lancet 1: 231
Bell E T 1933 Amyloid disease of kidneys. Amer J Path 9: 185
Bladen H A, Nylen M U, Glenner G G 1966 The ultrastructure of human amyloid as revealed by negative staining technique. J Ultrastruct Res 14: 449
Durie B G M, Persky B, Soehnlen B J et al 1982 Amyloid production in human myeloma stem-cell culture, with morphologic evidence of amyloid secretion by associated macrophages. New Eng J Med 307: 1689
Editorial 1980 Treatment of renal amyloidosis. Lancet 1: 1062
Heptinstall R H 1974 Amyloidosis, multiple myeloma, Waldenstrom's macroglobulinaemia, mixed IgG–IgM cryoglobulinaemia and benign monoclonal gammopathy. In: Pathology of the kidney. Little Brown, Boston, ch 20, p 737
McGekee H A, Gordon Walker W, Yardley J H 1963 Renal involvement in myeloma, amyloidosis, systemic lupus erythematosus and other disorders of connective tissue. In: Strauss M B, Welt L G (eds) Disorders of the kidney. Churchill, London, p 575

Metaxas P 1981 Familial mediterranean fever and amyloidosis. Kidney Int 20: 676

Rosenthal C J, Franklin E C 1975 Variation with age and disease of an amyloid A protein-related serum component. J Clin Invest 55: 746

Rosenthal C J, Sullivan L 1978 Serum amyloid A evidence for its origin in polymorphonuclear leukocytes. J Clin Invest 62: 1181

Ogg C S, Cameron J S, Williams D G et al 1981 Presentation and course of primary amyloidosis of the kidney. Clin Nephrol 15: 9

# 28

# Scleroderma

The generalised form of scleroderma not only affects the skin but also the gastro-intestinal tract, the lungs, the heart and the kidney.

*Pathology*

Renal lesions are uncommon. They consist mainly of a striking thickening of the intralobular arteries and afferent arterioles. One type of thickening consists of intimal proliferation. This may be found in renal biopsies obtained many years before death.

The other lesions develop in the last few weeks of life and rapidly cause the death of the patient from renal failure. The kidneys are swollen and pale, while the cut surface shows a mottled congestion of the cortex which is due to a patchy necrosis. The necrotic lesions are due to occlusion of the proximal portions of many intralobular arteries by a mucoid substance which lies in concentric layers in the intima. The distal parts of some of the intralobular arteries and the afferent glomerular arterioles also show necrosis and fibrinoid changes. These lesions are indistinguishable from those found in malignant hypertension and post-partum haemolytic uraemic syndrome. Isolated polyarteritic lesions and 'wireloop' lesions have also been described, but both changes are inconstant. There are no immunofluorescent deposits.

*Clinical features*

Proteinuria may be present for many years. This is usually associated with some reduction in renal blood flow but little impairment in renal function. Once renal function begins to deteriorate terminal renal failure usually follows within a few weeks. Some patients develop a catastrophic rise in blood pressure. They present with convulsions and rapidly go into coma. Other patients may develop renal failure without hypertension, and yet others may have hypertension and some degree of renal failure which does not progress. Occasionally, the acute deterioration of renal function appears to have been provoked by the use of adrenal steroids, when these have been used to alleviate some of the other symptoms of scleroderma.

## Treatment

It has been claimed that acute rapidly progressive renal failure can sometimes be reversed by intensive efforts to control the blood pressure. This has been done with a variety of drugs including methyldopa, reserpine, guanethedine, hydrallazine and propranolol. More recently it has been reported that the task is made easier with captopril. Once irreversible renal failure has occurred treatment with haemodialysis and transplantation has been singularly disastrous due to the intense vasoconstriction which has made the blood pressure uncontrollable and vascular access difficult. Bilateral nephrectomy followed by maintenance haemodialysis seems to offer the best available treatment.

### BIBLIOGRAPHY

Goldsmith H J, Peters J H, Zomeno M 1963 The evolution of renal disease in scleroderma. (A clinico-pathological study based on renal biopsies.) II Int Nephrology Congress, Excerpta Medica, International Congress Series 67
Hannigan C A, Hannigan M H 1956 Scleroderma of the kidneys. Amer J Med 20: 793
Heptinstal R H 1983 Scleroderma (progressive systemic sclerosis). In: Pathology of the kidney. Little Brown, Boston, p 696
LeRoy E C, Fleischmann R M 1978 The management of renal scleroderma. Amer J Med 64: 974
Moore H C, Sheehan H L 1952 The kidney of scleroderma. Lancet 1: 68
Urai L, Nagy Z, Szinay G et al 1958 Renal function in scleroderma. Brit Med J 2: 1264 2: 1264
Wasner C, Cooke C R, Fries J F 1978 Successful medical treatment of scleroderma renal crises. New Eng J Med 299: 873

# 29

# Radiation nephritis

With the precision now available with irradiation techniques radiation nephritis is rarely seen. It has only been described in patients with malignant tumours of the testicle following irradiation of the periaortic abdominal glands, and, many years ago, after irradiating the stomach to treat peptic ulceration.

## Pathology

There is little to see with the naked eye except some fibrous tissue between the kidney and the peritoneum. The capsule, however, is free and the kidney normal in size.

Microscopically the capsule shows considerable fibrous thickening. The glomeruli are smaller than normal and the glomerular loops show replacement with variable quantities of an eosin-staining material. Many of the tubules are atrophic and they are separated by large amounts of intertubular material which in some places includes fibrous tissue.

The larger vessels show no changes, the intralobular arteries and the arterioles may show sclerotic changes, and the glomerular capillaries occasionally show necrotic lesions similar to those found in malignant hypertension. These necrotic lesions may be present in the kidney even though they are absent from other organs, and the patient has not suffered from malignant hypertension clinically.

Following irradiation of the kidneys in animals the blood pressure rises before any abnormal microscopical changes are evident. It seems probable, therefore, that the vascular lesions that are seen later are due to the hypertension; the cause of the hypertension is unknown.

## Acute radiation nephritis

### Clinical features

The onset of symptoms attributable to changes in the kidney occurs after a latent period of six to twelve months from the start of radiotherapy. The reason for this interval is not known; it is one of the most interesting points about the disease.

Symptoms develop gradually; they include oedema, dyspnoea, hypertension, headache, nausea and vomiting, lassitude, and nocturia. In most instances the patient has to retire to bed within a month. There is no clear-cut acute nephritic syndrome or nephrotic syndrome. The condition usually appears as chronic renal failure of rapid onset. In all cases there is proteinuria and hypertension, but widespread oedema and cardiac failure seem rather to follow a hypertension of increasing severity than to be an integral part of the initial disturbance. Proteinuria is rarely greater than 5 g/day and hypoproteinaemia has not been recorded. Some degree of renal failure occurs in all cases and is characteristically associated with severe anaemia.

## Course

A third to a half of the cases reported in one series died within 4–12 months of the onset of symptoms. Death was due to hypertensive cardiac failure, hypertensive fits and renal failure. The remainder survived, but continued to have proteinuria, hypertension and some diminution in glomerular filtration rate.

## Prognosis

A rise in blood urea above 33 mmol/l (200 mg per 100 ml) at some time during the first three months or the development of pleural effusions without generalised oedema are stated to be signs indicative of a poor prognosis.

The duration of the latent period, the age of the patient, and the height of the blood pressure in the first five months, have no prognostic significance.

## Treatment

It is imperative to decide if the renal damage is unilateral or bilateral, for if it is unilateral the blood pressure can be lowered by nephrectomy.

Otherwise treatment is symptomatic and includes the control of hypertension, cardiac failure, oedema and renal failure. The necessity for blood transfusions appear to be greater than in other forms of renal failure; their administration is frequently accompanied by generalised reactions.

## Chronic radiation nephritis

Some patients never develop a period of acute renal disorder, but 18 months to several years after irradiation they are found to be suffering from proteinuria, hypertension and some impairment of renal function. The cause of this form of radiation nephritis is obscure. Some cases have shown no tendency to further deterioration.

## Malignant hypertension

Occasionally there is a sudden onset of malignant hypertension. It may or may not be accompanied by renal failure. Death occurs within a few weeks.

BIBLIOGRAPHY

Hartman F W, Bolliger A, Doub H P 1927 Functional studies throughout the course of roentgen-ray nephritis in dogs. J Amer Med Ass 88: 139
Luxton R W 1953 Radiation nephritis. Quart J Med N S 22: 215
Page I H 1936 Production of nephritis in dogs by roentgen rays. Amer J Med Sci 191: 251
Thompson P L, Mackay I R, Robson G S M et al 1971 Late radiation nephritis after gastric x-irradiation for peptic ulcer. Quart J Med 40: 145
Wilson C, Ledingham J M, Cohen M 1958 Hypertension following X-irradiation of the kidneys. Lancet 1: 9

# 30

# Thrombosis of the renal artery and vein

## RENAL ARTERY THROMBOSIS

An uncommon condition which occurs in elderly patients with advanced atheromatous vascular disease who have previously suffered from cerebral or coronary thrombosis, or peripheral arterial disease or in patients with long standing auricular fibrillation who have not been placed on anticoagulants.

### Pathology

The thrombus is either in the main renal artery or it may be confined to one or two of its branches. With occlusion of the main vessel the kidney becomes smaller, pale and bloodless. If, however, some of the renal veins become thrombosed at the same time there will be localised areas of congestive and interstitial oedema.

### Clinical features

In contrast to renal vein thrombosis the outstanding presenting symptom is severe pain. The patient usually presents as an acute emergency, either abdominal, if the pain is in the flank or hypochrondrium, or cardiac or respiratory if it radiates to the lower chest. Nausea and vomiting are common.

There is acute tenderness in the renal angle and flank, but there may be no rigidity. Haematuria sometimes occurs, presumably if there is a concomitant thrombosis of the renal veins; usually there is only a modest proteinuria.

A straight X-ray of the abdomen often shows a calcified abdominal aorta and radiological or radionuclide investigations confirm that the condition is renal, for there is no evidence of renal function on the side of the pain and tenderness. At cystoscopy no urine is seen emerging from the ureteric orifice, but a retrograde pyelogram shows a normal pelvis and calcyces. Subsequently the affected kidney becomes smaller while the normal kidney becomes larger. An aortogram reveals an obstructive lesion of the renal arterial tree.

*Prognosis*

The immediate prognosis is more concerned with the functional integrity of the other organs, e.g. whether cardiac failure was present before the renal arterial thrombosis occurred.

Usually when the patient survives, the artery recanalises and renal function returns to normal. Very occasionally there is only a partial recanalisation, this produces a renal artery stenosis with the sudden onset of severe hypertension. In other patients hypertension may develop many weeks later.

*Treatment*

The patient's general condition usually precludes any measures other than those of anticoagulant therapy, rest and symptomatic treatment. Occasionally it may be necessary to remove the kidney to control the blood pressure. In a few patients, however, the renal artery has been successfully revascularised several weeks after the thrombosis has occurred. Renal function has returned, the blood pressure has fallen and the kidney has increased in size.

## RENAL VEIN THROMBOSIS

Thrombosis of the renal veins is a rare condition. The thrombus may either originate in the inferior vena cava and spread laterally into the renal veins, or more usually it begins in the smaller veins within the parenchyma of a diseased kidney and spreads medially.

*Pathology*

The usual biopsy specimen, obtained several weeks or months after the onset of the thrombosis, merely shows a few insignificant and unspecific changes. Renal biopsies performed a few days after the onset, show extensive interstitial oedema with tubular separation. The presence of fibrin within small veins is very rare.

At autopsy the diagnostic feature is the finding of a thrombus in the renal vein with, in long-standing cases, the presence of large collateral venous channel between the capsule of the kidney and the surrounding tissues. Microscopically the glomeruli appear normal and the tubules are unchanged unless there has been much proteinuria, when the tubule cells will contain lipoid material and collections of an eosin staining substance, though in some long-standing cases there is considerable tubular atrophy, tubular separation and interstitial nephritis.

Inferior vena caval thrombosis may be spontaneous, or may be due to invasion by neoplasm, or to external compression. The most common renal disease to give rise to intrarenal venous thrombosis in adults is renal amyloidosis. In infants renal vein thrombosis is often associated with acute pyelonephritis.

## Clinical features

These depend on the rapidity of the thrombotic process, whether it is unilateral or bilateral, and if it is secondary to inferior vena caval thrombosis.

When the thrombosis is rapid, bilateral, and has spread from the inferior vena cava, there is sudden back pain extending into the flanks with oliguria, proteinuria and haematuria leading to renal failure with oedema of the lower limbs and the anterior abdominal wall. Death may occur rapidly from acute renal failure.

If the thrombosis is bilateral but the inferior vena cava is unobstructed there is no oedema of the lower limbs. In adults this is usually due to renal disease. In infants acute bilateral renal vein thrombosis often follows acute gastroenteritis, when the thrombosis is presumably caused by intense renal ischaemia in otherwise normal kidneys; or it may be associated with acute pyelonephritis; there is usually sepsis elsewhere, and the sudden onset of flank tenderness and pyuria with a swing fever may suggest the diagnosis. Acute renal failure and death are the usual outcome. An intravenous pyelogram usually shows a delayed and diminished density of contrast on the affected side. Very occasionally, however, there may be a dense nephrogram lasting up to 24–36 hours. This probably occurs if the renal vein thrombosis causes severe renal damage. Notching of the upper ureter by enlarged collateral veins is often seen. These may disappear as the thrombus dissolves.

Chronic renal vein thrombosis occurs in patients who have some form of chronic renal disease usually when they are suffering from a nephrotic syndrome. At one time it was thought that it was the renal vein thrombosis that had led to various forms of chronic renal disease such as membranous glomerular nephritis. The onset of the thrombosis is often silent particularly in the elderly when it is more likely to be associated with some other form of thrombo embolic disease such as a pulmonary embolus.

The findings which suggest chronic renal vein thrombosis are, sterile pyuria, intermittent microscopic haematuria, glycosuria, renal tubular acidosis and a raised urinary excretion of fibrin degredation products.

The radiological techniques used to verify the diagnosis of renal vein thrombosis vary as described on page 18.

The clinical course probably depends on the ability to recanalise the thrombus and establish a collateral venous circulation.

## Diagnosis

The sudden onset of oliguria, proteinuria, raised blood urea, and severe oedema confined to the lower limbs, without evidence of cardiac failure or hypoproteinaemia, should make one suspect that the inferior vena cava and renal veins are thrombosed. Collateral venous channels on the anterior abdominal wall do not appear until several weeks or months after the onset, but once they are evident they greatly simplify the diagnosis in those cases of inferior vena caval and renal vein thrombosis who have survived the acute phase. Sometimes with acute thrombosis the sudden onset of flank pain and pyuria has led to a diagnosis of acute pyelonephritis. Chronic thrombosis should be suspected if a patient with a nephrotic syndrome has a sterile pyuria, glycosuria and an excess of fibrin degradation products in the urine.

## Treatment

If the onset is recognised in adults it is reasonable to give anticoagulants; otherwise treatment is usually symptomatic. There are, however, some reports of the successful surgical removal of the clot.

In infants with severe pyelonephritis a nephrectomy may prevent the spread of the septic thrombus into the inferior vena cava and across to the other kidney.

BIBLIOGRAPHY

Ehrlich A, Brodoff B N, Rubin I L et al 1953 Malignant hypertension in a patient with renal artery occlusions. Arch Intern Med 92: 591

Fergus J N, Jones N F, Lea Thomas T 1969 Kidney function after renal arterial embolism. Brit Med J 4: 587

Knorring J von, Fyhrquist F, Lindfors O et al 1976 Renin/angiotensin system in hypertension after traumatic renal artery thrombosis. Lancet 1: 934

**Renal vein thrombosis**

Barenberg L H, Greenstein N M, Levy W et al 1941. Renal thrombosis with infarction complicating diarrhoea of the new born. Amer J Dis Child 62: 362

Blainey J D, Hardwicke J, Whitfield A G 1954 The nephrotic syndrome associated with thrombosis of the renal veins. Lancet 2: 1208

Cade R, Spooner G, Juncos L et al 1977 Chronic renal vein thrombosis. Amer J Med 63: 387

Cornog J L, Rawson A J, Karp L A et al 1970 Immunofluorescent and ultrastructural study of the renal glomerulus in renal vein thrombosis. Lab Invest 22: 101

Duncan A W, Schorr E, Clark F et al 1970 Unilateral renal vein thrombosis and nephrotic syndrome. J Urol 104: 502

Llach F, Papper S, Massry S G 1980 The clinical spectrum of renal vein thrombosis. Acute and chronic. Amer J Med 69: 819

McClelland C Q, Hughes J P 1950 Thrombosis of the renal vein in infants. J Paediat 36: 214

Morris J F, Ginn H E, Thompson D D 1963 Unilateral renal vein thrombosis associated with the nephrotic syndrome. Amer J Med 34: 867

Richet G, Gillot C, Vaysse J et al 1965 La thrombose isolée de la veine rénale Presse Medicale 73: 2035

Rosenmann E, Pollak V E, Pirani C L 1968 Renal vein thrombosis in the adult. A clinical and pathological study based on renal biopsies. Medicine 47: 269

# 31

# Porphyria

Porphyria is a rare and often familial disorder of porphyrin metabolism which results in widespread abnormalities, particularly in the skin, gastrointestinal tract and central nervous system. Frequently there are acute exacerbations which may be associated with renal disturbances.

*Pathology*

Porphyrins form part of the haemoglobin molecule. In porphyria their metabolism is disturbed, so that their concentration in the blood rises and they are excreted in increased quantities both in the urine and faeces. Several types of porphyrins are involved, but during an acute attack there is one, porphobilinogen, which is always present in large amounts.

Porphobilinogen is a colourless chromogen. Its presence, however, can sometimes be suspected on naked eye examination of the urine, for its breakdown products on standing give the urine an orange or nectarine-like colour; this is usually overlooked for it is confused with the appearance of a concentrated urine. The presence of prophobilinogen is confirmed with Ehrlich's reagent (the same which is used for detecting the presence of urobilinogen). Both urobilinogen and porphobilinogen give a red colour within 20 sec; they are then differentiated by adding chloroform; if the red colour remains outside the chloroform the colour is due to porphobilinogen; if it goes into the chloroform the colour is due to urobilinogen.

Frequently, acute prophyria is associated with an increased excretion of other porphyrins which may turn the urine dark purple.

At autopsy large amounts of porphyrins can be identified in the tubule cells. These probably account for the disturbance of tubular function.

*Clinical features of acute porphyria*

Acute prophyria is often provoked by the administration of barbiturates. Its main clinical features are abdominal pain, constipation, tachycardia, hypertension and peripheral neuritis. Later, there may be coma, generalised flaccid paralysis and jaundice. In addition the most advanced cases develop an uncontrolled diuresis with extensive loss of sodium, potassium, chloride and water which may cause circulatory collapse and death. Acute intermittent porphyria is one cause of 'inappropriate secretion of antidiuretic hormone'.

## Treatment

It is imperative that barbiturates, methyl dopa, sulphonamides and griseofulvin should not be given to patients who suffer from porphyria. To make sure of this the patient should be given a card on which it is clearly stated that she is suffering from porphyria and that these drugs, particularly barbiturates, must not be administered, however anxious and mentally disturbed the patient may appear.

Haemodialysis is a useful way to treat acute porphyria whether or not there is an associated acute renal failure, for it lowers the concentration of circulating porphyrins. Otherwise it is important to replace rapidly the water and electrolytes which may be aggravating the deterioration of renal function.

BIBLIOGRAPHY

Eales L et al 1963. The porphyrias. South African J Clin and Lab Med 9: 5, 81, 126, 143, 151, 162, 190, 347
Goldberg A, Rimington C 1955 Experimentally produced porphyria in animals. Proc Roy Soc B 143: 257
Linder G C 1947 Salt metabolism in acute porphyria. Lancet 2: 649
Nielsen B, Thorn N A 1965 Transient excess urinary excretion of antidiuretic material in acute intermittent porphyria with hyponatraemia and hypomagnesaemia. Amer J Med 38: 345
Prunty F T G 1949 Sodium and chloride depletion in acute porphyria with reference to the status of adrenal corticol function. J Clin Invest 28: 690
Rees H A, Goldberg A, Cochrane A L et al 1967, Renal haemodialysis in porphyria. Lancet I: 919
Watson C J, Schwartz S 1941, Simple test for urinary porphobilinogen. Proc Soc Exp Biol Med (NY) 47: 393
Whittaker S R F, Whitehead T P 1956 Acute and latent porphyria. Lancet 1: 547

# 32

# Haemoglobinuria and myoglobinuria

Haemoglobinuria is the term used for the appearance of free haemoglobin in the urine. It follows haemolysis of red cells, either in the blood stream or in the urine.

Free haemoglobin is about the biggest naturally occurring molecule that can pass freely through the normal glomerular membrane (mol wt 68 000). Haemoglobin in plasma is normally bound to protein and is present in a concentration of about 50 mg/l. In a normal individual there is sufficient haemoglobin binding protein (haptoglobins) to bind concentrations of haemoglobin up to 1.0–1.25 g/l. The bound haemoglobin does not pass through the glomerulus. The unbound or free form of haemoglobin passes readily through the glomerulus, some is reabsorbed in the proximal tubule, and the rest promptly appears in the urine. Tubular reabsorption of haemoglobin is always associated with haemosiderinuria, for as the haemo-globin is processed through the tubule cell some of the molecule is converted into haemosiderin and excreted into the urine. Haemosiderinuria will there-fore be present when there is free haemoglobin in the plasma whether or not there is haemoglobinuria.

Myoglobin is a muscle protein with a molecular weight of 17 000; it is freely filtered through the glomerulus, and little seems to be reabsorbed by the tubule; it first appears in the urine when the plasma concentration is about 100 mg/l, and its rate of excretion is extremely rapid. For this reason it is rarely detected in the blood.

## Methods of Identification

### Haemoglobin and myoglobin

These can be identified in solution, either spectroscopically or by the colour that is produced when they react with toluidine. A few milligrammes of purified toluidine hydrochloride are dissolved in 5 ml of glacial acetic acid; 1 ml of this solution and 1 ml of freshly prepared hydrogen peroxide are added to 2 ml of urine. The presence of haemoglobin or myohaemoglobin in considerable amounts will turn the urine blue; a lesser amount will only produce a green colour. If, in the presence of such a positive test in the urine, a simultaneous sample of blood is obtained and centrifuged and the supernatant plasma is pink the material in the urine is haemoglobin whereas if the plasma is not pink the urine contains myoglobin. False positive tests may occur if the urine is highly infected, and false negative tests may be due to the urine containing large amounts of ascorbic acid.

## Haemosiderin

In contrast to haemoglobin and myohaemoglobin which are in solution, haemosiderin in the urine is present in particulate form, either in disintegrating tubule cells or as amorphous debris. The test for haemosiderinuria consists, therefore, in using the Prussian blue reaction to stain the urine sediment. About 20 ml of urine is centrifuged and all but 1 ml of the supernatant fluid is discarded. 1 ml of 5% hydrochloric acid and 0.5 ml of a 10% aqueous solution of potassium ferrocyanide are then added to the 1 ml of urine in which the deposit has been resuspended. A drop is then examined under the microscope, when haemosiderin will appear as deep blue flecks lying free or within the tubule cells and casts.

## Renal changes associated with haemoglobinuria

### Changes associated with acute haemoglobinuria

Large amounts of haemoglobin have been given experimentally both to normal man and animals. There are either no adverse effects on the kidneys or a transient reduction in glomerular filtration rate. Renal blood flow is unchanged through PAH clearance falls. There is also a tansient fall in urine flow.

Under clinical conditions, however, haemoglobinuria is occasionally associated with acute renal failure. This is because the most common cause of acute renal failure associated with haemoglobinuria is the administration of incompatible blood. Though the associated haemoglobinuria facilitates the onset of the acute renal failure by blocking the collecting ducts (see below) the main determinant of the failure is the presence of the stroma of the destroyed incompatible red cells in the circulation. The patient's antibody fixes onto the blood group antigen on the membrane of the incompatible erythrocyte membrane to form a complex which causes intense renal ischaemia and acute renal failure. In addition to this immunological disturbance several other closely connected factors are responsible for the renal failure that follows clinical haemoglobinuria. Pre-existing oligaemia or dehydration are usually present, which causes renal vasoconstriction with an acute reduction in glomerular filtration rate. There is also a high concentration of circulating anti-diuretic hormone (ADH). This combination causes a maximal reabsorption of water from the glomerular filtrate so that the haemoglobin in the tubule lumen is highly concentrated; it then precipitates and causes obstruction of the nephron.

The pathological changes have been described in Chapter 11. There are focal areas of tubular necrosis, haemcasts and occasional collections of interstitial inflammatory cells. Large amounts of haemosiderin may be found in the tubule cells.

### Changes associated with chronic haemoglobinuria

There are two functional changes; proteinuria and persistent haemosiderinuria. Structurally the accumulation of haemosiderin in the tubule cell appears to be the only change which is specifically due to the haemoglobinuria. In addition, haemoglobin appears in the urine at lower plasma concentration of haemoglobin than in acute haemoglobinaemia. Following several haemoglobinuric crises haemoglobin may appear in the urine when the plasma concentration is only 250 mg/l. This is because the normal rate of production of haemoglobin binding protein is insufficient to keep up with the large quantities of haemoglobin that are liberated.

### Aetiology

The following conditions may cause haemoglobinuria:
   *Following intravascular haemolysis*:
1. Exercise:
   a. very strenuous exercise
   b. march haemoglobinuria
2. Mismatched transfusion
3. Paroxysmal nocturnal haemoglobinuria
4. Blackwater fever
5. Hypotonicity of the plasma (prostatic surgery)
6. Thermal and chemical injuries
7. Paroxysmal cold haemoglobinuria
8. Heat stress.

Other common causes of haemolysis, such as congenital spherocytosis or acquired haemolytic anaemia due to abnormal serum antibodies, rarely cause haemoglobinuria, for the rate of destruction is slower and the site of haemolysis is in the reticulo-endothelial system.

   *Following haemolysis in the urine*:
1. Any cause of haematuria when the specific gravity of the urine is below 1.007
2. Renal infarction.

# HAEMOGLOBINURIA FOLLOWING INTRAVASCULAR HAEMOLYSIS

## Exercise

Any normal person who undergoes sufficiently severe and prolonged strenuous exercise will have haemoglobinuria and proteinuria. This has been shown particularly in marathon runners. It is a benign complication of strenuous exercise, with no late sequelae.

There are in addition certain individuals who develop considerable haemoglobinuria and proteinuria upon performing any moderate exercise, e.g. a brisk walk, or a short run. The cause of the phenomenon is unexplained. It is due to intravascular haemolysis which only occurs in the upright posture; vigorous exercise taken in the horizontal posture does not produce haemoglobinuria. It is a benign condition sometimes associated with increased aminoaciduria, and is known as march haemoglobinuria. There is no treatment. There are spontaneous fluctuations in the tendency to haemolyse; when relapses occur physical exercise should be curtailed. They can sometimes be prevented by putting sponge rubber insoles into the shoes, the implication being that haemolysis may result from damage to red cells in the soles of the feet.

## Mismatched transfusion

In temperate climates, this is the most common cause of haemoglobinuria to be followed by acute renal failure. Plasma concentrations of haemoglobin may rise to 10 g/l or more; there is fever, shivering, severe pains in the back, hypotension and discoloured urine.

Transfusions are most frequently given because of recent loss of blood. If, when blood is being administered, the patient develops symptoms which suggest that haemolysis is taking place, the transfusion should be stopped immediately. A sample of the *patient's blood* is then centrifuged and the supernatant plasma examined by naked eye for the presence of haemoglobin. If the plasma is not pink, then haemolysis is not the cause of the patient's symptoms and the administration of blood should be continued with a fresh bottle of blood. The previous bottle may have contained some other protein which caused the patient's reaction; it may, for example, have been infected. This is insufficient reason for abandoning the attempt to replace the lost blood.

If, however, the plasma clearly contains haemoglobin, then no further blood transfusions should be given. It is essential nevertheless to try and overcome the renal vasoconstriction of the oligaemia, and a plasma expander such as Dextran should be given in as large amounts as possible, e.g. about one to two litres. If this causes severe anaemia (as opposed to oligaemia) the patient should be placed in an oxygen tent, for by increasing the plasma oxygen tension there may be sufficient improvement in his general condition to influence the extent of renal damage. It has been claimed that acute renal failure following mismatched transfusion can be avoided or cut short by immediate exchange transfusion. Cannulae are placed in the radial artery and cephalic vein, and the exchange begun with a litre of a plasma expander. It is continued with properly cross-matched blood. The duration of the exchange is determined by the concentration of the circulating haemoglobin in the plasma. An exchange of 5 to 8 litres can reduce the circulating concentration from about 8 g to 1 g/l. In addition to eliminating the haemoglobin, exchange transfusion has added advantages in that it removes the circulating immune complexes and it supplies large quantities of fresh haemoglobin binding protein, so that a high proportion of the haemoglobin that remains is bound to protein and not filtrable.

## Paroxysmal nocturnal haemoglobinuria

This is a rare disease characterised by an acquired abnormality of the red cells which greatly shortens their survival. Unlike most other causes of abnormal red cell destruction the cells in paroxysmal nocturnal haemoglobinuria are destroyed in the plasma, as opposed to the reticulo-endothelial system. This gives rise to high plasma concentrations of haemoglobin. The haemolytic process is particularly severe during sleep, so that the urine may be purple in the morning but a normal colour by evening. If the patient sleeps during the day the process is reversed. It has been demonstrated that the acceleration of haemolysis that occurs during sleep is not due to any accompanying change in plasma pH that may occur at that time.

The disease becomes manifest usually between the ages of 20 and 40, and occurs equally in both sexes. The tendency to haemolyse fluctuates, and during relapses haemoglobinaemia is continuous, though haemoglobinuria comes on in sudden sharp attacks. In addition to the discoloured urine these acute episodes are associated with headache, backache, muscular and abdominal pains. Acute haemolytic crises are sometimes brought on by mild infections. There may be severe anaemia and there is a continuous reticulocytosis; eventually the patient develops a pale brown pigmentation. Occasionally there may be remissions of a few weeks or months when the total blood haemoglobin concentration returns to normal, but haemosiderinuria continues uninterruptedly. Death usually occurs from thrombosis of visceral veins including the mesenteric, splenic and renal.

The anaemia cannot be treated with transfusions of ordinary blood, for these cause an intense haemolysis of the *patient's* red cells. This reaction is due to some substance present in the donated plasma, and can be avoided by giving red cells washed and suspended in saline.

## Blackwater fever

This complication of malignant tertian malaria usually occurs in those who have previously been treated with antimalarial drugs, particularly quinine, either prophylactically or for recurrent attacks of malaria. There is a sudden and severe haemolysis of unknown cause, sometimes followed by acute renal failure.

## Hypotonicity of plasma

Transurethral resections of the prostate are usually carried out with intermittent washouts of the bladder and urethra with water. If much water is absorbed during this procedure there may be haemolysis near the site of absorption, where the plasma osmolality is grossly reduced; there is haemoglobinaemia and, occasionally, haemoglobinuria; sometimes acute renal failure may develop.

## Thermal and chemical injuries

Patients with severe burns may develop haemoglobinaemia and haemoglobinuria from destruction of the red cells contained in or near the affected areas. Acute renal failure occurs quite frequently and, though this is mainly due to renal ischaemia from the reduced blood volume, it is obvious that a superimposed haemoglobinaemia will only make its development more likely.

Arsine causes spherocytosis and acute haemolysis. Death from severe anaemia may occur a few hours later. The gas is produced when certain metals and acids containing arsenic come into contact.

Other chemicals which sometimes cause severe haemolysis and haemoglobinuria include naphthalene (moth balls), sulphonamides, mephanesin, quinine, fava beans, sodium chlorate and phenol.

## Paroxysmal cold haemoglobinuria

This condition is characterised by sudden attacks of haemolysis which follow the cooling of a part or the whole of the body. It is due to an autohaemolysin which only becomes attached to the red cells at body temperatures below normal. When such red cells circulate to parts of the body with a normal temperature they are haemolysed. Severe attacks are associated with rigors, fever and anaemia; acute renal failure can occur.

This disorder occurs in congenital and aquired syphilis, and sometimes follows certain acute infections such as 'virus pneumonia'.

## Heat stress

This condition is due to a combination of heat stress and physical exercise. It is most often seen in recruits training in the summer. There is diffuse destruction of muscle with raised serum creatine kinase, aldolase, lactic dehydrogenase and serum glutamic oxaloacetic transaminase, with normal liver function tests. Acute renal failure develops together with persistent fever, in the absence of infection. Hypercatabolism and hyperkalaemia during the period of anuria are particularly striking. The kidneys are enlarged but show no lesions of the glomeruli or of tubular necrosis. The most consistent finding is the presence of pigmented casts in the lumina of the distal tubules, the collecting ducts and the thin limb of the loops of Henle.

## HAEMOGLOBINURIA FOLLOWING HAEMOLYSIS IN THE URINE

If there is haematuria and the urine concentration falls below approximately SG 1.007 the red cells will haemolyse and there will be free haemoglobin in the urine. This is only important as a diagnostic trap. It will be recognised if the urine specific gravity is measured, and the deposit examined microscopically for red cells and casts.

It has been reported that acute renal infarction may be associated with unilateral haemoglobinuria.

## MYOGLOBINURIA

### Renal changes associated with myoglobinuria

There is no doubt that myoglobinuria may by itself cause acute renal failure. This has been clearly demonstrated in a patient who was being extensively investigated in hospital. Myoglobinuria could be induced by exercise. Following a particularly severe bout of exercise the patient developed acute renal failure and was oliguric for 14 days. Fortunately he recovered.

Usually when acute renal failure develops in combination with myoglobinuria the cause of the failure is as obscure and complicated as in haemoglobinuria. For instance, myoglobinaemia, myoglobinuria and acute renal failure can occur in crush injuries. But injuries are associated with acute renal failure in the absence of myoglobinuria. The importance of the myoglobinuria in the aetiology of acute renal failure following injury has always been, and is likely to remain, problematical.

The cause of the renal failure which follows myoglobinuria is not clear. Widespread tubular obstruction must be one of the factors, for casts of precipitated myoglobin can be seen in the tubular lumens.

### Clinical features

Myoglobinuria results from rapid destruction of muscle. This may follow some obvious cause such as crush injuries, high voltage shock or localised muscle necrosis due to postural pressure during coma (e.g. barbiturate overdose, alcoholic intoxication, or hypothermia); it has also been described with sudden arterial occlusion and after severe convulsions. The other causes of acute muscle destruction are various biochemical disturbances which are not understood. One is said to be due to allergy to sea food, another is a variant of muscular dystrophy; and the most common is that known as idiopathic paroxysmal myoglobinuria.

## Idiopathic paroxysmal myoglobinuria

The tendency to attacks fluctuates, but it is unusual to have more than one attack a year. They are usually precipitated by strenuous exercise. The patient wakes up complaining of severe pain and stiffness in those muscles which were involved in the exercise, and that his urine is dark brown. On examination, the affected muscles are firm, tender and exquisitely painful upon being stretched. Walking may not be possible. The urine is dark but clear. The diagnosis can be made in the ward by finding that the substance in the urine is toluidine positive, i.e. that the urine contains large quantities of either haemoglobin or myohaemoglobin, when the plasma has a normal colour. It follows that the substance in the urine is myoglobin for if it were haemoglobin the plasma would be pink from haemoglobinaemia. Myoglobin is never present in the plasma in sufficient quantities to discolour it, for as it is not bound to protein and easily filtered at the glomerulus, it is rapidly excreted.

BIBLIOGRAPHY

**Haemoglobinuria**
Blackburn C R B, Hensley W J, Kerr Grant D et al 1954 Studies on intravascular haemolysis in man. The pathogenesis of the initial stages of acute renal failure. J Clin Invest 33: 825
Crosby W H 1953 Paroxysmal nocturnal haemoglobinuria. Relation of the clinical manifestations to underlying pathogenic mechanisms. Blood 8: 769
Goldberg M 1962 Studies on the acute renal effects of hemolyzed red blood cells in dogs including estimations of renal blood flow with krypton. J Clin Invest 41: 2112
Goldberg M 1962 Acute haemoglobinuric renal failure without ischaemia. J Clin Invest 41: 2112
Ham T H 1955 Haemoglobinuria. Amer J Med 18: 990
Hutt M P, Reger J F, Neustein H B 1961 Renal pathology in paroxysmal nocturnal haemoglobinuria. Amer J Med 31: 736
Landsteiner E K, Finch C A 1947 Haemoglobinaemia accompanying transurethral resection of the prostate. New Engl J Medicine 237: 310
Lathem W 1959 The renal excretion of haemoglobin; regulatory mechanisms and the differential excretion of free and protein-bound haemoglobin. J Clin Invest 38: 652
Lippman R W 1957 Urine and the urinary sediment, 2nd edn. Thomas, Springfield
McDonald R K, Miller J H, Roach E B 1951 Human glomerular permeability and tubular recovery values for haemoglobin. J Clin Invest 30: 1041
MacKenzie G M 1929 Paroxysmal haemoglobinuria, a review. Medicine 8: 159
Miller J H, McDonald R K 1951 The effect of haemoglobin on renal function in the human. J Clin Invest 30: 1033
Schmidt P J, Holland P V 1967 Pathogenesis of the acute renal failure associated with incompatible transfusion. Lancet 2: 1169

Schrier R W, Henderson H S, Tisher C G et al 1967 Nephropathy associated with heat stress and exercise. Ann Intern Med 67: 356

Spicer A J 1970 Studies on March haemoglobinuria Brit Med J 1: 155

Sussman R M, Kayden H J 1948 Renal insufficiency due to paroxysmal cold hemoglobinuria. Arch Intern Med 82: 598

Yuile C L, Van Zandt T F, Ervin D M et al 1949 Haemolytic reaction produced in dogs by transfusion of incompatible dog blood and plasma. Blood 4: 1232

**Myoglobinuria**

Blondheim S H, Margoliash E, Shafir E 1958 A simple test for myohemoglobinuria. J Amer Med Ass 167: 453

Hed R 1955 Myoglobinuria in man with special reference to familial form. Acta Med Scand Suppl 303, 151: 1

Spaet T H, Rosenthal M C, Damesher W 1954 Idiopathic myoglobinuria in man. Blood 9: 881

Wheby M S, Miller H S Jr 1960 Idiopathic paroxysmal myoglobinuria. Amer J Med 29: 599

# 33

# Congenital macroscopic structural lesions of the kidney

The term 'macroscopic' is inserted in the title of this section in order to exclude the congenital microscopic structural lesions of the tubules which are associated with innate functional defects (p. 350).

The following malformations will be discussed:

Renal agenesis
  a. bilateral
  b. unilateral
Renal hypoplasia
  a. bilateral
  b. unilateral (dwarfed kidney)
Renal ectopia
Anomalies due to fusion
  a. Horseshoe kidneys
  b. unilateral fused kidney, crossed renal ectopia
Duplication of pelvis and ureter
Cystic disease of the kidneys
  a. polycystic kidneys
  b. solitary cysts
  c. cystic disease of the medulla
  d. sponge kidneys.

## RENAL AGENESIS

### Bilateral agenesis

Bilateral agenesis is not compatible with life, though occasionally the infant may live for two to three days. Not only are the kidneys absent but the ureters are often rudimentary. Other congenital abnormalities, such as spina bifida, are always present. Bilateral agenesis can sometimes be suspected during pregnancy for it is often associated with oligohydramnios.

*Clinical note.* Unilateral congenital renal structural abnormalities are often associated with a homolateral illshaped external ear. There may only be some prominence, shortening or absence of the lobe, or there may be severe distortion. This can sometimes be a useful clue in a child with a fever of unknown origin.

### Unilateral agenesis

Unilateral agenesis (Fig. 33.2) is more common than bilateral agenesis and may not be discovered until autopsy for some other disease. It occurs equally in both sexes and is more frequent on the left side. The remaining kidney hypertrophies and often weighs as much as a normal pair of kidneys. Other associated congenital abnormalities may be found; in children gross abnormalities, such as meningocoele are not infrequent; in adults they are found less often and occur mainly in the genital tract, for instance, there may be a bicornuate or a double uterus.

## RENAL HYPOPLASIA

### Bilateral hypoplasia

Bilateral hypoplasia usually causes death shortly after birth. Very rarely it may produce a state of chronic renal failure after two to three years of life.

### Unilateral hypoplasia

Unilateral hypoplasia has to be differentiated from acquired unilateral disease, for chronic urinary obstruction or infection may also result in a remarkably small kidney. As this differentiation is sometimes very difficult, the term *unilateral dwarfed kidney* is used to include those kidneys which are unequivocally hypoplastic, and those in which hypoplasia is the most likely diagnosis.

By combining the incidence of unilateral agenesis and hypoplasia, Bell calculated from his autopsy records that in persons over one year of age the chance of there being only one kidney capable of sustaining life is about 1/200.

## RENAL ECTOPIA

Ectopic kidneys are usually situated either in the iliac fossae, including the brim of the pelvis, or in the pelvic cavity (Fig. 33.1). They occur equally in the two sexes, and are rather more common on the left side. In the iliac fossae they show no major structural alteration, but when they are in the pelvis they may be seriously distorted. Frequently the kidney is hypoplastic; the renal pelvis is usually directed forward and the ureter is often dilated and tortuous. The renal artery arises from the nearest part of the aorta or the common iliac artery.

Ectopic kidneys may function normally, but they are liable to hydronephrosis and pyelonephritis.

### Clinical features

Lower abdominal pain or discomfort, dysuria, frequency and haematuria

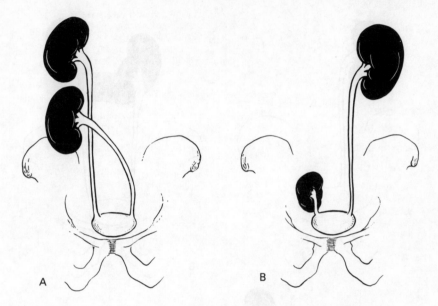

**Fig. 33.1** Renal ectopia: (A) Both kidneys on the same side, and (B) Unilateral pelvic kidney.

are the presenting symptoms; or proteinuria may be found during a routine examination. Occasionally an ectopic kidney may first be diagnosed during pregnancy and may be confused with a tumour or pelvic abscess; an intravenous pyelogram allows the right diagnosis to be made only if the kidney can excrete the radio opaque material; at other times a retrograde pyelogram or laparotomy is necessary.

Often there are other congenital abnormalities.

### Movable kidney

The mobility of the kidney may be greater than normal but it is extremely doubtful if excess mobility is ever the cause of symptoms, or makes the kidney more liable to infection or other disorders. At one time, however, numerous operations were performed to secure errant kidneys into more conventional sites. Most of the operations were performed in that notorious group of middleaged women who complain of vague abdominal pains.

## ANOMALIES DUE TO FUSION

### Horseshoe kidney

This malformation consists in the fusion of two poles of the kidneys, usually the lower poles, across the midline. The two pelves are always separate and

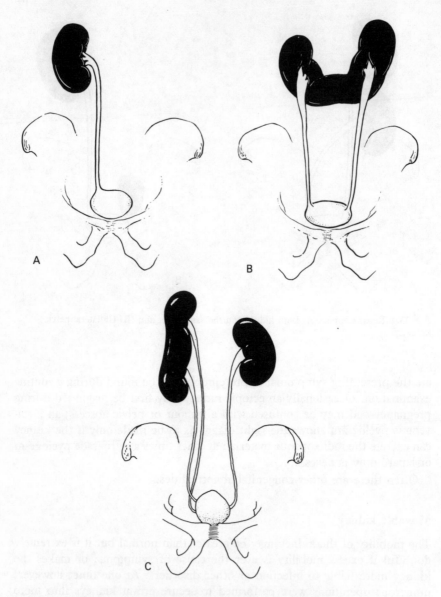

**Fig. 33.2** (A) Unilateral agenesis, (B) horsehoe kidney, (C) double ureter.

point in a forward direction, the two ureters travelling anteriorly over the surface of the lower poles (Fig. 33.2).

Horseshoe kidneys occur more frequently in males; and in persons over one year of age Bell found the incidence to be 1 : 400. There is no conclusive evidence that this abnormality is associated with a greater frequency of renal diseases than are normal kidneys.

### Unilateral fused kidney

Very rarely both kidneys may be fused together on one side of the body. Both ureters enter the bladder in their normal sites, so that one ureter has to travel across the midline and is thus more liable to cause hydronephrosis and infection.

## DUPLICATION OF PELVIS AND URETER

This anomaly is more common in women and is found most frequently on the left side; it is not unusual for it to be bilateral, when it is more extensive on one side than the other. The two ureters from one kidney may be completely separate in their course to the bladder, so that there are two ureteric orifices to one side of the midline (Fig. 33.2). At other times the two ureters fuse together either in the bladder wall or somewhere between the pelvis and the bladder. Occasionally one ureter may enter the vagina, the urethra, the seminal vesicles or the vas deferens. This is often the ureter from the upper part of the kidney while the ureter from the lower part enters the bladder in the normal place.

Duplication of the pelves and ureters is often associated with pain, hydronephrosis and recurrent urinary infection.

## CYSTIC DISEASE OF THE KIDNEYS

A malformation which may be unilateral or bilateral. Bilateral cystic disease of the kidneys is far more frequent and important clinically.

### Bilateral polycystic kidneys

This is a hereditary condition which declares itself clinically either in infancy (the neonatal form), or in middle age (the adult form); in childhood and up to the age of 20 incidence fall off to negligible proportions. The reason for this remarkable division of incidence is not known. It is possible that the two forms of the disease, though they appear almost indistinguishable structurally, may stem from different aetiologies. In favour of this theory is the fact that the adult form appears to be inherited as an autosomal dominant in families in which there are a number of other cases, whereas the neonatal form appears to be due to an autosomal recessive. There are no records of adult and neonatal cases occurring in the same family.

Both forms occur equally between the two sexes.

*Pathology*

Both kidneys tend to be considerably enlarged, though the degree of enlargement may be unequal (Fig. 33.3). Each consists of a compact mass

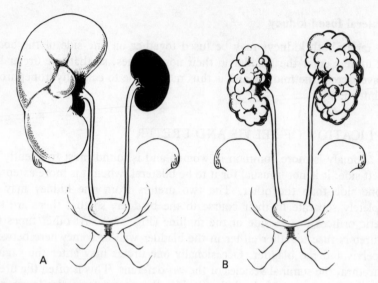

**Fig. 33.3** (A) Solitary cyst, (B) polycystic kidneys.

of cysts. On section the cysts are seen to be scattered equally in the cortex and medulla, and usually there does not seem to be any intact parenchyma. On rare occasions the cysts may be limited to one pole. In the neonatal disease all the cysts tend to be of a similar size, whereas in adults they vary considerably and some may be exceedingly large.

The cysts are filled with a watery fluid which may be clear, blood-stained from recent haemorrhage, or brown from an old haemorrhage; some may be filled with pus. They are lined by a single layer of epithelium and occasionally a normal glomerular tuft may be found invaginated into the cavity of a cyst, when the cyst is then considered to be the distended capsular space of that glomerulus. Cysts do not often communicate with the pelvis of the kidney.

It can be demonstrated that the contents of some cysts are in a continuous flux with the circulation, e.g. inulin placed in the cysts will appear in the blood and vice versa. It has been suggested therefore that the cysts have some renal 'functional' capacity, however trivial. Unless the cysts are joined to the pelvis, however, this is of no consequence whatever its extent.

Liver cysts are found in one-third of patients with polycystic kidneys and there is also a significant association with aneurysms of the cerebral arteries.

*Pathogenesis*

There are many theories but 'nothing certain is known' (Dalgaard, 1957). The identical abnormalities can be induced experimentally in animals chronically fed certain injurious substances. It is possible therefore that the disease is due to the inheritance of a metabolic defect that causes the endogenous production of such a substance.

## Clinical features

*Neonatal form.* Usually neonatal bilateral cystic kidneys cause stillbirth, and sometimes their size may cause serious difficulties during delivery. The infant may live for a few months or one to two years, only to succumb to chronic renal failure.

*Adult form.* The onset of the presenting symptoms usually occurs when the patient is about 40 years old, but the age of onset may range from 8 years to 77 years. These may be entirely renal with haematuria, clot-colic, or acute pyelonephritis, or they may be more generalised, when they are due to renal failure or hypertension. Sometimes the patient complains of abdominal distension, or pain following some relatively minor trauma. Proteinuria is always present and may be the first abnormality to draw attention to the renal disease.

Hypertension develops in about 75% of cases and is rarely malignant. As renal failure develops the usual fall in haemoglobin tends to be less pronounced than in other forms of renal disease. In some patients there is no significant fall in haemoglobin, or there may be polycythaemia. The ability to concentrate and acidify the urine is impaired early in the disease.

By the time the patient begins to complain of symptoms the kidneys are usually easily palpable and have a characteristic 'knobbly' feel. The diagnosis is confirmed by an intravenous pyelogram and an ultrasound examination. The pyelogram shows the pelvis to be elongated with the calyces stretched out, and their peripheral ends shaped into crescents of varying sizes (Fig. 33.4). Early disease with only unilateral abnormalities may be difficult to differentiate from solitary cysts or a tumour. An ultrasound examination is a considerably more sensitive technique for picking up small cysts before they are evident on a pyelogram. Renal cell carcinoma occurs in a few patients and is often bilateral. Therefore if a tumour is found on one side a thorough search should be made of the other at repeated intervals.

## Prognosis

The rate of renal impairment and the pattern of events varies enormously from patient to patient, but certain families show a tendency towards a recurring pattern.

Death is due either to chronic renal failure from compression of the renal parenchyma by the enlarging cysts, and chronic renal infection; or from hypertensive cardiac failure, and cerebrovascular accidents. Hypertensive cardiac failure is the most common immediate cause of death.

The average age of death (without the intervention of dialysis) is about 50

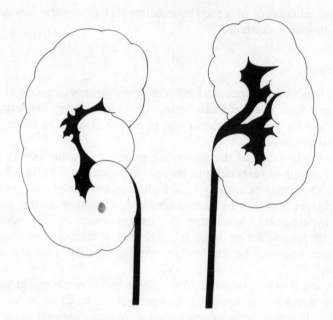

**Fig. 33.4** Polycystic kidneys. An intravenous pyelogram, illustrating the distortion of the pelvis and calyces by the cysts.

years, i.e. the average duration of the disease once it has become manifest is 5 to 10 years. There are wide variations around these means, however. If renal infections are promptly treated some patients live many years without appearing to deteriorate.

## Treatment

If the disease is almost confined to one kidney which is subject to recurrent infections and is functionally useless it may be wise to remove it, after first establishing that the function of the other kidney is adequate.

When the disease is bilateral the only measure which may cause any improvement is the evacuation of some of the larger cysts in order to relieve the pressure upon the residual parenchyma. The functional results of such operations, however, have not often been investigated; attention has been paid rather to the improvement in appearance of the intravenous pyelogram, and the continued survival of the patient. Until now there has not been a convincing demonstration that the operation will in fact prolong life; some authorities categorically deny that renal function is improved. Nevertheless, there is general agreement that the operation is sometimes useful in the relief of recurrent pain and haematuria and that occasionally it has lowered the blood pressure. It is considered that the operation should only be performed on one side at a time, for there is often a relatively severe transient post-operative deterioration in renal function.

Otherwise, treatment is symptomatic and is that of renal failure, renal infection, hypertension and cardiac failure.

If the patient suffers from migraine or has a cerebrovascular accident special attention should be given to the possibility of cerebral aneurysm. If renal function is good, prompt treatment of the aneurysm may extend life.

Patients with polycystic kidneys do exceptionally well on maintenance haemodialysis due to their tendency to pass considerable amounts of urine and to have much higher haemoglobins than patients with other renal disease. It is probably wise to perform arteriography on any patient who is being considered for transplantation. If a tumour is found, both kidneys should be removed and the patient should be kept on maintenance haemodialysis for one to three years before the transplant is performed.

## Solitary renal cysts

Small cysts are frequently found during routine autopsies; their size usually precludes them from having caused any ill effects.

Large 'solitary' cysts are rarely single, but occur in clusters of two or three (Fig. 33.3). They are more common on the right side, and more often seen in women. They may be situated in either pole, or in the middle of the kidney; nearly always they spring from the parenchyma, but occasionally they may be entirely sub-or extracapsular. The parenchyma near the cyst is always considerably compressed. They only rarely have a connection with the pelvis. The contents of the cysts contain 500–1000 ml of yellow or bloodstained fluid and sometimes considerably more. The walls of the cysts are composed of thin fibrous tissue in which a few atrophic tubules may be seen.

### Clinical features of large cysts

The main complaint is of intermittent attacks of abdominal pain interspersed by long remissions. The attacks tend to become more frequent as the years go by and the total duration of the history may be 20–30 years. The pain may be associated with fever, dysuria and occasionally with haematuria. Painless haematuria is sometimes the first symptom.

Cysts in the upper poles are particularly difficult to palpate and when on the right side may cause symptoms resembling cholecystitis. Lower-pole cysts cause gastric and intestinal symptoms, with nausea or diarrhoea; they are also liable to obstruct the ureter and cause renal infections.

The diagnosis should be evident from an intravenous pyelogram, which may show compression of the calyces and elongation of the pelvis. Often the appearances are difficult to differentiate from those of a tumour, and sometimes the radiological appearances are normal.

*Treatment*

This is surgical. If possible, a heminephrectomy is performed, otherwise a total nephrectomy is necessary.

## Cystic disease of the renal medulla

This condition is also known as familial juvenile nephronophthisis. The medulla is filled with cysts which vary in size from 100 microns to 1 cm. Eventually the cortex atrophies. Polyuria and nocturia are usually present from soon after birth but patients are often so used to these symptoms that they rarely complain of them. More frequently the presenting complaint is anaemia which is found to be is due to renal failure. Hypertension is unusual because there is a difficulty retaining sodium, which occasionally is so severe that all the features of salt wasting develop. There is a gross inability to concentrate and acidify the urine. There are no characteristic radiological findings.

Medullary cystic disease usually destroys the patient either in adolescence or early adult life. Treatment is that appropriate to chronic renal failure with particular attention to the adequacy of sodium intake.

## Sponge kidney

This is a radiological diagnosis of a relatively benign condition which is not usually diagnosed until adulthood. The I.V.P. may be performed because of a urinary infection or haematuria. The preliminary picture may show areas of calcification in the medulla. After the dye has been injected the I.V.P. shows multiple discrete opacifications in the pyramidal areas before the pelvis and calyces become opacified. The medullary opacities are grouped at the tips of the calyces and appear to branch away from them like a bouquet of flowers. It is characteristic that a retrograde pyelogram shows a completely different picture, for most of the cysts have such small connections into the calyces that they are not filled from below. There are very few descriptions of the structural changes and these are mainly from surgical specimens. They show collections of small cysts in the pyramids and medulla but the cortex is normal.

## BIBLIOGRAPHY

Baxter T J 1965 Polycystic kidney of infants and children. Nephron 2: 15
Bell E T 1946 Renal disease. Henry Kimpton, London
Bricker N S, Patton J F 1955 Cystic disease of the kidneys. Amer J Med 18: 207
Dalgaard O Z 1971 Polycystic disease of the kidneys. In: Strauss M B, Welt L G (eds) Diseases of the kidney, 2nd edn. Little Brown, Boston, p 1223
Darmady E M, Offer J, Woodhouse M A 1970 Toxic metabolic defect in polycystic disease of kidney. Lancet i: 547

De Bono D P, Evans D B 1977 The management of polycystic kidney disease with special reference to dialysis and transplantation. Quart J Med 46: 353

Friend D G, Hoskins R G Kirkin M W 1961 Relative erythrocythemia (polycythemia) and polycystic kidney disease, with uraemia. New Eng J Med 264: 17

Lambert P P 1947 Polycystic disease of the kidney. A review. Archives of Pathology 44: 34

Lufkin E G, Alfrey A C, Truckess M E et al 1974 Polycystic kidney disease. Earlier diagnosis using ultrasound. Urology 4: 5

Osathanondh V, Potter E L 1964 Pathogenesis of polycystic kidneys. Arch Path 77: 510

Potter E L 1946 Bilateral renal agenesis. J Pediat 29: 68

Rubin E L, Ross J C, Turner D P 1959 Cystic disease of the renal pyramids (sponge kidney). J Fac Radiol Lond 10: 134

Safouh M, Crocker J F S, Vernier R L 1970 Experimental cystic disease of the kidney. Sequential functional and morphologic studies. Lab Invest 23: 392

Simon H B, Thompson G J 1955 Congenital renal polycystic disease. A clinical and therapeutic study of three hundred and sixty-six cases. J Amer Med Ass 159: 657

Strauss M B 1963 Cystic disease of the renal medulla. In: Strauss M B, Welt L G J (eds) Disorders of the kidney. Churchill, London, p. 938

Suki W N 1982 Polycystic kidney disease. Kidney Int 22: 571

Whelton A 1978 Seat belts and polycystic kidneys. Lancet 2: 273

# 34

# Drugs and the kidney

The relation between drugs and the kidney is complex. The two most important aspects are that drugs may be nephrotoxic and that they may accumulate to toxic levels in renal failure.

**Nephrotoxic drugs** (Table 34.1)

There are many substances which are potentially nephrotoxic even when renal function is normal. If renal function is impaired and the excretion of the substance is so reduced that the plasma concentration of the drug rises the danger is greater. The kidney's vulnerability stems from the fact that the concentration of most substances excreted in the urine rises considerably as the urine becomes concentrated, and that the kidney often gets rid of foreign substances by tubular secretion, a process which raises the tubular intracellular concentration of the substance. The kidney is particularly at risk from any potentially toxic substance present in the blood because the renal blood flow is very great (approximately a quarter of the cardiac output), the kidney's metabolic rate is high, its endothelial surface large and its enzymatic system multitudinous. In addition, patients with renal diseases are liable to be treated with a wide variety of drugs for hypertension, bone disease, immunological disturbances, infections, gastrological upsets and neurological disturbances.

Some drugs may not be nephrotoxic but their use inevitably entails the administration of some accompanying electrolyte which may be dangerous when given in large quantities to patients with renal failure (Table 34.2).

**Drug administration in renal failure**

The majority of drugs are excreted at least in part by the kidney. If such drugs are administered in normal doses to patients with renal failure, they will, as their concentration inevitably rises to toxic levels, cause serious side effects. The dangers of giving drugs to patients with chronic renal failure can only be minimised by self-discipline, experience, and not being shy about either looking up the information, or asking the appropriate person

**Table 34.1** Nephrotoxic drugs

| Functional or structural impairment | Agent |
|---|---|
| GFR | Non steroidal inflammatory drugs e.g. indomethacin |
| Polyuria | Lithium, demeclocycline, methoxyflurane |
| *Structural and functional damage*<br>*Persistent*<br>  Arteritis | Diphenyl-hydantoin, gold salts, penicillin, propylthioracil, thiazides and sulphonamides |
| Glomerular changes<br>  Focal necrotising glomerulitis<br>  Diffuse proliferative glomerular nephritis | Hydrallazine, phenylbutazone, sulphonamides |
| Acute tubular necrosis | Many drugs including carbon tetrachloride, paraquat, ethylene glycol, amino-glycosides, ferrous sulphate, penicillin, quinine, salicylates, paracetamol, cephaloridine and cephalotin especially when given with frusemide. |
| Acute interstitial nephritis | A great many drugs including methicillin, penicillin, ampicillin, rifampicin, phenindione, sulphonamides (including Co-trimoxazole), thiazides, phenytoin. More rarely, frusemide, allopurinol, phenobarbitone, gentamicin, paracetamol etc. |
| *Acute*<br>Nephrotic syndrome with wide variety of histological changes from minimal to membranous glomerular nephritis | Penicillamine, captopril, gold salts, troxidone, tolbutamide, probenecid, phenindione, perchlorate, heroin addiction etc. |
| Systemic lupus erythematosus | Hydrallazine, isoniazid, procainamide and less frequently methylthiouracil, troxidone, reserpine, methyldopa, oral contraceptives, sulphonamides, griseofulvin, etc. |
| Papillary necrosis | Phenacetin |
| Obstructive uropathy<br>  Retroperitoneal fibrosis<br>  Intrarenal obstruction with urate cystitis | Methysergide, ergotamine, hydrallazine, dexamphetamine and methyldopa<br>Hyperuricaemia from treatment of malignancy with cytotoxic drugs or radiotherapy |

for advice. Unless one has already acquired the necessary knowledge one must be wary of giving any drug to a patient with renal failure. The following points based on Anderson, Gambertoglio and Schrier's several contributions on this subject are useful guidelines:

1. Do not use a drug in renal failure unless there is a definite indication.
2. Stop it's use as soon as possible. It is remarkable easy to continue a drug, for no better reason than that the patient is already on it.

**Table 34.2** Incidental load of electrolytes when giving drugs

| Electrolyte | Drug |
| --- | --- |
| Aluminium | Antacids used as phosphate binders |
| Magnesium | Antacids<br>Laxatives |
| Potassium | Salt substitutes |
| Sodium | Antacids, sodium-potassium exchange resins, large dose of penicillin G (sodium salt), carbenicillin, ampicillin |
| Calcium | Antacids, calcium exchange resins |
| Phosphate | Enemas, antacids |

3. If the appropriate dose has been determined in a well controlled study, its findings should be followed in preference to the use of a general formula.

Assuming a drug is totally excreted unchanged in the urine (e.g. streptomycin) the dose for a patient with renal failure can be calculated from the following formula.

$$\text{Dose for renal failure patient} = \text{Normal dose} \times \frac{\text{Patient's creatinine clearance}}{\text{Normal creatinine clearance}}$$

But most drugs are not totally excreted unchanged in the urine. Their elimination usually increases some metabolic process. In that case a reduction in renal function will obviously have less effect on the half-life of the drug. To calculate the altered dose interval if the same dose is given, or how much the dose should be reduced if the drug continues to be given at same time interval, the following modifications of the formula give useful approximations. In order to give the normal dose and change the time interval of its administration:

$$\text{Dose interval for renal failure patient} = \frac{\text{Normal dose interval}}{} \times \frac{1}{f(K_s - 1) + 1}$$

where f equals the fraction of the absorbed dose normally eliminated in an unchanged form by the kidney, and $K_s$ is a measure of the patient's renal function compared with normal renal function i.e.

$$\frac{\text{Patient's creatinine clearance}}{\text{Normal creatinine clearance}}$$

In order to change the dose and maintain the normal time interval of its administration the formula is inverted:-

$$\text{Dose for renal failure patient} = \frac{\text{Normal dose} \times f(K_s - 1) + 1}{1}$$

The dosage modification and contraindications of certain antimicrobial in patients with renal failure have been described in Table 22.2 in section 22 when discussing infection of the urine. Table 34.3 gives some information about the use of other types of drugs in renal failure.

**Table 34.3**

| Drug | Normal Dose | Route of administration | Comment | Modification of dose in renal failure |
|------|-------------|-------------------------|---------|----------------------------------------|
| *Anti tuberculous therapy* | | | | |
| Streptomycin | 1 g per day | Parenteral | Very toxic, vestibular toxity, nephrotoxicity | Avoid if possible |
| Rifampicin | 450–600 mg —per day | Oral | Relatively non toxic | None |
| INAH | 100–300 mg —per day | Oral | Toxic + peripheral neuropathy. | Modified dosage |
| Ethambutol | 1.5 g od | Oral | Optic neuritis | Avoid if possible |
| Pyrazinamide | 500 mg qds | Oral | Liver damage | Modified dosage |
| Ethionamide | 500 mg bd | Oral | Vomiting, peripheral neuropathy, liver damage | None |
| *Antifungal therapy* | | | | |
| Amphotericin B | 200 mg qds | Oral | Nausea, hypokalaemia | None |
| Flucytosine | 500 mg tds | Oral | Thrombocytopenia Leucopenia | Modified dosage |
| *Hypertensive therapy* | | | | |
| Propranolol | 100 mg tds | Oral | Cold hands | None or larger doses needed |
| Hydrallazine | 50 mg qds | Oral | SLE | Modified dosage |
| Minoxidil | 5–50 mg/day | Oral | Hirsutism Oedema | None |
| Captopril | 25 mg tds | Oral | Decrease in GFR (p. 123) | None |
| Nifedipine | 80–160 mg tds | Oral | Flushing, headaches | None |
| Verapamil | 80–160 mg tds | Oral | Flushing, headaches | None |

**Table 34.3** (contd)

| Drug | Normal Dose | Route of administration | Comment | Modification of dose in renal failure |
|---|---|---|---|---|
| *Diuretic therapy* | | | | |
| Bendrofluazide | 5–10 mg/day | Oral | Loss of potassium Impotence | Not effective with Ca > 30 ml/min |
| Frusemide | 20–40 mg | Oral | Loss of potassium | Increase dose + + with renal failure |
| Ethacrynic Acid | 50–150 mg/day | Oral | Deafness | Avoid |
| Spironolactone Triampterene Amiloride | 100–200 mg/day 150–250 mg/day 5–10 mg/day | Oral | Hyperkalaemia | Avoid |
| 70% Sorbitol | 50–100 ml 2 hourly until diarrhoea | Oral | | Most useful in an emergency |
| *Thrombo-embolic and cardiovascular therapy* | | | | |
| Heparin | — | Parenteral | Haemorrhage | N.B. drug interaction table |
| Warfarin | 3–10 mg/day | Oral | Haemorrhage | N.B. drug interaction table |
| Digoxin | — | Oral | Vomiting | Avoid |
| Digitoxin | — | Oral | Vomiting | Avoid |
| Procainamide | 250 mg 4–6hrly | Oral | Nausea, diarrhoea | None |
| Quinidine Sulphate | 200–400 mg tds | Oral | Nausea, diarrhoea | None |
| Lignocaine | 1.5–4 mg/min | Parenteral | Confusion, convulsions | None |
| *Anticonvulsants* | | | | |
| Phenytoin | 150–300 mg/day | Oral | Osteomalacia | None |
| Diazepam | 2–5 mg/day | Oral | Lethargy | None |

### Hypnotics

| Drug | Dose | Route | Side effects / Notes | Dose modification |
|---|---|---|---|---|
| Nitrazepam | 5–10 mg/day | Oral | Drowsiness, Ataxia | None |
| Chloral Hydrate | 250 mg tds | Oral | Ataxia | None |

Avoid short and medium acting barbiturates for patients with renal failure because of contamination with Barbital which accumulates when patient is on maintenance haemodialysis.

### Drugs used in psychiatry

| Drug | Dose | Route | Side effects / Notes | Dose modification |
|---|---|---|---|---|
| Tricyclic antidepressants (Amitryptyline) | 50–75 mg/day | Oral | Anticholinergic Tremor Tachycardia, hypotension | None |
| Phenothiazines (Chlorpromazine) | 25 mg/tds | Oral | Hypotension Anticholinergic | Start with low dose |
| Lithium | 0.25–2 g/day | Oral | Polyuria | Modified dose |

### Drugs used for gout

| Drug | Dose | Route | Side effects / Notes | Dose modification |
|---|---|---|---|---|
| Probenecid | — | Ineffective in renal failure | | — |
| Sulphinpyrazone | — | Ineffective in renal failure | | — |
| Allopurinol | 100–300 mg/day | Oral | | Modified dose |
| Colchicine | 0.5 mg tds | Oral | Diarrhoea | Modified dose |

### Oral Hypoglycaemic drugs

| Drug | Dose | Route | Side effects / Notes | Dose modification |
|---|---|---|---|---|
| Metformin | — | Avoid in renal failure because of lactic acidosis | | AVOID |
| Chlorpropamide | — | Oral | | Avoid |
| Tolbutamide | 0.5–2 g/day | Oral | | None |

### Analgesic and soporific drugs

| Drug | Dose | Route | Side effects / Notes | Dose modification |
|---|---|---|---|---|
| Aspirin | 300 mg/rds | Oral | | None |
| Paracetamol | 500 mg/rds | Oral | | None |
| Dextropropoxyphene | 65 mg tds | Oral | | Modified dose |
| Pentazocine | 25–100 mg 4hrly | Oral | | None |
| Opiates | — | Oral | Enhanced and prolonged activity in renal failure | Modified dose |

## Drug interactions

This is a wide subject. The following are particularly relevant to patients who suffer from renal disease:

1. Heparin inactivates hydrocortisone
2. Cimetidine, co-trimoxazole, clofibrate and allopurinol potentiate the anticoagulant effect of warfarin
3. Corticosteroids and rifampicin reduce the anticoagulant effect of warfarin
4. Rifampicin reduces the plasma concentration of corticosteriods
5. Antacids and iron depress the absorption of doxycycline
6. Azathioprine and allopurinol given together to patients with renal failure may depress the bone marrow
7. IV amino acid solutions inactivate all antibiotics in the solution
8. IV 5% dextrose inactivates the following antibiotics in the solution
   a. ampicillin
   b. kanamycin
   c. novobiocin
9. IV solutions containing dextrose, sucrose or dextran + bicarbonate rapidly inactivate penicillin
10. Heparin inactivates
    a. erythromycin
    b. kanamycin
    c. vancomycin
    d. tetracycline
    e. gentamicin
    f. streptomycin
11. Hydrocortisone sodium succinate inactivates
    a. vancomycin
    b. tetracycline
    c. kanamycin
    d. colistin
12. Vit B preparations inactivate tetracyclines.

# Appendix 1

# Some reference values

Since the previous edition was published, most laboratories in the UK have adopted SI units (Systeme International d'Unites) for the reporting of results. Accordingly, reference values for many constituents are given in SI units followed by the traditional units in the parentheses. This does not apply to monovalent ions (numerically the same in both systems) and the phosphatases for which the older units are still widely used and therefore given priority.

It must be emphasized that these reference ranges can only be regarded as a rough guide, since levels of many substances are affected by such variables as age, sex, race and diet. Furthermore, differences in analytical techniques mean that values quoted by one laboratory are not necessarily applicable to another. This is particularly true of enzyme determinations for which measured activity will depend on the choice of assay conditions.

## PLASMA CONTENTS

|  |  | Useful average |
|---|---|---|
| Albumin | 35 to 50 g/l | 40 g/l |
| Amylase (Phadebas)* | 70 to 300 iu/l | |
| Bicarbonate | 22 to 32 mmol/l | 27 mmol/l |
| Bilirubin (total) | 5 to 17 $\mu$mol/l (0.3 to 1.0 mg/100 ml) | |
| Calcium: total | 2.1 to 2.6 mmol/l (8.5 to 10.5 mg/100 ml) | 2.4 mmol/l |
| ionized | 1.09 to 1.24 mmol/l (4.4 to 5.0 mg/100 ml) | |
| Chloride | 95 to 105 mmol/l | 102 mmol/l |
| Cholesterol: total | 3.6 to 7.8 mmol/l (140 to 300 mg/100 ml) | 5.2 mmol/l |
| ester | 60 to 80% of total | |
| Complement: $C_3$ | 0.8 to 1.8 g/l | |
| $C_4$ | 0.13 to 0.43 g/l | |

| | | |
|---|---|---|
| Creatine | 15 to 46 μmol/l (0.2 to 0.6 mg/100 ml) | 30 μmol/l |
| Creatinine | 45 to 120 μmol/l (0.5 to 1.4 mg/100 ml) | 88 μmol/l |
| Fibrinogen | 2 to 4 g/l | |
| Globulin | 20 to 35 g/l | |
| Glucose (fasting) | | 4.0 mmol/l |
| capillary | 2.8 to 5.0 mmol/l (50 to 90 mg/100 ml) | |
| venous | 2.5 to 5.3 mmol/l (45 to 95 mg/100 ml) | |
| Immunoglobulins: IgA | 0.5 to 3.2 g/l | |
| IgG | 5.5 to 14.5 g/l | |
| IgM | 0.5 to 3.1 g/l | |
| Magnesium | 0.7 to 0.95 mmol/l (1.7 to 2.3 mg/100 ml) | 0.8 mmol/l |
| Osmolality | 275 to 285 mosmol/kg $H_2O$ | 280 mosmol/kg $H_2O$ |
| pH | 7.37 to 7.45 | 7.40 |
| Hydrogen ion concentration | 35.5 to 42.7 mmol/l | |
| Phosphatase: | | |
| alkaline (King Armstrong) | 3 to 13 units (21 to 94 iu/l) | |
| (Bodanski) | 1.5 to 5 units (8 to 27 iu/l) | |
| acid | | |
| a. total (King Armstrong) | 1 to 4 units (2 to 7 iu/l) | |
| b. formaldehyde stable (King Armstrong) | 0 to 2 units (0 to 4 iu/l) | |
| Phosphorus (inorganic) | 0.75 to 1.4 mmol/l (2.4 to 4.5 mg/100 ml) | 1.0 mmol/l |
| Potassium | 3.5 to 5.0 mmol/l | 4.5 mmol/l |
| Sodium | 135 to 145 mmol/l | 140 mmol/l |
| Sulphate | 0.25 to 0.5 mmol/l | |
| Urate | 100 to 300 μmol/l (2 to 5 mg/100 ml) | |
| Urea | 2.0 to 6.0 mmol/l (15 to 35 mg/100 ml) | 5.0 mmol/l |
| 25 OH Vit D | 15 to 85 nmol/l (6 to 34 ng/ml) | |
| 1,25(OH)₂Vit D | 55 to 140 pmol/l (23 to 58 pg/ml) | |

* Pharmacia diagnostics

## RENAL FUNCTIONAL CAPACITY

### Some reference values for young subjects, 1.73 m$^2$ surface area

| | |
|---|---|
| Renal plasma flow | 612 ± 68 ml/min |
| Renal blood flow | Approximately 1200 ml/min |
| Glomerular filtration rate: | |
| 1. Inulin clearance | 112 ± 15 ml/min |
| | Adult males by age groups*: |
| | 20–29 yr 123 ± 16 ml/min |
| | 50–59 yr 99 ± 15 ml/min |
| | 80–89 yr 65 ± 20 ml/min |
| 2. Creatinine clearance | Approximately the same as inulin |
| Urea clearance (at urine flows greater than 2 ml/min) | 75 ml/min |
| Maximal Tubular capacity (Tm): | |
| 1. To reabsorb glucose | 1.8 ± 0.36 mmol/min (323 ± 64 mg/min) |
| 2. To secrete PAH | 350 ± 57 $\mu$mol/min (68 ± 11 mg/min) |
| Ability to concentrate (Fluid deprivation) | 800 to 1200 mosmol/kg $H_2O$ (i.e. SG 1.022 to 1.032) |
| Ability to dilute | 40 to 80 mosmol/kg $H_2O$ (i.e. SG 1.002) |
| Ability to excrete a water load of 1 litre | 0.8 litres excreted in next 4 hours. |

* Shock NW 1946 Kidney function tests in aged males. Geriatrics I: 232

## DAILY URINARY EXCRETIONS

Twenty-four-hour output, on a mixed diet.

| | |
|---|---|
| Ammonia | 30 to 60 mmol |
| Amylase (Phadebas)* | 170 to 2000 iu/l |
| Calcium | 2.0 to 10.0 mmol (80 to 400 mg) |
| Coproporphyrin, total | 0.1 to 0.4 $\mu$mol (65 to 260 $\mu$g) |
| Chloride | 80 to 200 mmol |
| Creatine: | |
| Children | up to 1100 $\mu$mol (up to 150 mg) |
| Women | small amounts |
| Men | nil |
| Creatinine | 7 to 16 mmol (0.8 to 1.8 g) |
| Glucose | 0.1 to 0.7 mmol (16 to 132 mg) |
| Magnesium | 3 to 5 mmol (70 to 120 mg) |

| | |
|---|---|
| Phosphorus (inorganic) | 15 to 50 mmol (0.5 to 1.6 g) |
| Potassium | 30 to 100 mmol |
| pH | 4.8 to 7.4 |
| Sodium | 80 to 200 mmol |
| Titratable acid (Hydrogen ion) | 20 to 30 mmol |
| Urate | 0.6 to 12.0 mmol (0.1 to 2.0 g) |
| Urea | 270 to 580 mmol (16 to 35 g) |
| Urobilinogen | Less than 3.4 umol (Less than 2 mg) |
| Volume | 1.0 to 2.0 litres |

* Pharmacia diagnostics

## BODY CONTENTS OF SODIUM AND POTASSIUM, RED CELL MASS AND FLUID VOLUMES IN WHITE SUBJECTS OF AVERAGE HEIGHT AND WEIGHT

| | Males | Females |
|---|---|---|
| Total exchangeable sodium | 3010 mmol | 2295 mmol |
| Total exchangeable potassium | 3395 mmol | 2310 mmol |
| Plasma volume. | 2.95 l | 1.92 l |
| Red cell mass. | 1.97 l | 1.12 l |
| Extracellular fluid | 17.5 l | 13.6 l |
| Intracellular fluid | 22.2 l | 15.0 l |
| Total body water | 39.7 l | 28.6 l |

## APPROXIMATE COMPOSITION OF VARIOUS BODY FLUIDS

| Fluid | $HCO_3$ mmol/l | Cl mmol/l | P mmol/l | Na mmol/l | K mmol/l | Protein g/l | Water g/l |
|---|---|---|---|---|---|---|---|
| Serum | 27 | 102 | 1.0 | 140 | 4.5 | 70 | 940 |
| Interstitial fluid | 28 | 111 | — | 145 | 3.3 | trace | 993 |
| Spinal fluid | 21 | 125 | — | 140 | 2.8 | 0.3 | 993 |
| Gastric juice | — | 145 | — | 50 | 12.0 | mucus | 993 |
| Bile | 38 | 108 | — | 150 | 5.0 | mucus | 990 |
| Pancreatic juice | 110 | 40 | — | 140 | 5.0 | mucus | 993 |
| Jejunal juice | 30 | 110 | — | 138 | 5.0 | mucus | 993 |
| Sweat | — | 40 | — | 42 | — | — | 993 |
| Intracellular fluid: skeletal muscle; | | mmol/kg | mmol/kg | mmol/kg | mmol/kg | g/kg | |
| amounts per kg of intracellular water | — | 3 | 50 | 7 | 155 | 306 | |

The composition of sweat may vary considerably

## CONVERSION OF TRADITIONAL INTO SI UNITS

|  | Mol/atomic weight | Traditional units | SI units | Conversion factor |
|---|---|---|---|---|
| Bilirubin | 585 | mg/100 ml | $\mu$mol/l | 17.1 |
| Calcium | 40 | mg/100 ml | mmol/l | 0.25 |
| Cholesterol | 387 | mg/100 ml | mmol/l | 0.0258 |
| Creatine | 131 | mg/100 ml | $\mu$mol/l | 76.3 |
| Creatinine | 113 | mg/100 ml | $\mu$mol/l | 88.4 |
| Glucose | 180 | mg/100 ml | mmol/l | 0.056 |
| Magnesium | 24 | mg/100 ml | mmol/l | 0.411 |
| Phosphorus | 31 | mg/100 ml | mmol/l | 0.323 |
| Urate | 168 | mg/100 ml | mmol/l | 0.0595 |
| Urea | 60 | mg/100 ml | mmol/l | 0.167 |
| 25 OH Vit D | 400 | ng/ml | nmol/l | 2.5 |
| 1,25(OH)$_2$Vit D | 416 | pg/ml | pmol/l | 2.4 |

## EQUIVALENT AND MOLECULAR WEIGHTS

Equivalent weights:

| N | 14 | Mg | 12 |
|---|---|---|---|
| K | 39 | P | 16 (variable) |
| Ca | 20 | Cl | 35.5 |
| Na | 23 | O | 8 |

Molecular weights:

| | |
|---|---|
| Na$_3$ Citrate (2H$_2$O) | 294.1 |
| NaCl | 58.5 |
| Na Lactate | 112.0 |
| NaHCO$_3$ | 84.0 |
| Na$_2$HPO$_4$ (12H$_2$O) | 358.2 |
| NaH$_2$PO$_4$ (H$_2$O) | 156.0 |
| KHCO$_3$ | 100.1 |
| KCl | 74.6 |
| K$_3$ Citrate (H$_2$O) | 324.4 |
| K Acetate | 98.1 |
| K$_2$HPO$_4$ | 174.2 |
| NH$_4$Cl | 53.5 |
| CaCO$_3$ | 100.1 |
| Ca gluconate (H$_2$O) | 448.4 |
| CaCl$_2$ | 111.0 |
| Ca Lactate (5H$_2$O) | 308.3 |
| Mannitol | 180.0 |
| Glucose | 180.2 |

# Appendix 2

# Diets

It is impossible to give exhaustive information about the dietary management of the patient with renal failure in such a limited space. The points detailed in this appendix are intended to highlight some of the considerations which are necessary.

Patients with renal failure rarely feel hungry at the time when they need nutrition most. Lack of appetite can arise for many reasons including the underlying medical and psychosocial condition as well as the commoner problem of acute anxiety — a powerful appetite depressant. It is necessary to understand this and explain any problems carefully. Only then is it possible to succeed with the implementation of a dietary regimen which may be complicated and difficult to follow. Ideally a dietitian should be closely involved in the management of the patient at this stage.

## GENERAL INFORMATION ABOUT LOW SODIUM DIETS

1. These regimens can be very unpalatable unless care is taken during preparation.
    a. make liberal use of alternative flavourings:
       herbs, e.g. bay leaves, thyme, sage, rosemary, etc. spices, e.g. paprika, cloves, mace, nutmeg and curry spices including ginger, coriander, cumin, etc.
       mustard, pepper, vinegar and lemon juice
       home made unsalted pickles and chutneys
    b. use different and varied cooking methods, e.g. casseroles, stir-fry, marinading, etc.
2. Some specially prepared foods are prescribable in certain conditions (FP10). The prescription should be endorsed ACBS and currently available products are listed in MIMS and the British National Formulary (BNF) as Borderline Substances.
3. MAXIPRO HBV (Scientific Hospital Supplies) is an 88% protein powder which contains some sodium. It is prescribable for proven hypoproteinaemia.

4. CASILAN (Farley) is a 90% protein powder made from calcium caseinate. It is prescribable for proven hypoproteinaemia. Care should be taken when using this product because it has a distinctive strong flavour which can be unacceptable to the patient. It has a low sodium content.

5. FORTIMEL (Cow and Gate) is presented in a variety of flavours in 200 ml cartons. It is a high protein drink but is not prescribable.

6. It may be necessary to impose a fluid restriction — many types of food, e.g. soups, milk puddings, sauces, etc. contain fluid and should, therefore, be restricted.

7. There are several degrees of sodium restriction in current use:
   a. *No added salt — approximately 80–100 mmol Na$^+$*
      (i) No salt added at table
      (ii) No foods are allowed which contain large quantities of sodium (see list below)
      (iii) Salt is allowed in moderation in cooking
   b. *\*Low Salt — 40–50 mmol Na$^+$*
      (i) No salt added at table
      (ii) No foods are allowed which contain large quantities of sodium (see list below)
      (iii) No salt is allowed in cooking
      (iv) The use of ordinary bread and butter is restricted
      (v) The use of milk is restricted
   c. *\*Low sodium — 20–25 mmol Na$^+$*
      (i) No salt added at table
      (ii) No foods are allowed which contain large quantities of sodium (see list below)
      (iii) No salt is allowed in cooking
      (iv) No ordinary butter is allowed
      (v) The use of ordinary bread is restricted
      (vi) The use of milk is restricted.

## Foods to be avoided on a low sodium diet

1. Breads, cereal foods, etc.
   all breads unless specially made without salt
   all cakes and biscuits unless salt-free
   all crispbreads (e.g. Ryvita, Vita Wheat, etc.)
   any other foods containing baking power, baking soda or self-raising flour
   all breakfast cereals containing salt/sodium
   (Puffed Wheat, Shredded Wheat and porridge cooked without salt are allowed).

*It is *extremely* difficult to achieve this level if a high intake of protein is required.

2. Dairy products
   all cheese except home-made unsalted cheese
   salted butter and margarine
   yoghurt (all varieties)
   evaporated or condensed milk
   dried milk powders
   commercially manufactured desserts; ice-cream.
3. Meat and fish
   bacon, ham and all similar preserved meats
   commercially prepared 'made-up' products, e.g. sausages, meat pies, hamburgers, etc.
   salty fish and smoked fish, e.g. kippers, smoked haddock, anchovies, etc.
   all fish and meat pastes
   all tinned meats and tinned fish.
4. Miscellaneous
   tinned and packet vegetables and soups
   soy sauce and any products containing monosodium glutamate
   commercial pickles, chutneys, sauces, salad cream, etc.
   culinary salts, e.g. garlic salt, celery salt and other
   flavourings, e.g. Aromat, bouillon cubes, stock cubes, etc.
   Bovril, Oxo and Marmite and other meat or yeast extracts,
   all gravy mixes
   tinned tomato juice
   spinach, celery
   dried fruits
   potato crisps and salted nuts
   golden syrup, black treacle
   chocolate, cocoa and any products containing them
   toffees and licorice
   Ovaltine, Horlicks and other similar beverages
   rennet
   Lucozade, soda water
   beers, lagers and stouts
   health salts and indigestion powders or tablets.

## Foods allowed freely on a low sodium diet

1. Fats and oils including unsalted butter, unsalted margarine (Tomor), lard, suet, dripping, all cooking oils, double cream
2. Unsalted crackers, e.g. salt free Ryvita, Matzos, Rakusen's unsalted crackers
3. Shredded Wheat, Puffed Wheat, porridge cooked without salt
4. All fresh or frozen vegetables except spinach and celery
5. All fresh or frozen fruit and fruit juices
6. Low sodium canned vegetables, e.g. peas, baked beans, etc. These are

widely available in larger chemists, e.g. Boots and most health food stores. Remember to check the label first

7. Sugar, glucose and specially produced preparations, e.g. Hycal, Caloreen, Maxijul, etc. (see Borderline Substances list in MIMS or BNF)

8. Jams, marmalades and honey

9. Boiled sweets and peppermints

10. Plain flour, cornflour and wheatstarch and products made from these, some of which are prescribable (see Borderline Substances list in MIMS or BNF).

## Low sodium baking powder

This recipe can be made up by any chemist and should be used with plain flour in the same way as ordinary baking powder.

| | |
|---|---|
| Starch | 28 g |
| Potassium bicarbonate | 40 g |
| Tartaric acid | 8 g |
| Potassium bitartrate | 56 g |

## GENERAL INFORMATION ABOUT LOW PROTEIN DIETS

1. It is important to ensure that positive nitrogen balance is achieved and that the protein which is taken is not used to provide energy. It is also important to attempt to achieve and maintain ideal weight for height (remembering to make appropriate allowances for oedematous weight). Suggested initial guidelines are:

Protein: 0.5 g per kg body weight

Energy: 35–40 kcal per kg body weight

This can then be modified appropriately.

2. Several products are available on prescription (FP10) for use in conjunction with low protein diets. The prescription should be endorsed ACBS and the relevant products are listed as Borderline Substances in MIMS or the British National Formulary (BNF).

3. If there is a sodium restriction all foods should be cooked without salt and all salty foods listed on p 571 should be avoided appropriately.

4. If there is a potassium restriction all foods listed on page 575 should be avoided appropriately.

## Foods containing large amounts of protein

1. Meat and fish
   all types including preserved, tinned, frozen and made up
   products, e.g. pies, sausages, burgers, fish fingers, etc.

2. Eggs

3. Cheese

all types except cottage cheese (although this does contain some protein)
4. Milk
all types including tinned and dried milks
milk products including yoghurt, ice cream, milk puddings, etc.
5. Nuts
all types
peanut butter and marzipan
6. Pulses
all types including peas (especially dried peas, e.g. chick peas) lentils and beans including broad beans, baked beans, soy beans, red kidney beans, etc.

## Foods containing significant quantities of protein

1. Bread
all types unless specially prepared with protein free flour
2. Cereals
all types including
breakfast cereals
pudding cereals, e.g. rice, sago, semolina, etc.
3. Flour
and all other products made with flour including
biscuits
cakes
pastries
sauces
(It is possible to modify many recipes to use protein free flour)
4. Potatoes
all types
5. Chocolates, toffees, fudge, licorice

## Foods allowed freely on a low protein diet

1. Fats and oils including butter, margarine, lard, suet, dripping, all cooking oils and double cream
2. Sugars including sugar, glucose, honey, jams, marmalades, boiled sweets, soft drinks
3. Starches including cornflour, wheatstarch and products made from these
4. Prescribable foods (see Borderline Substances list in MIMS or BNF) including
   a. Sugar – substitutes, e.g. Hycal, Fortical Caloreen, Maxijul, Calonutrin
   b. Starches including pasta (Aproten/Aglutella range) and breads, bread mixes and biscuits (Juvela, Aproten and Rite–Diet ranges).

## GENERAL INFORMATION ABOUT LOW POTASSIUM DIETS

Potassium is widely distributed in foods, particularly fruit and vegetables. It is soluble in water and so methods of cooking should be used (particularly for potatoes) which enable the potassium to leach into the cooking water — which should then be discarded. Patients on low potassium diets should avoid using pressure cookers, microwave ovens and other similar items of equipment for preparing vegetables.

It may be necessary to prescribe supplements of Vitamin B complex and Vitamin C to counteract the loss of these vitamins during the leaching process.

Meat, fish, milk, cheese and eggs also contain significant quantities of potassium and should only be allowed in limited amounts as indicated:

Meat and fish — approximately 6 oz. daily

Milk — $\frac{1}{2}$ pint daily

Eggs and cheese — at one meal only

In addition, foods which contain exceptionally high amounts of potassium should be eliminated completely from the diet.

### Foods containing large amounts of potassium

1. Nuts
   *all* types
   any products made from nuts, e.g. peanut butter, marzipan, etc.
   any products containing nuts, e.g. cakes, biscuits,
   confectionery, etc.
2. Instant coffee powders/granules, e.g. Maxwell House, Nescafe, Gold Blend, etc. (Percolated or filtered coffees are allowed). Instant tea powders, e.g. Nestea, Lemsip, Lift, etc. (Leaf tea and tea bags are allowed)
3. Chocolate
   all types
   any products made from or containing chocolate
4. Dried fruits, e.g. raisins, prunes, dates, etc.
   *any* products containing dried fruit, e.g. cakes, puddings, etc.
5. Dried vegetables, e.g. peas, onions
   *any* products containing dried vegetables, e.g. packet soup mixes, rehydrated meals, etc.
6. Salt substitutes, e.g. Selora, Ruthmol, etc. (These are made from potassium chloride.)
7. Wholegrain cereals including
   breakfast cereals, e.g. Weetabix, All Bran, Shredded Wheat, muesli etc.
   wholemeal and other similar breads
   brown rice
   wholegrain biscuits and crackers, e.g. digestive, Ryvita, etc.
8. Malted milk drinks, e.g. Ovaltine, Horlicks, etc.

9. Concentrated fruit drinks, e.g. blackcurrant cordials, canned or frozen fruit juices
10. Fruit squashes
11. Beers, stouts, lager and cider
12. Meat extracts, e.g. Bovril, Oxo
13. Molasses and black treacle.

## GENERAL INFORMATION ABOUT HIGH PROTEIN DIETS

1. Large amounts of dietary protein are required to counteract protein losses. These may be urinary losses, e.g. Nephrotic Syndrome or dialysate losses e.g. CAPD. It is vital that these losses are replaced otherwise the patient will go into negative nitrogen balance.

2. Dietary protein should be utilised as effectively as possible and should not be used as an energy source. The patient's energy requirements should be provided by fats and carbohydrates. In order to ensure effective protein utilisation a high calorie diet *must* also be given.

3. It may be necessary to suggest supplementary feeding regimens to patients who are either anorexic or are unable to cope with large quantities of food:

    a. Fortified food i.e. the addition of high protein/high calorie items to regular foodstuffs (eggs, milk powder, cream, etc.) can be useful

    b. Commercially available supplements, e.g. Complan, Express Supplement, Fortimel, Carnation Build-Up etc.

    c. Specially formulated powder supplements, e.g. Caloreen, Maxijul, Maxipro HBV, Forceval Protein, etc.

    d. Specially formulated tube feeding products which can be used as overnight supplements to the regular diet.

4. Foods which contain large amounts and significant amounts of protein are listed on page 573, 574. A selection of supplements which are currently available are listed on page 583.

The following meal patterns are only suggested ways of introducing dietary modifications. They may not be suitable for individual patients in which case they should be modified appropriately. A dietitian would be able to advise on such modifications.

Each meal plan should be used in conjunction with the information about specific nutrient contents given on pages 580–582 and 583.

1 oz (30 g) meat = 1½ oz (45 g) fish *or*
                 ¾ oz (20 g) cheese — if allowed, *or*
                 1 egg

## 1. 160–165 g protein 30–35 mmol sodium diet
*(High protein, low sodium)*

# ALL FOODS TO BE COOKED WITHOUT ADDED SALT

| Meal | oz | g | Food | Protein (g) | Sodium (mmol) |
|------|----|----|------|-------------|---------------|
| Breakfast | 5 | 140 | Porridge | 2.0 | 0.2 |
| | 4 | 115 | 2 eggs (boiled, poached or fried) | 14.0 | 7.0 |
| | 2 | 60 | Unsalted bread | 4.6 | — |
| | | | Unsalted butter or margarine* | TR | TR |
| | | | Marmalade or honey* | — | — |
| | | | Tea or coffee | | |
| | | | Sugar* | — | — |
| | | | Milk (ordinary) from daily allowance | — | — |
| Mid morning | 2 | 60 | Unsalted bread | 4.6 | |
| | | | Unsalted butter or margarine* | — | — |
| | 2 | 60 | Lean meat as sandwich filling | 12.5 | 1.2 |
| | | | Tea or coffee with milk from daily allowance | — | — |
| | | | Sugar* | | |
| Main meal | 6 | 170 | Grilled fish (cooked weight) | 33.6 | 6.35 |
| | 4 | 115 | Potatoes (boiled, fried or sautéed) | 1.6 | TR |
| | | | Vegetables or salad (average helping) | 0.6 | 0.2 |
| | | | Fresh, tinned or stewed fruit (average helping) | 0.4 | 0.2 |
| | | | Pudding using cereal and milk from allowance | — | — |
| Mid-afternoon | 2 | 60 | Unsalted bread | 4.6 | — |
| | | | Unsalted butter or margarine* | TR | TR |
| | 2 | 60 | Lean meat as sandwich filling | 12.5 | 1.2 |
| | 1 | 30 | Cake made from low sodium ingredients (see general instructions) | 2.0 | 0.4 |
| | | | Tea with milk from daily allowance | — | — |
| | | | Sugar* | | |
| Light meal | 3 | 90 | Lean meat (cooked weight) | 18.8 | 2.0 |
| | 4 | 115 | Potatoes (boiled, roasted, etc.) | 1.6 | TR |
| | | | Vegetables or salad (average helping) | 0.6 | 0.2 |
| | | | Fresh, tinned or stewed fruit (average helping) | 0.4 | 0.2 |
| Daily | 10 | 300 | Ordinary milk for tea etc | 3.8 | 6.5 |
| | 3 | 90 | Double cream for puddings | 1.3 | 0.8 |
| | 1 | 30 | Rice for puddings | 0.5 | TR |
| | 7 | 200 | Fortimel (any flavor) | 9.7 | 2.2 |
| | 1 | 30 | Maxipro 1 + BV to use in drinks, puddings etc | 26.4 | 3.0 |
| | | | TOTALS | 162.2 | 31.65 |

* These foods are allowed freely

## 2. *40 g protein 35–40 mmol sodium diet*
### *(Low protein, low sodium)*

# ALL FOODS TO BE COOKED WITHOUT ADDED SALT

| Meal | oz | g | Food | Protein (g) | Sodium (mmol) |
|---|---|---|---|---|---|
| Breakfast | 4 | 115 | Fresh, tinned or stewed fruit & sugar | 0.4 | 0.2 |
| | 2 | 55 | Egg (boiled, poached or fried) | 6.8 | 3.3 |
| | 1 | 30 | Bread (ordinary) | 2.3 | 7.0 |
| | ½ | 15 | Butter or margarine (ordinary) | TR | 5.6 |
| | | | Marmalade or honey* | | |
| | | | Tea or coffee | — | — |
| | | | Sugar* | — | — |
| | | | Milk from daily allowance | — | — |
| Mid morning | | | Unsalted protein free bread* | — | — |
| | | | Unsalted butter or margarine* | — | — |
| | | | Jam or honey* | — | — |
| | | | Tea or coffee with milk from daily allowance | — | — |
| | | | Sugar* | — | — |
| Main meal | 1½ | 45 | Lean meat (cooked weight) | 11.3 | 3.3 |
| | 4 | 115 | Potatoes (boiled, fried, roast, etc.) | 1.6 | TR |
| | | | Green vegetables or salad (average helping) | 0.6 | 0.2 |
| | | | 'Milk' pudding made with cereal, double cream and water | 1.6 | TR |
| Mid afternoon | 1 | 30 | Bread (ordinary) | 2.3 | 7.0 |
| | ½ | 15 | Butter or margarine (ordinary) | TR | 5.6 |
| | | | Jam or honey* | — | — |
| | | | Tea with milk from daily allowance | — | — |
| | | | Sugar* | — | — |
| Light meal | 1 | 30 | Lean meat or poultry | 7.5 | 2.2 |
| | 3 | 90 | Potatoes (boiled, fried, roast, etc.) | 1.3 | TR |
| | | | Green vegetables or salad (average helping) | 0.6 | 0.2 |
| | | | Fresh, tinned or stewed (average helping) | 0.4 | 0.2 |
| | | | Double cream from daily allowance | — | — |
| Daily allowances | 2 | 60 | Milk (ordinary) for tea and coffee | 2.0 | 1.3 |
| | 4 | 100 | Double cream for puddings | 1.5 | 0.9 |
| | | | TOTALS | 40.2 | 37.0 |

* These foods are allowed freely

## 3. *20 g protein, 20 mmol sodium diet*
*(Very low protein, low sodium)*

## ALL FOODS TO BE COOKED WITHOUT ADDED SALT

| Meal | oz | g | Food | Protein (g) | Sodium (mmol) |
|------|----|----|------|------------|---------------|
| Breakfast | 4 | 115 | Fresh, tinned or stewed fruit & sugar | 0.4 | 0.2 |
| | 1 | 30 | Bread (ordinary) | 2.3 | 7.0 |
| | | | Unsalted butter or margarine* | TR | — |
| | | | Marmalade or honey* | — | — |
| | | | Tea or coffee | — | — |
| | | | Sugar* | — | — |
| | | | Milk from daily allowance | — | — |
| Mid morning | | | Unsalted protein free bread* | — | — |
| | | | Unsalted butter or margarine* | — | — |
| | | | Jam or honey* | — | — |
| | | | Tea or coffee with milk from daily allowance | — | — |
| | | | Sugar* | — | — |
| Main meal | 1 | 30 | Lean meat (cooked weight) | 7.5 | 2.2 |
| | 2 | 60 | Potatoes (boiled, fried, roast, etc.) | 0.8 | TR |
| | | | Green vegetables or salad (average helping) | 0.6 | 0.2 |
| | | | Fresh, tinned or stewed fruit (average helping) | 0.4 | 0.2 |
| | | | Double Cream from daily allowance | — | — |
| Mid afternoon | 1 | 30 | Bread (ordinary) | 2.3 | 7.0 |
| | ½ | 15 | Unsalted butter or margarine* | TR | — |
| | | | Unsalted bread* | — | — |
| | | | Jam or honey* | — | — |
| | | | Tea with milk from daily allowance | — | — |
| | | | Sugar* | — | — |
| Light meal | | | NO MEAT, FISH, ETC. | | |
| | | | Protein free, salt free pasta* | 0.4 | — |
| | 2 | 60 | Potatoes (boiled, fried, roasted, etc.) | 0.8 | TR |
| | | | Green vegetables or salad (average helping) | 0.6 | 0.2 |
| | | | Fresh, tinned or stewed fruit (average helping) | 0.4 | 0.2 |
| | | | Double cream from daily allowance | — | — |
| Daily allowances | 2 | 60 | Milk (ordinary) for tea and coffee | 2.0 | 1.3 |
| | 3 | 90 | Double cream for puddings | 1.3 | 0.8 |
| | | | TOTALS | 19.8 | 19.3 |

* These foods are allowed freely

*Selected nutrient composition of various foods*
*(analysis per 100 g foodstuff)*

| Food<br>(100 g) | Energy<br>(kcal) | Protein<br>(g) | Sodium<br>(mmol) | Potassium<br>(mmol) |
|---|---|---|---|---|
| **BREAD AND CEREALS** | | | | |
| Bread — brown | 223 | 8.9 | 23.91 | 5.38 |
| white | 233 | 7.8 | 23.48 | 2.56 |
| wholemeal | 216 | 8.8 | 23.48 | 5.64 |
| Starch reduced rolls | 384 | 44.0 | 28.25 | 3.33 |
| Cream Crackers | 440 | 9.5 | 26.52 | 3.07 |
| Crispbread — rye | 321 | 9.4 | 9.56 | 12.82 |
| Chocolate — full coated | 524 | 5.7 | 6.96 | 5.90 |
| Digestive — plain | 471 | 9.8 | 19.30 | 4.10 |
| Semi-sweet biscuits | 457 | 6.7 | 17.83 | 3.59 |
| Cornflakes | 368 | 8.6 | 50.43 | 2.54 |
| Puffed Wheat | 325 | 14.2 | 0.17 | 10.00 |
| Rice Krispies | 372 | 5.9 | 48.26 | 3.85 |
| Shredded Wheat | 324 | 10.6 | 0.35 | 8.46 |
| Porridge (cooked) | 44 | 1.4 | 25.22 | 1.08 |
| Flour — wholemeal | 318 | 13.2 | 0.13 | 9.23 |
| white | 337 | 11.3 | 0.13 | 3.33 |
| Rice — boiled | 123 | 2.2 | 0.9 | 0.97 |
| Spaghetti — boiled | 117 | 4.2 | 0.9 | 1.28 |
| **MILK AND MILK PRODUCTS** | | | | |
| Milk (cow's) — whole | 65 | 3.3 | 2.17 | 3.85 |
| skimmed | 33 | 3.4 | 2.26 | 3.85 |
| dried-whole | 490 | 26.3 | 19.13 | 32.56 |
| dried-skimmed | 355 | 36.4 | 23.91 | 42.31 |
| Butter — salted | 740 | 0.4 | 37.83 | 0.38 |
| Cream — single | 212 | 2.4 | 1.83 | 3.08 |
| double | 447 | 1.5 | 1.17 | 2.03 |
| *Cheese* | | | | |
| Camembert type | 300 | 22.8 | 61.30 | 2.82 |
| Cheddar type | 406 | 26.0 | 26.52 | 3.08 |
| Stilton | 462 | 25.6 | 50.00 | 4.10 |
| Cottage Cheese | 96 | 13.6 | 19.57 | 1.38 |
| Cheese spread | 283 | 18.3 | 50.87 | 3.85 |
| Yoghurt — natural | 52 | 5.0 | 3.30 | 6.15 |
| flavoured | 81 | 5.0 | 2.78 | 5.64 |
| fruit | 95 | 4.8 | 2.78 | 5.64 |
| **FATS AND OILS** | | | | |
| Butter — salted | 740 | 0.4 | 37.83 | 0.38 |
| Lard | 891 | TR | 0.09 | 0.03 |
| Low fat spread | 366 | 0.0 | 30.00 | TR |
| Margarine | 730 | 0.1 | 34.78 | 0.13 |
| Vegetable oils | 899 | TR | TR | TR |
| **EGGS, MEAT AND FISH** | | | | |
| **EGGS** | | | | |
| whole raw | 147 | 12.3 | 6.09 | 3.59 |
| fried | 232 | 14.1 | 9.57 | 4.62 |
| poached | 155 | 12.4 | 4.78 | 3.08 |

| Food (100 g) | Energy (kcal) | Protein (g) | Sodium (mmol) | Potassium (mmol) |
|---|---|---|---|---|
| **MEATS** | | | | |
| Bacon — grilled | | | | |
|     back rashers | 405 | 25.3 | 87.83 | 7.44 |
|     streaky rashers | 422 | 24.5 | 86.52 | 7.44 |
| Beef — mince (stewed) | 229 | 23.1 | 13.91 | 7.44 |
|     steak including fat (grilled) | 218 | 27.3 | 2.39 | 9.74 |
|     sirloin including fat (roast) | 284 | 23.6 | 2.35 | 7.69 |
|     stewed including fat | 223 | 30.9 | 15.65 | 5.90 |
| Lamb — chops including fat (grilled) | 335 | 23.5 | 3.13 | 8.21 |
|     leg including fat (roast) | 266 | 26.1 | 2.83 | 7.95 |
| Pork — chop including fat (grilled) | 332 | 28.5 | 3.65 | 9.74 |
|     leg including fat (roast) | 286 | 26.9 | 3.43 | 8.97 |
| Chicken — boiled | 183 | 29.2 | 3.57 | 7.69 |
|     roast | 148 | 24.8 | 3.52 | 7.95 |
| Liver — calf (fried) | 254 | 26.9 | 7.39 | 11.79 |
|     lamb (fried) | 232 | 22.9 | 8.26 | 7.69 |
|     ox (stewed) | 198 | 24.8 | 4.78 | 6.41 |
| Tongue — ox (boiled) | 293 | 19.5 | 43.48 | 3.85 |
| Beef — corned | 217 | 26.9 | 41.30 | 3.59 |
| Ham | 120 | 18.4 | 54.35 | 7.18 |
| Luncheon Meat | 313 | 12.6 | 45.65 | 3.59 |
| Sausages — | | | | |
| Beef — fried | 269 | 12.9 | 47.39 | 4.62 |
|     grilled | 265 | 13.0 | 47.83 | 4.87 |
| Pork — fried | 317 | 13.8 | 45.65 | 5.13 |
|     grilled | 318 | 13.3 | 43.48 | 5.13 |
| **FISH** | | | | |
| Cod — fried in batter | 199 | 19.6 | 4.35 | 9.49 |
|     grilled | 95 | 20.8 | 3.96 | 9.74 |
|     poached | 94 | 20.9 | 4.78 | 8.46 |
| Plaice — fried in batter | 279 | 15.8 | 9.57 | 5.90 |
|     steamed | 93 | 18.9 | 5.22 | 7.18 |
| Herring — fried | 234 | 23.1 | 4.35 | 10.77 |
|     grilled | 199 | 20.4 | 7.39 | 9.49 |
| Salmon — steamed | 197 | 20.1 | 4.78 | 8.46 |
|     canned | 155 | 20.3 | 24.78 | 7.69 |
| Sardines — canned | 217 | 23.7 | 28.26 | 11.03 |
| Shrimps — boiled | 117 | 23.8 | 166.96 | 10.26 |
|     canned | 94 | 20.8 | 42.61 | 2.56 |
| **MISCELLANEOUS** | | | | |
| Ice Cream — dairy | 167 | 3.7 | 3.48 | 4.62 |
|     non dairy | 165 | 3.3 | 3.04 | 3.85 |
| Boiled sweets | 327 | TR | 1.09 | 0.21 |
| Chocolate — assorted | 460 | 4.1 | 2.61 | 6.15 |
|     milk | 529 | 8.4 | 5.22 | 10.77 |

| Food (100 g) | Energy (kcal) | Protein (g) | Sodium (mmol) | Potassium (mmol) |
|---|---|---|---|---|
| Toffees — mixed | 430 | 2.1 | 13.91 | 5.38 |
| Horlicks | 396 | 13.8 | 15.22 | 19.23 |
| Ovaltine | 378 | 9.8 | 6.52 | 21.79 |
| Casilan* | 376 | 90.0 | 0.30 | — |
| Complan (flavoured)* | 445 | 20.0 | 15.90 | 21.30 |

N.B. 100 g food is not necessarily a standard portion which would be consumed

Data obtained from: McCance & Widdowson 1978 Composition of Food, 4th revised edn. Paul & Southgate, HMSO, London.

* Data obtained from manufacturers's information

*Supplements for use in high protein, high energy diets*
A selection of products currently available
Some further information about the protein/energy content in foods is on page 580–592

| Product | Use | Manufacturer | ACBS* | Quantity | Energy (kcal) | Protein (g) | Sodium (mmol) | Potassium (mmol) |
|---|---|---|---|---|---|---|---|---|
| Build-up | 4 | Carnation Foods | No | 100 g | 349 | 22.67 | 14.5 | 26.2 |
| Caloreen | 1 | Roussel | Yes | 100 g | 400 | — | 0.1 | 0.1 |
| Casilan | 1 | Farley | Yes | 100 g | 376 | 90.0 | 0.3 | — |
| Clinifeed Protein Rich | 3 | Roussel | Yes | 375 ml | 500 | 30.0 | 12.7 | 21.5 |
| Clinifeed Select | 2 | Roussel | Yes | 375 ml | 500 | 22.5 | 7.0 | 14.4 |
| Complan-flavoured‡ | 4 | Farley | No | 100 g | 445 | 20.0 | 15.9 | 21.3 |
| Duocal | 1 | Scientific Hospital Supplies | No | 100 g | 197 | — | 0.5 | TR |
| Ensure Plus | 2 | Abbott Labs | Yes | 235 ml | 340 | 13.0 | 11.0 | 11.0 |
| Express High Energy | 3 | Express Nutrition | No | 500 ml | 750 | 29.5 | 20.0 | 22.5 |
| Express Supplement | 4 | Express Nutrition | No | 200 ml | 315 | 11.4 | 8.0 | 9.0 |
| Forceval Protein | 1 | Unigreg | Yes | 100 g | 366 | 55.0 | 5.0 | 1.3 |
| Fortical‡ | 1 + 4 | Cow and Gate | No | 200 ml | 492 | — | 0.6 | 0.4 |
| Fortimel | 4 | Cow and Gate | No | 200 ml | 200 | 19.4 | 4.4 | 10.2 |
| Fortisip Energy Plus | 4 | Cow and Gate | No | 200 ml | 250 | 10.0 | 7.0 | 7.6 |
| Fortison Energy Plus | 4 | Cow and Gate | No | 500 ml | 750 | 25.0 | 17.5 | 19.2 |
| Hycal | 1 + 4 | Beecham Products | Yes | 171 ml | 425 | — | 1.0 | TR |
| Maxipro HBV | 1 | Scientific Hospital Supplies | Yes | 100 g | 352 | 88.0 | 10.0 | — |
| Nutrauxil | 2 | Kabi Vitrum | Yes | 500 ml | 500 | 19.0 | 16.5 | 16.0 |

N.B. Many companies listed above produce supplements in addition to those listed. Details can be obtained from the manufacturers.

*Key:*

*ACBS = check the prescribing constraints listed in MIMS or BNF: these are modified continuously

‡ = average analysis

*Uses:* 1 = Powder or liquid supplement — can be added to food

2 = Tube feed or sip feed

3 = Tube feed

4 = Sip feed — may need to be reconstituted according to manufacturer's directions

# Index